SYNAPTIC PLASTICITY: NEW RESEARCH

SYNAPTIC PLASTICITY: NEW RESEARCH

TIM F. KAISER
AND FELIX J. PETERS
EDITORS

Nova Science Publishers, Inc.
New York

For permission to use material from this book please contact us:
Telephone 631-231-7269; Fax 631-231-8175
Web Site: http://www.novapublishers.com

LIBRARY OF CONGRESS CATALOGING-IN-PUBLICATION DATA

Synaptic plasticity : new research / Tim F. Kaiser and Felix J. Peters (editors).
p. ; cm.
Includes bibliographical references and index.
ISBN 978-1-60456-732-8 (hardcover)
1. Neuroplasticity. I. Kaiser, Tim F. II. Peters, Felix J.
[DNLM: 1. Neuronal Plasticity--physiology. 2. Synapses--physiology. 3. Brain Chemistry. 4. Synaptic Transmission--physiology. WL 102.8 S992565 2008]
QP363.3.S966 2008
612.8--dc22

2008018269

Published by Nova Science Publishers, Inc. ✝ New York

CONTENTS

Preface vii

Chapter 1 Synaptic Plasticity : Physiology and Neurological Disease **1**
Stephen D. Skaper

Chapter 2 Molecular Mechanisms of Learning and Memory Based on Research on Ca2+/Calmodulin-Dependent Protein Kinase II **45**
Takashi Yamauchi and Hiroko Sugiura

Chapter 3 Synaptic Plasticity: Emerging Role for Endocannabinoid System **77**
Balapal S. Basavarajappa and Ottavio Arancio

Chapter 4 The Presence of PErforated Synapses in the Striatum after Dopamine Depletion: Is This a Sign of Negative Brain Plasticity? **113**
Maria Rosa Avila-Costa, Ana Luisa Gutierrez-Valdez, Jose Luis Ordoñez-Librado, Verónica Anaya-Martínez, Laura Colin-Barenque, César Sánchez Vázquez del Mercado, Leonardo Reynoso-Erazo

Chapter 5 Synaptic Plasticity and Motor Learning in the Cerebellum **143**
Shun Tsuruno and Tomoo Hirano

Chapter 6 Seizure-Induced Synaptic Plasticity: Understanding Synaptic Reorganization **163**
Benedict C. Albensi

Chapter 7 Synaptic Plasticity in Cocaine Addiction **177**
Margarida Corominas, Carlos Roncero, Xavier Castells, Miquel Casas

Chapter 8 Synaptic Plasticity in the Medial Prefrontal Cortex **221**
E.S. Louise Faber

Chapter 9 Cellular Cognition: A Focus on LTP and LTD in the Lateral Nucleus of the Amygdala **269**
Doris Albrecht and Oliver von Bohlen und Halbach

Chapter 10 Synaptic Plasticity and Mnemonic Encoding by Hippocampal Formation Place Cells **309**
M. Tsanov, J. R. Brotons-Mas, M. V. Sanchez-Vives and S. M. O'Mara

Chapter 11 Regulation of Synaptic Plasticity by the Scaffolding Protein Spinophilin **345**
D. Sarrouilhe and T. Métayé

Chapter 12 Dopamine-Dependent Synaptic Plasticity in The Cortico-Basal Ganglia-Thalamocortical Loops as Mechanism of Visual Attention **361**
Isabella Silkis

Index **379**

PREFACE

Synaptic plasticity is the ability of the connection, or synapse, between two neurons to change in strength. There are several underlying mechanisms that cooperate to achieve synaptic plasticity, including changes in the quantity of neurotransmitter released into a synapse and changes in how effectively cells respond to those neurotransmitters. Since memories are postulated to be represented by vastly interconnected networks of synapses in the brain, synaptic plasticity is one of the important neurochemical foundations of learning and memory. In this book the discussion of synaptic plasticity that effects both physical and mental behavior of organisms is discussed including the physical performance of an organism that resulted in a stroke, drug addiction, or the mechanisms of brain plasticity that forms mental disorders such as depression.

Chapter 1 - Neuroplasticity is both a substrate of learning and memory and a mediator of responses to neuronal cell attrition and injury (compensatory plasticity). It is a continuous process in reaction to neuronal activity and neuronal injury, death, and genesis, which involves modulation of structural and functional processes of axons, dendrites, and synapses. The varied structural elements that embody plasticity include long-term potentiation (a cellular correlate of learning and memory), synaptic efficacy, synaptic remodelling, synaptogenesis, neurite extension including axonal sprouting and dendritic remodelling, and neurogenesis and recruitment. Degenerative diseases of the human brain have long been viewed as among the most enigmatic and intractable problems in biomedicine. As research on human neurodegeneration has moved from descriptive phenomenology to mechanistic analysis, it has become increasing apparent that the morphological lesions long used by neuropathologists to confirm a clinical diagnosis after death might provide an experimentally tractable handle to understand causative pathways. For example, Alzheimer's disease (AD) is an aging-dependent neurodegenerative disorder that is characterised by neuropathologically by the deposition of insoluble amyloid β-peptide (Aβ) in extracellular plaques and aggregated tau protein, which is found largely in the intracellular neurofibrillary tangles. There is growing evidence that mild cognitive impairment in early AD may be due to synaptic dysfunction caused by the accumulation of non-fibrillar, oligomeric Aβ, long before widespread synaptic loss and neurodegeneration occur. Soluble Aβ oligomers can adversely affect synaptic structure and plasticity at extremely low concentrations, although the molecular substrates by which synaptic memory mechanisms are disrupted remain poorly understood. A primary locus of excitatory synaptic transmission in the mammalian central nervous system is the dendritic spine. These protrusions from dendritic shafts exhibit dynamic changes in number, size and shape in response to variation in hormonal status, developmental stage, and changes in afferent input. Not surprisingly, loss of spine density has been linked to cognitive and memory impairment in AD, but the underlying mechanism(s) in this case is uncertain, as well. Intriguingly, findings in other neurodegenerative diseases indicate that a broadly similar process of synaptic dysfunction is induced by diffusible oligomers of misfolded proteins. This chapter will present a critical review of current knowledge on the bases of synaptic dysfunction in neurodegenerative diseases, with a focus on AD, and will encompass both amyloid- and non-amyloid-driven mechanisms. Where appropriate, consideration will also be given to emerging data which point to potential therapeutic approaches for ameliorating the cognitive and memory deficits associated with these disorders.

Chapter 2 - In the central nervous system (CNS), changes in the efficiency of synaptic transmission are important for a number of aspects of neural function. Much has been learned about the activity-dependent synaptic modifications, namely synaptic plasticity, that are thought to underlie memory storage, but these modifications are largely unknown at the molecular level.It is important to find and characterize the "memory molecules", and "memory apparatus or memory forming apparatus" in the brain. One of the best candidates for a molecular component of the memory apparatus is Ca^{2+}/calmodulin-dependent protein kinase II (CaMKII). The postsynaptic density (PSD) is also a good candidate for a body of the memory apparatus.

CaMKII is one of the most prominent protein kinases, and plays a multifunctional role in many intracellular events. CaMKII activity is regulated by autophosphorylation. It is present in essentially every tissue but most concentrated in the brain. Neuronal CaMKII is present in both presynapses and postsynapses, and is also the major component of the PSD. The PSD serves as a general organizer of the postsynaptic signal transduction machinery, which links regulatory molecules to their targets. Dysfunction of CaMKII may relate to neuronal disorders.

This review covers the molecular basis of learning and memory taking into consideration research on CaMKII, a major component of neurons.

Chapter 3 - Changes in synaptic strength are thought to be crucial to experience-dependent modifications of neural function. The diversity of mechanisms underlying these changes is far greater than previously expected. In the last few years, a new class of use-dependent synaptic plasticity that requires endocannabinoid signaling system has been identified in several brain regions. The endocannabinoid signaling system is composed of the cannabinoid receptors; their endogenous ligands, the endocannabinoids; the enzymes that produce and inactivate the endocannabinoids; and the endocannabinoid transporters. Endogenous cannabinoids (endocannabinoids) (ECs) are lipid mediators that activate these same cannabinoid receptors. Elegant work from several laboratories over the past 6 years has established that ECs are produced on demand in activity-dependent manners and released from postsynaptic neurons. The released ECs travel backward across the synapse, activate presynaptic CB1 receptors, and modulate presynaptic functions. Retrograde EC signaling is crucial for certain forms of short-term and long-term synaptic plasticity at excitatory or inhibitory synapses in many brain regions, and thereby contributes to various aspects of brain function including learning and memory. Thus, the EC system is emerging as a major player in synaptic plasticity. In this review, the authors describe molecular mechanisms of the endocannabinoid-mediated synaptic modulation and its possible physiological significance.

Chapter 4 - Synaptic plasticity is the process by which long-lasting changes take place at synaptic connections. The concept of plasticity can be applied to molecular as well as to environmental events. The phenomenon itself is complex and can involve many levels of organization. Some authors separate forms into adaptations that have positive or negative consequences for the animal. For example, if an organism, after a stroke, can recover to normal levels of performance, that adaptiveness could be considered an example of "positive plasticity". An excessive level of neuronal growth leading to spasticity or tonic paralysis, or an excessive release of neurotransmitters in response to injury, which could kill nerve cells, would have to be considered perhaps as a "negative or maladaptive" plasticity.

The striatum is the point of entry of information into the basal ganglia, and it has important roles in motor control and habit learning. The neocortex provides the major excitatory inputs to striatal medium spiny projection neurons. Morphological studies have demonstrated that the majority of these afferent terminals impinge on the head of the spines on the dendrites of these striatal neurons, whereas most dopaminergic afferent fibers coming from the substantia nigra make synapses on the necks of the same dendritic spines. This close anatomical localization of these two types of synapses suggests that dopamine released from the nigrostriatal afferent terminals may have modulatory effects on the excitatory signals generated from the cortex.

The importance of dopamine in normal striatal function is evidenced by the severe disruption of behavior observed in Parkinson's disease and after chemical lesions of nigral dopaminergic inputs to striatum. In recent years attention has been focused on perforated synapses considering their possible involvement in synaptic plasticity in the nervous system. It has been hypothesized that an increase in the number of synapses may represent a structural basis for the enduring expression of synaptic plasticity during some events that involve memory and learning; also it has been suggested that perforated synapses increase in number after some experimental situations. The aim of this chapter was to analyze whether the dopamine depletion produces changes in the synaptology of the corpus striatum of rats after the unilateral injection of 6-OHDA. The findings suggest that after the lesion, both contralateral and ipsilateral striata present a significant increment in the number of perforated synapses, suggesting brain plasticity that might be deleterious for the spines, because this type of synaptic contacts are excitatory, and in the absence of the modulatory effects of dopamine, the neuron could die by excitotoxic mechanisms. Thus, the authors conclude that the presence of perforated synapses after striatal dopamine depletion might be a form of negative synaptic plasticity.

Chapter 5 - The cerebellum plays a key role in motor learning. Since Marr and Albus proposed the perceptron model of cerebellar cortex, extensive study has been performed to clarify the mechanism of motor learning. The cerebellar long-term depression (LTD) is a type of synaptic plasticity occurring at the parallel fiber–Purkinje cell synapses, which was predicted by Albus and has been regarded as a cellular basis of motor learning. Not only its involvement in motor learning but also its regulation mechanisms at a molecular level have been clarified. On the other hand, other forms of synaptic plasticity have been reported in the cerebellum. Long-term potentiation (LTP) and LTD occur at both excitatory and inhibitory synapses in the cortex and also in the cerebellar nuclei. Their molecular mechanisms and implication in motor learning have also been studied.

In this chapter, the authors begin by reviewing research on the regulatory molecular mechanisms of the cerebellar LTD. Then, they turn to other forms of synaptic plasticity.

Finally, the authors summarize the involvement of cerebellar synaptic plasticity in several motor learning tasks by reviewing studies on animals with surgical lesion, chemical inactivation or genetic manipulation of a specific region of the cerebellar circuit.

Chapter 6 - The hippocampus in epilepsy patients exhibits brain plasticity in response to seizure activity. Experimentally, brain plasticity in animals subjected to kindling, or chemically-induced epilepsy, appears to be related to a long-term potentiation (LTP)-like reorganization of the neural networks. LTP is a widely accepted model of plasticity that results in activity-dependent long-term synaptic change and possibly memory encoding. Studies have further suggested that LTP induction and other activity-induced changes up-regulate various growth factors and may underlie hippocampal mossy fiber sprouting, which occurs frequently after repeated seizure activity. This chapter will highlight important background information, and discuss experimental models and methods that are currently being used for modeling plasticity/epilepsy and for profiling gene expression.

Chapter 7 - Addiction has been described as a pathological usurpation of the neuronal mechanisms involved in reward, motivation and reinforcement. Nevertheless, environmental stimuli closely associated with the drug can acquire the ability to elicit the emotional responses that were induced by the drug. From this perspective, addiction has something to do with long-term associative learning and memory. These effects induced by cocaine consumption account for the chronic relapse which characterizes addiction. Long-term potentiation (LTP) and long-term depression (LTD) are forms of synaptic plasticity by which chronic cocaine induces changes in the mesocorticolimbic system primarily through dopamine and glutamate transmission. Recent evidence suggests that brain-derived neurotrophic factor (BDNF) and its intracellular pathways are involved in the molecular mechanisms that modify synaptic plasticity underlying addiction.

A single dose of cocaine induces an enhancement in locomotor activity that correlates with an increase in synaptic strength (the ratio AMPAR/NMDAR) in the VTA. This effect was not increased after repeated cocaine doses, indicating that cocaine-induced synaptic plasticity in the VTA is transient and also has a ceiling effect. Adaptations in downstream circuitry, such the nucleus accumbens (NAc), are likely to be more important for the longer-lasting behavioral changes associated with drug addiction. EPSC is decreased (LTD was induced) at synapses made by prefrontal cortical afferents in spiny neurons of the NAc shell, but not in the core. This inhibitory effect appears to be induced by D1 receptor activation. These changes in synaptic plasticity disrupt goal-directed behavior. In the dorsal striatum, LTP can be induced in physiological conditions as well as after chronic cocaine treatment. However, saline treated rats are able to reverse LTP, whereas cocaine treated rodents do not. In the dorsal striatum, LTP is induced by D1 receptor activation and enhanced by D2 receptor antagonists. In physiological conditions, the ability to reverse LTP at striatal synapses functions as a mechanism for "forgetting" maladaptive habits, thus the lack of ability to reverse LTP may have important consequences in drug addiction. Increased BDNF levels in VTA neurons during withdrawal from cocaine plays a role in synaptic remodeling. BDNF also promotes long-lasting changes in the mesolimbic dopamine system by activating mechanisms of associative learning that underlie persistent addictive behavior.

Chapter 8 - Synaptic plasticity in the medial prefrontal cortex is essential for shaping the responsiveness of neuronal networks involved in executive and cognitive functions. This chapter will review the current literature on synaptic plasticity in this brain region. It will begin with an overview of the basic circuitry in the medial prefrontal cortex. It will then describe the multiple forms of short-term plasticity exhibited by pyramidal neurons in the medial prefrontal cortex. The cellular and molecular mechanisms underlying long-term synaptic changes will next be described, including long-term potentiation, long-term depression and spike timing-dependent plasticity, in addition to how these forms of long-term synaptic changes are modulated by neuromodulators such as dopamine. Synaptic plasticity at connections between the hippocampus and the medial prefrontal cortex will be examined, together with a discussion on the role of interactions between the medial prefrontal cortex and the amygdala. Finally, the author will explore the physiological function of synaptic plasticity in the medial prefrontal cortex, including the role it plays in working memory, in determining rules to shape behavioural patterns, in consolidation of memories, in neurological disorders, and in drug addiction.

Chapter 9 - Synaptic plasticity is a fundamental process underlying learning and memory formation. Long-term potentiation (LTP) and long-term depression (LTD) are the predominant experimental models used for studying the mechanisms of synaptic plasticity. This chapter focuses on signal molecules and signaling cascades involved in pre- and postsynaptic mechanisms that contribute to the induction of LTP and LTD in a key structure of the limbic system, the lateral nucleus of the amygdala (LA). The amygdala is a component of the limbic system that plays a central role in emotional behavior predominantly in fear conditioning. Moreover, the amygdala is involved in certain psychopathologies, like epilepsy or major depression. The amygdala is a complex structure, composed of different brain nuclei, whereby the LA seems to play an essential role for the amygdala, since the LA represents the main input station of the amygdala. Since a large body of literature highlights the role of the amygdala in fear learning, the authors therefore focus primarily on differences and similarities in long-term transmission changes recorded in coronal and horizontal brain slices of mice and rats. Topics include the four cardinal features of synaptic plasticity in the LA (cooperativity, associativity, persistence, and input-specificity). Further topics include the modulatory actions of various transmitter systems on amygdaloid plasticity, evidences for upregulated postsynaptic mechanisms in LTP, and the role of gene expression regulation in the maintenance of LTP. Moreover, the authors will shed light onto the paradigms used to induce synaptic plasticity, since, depending on the used stimulation protocols, multiple, different forms of LTP and LTD can be induced in the LA. Furthermore, it is known that the efficiency of transmission across synapses can be potentiated or depressed in response to a prior history of stimulation. The authors will present data that support the finding that this phenomenon, called metaplasticity, is not restricted to the cortex and hippocampus, but can also be observed at the level of the amygdala. Last, but not least, the authors briefly discuss the impact of age and gender on LTP and LTD within the LA.

Chapter 10 - In order to guide behavior, sensory information has to be analyzed in the context of previous memory and attention-related episodes. Such episodes can represent sequences of sensory items in space and time and the learning of such sequences is known as episodic memory. The formation of this memory is believed to be mediated in the hippocampal region, and is generated by the changes in neuronal efficacy known as long-term synaptic plasticity. In this chapter the authors will review some of the up-to-date models of synaptic plasticity and their relation to the structural and functional memory processes demonstrated by behavioral and electrophysiological experiments. The main aim of this chapter is to describe how neuroplastic mechanisms work together to create network representations of previous experiences. Here, the authors specifically consider experience-dependent modulation of hippocampal cell firing in the context of spatial memory formation. The information encoded by the firing patterns of these neurons represents sequences of events and places that will be stored in a long-term manner. However, the precise connection between the neuronal firing rate changes and long-term synaptic plasticity is still controversial. A significant challenge remains to reveal how the processing, encoding and storage of highly-integrated sensory information occurs within the circuitry of the hippocampus. Recent electrophysiological findings in combination with computational memory models allow researchers to obtain closer insights into how information is represented in the hippocampal formation and how this information is encoded. To gain a better understanding of hippocampal experience-dependent synaptic plasticity, the authors also will create parallels between the synaptic alterations in the declarative memory system and the equivalent synaptic changes throughout the functionally well-known perceptual and procedural memory systems. The authors review the development of hippocampus-dependent memory models and stress the importance of functional patterns that characterize the remodeling of the neural connectivity.

Chapter 11 - Spinophilin/neurabin 2 is a protein scaffold that targets protein phosphatase 1 catalytic subunit (PP1c) close to some of its substrates. Gene analysis and biochemical approaches have contributed to define in spinophilin a number of distinct modular domains, such as one F-actin-, a receptor- and a PP1c-binding domains, a PSD95/DLG/zo-1 (PDZ) and three coiled-coil domains, that govern protein-protein interactions. Spinophilin plays important functions in the nervous system where it is implicated in spine morphology and density regulation, neuronal migration and synaptic plasticity. Morphological studies and subcellular distribution analysis indicated that spinophilin was enriched in dendritic spines in the postsynaptic density (PSD). The spinophilin interactome includes the glutamatergic α-amino-3-hydroxy-5-methylisoxazole-4-propionic acid (AMPA) and N-methyl-D-aspartic acid (NMDA) receptors that interact with the PDZ domain of the scaffolding protein. Studies using spinophilin Knockout (KO) mice suggested that spinophilin serves to regulate excitatory synaptic transmission and plasticity by targeting PP1c in the proximity of AMPA and NMDA receptors, promoting their down-regulation by dephosphorylation and thus regulating the efficiency of post-synaptic glutamatergic neurotransmission. The use of spinophilin KO mice also provides evidence that spinophilin is a good candidate to serve as a link between excitatory synapse transmission and changes in spine morphology and density. The molecular mechanism that controls spine morphology was in part recently elucidated and involved another spinophilin partner protein, the Rho-guanine nucleotide exchange factor Lfc. This review presents the available data that are contributing to the appreciation of spinophilin functions in synaptic plasticity and compares these functions to those of the related structural protein neurabin 1.

Chapter 12 - A hypothesis is advanced that dopamine-dependent synaptic plasticity (LTP, LTD) and subsequent activity reorganization in the cortico-basal ganglia-thalamocortical loops underlies attentional selection and processing of a visual stimulus. Both effects are the result of opposite modulatory action of dopamine on strong and weak cortico-striatal inputs that synergistically leads to disinhibition and inhibition via the basal ganglia of thalamic cells projected to those neocortical neurons, in which initial visual activation was strong and weak, respectively. Thus, the output basal ganglia projections to the thalamus could play a role of "attentional filter" that amplifies cortical responses to attended stimulus, and suppresses reactions to ignored stimuli. A proposed model based on cortico-striatal synaptic plasticity allows explaination of some experimentally revealed effects of which mechanisms were unclear from points of view of commonly accepted models that are based on feedback connections from higher to lower cortical areas and to the thalamus. The authors assume that proposed necessity of sensory activation of dopaminergic cells for switching the attentional part of processing and known latency of sensory activation of dopaminergic cells (which is about 100 ms) explain experimentally-obtained absence of attentional modulation of neocortical responses with latencies that do not exceed 100 ms. This model can also help the understanding of the mechanisms underlaying attentional disorders.

In: Synaptic Plasticity: New Research
Editors: Tim F. Kaiser and Felix J. Peters

ISBN: 978-1-60456-732-8

Chapter 1

SYNAPTIC PLASTICITY: PHYSIOLOGY AND NEUROLOGICAL DISEASE

Stephen D. Skaper *

Neurology Centre of Excellence for Drug Discovery, GlaxoSmithKline Research and Development Limited, New Frontiers Science Park.Third Avenue,CM19 5AW, Harlow, Essex, United Kingdom

ABSTRACT

Neuroplasticity is both a substrate of learning and memory and a mediator of responses to neuronal cell attrition and injury (compensatory plasticity). It is a continuous process in reaction to neuronal activity and neuronal injury, death, and genesis, which involves modulation of structural and functional processes of axons, dendrites, and synapses. The varied structural elements that embody plasticity include long-term potentiation (a cellular correlate of learning and memory), synaptic efficacy, synaptic remodelling, synaptogenesis, neurite extension including axonal sprouting and dendritic remodelling, and neurogenesis and recruitment. Degenerative diseases of the human brain have long been viewed as among the most enigmatic and intractable problems in biomedicine. As research on human neurodegeneration has moved from descriptive phenomenology to mechanistic analysis, it has become increasing apparent that the morphological lesions long used by neuropathologists to confirm a clinical diagnosis after death might provide an experimentally tractable handle to understand causative pathways. For example, Alzheimer's disease (AD) is an aging-dependent neurodegenerative disorder that is characterised by neuropathologically by the deposition of insoluble amyloid β-peptide (Aβ) in extracellular plaques and aggregated tau protein, which is found largely in the intracellular neurofibrillary tangles. There is growing evidence that mild cognitive impairment in early AD may be due to synaptic dysfunction caused by the accumulation of non-fibrillar, oligomeric Aβ, long before widespread synaptic loss and neurodegeneration occur. Soluble Aβ oligomers can adversely affect synaptic structure and plasticity at extremely low concentrations, although the molecular

* Tel: 0044-1279-622350 / Fax: 0044-1279-622555. E-mail: Stephen_d_Skaper@gsk.com

substrates by which synaptic memory mechanisms are disrupted remain poorly understood. A primary locus of excitatory synaptic transmission in the mammalian central nervous system is the dendritic spine. These protrusions from dendritic shafts exhibit dynamic changes in number, size and shape in response to variation in hormonal status, developmental stage, and changes in afferent input. Not surprisingly, loss of spine density has been linked to cognitive and memory impairment in AD, but the underlying mechanism(s) in this case is uncertain, as well. Intriguingly, findings in other neurodegenerative diseases indicate that a broadly similar process of synaptic dysfunction is induced by diffusible oligomers of misfolded proteins. This chapter will present a critical review of current knowledge on the bases of synaptic dysfunction in neurodegenerative diseases, with a focus on AD, and will encompass both amyloid- and non-amyloid-driven mechanisms. Where appropriate, consideration will also be given to emerging data which point to potential therapeutic approaches for ameliorating the cognitive and memory deficits associated with these disorders.

Keywords: plasticity, synapse, dendrites, spines, glutamatergic, neurodegeneration, memory, cognition, Alzheimer's disease, Parkinson's disease

INTRODUCTION

Neuroplasticity comprises a spectrum of structural elements: long-term potentiation (LTP), synaptic efficacy and remodeling, synaptogenesis, neuritogenesis including axonal sprouting and dendritic remodeling, and neurogenesis. Synaptic strengthening, which requires activation of pre- and postsynaptic elements underlies the phenomenon of LTP as a model of memory formation, and which is associated with synapse dynamics including formation and removal of synapses and changes in synapse morphology [Chang and Greenough, 1984; Martin *et al.,* 2000]. Signals of plasticity include intraneuronal (anterograde and retrograde), interneuronal (transsynaptic and extra/parasynaptic) as well as intercellular signaling through glia [Cotman and Nieto-Sampedro 1984]. Those neuronal systems playing a crucial role in higher brain functions (e.g. learning, memory, cognition) such as hippocampus, neocortical association areas, and the cholinergic basal forebrain neurons, retain a high degree of structural plasticity throughout life [Arendt, 2004]. A number of molecules acting as such signals will be discussed in the course of this article.

The adult central nervous system (CNS) responds to injury with limited yet sometimes effective restoration of synaptic circuitry. Whether compensatory growth is widespread and whether it reverses cognitive deficits is a subject still debated [Cotman *et al.,* 1991; Masliah *et al.,* 1995]. Functional recovery requires that reactive synaptogenesis not exacerbate circuitry dysfunction [Cotman *et al.,* 1991; Masliah et al., 1991]. Brain self-reorganization continuously balances synapse formation and removal as well as neurite sprouting and retraction, and in some conditions, inhibition of sprouting may actually be protective by sequestering dysfunctional neurons [Mesulam, 2000]. At the other end of the spectrum, mechanisms that regulate neuronal plasticity might be instrumental in neurodegenerative diseases. Intriguingly, brain regions with the highest degree of structural plasticity are those that take longest to mature during childhood [Braak and Braak, 1996] and are the same regions with the highest degree of vulnerability during aging and in Alzheimer's disease (AD) [Braak and Braak, 1991; Arendt, 2004].

Neuroplasticity and synapses: Alzheimer's disease as a case in point

Twenty-five percent of individuals over 65 years of age have sufficient cognitive problems, short of dementia, to affect the quality of their lives [Unverzagt et al., 2001]. The ability to learn consciously and recall new information is one of the areas most affected during aging. Yet, our knowledge about the factors that predispose a person to age-associated cognitive problems remains fragmented. The balance between dynamic stabilization and destabilization of synapses may provide the basis for failure of plasticity with age and disease. In vivo, synaptogenesis rates decline with developmental age, and there is recapitulation of developmental gene expression responses in adult lesion [Styren *et al.,* 1999] and aging, including AD [Kondo *et al.,* 1996]. If mechanisms controlling developmental plasticity were to be defective and later reactivated (e.g. in aging, mild cognitive impairment in early AD, or clinically diagnosed AD), they might contribute to ineffective plasticity responses and exacerbate the plasticity burden of aging and AD. The differential susceptibility of AD-specific regions and neurons may, indeed, be related to the degree of retained capacity for plastic remodeling [Arendt *et al.,* 1998].

AD is an aging-dependent neurodegenerative disorder characterized by two main neuropathological hallmarks in the brain: deposition of insoluble fibrillar Aβ (amyloid β-peptide) in extracellular plaques; aggregated hyperphosphorylated tau protein, which is found largely in the intracellular neurofibrillary tangles [Selkoe and Schenk, 2003]. Aβ is generated by sequential proteolytic cleavage of amyloid precursor protein (APP). The non-amyloidogenic pathway involves cleavage by α-secretases, while the amyloidogenic pathway involves cleavage by β- and γ-secretases [Jarrett *et al.,* 1993; De Strooper *et al.,* 2000]. Aβ generated by γ-secretase activity can vary in length: the most common forms contain 38, 40 or 42 amino acids. Because of the two additional amino acids isoleucine and alanine, $A\beta_{1\text{-}42}$ aggregates more quickly than $A\beta_{1\text{-}40}$ [Grimm *et al.,* 2007] and is the major component of neuritic plaques in AD. The relevance of $A\beta_{1\text{-}42}$ in AD is further supported by familial forms of AD. Most of the missense mutations in the genes encoding APP and presenilin increase the production of $A\beta_{1\text{-}42}$. There is now extensive evidence that abnormal processing of Aβ, as a result of altered production by β-secretase and γ-secretase cleavage of amyloid precursor protein (APP) or impaired Aβ clearage mechanisms, leading to the accumulation of toxic aggregates, is a causal factor in AD [Hardy and Selkoe, 2002]. The thesis that synaptic memory mechanisms are a consequence of Aβ-induced dysfunction will be discussed further on.

Synaptic loss in the hippocampus and neocortex is an early event and is the major structural correlate of cognitive dysfunction in AD [Gonatas *et al.,* 1967; Davies *et al.,* 1987; Scheff *et al.,* 1990; Terry *et al.,* 1991; DeKosky *et al.,* 1996; Masliah, 1998; reviewed in Arendt, 2001]. Synaptic pathology is reflected by a loss of all major components of small synaptic vesicles and most peptides, accompanied by extensive aberrant changes of the synapse [Lassmann *et al.,* 1993]. The bulk of neocortical synaptic loss most likely derives from loss of cortico-cortical associational fibers [Morrison *et al.,* 1990], rather than degeneration of subcortical input [Arendt *et al.,* 1995b]. Synapse and dendrite loss in AD exceeds that seen with normal aging [Terry *et al.,* 1994]. AD is a slowly progressing disorder, Synaptic degeneration, like early AD, is a slow process progressing from an initially reversible functionally responsive stage of down-regulation of synaptic function to stages irreversibly associated by marked synapse loss [Rapoport, 1999]. Memory loss in AD may result from synaptic dysfunction that precedes large-scale neurodegeneration, where the synapse-to-neuron ratio is decreased by about 50% [Chapman *et al.,* 1999; Chen *et al.,* 2000]. This is eventually accompanied by the loss of about 10-20% of cortical neurons [Masliah, 1998].

In contrast to a continuous growth during aging, both axonal and dendritic proliferation in AD is restricted to certain cell types and stages of the disease [Arendt *et al.,* 1995a, 1998], and is aberrant with respect to localization, morphology, cytoskeletal composition [Arendt *et al.,* 1986; McKee *et al.,* 1989; Phinney *et al.,* 1999], and synaptic protein expression [Geddes et al., 1985, Ihara, 1988]. Aberrant sprouts are detectable early in AD, precede tangle formation and occur in the absence of frank neuronal cell loss [Ihara 1988; Su *et al.,* 1993]. In AD, axon length correlates with dementia severity suggesting regressive axonal events may be more relevant than dendritic attrition or neuronal cell loss [Anderson, 1996]. This is consistent with degeneration of synaptic termini that then leads to secondary transneuronal degeneration of postsynaptic dendrites [Su *et al.,* 1997]. Dendritic extent in the hippocampus normally increases with age, perhaps as a compensatory response to loss of synaptic connections [Flood and Coleman, 1990]. This may not be sustainable, however, because enhanced dendritic growth in early aging is followed by regression of dendritic arbors in the latest age [Flood *et al.,* 1985]. Massive somatodendritic sprouting is seen also in neocortex and hippocampus in AD [Ihara, 1988], which may reflect unsuccessful remodeling in response to presynaptic or axonal damage [Scott, 1993]. Disturbed neuroplastic mechanisms might thus represent an event of primary significance, inherent to the pathobiology of AD, rather than a response triggered by ongoing degeneration.

Dendritic spines and synaptic degeneration

As discussed above, early AD almost solely comprises severely dysfunctional memory [Terry *et al.,* 1991; Selkoe, 2002; Coleman *et al.,* 2004], a specificity likely attributable to a vulnerability of particular memory-focused synapses to degeneration [Selkoe, 2002; Scheff and Price, 2003; Coleman *et al.,* 2004]. Recent evidence suggests that synapse degeneration begins at the level of dendritic spines, which are the loci of memory-initiating mechanisms [Harris and Kater, 1994; Carlisle and Kennedy, 2005; Segal, 2005]. During development, dendritic spines appear to begin as thin extensions called filopodia that then mature with an expanded mushroom-shaped "head" linked by a neck to the dendrites [Matus, 2005]. These protrusions from dendritic shafts exhibit dynamic changes in number, size, and shape in response to variation in hormonal status, developmental stage, and changes in afferent input [Fifkova, 1985; Muñoz-Cueto *et al.,* 1991; Wooley and McEwen, 1992; Moser *et al.,* 1994; Murphy and Segal, 1996]. Pathological loss of spines and their associated molecules is well documented for AD brain [Scheibel, 1983; Ferrer and Gullotta, 1990; Shim and Lubec, 2002; Scheff and Price, 2003] and transgenic AD mouse models [Lanz *et al.,* 2003; Calon *et al.,* 2004; Moolman *et al.,* 2004; Spires *et al.,* 2005; Jacobsen *et al.,* 2006], together with significant decreases in molecules involved in spine signaling [Sze *et al.,* 2001; Mishizen-Eberz *et al.,* 2004] and control of filamentous actin [Harigaya *et al.,* 1996; Shim and Lubec, 2002; Counts *et al.,* 2006]. Conceivably, AD dementia may be initiated before synapse degeneration by spine aberrations. In fact, spine shape distortions are evident in other severe cognitive diseases such as mental retardation and prionoses. Mechanisms which may affect dendritic spine formation and plasticity in neurodegenerative disorders will now be discussed.

Aβ-induced synaptotoxicity

In spite of their central importance to AD, the molecules responsible for spine pathology remain unknown. Involvement of insoluble Aβ fibrils has been considered a prime suspect for many years; however, abnormal neuropil in AD can occur in the absence of contiguous amyloid plaques [Einstein *et al.,* 1994; Lue *et al.,* 1999; Coleman *et al.,* 2004]. In transgenic mouse models, synapse abnormalities as well as memory impairments correlate poorly with plaque burden and can occur before plaque formation [Holcomb *et al.,* 1999; Hsia *et al.,* 1999; Larson *et al.,* 1999; Mucke *et al.,* 2000; Jacobsen *et al.,* 2006]. Although Aβ antibodies prevent synaptic degeneration in transgenic mice [Buttini *et al.,* 2005], memory impairment is reversed without plaque loss [Dodart *et al.,* 2002; Kotilinek *et al.,* 2002]. These findings suggest that a toxin from Aβ, not present in plaques, may be the culprit behind synapse degeneration. Indeed, AD brain [Gong *et al.,* 2003; Kayed *et al.,* 2003; Lacor *et al.,* 2004] and cerebrospinal fluid [Georganopoulou *et al.,* 2005; Haes *et al.,* 2005] contain small neurotoxins that comprise soluble Aβ oligomers, termed Aβ-derived diffusible ligands (ADDLs) [Lambert *et al.,* 1998]. Neuronal injury triggered by ADDLs is now viewed by many as a central feature of AD pathology [Standridge, 2006]. ADDLs are gain-of-function ligands that target dendritic spines [Lacor *et al.,* 2004] and disrupt synaptic plasticity [Lambert *et al.,* 1998; Wang *et al.,* 2002].

The cellular actions of ADDLs may be of particular relevance to neutropil damage [Klein, 2006] A recent study by Lacor *et al.* (2007) provides direct biological evidence for the hypothesis that synaptic damage is caused by ADDLs, establishing that the latter alter spine composition, morphology and density in highly differentiated cultures of hippocampal neurons (a widely accepted model for studies of synapse cell biology) (Fig. 1).

ADDLs bound to neurons with specificity, attaching to presumed excitatory pyramidal neurons but not GABAergic neurons [Lacor *et al.,* 2007]. Because ADDLs block LTP [Lambert *et al.,* 1998; Wang *et al.,* 2002] by binding directly to dendritic spines [Lacor *et al.,* 2004] and disrupt N-methyl-D-aspartate (NMDA) receptor-mediated CREB phosphorylation [Tong *et al.,* 2001], it is not unexpected that surface glutamate receptor levels would be altered by ADDLs [Gong *et al.,* 2003]. Additionally, ADDLs induce abnormal expression of Arc [Lacor *et al.,* 2004], a spine cytoskeletal protein that influences glutamate receptor trafficking [Mokin *et al.,* 2006], and cause a major loss of surface NMDA receptors [Lacor *et al.,* 2007]. Loss of NMDA receptors has been seen in AD brain [Sze *et al.,* 2001; Mishizen-Eberz *et al.,* 2004] and in a transgenic AD mouse model [Snyder *et al.,* 2005], and correlates with synaptic alterations and cognitive deficits [Terry *et al.,* 1991; Sze *et al.,* 1997; Counts *et al.,* 2006]. The large decrease in receptor expression reported by Lacor *et al.* (2007) occurred prior to changes in spine density, consistent with synaptic plasticity being compromised before onset of degeneration.

In addition to affecting NMDA receptors, ADDLs promoted a rapid decrease in membrane expression of EphB2. These two synaptic receptors physically interact via their extracellular domains [Dalva *et al.,* 2000] and are functionally related to plasticity. NMDA receptors play a central role in the induction of LTP [Morris and Davis, 1994], and EphB2 exerts control over NMDA-dependent LTP [Matynia *et al.,* 2002]. Moreover, both receptors influence dendritic spine morphology and maintenance [Carlisle and Kennedy, 2005]. Taken together, the observed disruption of dendritic spines links ADDLs to a major facet of AD pathology, and provides compelling evidence that ADDLs in AD brain cause neuropil damage believed to underlie dementia.

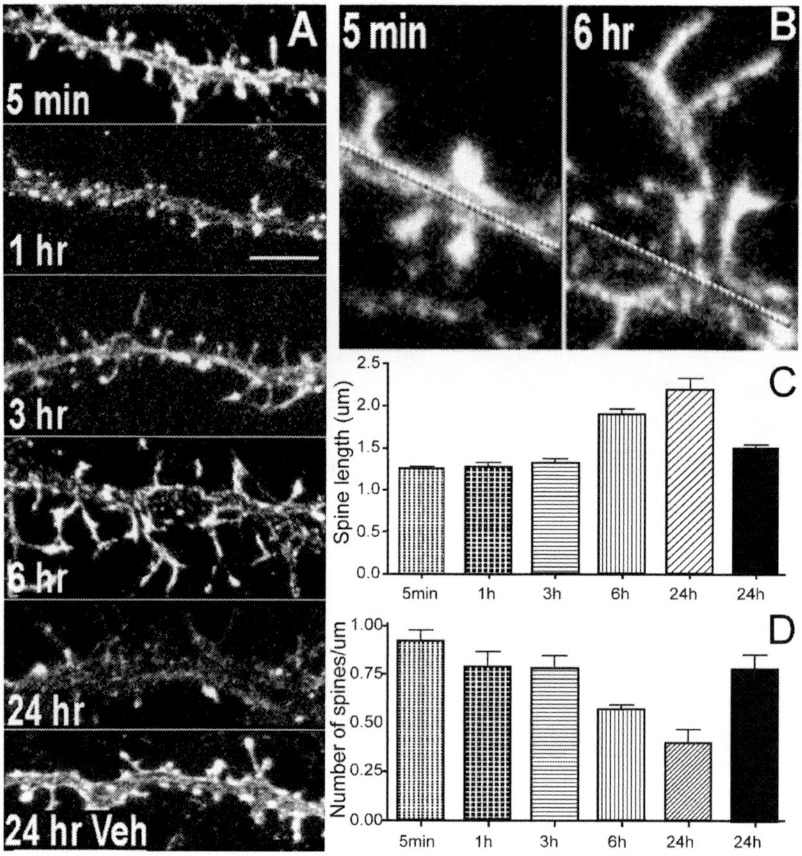

Figure 1. ADDL-induced aberrations in dendritic spine morphology and density. Cultured rat hippocampal neurons at 21 days in vitro were treated for the times indicated with 500 nM ADDL. ***A,*** Confocal microscopy images representative of individual dendrtitic branches decorated with spiny protrusions immunolabeled for drebrin after ADDL or vehicle (Veh) treatment. Longer and more irregularly shaped spines appear after as early as 3 hours treatment and are more pronounced after 6 hours. Also note the reduced number of dendritic spines after 24 hours ADDL. Scale bar, 5 μm. ***B,*** Illustration of zoomed dendritic branches harboring "spines" demonstrates the pronounced lengthening of dendritic protrusions after 6 hours of ADDL treatment. The line marks the dendritic shaft. ***C,D,*** Histograms represent average length and density of drebrin-labeled dendritic spines after ADDL (patterned bars) or vehicle (black bars) incubation at various times. See Lacor *et al.* (2007) for further details. [Reproduced from *The Journal of Neuroscience 27(4),* P.N. Lacor, M.C. Buniel, P.W. Furlow, A.S. Clemente, P.T. Velasco, M. Wood, K.L. Viola and W.L. Klein, Aβ oligomer-induced aberrations in synapse composition, shape and density provide a molecular basis for loss of connectivity in Alzheimer's disease, 796-807 (Fig. 5), Copyright (2007), with permission from The Society for Neuroscience].

The underlying cellular mechanism of Aβ oligomer-induced synaptic modifications has been examined using a recently described stable oligomeric Aβ preparation called "$A\beta_{1-42}$ globulomer", which localizes to hippocampal neurons and impairs LTP [Barghorn *et al.*, 2005]. The pathological relevance of $A\beta_{1-42}$ globulomer is supported by the observation that specific antibodies detect globulomer epitopes in brains of AD patients and Aβ-overproducing transgenic mice [Barghorn *et al.*, 2005]. In a subsequent studt, $A\beta_{1-42}$ globulomer was reported to suppress spontaneous synaptic activity by inhibition of P/Q-type calcium currents [Nimmrich *et al.*, 2008]. Because intact P/Q calcium currents are needed for synaptic plasticity, the disruption of such currents by $A\beta_{1-42}$ globulomer may cause deficits in cellular mechanisms of information storage in brains of AD patients. These data, however, do not unambiguously prove that $A\beta_{1-42}$ globulomer directly interacts with P/Q-channel subunits. It is also possible that binding occurs at other synaptic proteins, which then causes a modification of the P/Q current, perhaps by interacting with the auxiliary subunits of the channel [Nimmrich *et al.*, 2008].

A novel transgenic mouse model has recently been described, expressing a human APP with the Swedish and Arctic mutations (arcAβ mice) that produces a form of Aβ more prone to yield Aβ oligomers [Knobloch *et al.*, 2007a]. In these mice, expression of the mutant APP induces severe behavioral deficits before the onset of extracellular Aβ plaque formation. Overexpression of Arctic Aβ is associated with an age-dependent impairment in hippocampal LTP and synaptic plasticity in vitro that involves protein phosphatase 1-dependent mechanisms [Knobloch *et al.*, 2007b]. Futhermore, the pharmacologic and genetic inhibition of protein phosphatase 1 in vitro and in vivo reversed the defect in synaptic plasticity induced by Aβ oligomers. These findings support a role for protein phosphatase 1 in the mechanisms of Aβ oligomer-mediated synaptotoxicity.

Glucose tolerance and insulin

Poor glucose tolerance and memory deficits, short of dementia, often accompany aging. Indeed, there is a growing literature indicating that individuals with diabetes have impairments in recent memory [Richardson, 1990; Stewart and Liolitsa, 1999; Biessels *et al.*, 2001; Strachan *et al.*, 2000]. In addition, nondiabetic individuals with mild forms of impaired glucose tolerance (IGT) may also have cognitive impairments [Vanhanen *et al.*, 1997; Kaplan *et al.*, 2000]. The prevalence of memory problems and IGT rise with age [Harris *et al.*, 1987; Shimokata *et al.*, 1991; Unverzagt *et al.*, 2001]. In addition to genetic predisposition, obesity and low levels of physical activity have been identified as risk factors for IGT in adults and children [Fagot-Campagna, 2000; Astrup, 2001]. With life expectancy and obesity on the rise, the prevalence of memory dysfunction and IGT will likely continue to climb. Hypothalamus-pituitary-adrenal axis hyperactivity has been associated with hippocampal atrophy in aging [Lupien *et al.*, 1998]. Cortisol administration reduces glucose transport into neurons [Horner *et al.*, 1990] and causes reductions in hippocampal glucose utilization [de Leon *et al.*, 1997], which may explain why animals that have abnormal glucose metabolism have more hippocampal damage when exposed to high levels of corticosteroids [Magariños and McEwen, 2000]. In addition to the higher prevalence of memory problems and IGT mentioned above, age-associated reductions in hippocampal volumes have also been reported [Convit *et al.*, 1995]. Moreover, a recent study has shown that among nondiabetic, nondemented middle-aged and elderly individuals, decreased peripheral glucose regulation was associated with decreased general cognitive performance, memory impairments, and atrophy of the hippocampus, a brain area that is key for learning and memory [Convit *et al.*, 2003]. These findings support the view that metabolic substrate delivery may influence brain structure and function, and that better lifetime management of blood sugar may improve memory in old age and perhaps even reduce the risk of hippocampal damage and possibly AD.

There is increasing evidence that insulin has metabolic, neurotrophic and neuromodulatory actions in the brain [Gerozissis, 2003]. Although there is relatively little insulin produced within the brain, peripheral insulin has been shown to cross the blood-brain barrier via a receptor-mediated transport process [Plum *et al.*, 2005]. In the brain, insulin receptors are expressed by both astrocytes and neurons [Boyd *et al.*, 1985; Zhu *et al.*, 1990]. Neuronal insulin receptors are concentrated at synapses and are components of postsynaptic densities [Abbott *et al.*, 1999]. Such a localization of insulin receptors has suggested a role for insulin in learning and memory processes. For example, insulin receptors are upregulated and undergo translocation after spatial learning [Zhao and Alkon, 2001]. Insulin modulates the activity of excitatory and inhibitory receptors, including glutamate and GABA receptors and activates the Shc-Ras-MAPK (mitogen-activated protein kinase) pathway and the PI3K (phosphatidylinositol 3-kinase)/PKC (protein kinase C) pathway, both of which are involved in memory processing [Nelson and Alkon, 2005]. The incidence of insulin resistance, a symptom of Type II diabetes, is associated with a higher prevalence of AD [Ott *et al.*, 1996]. Many AD patients have abnormal insulin levels in the cerebrospinal fliud, suggesting altered insulin processing. Insulin also regulates the phosphorylation of tau, a major component of neurofibrillary tangles [Carro and Torres-Aleman, 2004]. Intracerebroventricular injection of streptozotocin or depletion of neuronal insulin receptors produces AD-like effects [Hoyer and Lannert, 1999]. Similarly, the insulin-related peptide insulin-like growth factor-1 is abundant in the CNS and is essential for normal brain development, promoting neuronal growth, dendritic arborisation and synaptogenesis [Bondy and Cheng, 2004]. A recent study has found that insulin and insulin-like growth factor-1 increase the expression of monocarboxylate transporter MCT2 in cultured cortical neurons via a common mechanism involving a translational regulation [Chenal *et al.*, 2007]. In this regard, MCT2 belongs, together with the dendritic scaffolding protein PSD-95, to a class of synaptic proteins regulated at the translational level under conditions leading to synaptic plasticity [Lee *et al.*, 2005]. Considering the primary function of MCT2 as a carrier of alternative energy substrates (lactate, pyruvate, ketone bodies) for neurons [Pierre and Pellerin, 2005], a possible role of insulin- and insulin-like growth factor-1-induced enhancement of MCT2 expression in neurons could be to constitute a reserve pool that is mobilized when necessary to ensure adequate supply of energy substrates to fuel active synapses.

Cholesterol and apolipoprotein E

Cholesterol, like insulin, plays an important role in basic metabolic processes in peripheral tissues and can act as a signaling molecule in the CNS in neuronal function [Dietschy and Turley, 2001]. Levels of cholesterol in the brain are critical for synapse formation and maintenance and recent studies indentify cholesterol as a limiting factor in synaptogenesis [Koudinov and Koudinova, 2001]. One of insulin's main effects in the periphery is to stimulate the activity of HMG-CoA reductase, which catalyses the rate-limiting step in cholesterol biosynthesis. Another link between cholesterol and insulin is that

Type II diabetes is associated with high synthesis and low absorption of cholesterol, and insulin-resistant patients have increased cholesterol synthesis [Pihlajamäki *et al.,* 2004]. Several lines of evidence have implicated a role for cholesterol in AD: elevated cholesterol is associated with increased risk for AD [Evans *et al.,* 2004]; AD patients have elevated levels of total serum cholesterol and LDL (low density lipoprotein)-associated cholesterol [Jarvik *et al.,* 1995]; the ε4 mutant in the gene for ApoE (apolipoprotein E), and important cholesterol transport protein associated with LDL, is a risk factor for AD [Breitner *et al.,* 1999]. Cholesterol may not only promote AD indirectly by promoting cardiovascular disease, but also more directly by interacting with APP. Cholesterol binds to APP and Aβ near the α-secretase cleavage site, and $A\beta_{1\text{-}42}$ competitively inhibits cholesterol binding to ApoE and LDL [Yao and Papadopoulos, 2002].

ApoE is a component of several classes of lipoproteins regulating lipid metabolism and distribution [Mahley and Huang, 1999]. ApoE isotype ε4 is a risk factor for familial and late-onset (>65 years) sporadic AD (LOAD) [Breitner *et al.,* 1999], and early-onset familial AD (FAD) (<65 years) [Roses *et al.,* 1995; Meyer, 1998]. The major epidemiological effect of ε4 in AD is to promote an earlier age of onset that ε3, typically by about 5 years but as much as 15 years [Meyer, 1998; Mesulam, 1999; Ashford and Mortimer, 2002]. Because AD is characterized by ongoing neurodegeneration, accelerated clinical onset could be caused by defects in ApoE-related compensatory mechanisms that repair circuitry [Mesulam, 1999; Teter, 2000]. Differential intracellular trafficking may underlie ApoE isotype effects on plasticity. ApoE isotypes localize differentially and accumulate in neurons and astrocytes [Xu *et al.,* 1998]. AopE isotypes may be sorted into late endosomes, escaping lysosomal hydrolysis, where they can differentially mediate intracellular processes [Mahley and Rall, 2000]. Several lines of transgenic mice have been developed that express the human AopE isotypes under the transcriptional control of various promoters [reviewed in Teter and Ashford, 2002]. In one such line, only female ε4 transgenic mice (under control of the neuron-specific NSE promoter) develop age-related progressive impairments in spatial learning and memory [Raber *et al.,* 1998], a finding consistent with the epidemiological interaction of Apoε4 and female gender on increased risk to develop AD.

Recently, the neuronal sortilin-related receptor SorLA/LR11 (LR11), a member of the ApoE/LDL receptor family, was identified as a probable risk factor for LOAD [Rogaeva *et al.,* 2007]. LR11 functions as a sorting and trafficking protein, guiding APP into the recycling endosome pathways that lead to a reduction of Aβ production [Offe *et al.,* 2006]. Polymorphisms associated with increased AD risk appeared to reduce LR11 mRNA in ~15% of AD cases. Furthermore, neuronal LR11 expression is reduced in the overall LOAD population but not in familial AD pathology [Dodson *et al.,* 2006]. This argues that LR11 deficits in LOAD are not simply secondary to pathology and might play a causal role. Because lipoprotein receptor family proteins are frequently lipid-regulated, for example by cholesterol or essential fatty acids [Zheng *et al.,* 2002], dietary lipids might be expected to increase LR11 expression and thereby reduce AD risk. The only plasma lipid predictive of AD risk in the Framingham study was docosahexaenoic acid (DHA), an essential ω-3 fatty acid related to reduced AD risk and reduced Aβ accumulation [Johnson and Schaefer, 2006]. Dietary DHA significantly improved cognitive deficits, protected synaptic protein loss and lowered insoluble Aβ in an aged DHA-depleted transgenic AD mouse model (Tg2576), apparently by reducing Aβ production [Calon *et al.,* 2004; Lim *et al.,* 2005]. DHA mediated reductions in Aβ have also been found in PS1 x APP mice [Oksman *et al.,* 2006] and in 3 x Tg mice [Green *et al.,* 2007]. In the study by Ma and colleagues (2007), DHA significantly increased LR11 protein levels in aged non-transgenic mice and in DHA-depleted transgenic (APPsw) AD mice. This observation may help explain epidemiology suggesting reduced AD risk associated with increased fish consumption and lower n-6/n-3 fatty acid ratios [Morris *et al.,* 2003; Kalmijn e*t al.,* 2004].

Protein trafficking

Endosomes are believed to be major sorting stations in the endocytotic process, sending proteins and lipids to multiple destinations including the cell surface, Golgi complex and lysosomes [Murk *et al.,* 2003]. Kennedy and Ehlers (2006) have described protein trafficking to and from the postsynaptic membrane as a key mechanism underlying various forms of synaptic plasticity. Ehlers (2000) demonstrated that AMPA receptor sorting occurs early in endosomes and is regulated by synaptic activity and activation of AMPA and NMDA receptors. It has also been suggested that stores of receptors are maintained intracellularly, in organelles capable of rapid delivery to synapses [Ehlers, 2000; Carroll e*t al.,* 2001; Sheng and Lee, 2001]. Endocytosis and exocytosis serve important roles in LTP and long-term depression at hippocampal synapses [Luscher *et al.,* 1999; Shi *et al.,* 1999; Cooney *et al.,* 2002]. Blocking exocytosis prevents the induction of LTP, whereas blocking endocytosis prevents the induction of long-term depression. Endosomes may indeed provide a local store of receptors at individual dendritic spines. However, relatively little is known about the distribution of endosomal organelles in distal dendrites where most synapses are located [Luscher and Frerking, 2001]. The recent observations of Park *et al.* (2006) that spine expansion is trafficked from recycling endosomes that reside locally at the spines themselves suggests that agents which stimulate endocytosis and dendritic spine structure [Popov *et al.,* 2008] may promote synaptic plasticity.

Kinases and synaptic plasticity

Extracellular signal-regulated kinases

Extracellular signal-regulated kinases (ERKs) are members of the MAPK superfamily and form a major signal transduction pathway mediating extracellular stimuli to the nucleus [Schaeffer and Weber, 1999]. Originally discovered as regulators of cell division and differentiation, an important role of the ERK signaling pathway is also evident in synaptic plasticity, learning and memory [Impey *et al.,* 1999; Sweatt, 2004; Thomas and Huganir, 2004]. For example, ERK activation is required for hippocampal LTP induction [English and Sweatt, 1996; Atkins *et al.,* 1998; Kanterewicz *et al.,* 2000]. Behavioral studies have also demonstrated a major role of ERK in long-term memory [Atkins *et al.,* 1998; Blum *et al.,* 1999]. These findings, however, lack a direct link which proves a relationship between LTP and memory. ERK1 and ERK2 display a high degree of sequence homology and share a similar substrate profile [Boulton *et al.,* 1991], and are solely activated by MAPK kinases (MEKs). In the analysis of ERK signaling, most experiments use MEK inhibitors because no specific ERK inhibitors are available, and these do not distinguish between MEK isoforms, making it difficult to dissect the specific contribution of each isoform to physiological function. ERK1 knockout mice do not show impairment in learning [Selcher *et al.*, 2001], but the embryonic lethality of ERK2 null knockout mice [Satoh *et al.*, 2007] precludes similar analyses. Utilizing a gene targeting technique, Satoh *et al.* (2007) have generated a series of mice in which ERK2 expression decreased in an allele dose-dependent manner. Knockdown mice in which ERK2 expression was partially (20-40%) reduced showed a deficit in long-term memory as well as learning impairments [Satoh *et al.*, 2007].

Long-term memory formation involves complex biochemical cascades leading to changes in gene expression, accomplished partly by epigenetic mechanisms that remodel chromatin [Tsankova *et al.*, 2004], These include post-translational modifications of histones, which regulate the dynamic interplay between the native inhibitory state of chromatin and a transcriptionally active state [Jenuwein and Allis, 2001]. A number of studies suggest that chromatin remodeling contributes to regulation of gene expression and neuronal function, particularly in memory and synaptic plasticity [Guan *et al.*, 2002; Korzus *et al.*, 2004; Levenson *et al.*, 2004]. The regulation of histone phosphorylation is especially intriguing, given the importance of the ERK/MAPK cascade in learning and memory. While ERK was shown to regulate histone phosphorylation in hippocampal CA1 neurons [Levenson *et al.*, 2004], the precise downstream molecular mechanisms were not defined. One important histone kinase that has been identified is mitogen- and stress-activated protein kinase-1 (MSK1), a nuclear kinase downstream of ERK/MAPK and p38/MAPK [Deak *et al.*, 1998]. Although MSK1 appears to affect multiple targets important for plasticity and memory, its role in role in behavioral learning remained largely unknown. A recent study now shows that mice lacking MSK1 have deficits in multiple hippocampus-dependent tasks, and a selective deficiency in histone H3 phosphorylation and acetylation, both markers of transcriptional activation [Chwang *et al.*, 2007].These results establish MSK1 as an important regulator of hippocampal chromatin remodeling in long-term memory.

Glycogen synthase kinase-3

Glycogen synthase kinase-3 (GSK-3) is a ubiquitously expressed serine/threonine kinase that is particularly abundant in the CNS [Woodgett, 1990]. GSK-3 phosphorylation substrates include cytoskeletal proteins, transcription factors, and metabolic regulators, thus leading to a prominent role for GSK-3 in cellular architecture, gene expression, and apoptosis among others [Jope and Johnson, 2004]. This kinase may also play an important role in AD. Up-regulation of GSK-3 by conditional induction [Hernandez *et al.*, 2002; Engel *et al.*, 2006] in mice or by simultaneous inhibition of PI3K and PKC [Liu *et al.*, 2003] in rats not only induces tau hyperphosphorylation, but also impairs spatial learning any memory. Moreover, two types of molecules approved for AD therapy, i.e. an inhibitor of acetylcholinesterase [Scarpini *et al.*, 2003] and an NMDA receptor antagonist [Reisberg *et al.*, 2003] can increase the serine inhibitory phosphorylation of GSK-3 in mouse brain and thus lead to the inhibition of the kinase [De Sarno et al., 2006]. Collectively, these findings suggest that activation of GSK-3 impairs learning and memory, whereas inhibition of GSK-3 reverses this effect. The mechanism by which GSK-3 regulates learning and memory is not understood, although impaired LTP may be a factor. Recent studies have shown that GSK-3 was inhibited during LTP but activated during long-term depression [Peineau *et al.*, 2007], and that conditional expression of GSK-3 in mouse brain inhibited LTP [Hooper *et al.*, 2007]. Using pharmacological and genetic manipulations of GSK-3 activity, Zhu *et al.* (2007) have now demonstrated that overactivation of GSK-3 inhibits the induction of LTP in rat hippocampus.

With activation of GSK-3, both presynaptic release of glutamate and expression of postsynaptic proteins decreased, and LTP-associated synaptic impairments were observed morphologically. These lesions were partially but significantly restored with a concomitant inhibition of the GSK-3 upregulation [Zhu *et al.,* 2007]. These results reveal that GSK-3 activation impairs synaptic plasticity both functionally and structurally, which may underlie the GSK-3-involved deficits in learning and memory.

The PI3K/Akt signaling pathway is of central importance for neuronal physiology. In addition to its role in neuronal cell survival [Brunet *et al.,* 2001] this pathway has been implicated in dendritic morphogenesis [Jaworski *et al.,* 2005], establishment of neuronal polarity [Jiang *et al.,* 2005], synaptic potentiation [Opazo *et al.,* 2003; Wang *et al.,* 2003] and memory formation [Lin *et al.,* 2001; Mizuno *et al.,* 2003]. In addition, PI3K/Akt signaling regulates translation by activating mTOR (mammalian target of rapamycin [Ruggero and Sonenberg, 2005] and suppresses the activity of GSK-3 [Cross *et al.,* 1995]. Presenilin-1 (PS1) is a ubiquitously expressed transmembrane protein that plays critical roles in development [Shen *et al.,* 1997; Wong *et al.,* 1997] and in FAD [Sherrington *et al.,* 1995]. Recent studies in fibroblasts implicate PS1 in the regulation of the PI3K/Akt signaling pathway [Baki *et al.,* 2004; Uemura *et al.,* 2007]. In this context, newly published data [Baki *et al.,* 2008] propose that wild-type PS1 prevents neuronal degeneration by promoting PI3K/Akt signaling, while PS1 FAD mutations increase GSK-3 activity and promote neuronal apoptosis by inhibiting the function of PS1 in this pathway. These observations suggest that stimulation of PI3K/Akt signaling may be beneficial to FAD patients.

Cyclin-dependent kinase 5

Cyclin-dependent kinase 5 (Cdk5) belongs to the family of serine/threonine cyclin-dependent kinases. Despite its high degree of homology to other cyclin-dependent kinases, Cdk5 stands alone in this family by virtue of not being activated by cyclins [Liu and Kipreos, 2000]. Cdk5 plays an important role in a range of physiological and pathological processes. This multifunctionality is best characterized in neurons and includes involvement in nervous system development, dopaminergic function and neurodegeneration, and is reviewed elsewhere [Dhavan and Tsai, 2001; Shelton and Johnson, 2004]. Cdk5 has been reported to affect pre-synaptic molecular mechanisms, including modulation of voltage-dependent calcium channels and vesicle cycling. Post-synaptically, Cdk5 plays a role in the clustering of proteins, modulation of ion channels and intracellular signaling by regulating PKA and the MAPK pathway, as well as protein phosphatases. Extra-synaptic processes affected by Cdk5 include cell adhesion, transcription and protein translation. In addition, Cdk5 has been implicated in the direct phosphorylation of numerous substrates relevant to synaptic plasticity [reviewed in Angelo *et al.,* 2006]. Collapsin response mediator protein (CRMP) is a signaling molecule of semaphorin3A (Sema3A) [Goshima *et al.,* 1995], one member of the semaphorin family of repellent axonal guidance cues [Raper, 2000]. Sema3A functions not only as a chemorepulsive cue but also in endocytosis, facilitation of axonal transport, and spine development [Nakamura *et al.,* 2000; Morita *et al.,* 2006] through the Fyn-Cdk5 cascade [Morita *et al.,* 2006]. How Sema3A regulates the cytoskeleton has remained unclear, although a new report [Yamashita *et al.,* 2007] suggests that regulation of spine development by Sema3A occurs through Cdk5 phosphorylation of CRMP1, one of the five CRMP family members [Wang and Strittmatter, 1996].

CELL ADHESION MOLECULES AND SYNAPTIC STRUCTURE

Cell adhesion molecules of the immunoglobulin and and cadherin superfamilies have a wide range of functions during development. For example, in the nervous system they play roles in cell migration, axonal growth and guidance, and synapse formation [Walsh and Doherty, 1997]. The neural cell adhesion molecule (NCAM), a member of the immunoglobulin superfamily is a membrane-associated glycoprotein expressed on the surface of neurons and glial cells, and plays a key role in nervous system development [Goodman, 1996] and synaptic plasticity in relation to learning and memory consolidation [Schachner, 1997; Benson *et al.,* 2000; Venero *et al.,* 2006]. Although initially thought to function by modulating adhesion between cells, it is now clear that some cell adhesion molecule functions require the activation of specific second messenger signaling cascades in cells. For example, there is now substantial evidence that NCAM, N-cadherin, and L1 signal via a direct interaction with the fibroblast growth factor receptor (FGFR) [Williams *et al.,* 1994, 2001; Saffell *et al.,* 1997; Sanchez-Heras *et al.,* 2006]. A number of studies have shown that FGFR and NCAM are involved in learning and memory consolidation [Cremer *et al.,* 1994; Sasaki *et al.,* 1999]. A peptide (FGL) mimicking the heterophilic binding of NCAM to FGFR1 has been identified [Kiselyov *et al.,* 2003] which increases the length of neurites from rat embryonic hippocampal neurons with a bell-shaped concentration-response curve characteristic of growth factor-induced neuritogenesis. This stimulatory response can be blocked with an antibody against FGFR, indicating that the NCAM-derived FGL peptide is an agonist of the FGFR [Kiselyov *et al.,* 2003; Neiiendam *et al.,* 2004]. FGL improves cognitive function through enhancement of synaptic function [Cambon *et al.,* 2004]. Whereas FGL mimetic did not affect synaptic or spine density in the hippocampus of aged rats, it did induce significant structural alterations in synapses and dendritic spines [Popov *et al.,* 2008]. These findings indicate that the behavioural changes reported previously following FGL peptide treatment may be at least partially driven by structural modifications in synapses and dendritic spines in hippocampus.

Neurotrophins, astrocytes and dendritic spine plasticity

Neurotrophic factors are secreted proteins that promote neurite outgrowth, neuronal cell differentiation and survival both *in vivo* and *in vitro*. The neurotrophins are a gene family of neurotrophic factors that were identified as promoters of neuronal survival, but it is now appreciated that they regulate many aspects of neuronal development and function, including synapse formation and synaptic plasticity [Sofroniew *et al.,* 2001; Chao *et al.,* 2003; Lu and Woo, 2005; Reichardt, 2006]. The first neurotrophin, nerve growth factor (NGF), was discovered during a search for survival factors that could explain the deleterious effects of deletion of target tissues on the subsequent survival of motor and sensory neurons [Levi-Montalcini, 1987]. NGF is part of the neurotrophin family of polypeptides which function as homodimers, and which share a high degree of structural homology and includes brain-derived neurotrophic factor (BDNF), neurotrophin-3 (NT-3), and neurotrophin-4 (NT-4) [Ibáñez, 1994]. The neurotrophins interact with two entirely distinct classes of receptors, $p75^{NTR}$ and Trks (tropomyosin receptor kinases). The former was initially identified as a low-affinity receptor for NGF, but was subsequently shown to bind each of the neurotrophins with approximately equal nanomolar affinity [Frade and Barde, 1998; Rodriguez-Tebár *et al.*, 1998]. In contrast to interactions with p75^{NTR}, the neurotrophins dimerise the Trk receptors, resulting in activation through transphosphorylation of the kinases present in their cytoplasmic domains. Activated neurotrophin Trk receptors trigger three signaling cascades, phospholipase Cγ-IP$_3$, Ras-Raf-ERK, and PI3K, all of which have been implicated in the varied actions of neurotrophins, ranging from modulation of gene expression, neuronal morphology, synaptic plasticity, and neurotransmitter release [Segal and Greenberg, 1996; Chao, 2003; Reichardt, 2006]. The four neurotrophins exhibit specificity in their interactions with the three members of this receptor family with NGF activating TrkA, BDNF and NT-4 activating TrkB, and NT-3 activating TrkC. In addition, NT-3 can activate the other Trk receptors with less efficiency [Esposito *et al.*, 2001].

Among the neurotrophins, BDNF in particular is a potent modulator of activity-dependent synaptic plasticity in the CNS [Akaneya *et al.*, 1997; Poo, 2001] (Fig. 2).

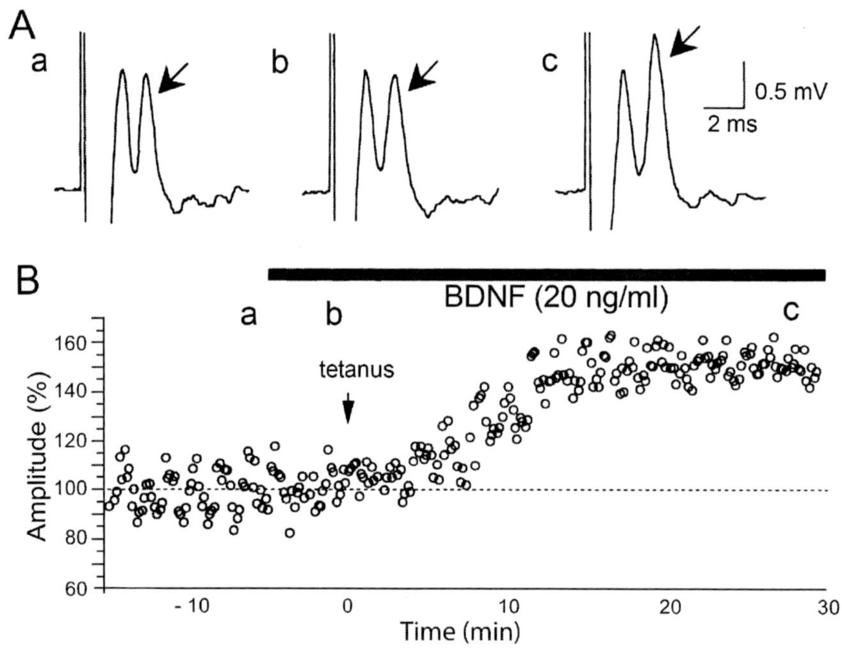

Figure 2. Enhancement of LTP by BDNF. *A*, Examples of layer II/III field responses to test stimulation of layer IV, recorded at the time points indicated by corresponding letters in *B*. Time course of the amplitude of postsynaptic component of responses to test stimulation of layer IV. Tetanic stimulation was given to layer IV at time point 0 (arrow). See Akaneya *et al.* (1997) for further details. [Reproduced from *The Journal of Neuroscience 17(17)*, Y. Akaneya, T. Tsumoto, S. Kinoshita and H. Hatanaka, Brain-derived neurotrophic factor enhances long-term potentiation in rat visual cortex, 6707-6716 (Fig. 6), Copyright (1997), with permission from The Society for Neuroscience].

BDNF acts via Rho GTPases to regulate the assembly of the actin cytoskeleton in developing neurons [Ozdinler and Erzurumlu, 2001; Gehler *et al.*, 2004], and aspects of these signaling pathways may be retained into adulthood in hippocampus [Rex *et al.*, 2007]. Indeed, long-term (minutes to hours) exposure to BDNF induces varied effects on hippocampal neurons, ranging from modulation of synaptic transmission and plasticity to structural changes of dendrites, spines, and presynaptic terminals [McAllister *et al.,* 1999; Poo, 2001; Tyler *et al.,* 2002; Lu, 2003; Amaral *et al.,* 2007]. Conversely, brief (<300 milliseconds) and highly targeted (<20 μm) BDNF pulses evoke fast Na^+ currents through direct activation of $Na_v1.9$ channels [Blum *et al.,* 2002] and slower non-selective cationic currents mediated by transient receptor potential canonical subfamily 3 (TRPC3) channels [Li *et al.,* 1999]. A recent study shows that BDNF elicits a nonselective cationic current (I_{BDNF}) in hippocampal CA1 pyramidal neurons that requires functional Trk receptors, phospholipcase C activity, IP_3 receptors, full intracellular Ca^{2+} stores, and extracellular Ca^{2+}, suggesting the involvement of TRPC channels [Amaral and Pozzo-Miller, 2007]. I_{BDNF} was absent in neurons loaded with anti-TRPC3 function-blocking antibodies or in those transfected with a siRNA construct designed to knockdown TRPC3 expression. BDNF also increased the levels of surface accessible TRPC3 in cultured hippocampal neurons with a requirement for PI3K and a time-course that paralleled the activation of I_{BDNF}, which was also blocked by a PI3K inhibitor [Amaral and Pozzo-Miller, 2007]. Moreover, siRNA-mediated TRPC3 channel knockdown prevented the BDNF-induced increase of dendritic spine density in CA1 pyramidal neurons. TRPC channels may represent novel mediators of BDNF-initiated dendritic remodeling through the activation of a slowly developing and sustained membrane depolarization [Amaral and Pozzo-Miller, 2007].

Neurons of the medial septum and diagonal band of Broca (MS-DBB) project to the hippocampus, modulating its activity and providing important input for cognitive functions such as memory [Winson, 1978]. In addition to cholinergic and GABAergic neurons, glutamatergic neurons [Colom *et al.,* 2005] and neurons that can release acetylcholine and glutamate simultaneously [Allen *et al.,* 2006] have recently been described in the basal forebrain. It is well known that NGF promotes synaptic function of cholinergic basal forebrain neurons [Hartikka and Hefti, 1988], and new findings indicate that NGF is capable of increasing both acetylcholine and glutamate transmission from cholinergic MS-DBB neurons [Huh *et al.,* 2008]. Intriguingly, the latter actions of NGF were mediated by its receptor $p75^{NTR}$, and not TrkA. Accumulating evidence suggests that dysfunctional NGF signaling is implicated in AD. Individuals with early to late stages of AD display reductions in TrkA and p75NTR expression that are correlated with their performance on memory tests [Salehi *et al.,* 2003]. In addition, NGF replacement therapy has emerged as a potential treatment for AD. In a recent phase I clinical trial, implanting NGF-producing fibroblasts into the basal forebrain of AD patients significantly slowed the rate of cognitive decline and increased cortical glucose uptake [Tuszynski *et al.,* 2005]. Conceivably, dysfunctional NGF signaling in AD may cause reductions in both acetylcholine and glutamate release from septal cholinergic neurons, and both changes may contribute to the cognitive deficits associated with AD. Conversely, increasing NGF levels in the brain may enhance both cholinergic and glutamatergic transmission in the septo hippocampal circuit, improving cognitive functions.

Brain development and function depend on glial cells, as they guide the migration of neuronal somata and axons [Silver *et al.,* 1982; Kuwada, 1986; Rakic, 1990], promote the survival and differentiation of neurons [Hosoya *et al.,* 1995; Jones *et al.,* 1995; Pfrieger and Barres, 1995], and insulate and nourish neurons [Tsacopoulos and Magistretti, 1996]. Glial processes ensheath most synapses in the brain [Pomeroy and Purves, 1988; Peters *et al.,* 1991], and a number of studies now support the notion that glial cells do indeed promote the formation and function of synapses. For example, retinal ganglion cells in vitro formed synapses with normal ultrastructure but displayed little spontaneous synaptic activity and high failure rates in evoked synaptic transmission unless cocultured with neuroglia [Pfrieger and Barres, 1997]. Moreover, the efficacy of adult synapses may also depend on their intimate partnership with glial cells [Pfrieger and Barres, 1996]. A subsequent report from this group demonstrated that the total number of synapses on a neuron is not an intrinsic property of that neuron, but can be regulated by extrinsic signals [Ullian *et al.,* 2001]. In the absence of glia, retinal ganglion cell neurons had only a limited ability to form synapses. Astrocytes markedly increased the number of mature, functional synapses and were required for synaptic maintenance in vitro [Ullian *et al.,* 2001] (Fig. 3).

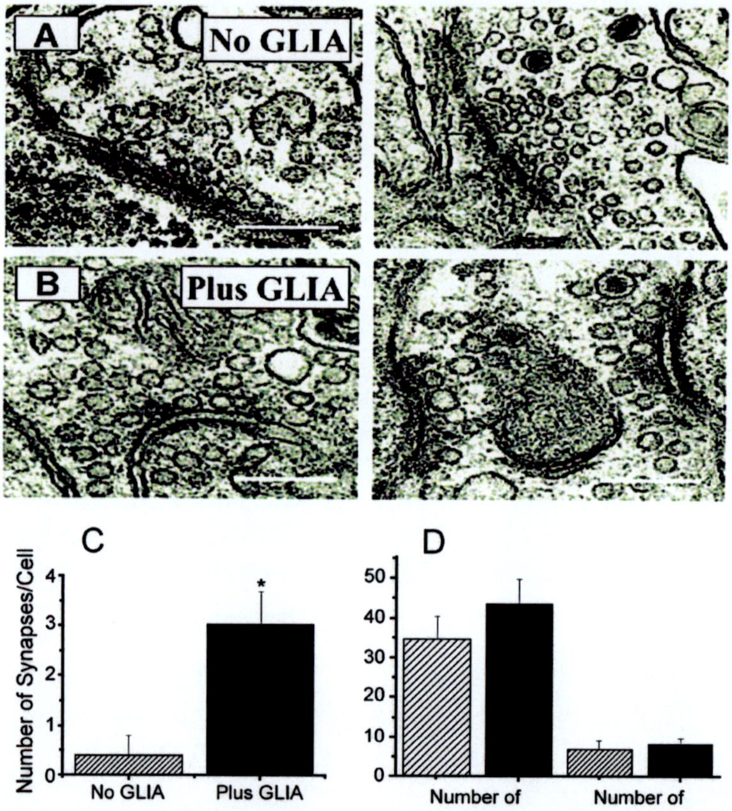

Figure 3. Astrocytes increase the number of synapses per neuron. (A and B) Electron micrographs of synapses between retinal ganglion cell neurons cultured in the absence of glia (A, left and right) and glia (B, left and right). No difference is noted in synaptic ultrastructure. Bar, 200 nm. (C) The number of synapses detected by electron microscopy increased 7-fold in the presence of glia (p=0.013, Student't t-test). (D) No differences in the total number of vesicles without glia or docked vesicles without glia, per synapse. [Reproduced from *Science, 291(657),* E.M. Ullian, S.K. Sapperstein, K.S. Christopherson and B.A. Barres, Control of synapse number by glia, 657-661 (Fig. 4), Copyright (2001), with permission from the American Association for the Advancement of Science].

Moreover, most synapses were generated concurrently with the development of glia in vivo, raising the possibility that glia may actively participate in synaptic plasticity [Ullian *et al.,* 2001]. Astrocyte-secreted proteins that promote CNS synaptogenesis include thrombospondins [Christopherson *et al.,* 2005]. While thrombospondins induce the formation of ultrastructurally normal synapses bearing pre- and postsynaptic specializations that are presynaptically active but postsynaptically silect, an unidentified astrocyte signal induces postsynaptic function by inserting functional AMPA receptors into postsynaptic sites [Christopherson *et al.,* 2005]. This is reminiscent of the two-step model for activation of silent synapses in the developing brain thought to be important for synapse refinement and and circuit modification wherein silent structural synapses are initially formed and some become postsynaptically functional in a second step involving an activity-dependent mechanism [Malenka and Nicoll, 1997]. The above findings implicate astrocytes as active players in both of these steps. Although thrombospondin levels are normally low in the adult brain, reemergence of thrombospondins in reactive astrocytes [Moller *et al.,* 1996; Lin *et al.,* 2003] could account for the formation of aberrant sysnapses that result in epilepsy at astrocytic scars as well as the tendency of axotomized axons to synaptically differentiate and fail to regenerate when they contact reactive astrocytes [Liuzzi and Lasek, 1987]. If so, pharmacological manipulation of thrombospondins may help to promote synaptic plasticity and repair in CNS diseases.

Intriguing new data also point to a role for the complement pathway components C1q and C3 in synaptic elimination, being upregulated when neurons were exposed to astrocytes [Stevens *et al.,* 2007]. Activated microglia secrete most complement cascade components, including particularly high amounts of C1q, and are localized in brain regions during a narrow window of postnatal development that coincides with the peak of synapse formation and elimination [Dalmau et al., 1998; Fiske and Brunjes, 2000]. Conceivably, pharmacological inhibition of the classical complement cascade may inhibit synapse loss and neurodegeneration in neurodegenerative diseases like AD, motor neuron disease and multiple sclerosis.

Estradiol (E_2) can promote dendritic outgrowth, spinogenesis, and synaptogenesis in several discrete loci within the developing and adult brain [Woolley and McEwen, 1992,1993,1994; Calizo and Flanagan-Cato, 2000; Sakamoto *et al.,* 2003]. Astrocytes are important in E_2-induced dendritic spine synapse formation and efficacy [Mong *et al.,* 1999]. Evidence now points to PGE_2 as a mediator of mediator cell-to-cell communication involving crosstalk between astrocytes and neurons [Rage *et al.,* 1997; Bezzi *et al.,* 1998]. Astrocytes release glutamate in response to PGE_2 [Bezzi *et al.,* 1998], which can activate glutamate receptors on neighboring neurons and modulate their dendritic spine density [McKinney *et al.,* 1999; Luthi *et al.,* 2001]. A novel mechanism of neuronal spine plasticity has recently been reported, in which E_2 induces PGE_2 synthesis that in turn increases the density of spine-like processes [Amateau and McCarthy, 2002]. This effect is region-specific in that it was observed in the preoptic area but not the hippocampus, and was dependent on the activation of AMPA-kainate receptors by glutamate that may originate from astrocytes.

Neuronal cell loss is a common feature of many neurological maladies that affect the brain including traumatic brain injury, stroke, and AD [Morrison and Hof, 1997]. Stem cell-based approaches have received considerable attention as a potential means of treatment [Oliveira and Hodges, 2005; Lindvall and Kokaia, 2006; Vora et al., 2006]. Transplanted cells may serve as a reservoir, providing trophic support to surviving cells and synapses, or they may actually replace and partially repopulate damaged areas. However, it remains to be determined whether stem cells can ameliorate memory dysfunction in these disorders. In this context, a recent study describes neural stem cell transplantation into the hippocampus of a transgenic model with targeted neuronal cell loss and consequent improvement in short-term memory on a spatial task in a time-dependent manner [Yamasaki *et al.,* 2007]. The fact that the stem cells localized to the hippocampus in induced mice is consistent with the selective improvement seen on the hippocamal-dependent task, but not on the corically dependent task [Yamasaki *et al.,* 2007]. Trophic mechanisms are likely to contribute to the improvement of memory in the last model. Increases in BDNF occur after brain injury [Kokaia *et al.,* 1998] and BDNF has also been shown to upregulate synapsin [Causing *et al.,* 1997]. The levels of synapsin seen in induced neural stem cell transplanted mice were significantly greater than those seen in lesioned vehicle-injected controls at the CA1 region of the hippocampus [Yamasaki *et al.,* 2007], and are consistent with neurotrophin-induced sprouting. Neurotrophins may contribute also to the neuronal sparing effect seen at both the dentate gyrus and CA1 region of neural stem cell transplanted mice resulting in memory improvement. Although these authors did not see an increase in endogenous neurogenesis with lesioning, neurotrophin-mediated augmentation of endogenous neurogenesis has been described by others [Zigova *et al.,* 1998; Yoshimura *et al.,* 2001].

Inflammation and synaptic plasticity

Recent evidence suggests an inflammatory component in AD, which is characterized by astrogliosis, microgliosis, cytokine elevation, and changes in acute phase proteins [Wyss-Coray, 2006]. Tumor necrosis factor-α (TNF-α) is a cytokine thought to play a central role in the self-propagation of neuroinflammation [Perry *et al.,* 2001]. Increased levels of TNF-α in the brain and plasma of AD patients and an upregulation of TNF receptor 1 have been detected in the AD brain [Fillit *et al.,* 1991; Li *et al.,* 2004]. As already discussed, synaptic dysfunction has gained increasing recognition as an important pathophysiological component of AD. TNF-α may well be involved in such dysfunction. In experimental models, TNF-α alters synaptic transmission in rat hippocampal slices [Tancredi *et al.,* 1992], and TNF-α released by glia controls synaptic strength [Beattie *et al.,* 2002; Stellwagen *et al.,* 2006]. This cytokine may also act as a mediator of Aβ oligomer disruption of memory processes [Wang *et al.,* 2005]. The underlying mechanism is not known, but may involve synaptic scaling. The latter has been suggested to be a key component in the synaptic dysfunction of AD [Small, 2004]. Synaptic scaling involves uniform adjustments in the strength of all synaptic connections for a neuron in response to changes in the neuron's electrical activity [Turrigiano and Nelson, 2004; Stellwagen and Malenka, 2006], and is a homeostatic mechanism which serves for the optimal functioning of neural networks. As synaptic scaling can be regulated by TNF-α [Stellwagen and Malenka, 2006], synaptic dysregulation produced by excess TNF-α [Fillit *et al.,* 1991; Ramos *et al.,* 2006; Álvarez *et al.,* 2007; Tan *et al.,* 2007] may contribute to cognitive and behavioral deficits in AD. Preliminary clinical studies investigating anatomically targeted anti-TNF-α treatment have been reported with encouraging [Tobinick *et al.,* 2006; Tobinick and Gross, 2008], albeit cautionary outcome. Intriguingly, a concentration-dependent duality effect has also been observed for interleukin-1, with the cytokine regulating hippocampal slice LTP under physiological conditions but inhibiting at higher doses [Ross *et al.,* 2003].

Other CNS disorders characterized by altered neuronal spine plasticity

Parkinson's disease

Parkinson's disease (PD) is a common neurodegenerative disorder that leads to difficulty in effectively translating thought into action [Savitt *et al.,* 2006]. PD symptoms are caused by the loss of nigral dopaminergic neurons that innervate the striatum [Albin *et al.,* 1989]. Nigrostriatal dopamine axons synapse onto striatal medium spiny neurons (MSNs) which comprise ~90% of all striatal neurons. These MSNs have radially projecting dendrites that are densely studded with spines [Wilson and Groves, 1980]. Postmortem studies of PD reveal a marked decrease in MSN spine density and dendritic length [McNeill *et al.,* 1988; Zaja-Milatovic *et al.,* 2005]. Similar morphological changes in MSNs are seen in animal models of parkinsonism [Arbuthnott *et al.,* 2000; Day *et al.,* 2006; Neely *et al.,* 2007; Solis *et al.,* 2007]. These changes in dendritic structure are enduring and do not appear to be reversed by levedopa [Zaja-Milatovic *et al.,* 2005].

Mechanisms underlying spine loss and the biochemical and functional consequences are poorly understood. Dopamine depletion increases serine/threonine phosphorylation of multiple synaptic proteins [Brown *et al.,* 2005]; increases in protein phosphorylation are accompanied by a decrease in protein phosphatase 1 (PP1) activity, more specifically decreased activity of the PP1γ_1 isoform. PP1γ_1 is targeted to synapses by interacting with spinophilin, an F-actin-targeting subunit. Total levels of spinophilin or PP1γ_1 were unaffected by striatal dopamine depletion in the 6-hydroxydopamine lesioned rat model of parkinsonism, while association of PP1γ_1 with spinophilin increased [Baucum *et al.,* 2007]. These authors are currently using proteomics to identify novel spinophilin interacting partners that are modulated by striatal dopamine depletion.

The prevailing model of PD asserts that dopamine depletion elevates the activity of striatopallidal neurons and lowers the activity of striatonigral neurons, which leads to an imbalance in the control of basal ganglia outflow to the thalamus and an inability to move effectively in response to higher motor commands [Savitt *et al.,* 2006]. How striatopallidal neurons are changing in ways that are critical to the emergence of PD motor symptoms has remained unknown. A new study now shows that dopamine depletion leads to a rapid and profound loss of spines and glutamatergic synapses on striatopallidal MSNs but not on neighboring striatonigral MSNs [Day *et al.,* 2006]. Moreover, this loss of connectivity was triggered by a novel mechanism—dysregulation of intraspine Cav1.3 L-type Ca^{2+} channels. The disconnection of striatopallidal neurons from motor command structures is likely to be a key step in the emergence of pathological activity that is responsible for symptoms in PD [Day *et al.,* 2006].

Fragile X Syndrome

Fragile X syndrome (FXS), a common form of inherited mental retardation, is caused by amplification of CGG-repeats in the gene [fragile X mental retardation 1 (*Fmr1*)] that encodes fragile X mental retardation protein (FMRP); this leads to gene silencing and an absence of FMRP. The fragile X protein associates with polyribosomes and functions as a negative regulator of protein synthesis [Todd and Malter, 2002], including that occurring in the vicinity of dendritic spines [Zalfa *et al.,* 2003; Weiler *et al.,* 2004; Muddashetty *et al.,* 2007]. A prominent anatomical feature of FXS is increased frequency of elongated apical dendritic spines of neocortical and hippocampal neurons in knockout mice [Comery *et al.*, 1997; Grossman *et al.*, 2006] and in patients with FXS [Rudelli *et al.*, 1985; Irwin *et al.*, 2001], suggesting an anatomical/physiological basis for the cognitive deficits associated with this disorder [Oostra and Hoogeveen, 1997]. It is possible that spine abnormalities found in FXS disrupt the production of LTP and thereby produce learning problems that characterize the syndrome. *Fmr1*-KO mice have deficits in types of learning that are dependent on the hippocampus. LTP elicited by threshold levels of theta burst afferent stimulation was severely impaired in the hippocampal field CA1 of young adult *Fmr1*-KO mice [Lauterborn *et al.*, 2007]. The LTP impairment was evident within 5 minutes of induction; BDNF infusion fully restored LTP in slices from fragile X mice and did so without causing evident changes to baseline physiological or theta burst responses [Lauterborn *et al.*, 2007]. The neurotrophin positively modulates the formation of LTP in normal rodents [Korte *et al.*, 1995; Patterson *et al.*, 1996; Kang *et al.*, 1997] and offset deficits in LTP in mouse models of Huntington's disease [Lynch *et al.*, 2007], possibly via effects on the actin cytoskeleton [Rex *et al.*, 2007]. These results raise the question of whether it will be possible to treat the plasticity deficits in FXS (and other disorders characterized by synaptic dysfunction) by upregulating expression of BDNF. An approach of this type, using positive modulators of AMPA-type glutamate receptors to stimulate neurotrophin production, was reported previously to reverse age-related impairments to LTP in rat [Rex *et al.*, 2006]. Because BDNF has a relatively long half-life, it was possible in those studies to stably increase neurotrophin levels using twice daily treatment with a short half-life compound [Rex *et al.*, 2006].

Conclusion

Neuroplasticity is both a substrate of learning and memory and a mediator of responses to neuronal cell attrition and injury. A primary locus of excitatory synaptic transmission in the mammalian central nervous system is the dendritic spine. This review has highlighted a number of factors which can impinge on synaptic plasticity and spine dysfunction, including Aβ, impaired glucose tolerance, lipid metabolism, kinase signaling cascades, cell adhesion molecules, neurotrophic factors, and astrocytes. Aging is associated with deficits in learning and memory, often called age-associated memory impairment. Although the various cognitive deficits included in the latter are often subtle, they nonetheless can impact the quality of life for those affected by them. Research on the cellular and molecular bases underlying these age-related cognitive deficits and on strategies to enhance/restore synaptic plasticity and/or cognitive capabilities may lead to effective treatments for both age-associated memory impairment and for other, more severe cognitive impairments (e.g. AD).

References

Abbott, M.A., Wells, D.G., and Fallon, J.R. (1999). The insulin receptor tyrosine kinase substrate p58/53 and the insulin receptor are components of CNS synapses. *Journal of Neuroscience 19,* 7300-7308.

Abruthnott, G.W., Ingham, C.A., and Wickens, J.R. (2000). Dopamine and synaptic plasticity in the neostriatum. *Journal of Anatomy, 196,* 587-596.

Akaneya, Y., Tsumoto, T., Kinoshita, S., and Hatanaka, H. (1997). Brain-derived neurotrophic factor enhances long-term potentiation in rat visual cortex. *Journal of Neuroscience, 17,* 6707-6716.

Albin, R.L., Young, A.B., and Penney, J.B. (1989). The functional anatomy of basal ganglia disorders. *Trends in Neuroscience, 12,* 366-375.

Allen, T.G., Abogadie, F.C., and Brown, D.A. (2006). Simultaneous release of glutamate and acetylcholine from single magnocellular "cholinergic" basal forebrain cholinergic neurons. *Journal of Neuroscience, 26,* 1588-1595.

Almonte, A.G., Hamill, C.E., Chhatwal, J.P., Wingo, T.S., Barber, J.A., Lyuboslavsky, P.N., Sweatt, J.D., Ressler, K.J., White, D.A., and Traynelis, S.F. (2007). Learning and memory deficits in mice lacking protease activated receptor-1. *Neurobiology of Learning and Memory, 88,* 295-304.

Álvarez, A., Cacabelos, R., Sanpedro, C., García-Fantini, M., and Aleixandre, M. (2007). Serum TNF-alpha levels are increased and correlate negatively with free IGF-1 in Alzheimer disease. *Neurobiology of Aging, 28,* 533-536.

Amaral, M.D., and Pozzo-Miller, L. (2007). TRPC3 channels are necessary for brain-derived neurotrophic factor to activate a nonselective cationic current and to induce dendritic spine formation. *Journal of Neuroscience, 27,* 5179-5189.

Amaral. M.D., Chapleau, C.A., and Pozzo-Miller, L. (2007). Transient receptor potential channels as novel effectors of brain-derived neurotrophic factor signaling: potential implications for Rett syndrome. *Pharmacology and Therapeutics, 113,* 394-409.

Amateau, S.K., and McCarthy, M.M. (2002). A novel mechanism of dendritic spine plasticity involving estradiol induction of prostaglandin-E_2. *Journal of Neuroscience, 22,* 8586-8596.

Anderson, B. (1996). Axonal length correlates with dementia severity in Alzheimer's disease. *Medical Science Research, 24,* 271-273.

Andreescu, C.E., Milojkovic, B.A., Haasdijk, E.D., Kramer, P., De Jong, F.H., Krust, A., De Zeeuw, C.I. and De Jeu, M.T.G. (2007). Estradiol improves cerebellar memory formation by activating estrogen receptor β. *Journal of Neuroscience, 27,* 10832-10839.

Angelo, M., Plattner, F., and Giese, K.P. (2006). Cyclin-dependent kinase 5 in synaptic plasticity, learning and memory. *Journal of Neurochemistry, 99,* 353-370.

Arendt, T., Zvegintseva, H.G., and Leontovich, T.A. (1986). Dendritic changes in the basal nucleus of Meynert and in the diagonal band nucleus in Alzheimer's disease—A quantitative golgi investigation. *Neuroscience, 19,* 1265-1278.

Arendt, T., Brückner, M.K., Bigl, V., and Marcova, L. (1995a). Dendritic reorganization in the basal forebrain under degenerative conditions and its defects in Alzheimer's disease. II. Ageing, Korsakoff's disease, Parkinson's disease, and Alzheimer's disease. *Journal of Comparative Neurology, 351,* 189-222.

Arendt, T., Brückner, M.K., Bigl, V., and Marcova, L. (1995b). Dendritic reorganization in the basal forebrain under degenerative conditions and its defects in Alzheimer's disease. III. The basal forebrain compared to subcortical areas. *Journal of Comparative Neurology, 351,* 223-246.

Arendt, T., Brückner, M.K., Gertz, H.J., and Marcova, L. (1998). Cortical distribution of neurofibrillary tangles in Alzheimer's disease matches the pattern of neurons that retain their capacity of plastic remodelling in the adult brain. *Neuroscience, 83,* 991-1002.

Arendt, T. (2001). Alzheimer's disease as a disorder of mechanisms underlying structural brain self-organization. *Neuroscience, 102,* 723-765.

Arendt, T. (2004). Neurodegeneration and plasticity. *International Journal of Developmental Neuroscience, 22,* 507-514.

Ashford, J.W., and Mortimer, J.A. (2002). Non-familial Alzheimer's disease is mainly due to genetic factors. *Journal of Alzheimer's Disease, 4,* 169-177.

Astrup, A. (2001). Healthy lifestyles in Europe: prevention of obesity and type II diabetes by diet and physical activity. *Public Health and Nutrition, 4,* 499-515.

Atkins, C.M., Selcher, J.C., Petraitis, J.J., Trzaskos, J.M., and Sweatt, J.D. (1998). The MAPK kinase cascade is required for mammalian associative learning. *Nature Neuroscience, 1,* 602-609.

Baki, L., Shioi, J., Wen, P., Shao, Z., Schwarzman, A., Gama-Sosa, M., Neve, R., and Robakis, N.K. (2004). PS1 activates PI3K thus inhibiting GSK-3 activity and tau overphosphorylation: effects of FAD mutations. *The EMBO Journal, 23,* 2586-2596.

Baki, L., Neve, R.L., Shao, Z., Shioi, J., Georgakopoulos, A., and Robakis, N.K. (2008). Wild-type but not FAD mutant presenilin-1 prevents neuronal degeneration by promoting phosphatidylinositol 3-kinase neuroprotective signaling. *Journal of Neuroscience, 28,* 483-490.

Barghorn, S., Nimmrich, V., Striebinger, A., Krantz, C., Keller, P., Janson, B., Bahr, M., Schmidt, M., Bitner, R.S., Harlan, J., Barlow, E., Ebert, U., and Hillen, H. (2005). Glubular amyloid β-peptide$_{1\text{-}42}$ oligomer-a homogeneous and stable neuropathological protein in Alzheimer's disease. *Journal of Neurochemistry, 95,* 834-847.

Baucum, II, A.J., Ham, A.-J. L., Brown, A.M., and Colbran, R.J. (2007). Proteomic analysis of spinophilin interacting partners. *Society for Neuroscience Abstract,* 45.14.

Beattie, E.C., Stellwagen, D., Morishita, W., Bresnahan, J.C., Ha, B.K., Von Zastrow, M., Beattie, M.S., and Malenka, R.C. (2002). Control of synaptic strength by glial TNFα. *Science, 295,* 2282-2285.

Benson, D.L., Schnapp, L.M., Shapiro, L., and Huntley, G.W. (2000). Making memories stick: cell-adhesion molecules in synaptic plasticity. *Trends in Cell Biology, 10,* 473-482.

Bezzi, P., Carmignoto, G., Pasti, L., Vesce, S., Rossi, D., Rizzini, B.L., Pozzan, T., and Volterra, A. (1998). Prostaglandins stimulate calcium-dependent glutamate release in astrocytes. *Nature, 391,* 281-285.

Biessels, G.J., ter Braak, E.W.M.T., Erkelens, D.W., and Hijman, R. (2001). Cognitive function in patients with type 2 diabetes mellitus. *Neuroscience Research Communications, 28,* 11-22.

Blum, S., Moore, A.N., Adams, F., and Dash, P.K. (1999). A mitogen-activated protein kinase cascade in the CA1/CA2 subfield of the dorsal hippocampus is essential for long-term spatial memory. *Journal of Neuroscience, 19,* 3535-3544.

Blum, R., Kafitz, K.W., and Konnerth, A. (2002). Neurotrophin-evoked depolarization requires the solium channel $Na_v1.9$. *Nature, 419,* 687-693.

Bondy, C.A., and Cheng, C.M. (2004) Signaling by insulin-like growth factor 1 in brain. *European Journal of Pharmacology, 490,* 25-31.

Boulton, T.G., Nye, S.H., Robbins, D.J., Ip, N.Y., Radziejewska, E., Morgenbesser, S.D., DePinho, R.A., Panayotatos, N., Cobb, M.H., and Yancopoulos, G.D. (1991). ERKs: a family of protein-serine/threonine kinases that are activated and tyrosine phosphorylated in response to insulin and NGF. *Cell, 65,* 663-675.

Boyd, F.T. Jr., Clarke, D.W., Muther, T.F., and Raizada, M.K. (1985). Insulin receptors and insulin modulation of norepinephrine uptake in neuronal cultures from rat brain. *Journal of Biological Chemistry,260,* 15880-15884.

Braak, H., and Braak, E. (1991). Neuropathological staging of Azheimer related changes. *Acta Neuropathologica (Berlin), 82,* 239-259.

Braak, H., and Braak, E. (1996). Development of Alzheimer-related neurofibrillary changes in the neocortex inversely recapitulates cortical myelogenesis. *Acta Neuropathologica (Berlin), 92,* 197-201.

Breitner, J.C.S., Wyse, B.W., Anthony, J.C., Welsh-Bohmer K.A., Steffens, D.C., Norton, M.C., Tschanz, J.T., Plassman, B.L., Meyer, M.R., Skoog, I., and A. Khachaturian, A. (1999). APOE-[small element of]4 count predicts age when prevalence of AD increases, then declines: The Cache County Study. *Neurology, 53,* 321-331.

Brown, A.M., Deutch, A.Y., and Colbran, R.J. (2005). Dopamine depletion alters phosphorylation of striatal proteins in a model of Parkinsonism. *European Journal of Neuroscience, 22,* 247-256.

Brunet, A., Datta, S.R., and Greenberg, M.E. (2001). Transcription-dependent and – independent control of neuronal survival by the PI3K-Akt signaling pathway. *Current Opinions in Neurobiology, 11,* 297-305.

Bruno, M.A., Clarke, P.B.S., Seltzer, A., Quirion, R., Burgess, K., Cuello, A.C., and Saragovi, H.U. (2004). Long-lasting rescue of age-associated deficits in cognition and the CNS cholinergic phenotype by a partial agonist peptidomimetic ligand of TrkA. *Journal of Neuroscience, 24,* 8009-8018.

Buttini, M., Masliah, E., Barbour, R., Grajeda, H., Motter, R., Johnson-Wood, K., Khan, K., Seubert, P., Freedman, S., Schenk, D., and Games, D. (2005). β-Amyloid immunotherapy prevents synaptic degeneration in a mouse model of Alzheimer's disease. *Journal of Neuroscience, 25,* 9096-9101.

Calizo, L.H., and Flanagan-Cato, L.M. (2000). Estrogen selectively regulates spine density within the dendritic arbor of rat ventromedial hypothalamic neurons. *Journal of Neuroscience, 20,* 1589-1596.

Calon, F., Lim, G.P., Yang, F., Morihara, T., Teter, B., Ubeda, O., Rostaing, P., Triller, A., Salem, Jr.N., Ashe, K.H., Frautschy, S.A., and Cole, G.M. (2004). Docosahexaenoic acid protects from dendritic pathology in an Alzheimer's disease mouse model. *Neuron, 43,* 633-645.

Cambon, K., Hansen, S.M., Venero, C., Herrero, A.I., Skibo, G., Berezin, V., Bock, E., and Sandi, C. (2004). A synthetic neural cell adhesion molecule mimetic peptide promotes synaptogenesis, enhances presynaptic function, and facilitates memory consolidation. *Journal of Neuroscience, 24,* 4197-4204.

Carlisle, H.J., and Kennedy, M.B. (2005).Spine architecture and synaptic plasticity. *Trends in Neuroscience, 28,* 182-187.

Carro, E., and Torres-Aleman, I. (2004).The role of insulin and insulin-like growth factor I in the molecular and cellular mechanisms underlying the pathology of Alzheimer's disease. *European Journal of Pharmacology, 490,* 127-133.

Carroll, R.C., Beattie, E.C., von Zastrow, M., and Malenka, R.C. (2001). Role of AMPA receptor endocytosis in synaptic plasticity. *Nature Reviews Neuroscience, 2,* 315-324.

Causing, C.G., Gloster, A., Aloyz, R., Bamji, S.X., Chang, E., Fawcett, J., Kuchel, G., and Miller, F.D. (1997). Synaptic innervation density is regulated by neuron-derived BDNF. *Neuron, 18,* 257-267.

Chang, F.L., and Greenough, W.T. (1984).Transient and enduring morphological correlates of synaptic activity and efficacy change in the rat hippocampal slice. *Brain Research, 309,* 25-46.

Chao, M.V. (2003). Neurotrophins and their receptors: a convergence point for many signalling pathways. *Nature Reviews Neuroscience, 4,* 299-309.

Chapman, P.F., White, G.L., Jones, M.W., Cooper-Blacketer, D., Marshall, V.J., Irizarry, M., Younkin, L., Good, M.A., Bliss, T.V.P., Hyman, B.T., Younkin, S.G., and Hsiao, K.K. (1999). Impaired synaptic plasticity and learning in amyloid precursor protein transgenic mice. *Nature Neuroscience, 2,* 271-276.

Chen, G., Chen, K.S., Knox, J., Inglis, J., Bernard, A., Martin, S.J., Justice, A., McConlogue, L., Games, D., Freedman, S.B., and Morris, R.G.M. (2000). A learning deficit related to age and β-amyloid plaques in a mouse model of Alzheimer's disease. *Nature, 408,* 975-979.

Chenal, J., Pierre, K.,and Pellerin, L. (2007). Insulin and IGF-1 enhance the expression of the neuronal monocarboxylate transporter MCT2 by translational activation via stimulation of the phosphoinositide 3-kinase-Akt-mammalian target of rapamycin pathway. *European Journal of Neuroscience, 27,* 53-65.

Christopherson, K.S., Ullian, E.M., Stokes, C.C., Mullowney, C.E., Hell, J.W., Agah, A., Lawler, J., Mosher, D.F., Bornstein, P., and Barres, B.A. (2005). Thrombospondins are astrocyte-secreted proteins that promote CNS synaptogenesis. *Cell, 120,* 421-433.

Chwang, W.B., Arthur, J.S., Schumacher, A., and Sweatt, J.D. (2007). The nuclear kinase mitogen- and stress-activated protein kinase 1 regulates hippocampal chromatin remodeling in memory formation. *Journal of Neuroscience, 27,* 12732-12742.

Coleman, P., Federoff, H., and Kurlan, R. (2004). A focus on the synapse for neuroprotection in Alzheimer's disease and other dementias. *Neurology, 63,* 1155-1162.

Colom, L.V., Castaneda, M.T., Reyna, T., Hernandez, S., and Garrido-Sanabria E. (2005). Characterization of medial septal glutamatergic neurons and their projections to the hippocampus. *Synapse, 58,* 151-164.

Comery, T., Harris, J., Willems, P., Oostra, B., Irwin, S., Weiler, I., and Greenough, W. (1997). Abnormal dendritic spines in fragile X knock-out mice: maturation and pruning deficits. *Proceedings of the National Academy of Sciences, USA 94,* 5401-5404.

Convit, A., de Leon, M.J., Hoptman, M.J., Tarshish, C., De Santi, S., and Rusinek, H. (1995). Age-related changes in brain: I. Magnetic resonance imaging measures of temporal lobe volumes in normal subjects. *Psychiatry Quarterly, 66,* 343-355.

Convit, A., Wolf, O.T., Tarshish, C., and de Leon, M. J. (2003). Reduced glucose tolerance is associated with poor memory performance and hippocampal atrophy among normal elderly. *Proceedings of the National Academy of Sciences, USA 100,* 2019-2022.

Cooney, J.R., Hurlburt, J.L., Selig, D.K., Harris, K.M., and Fiala, J.C. (2002). Endosomal compartments serve multiple hippocampal dendritic spines from a widespread rather than a local store of recycling membrane. *Journal of Neuroscience, 22,* 2215-2224.

Cotman, C.W., and Nieto-Sampedro, M. (1984). Cell biology of synaptic plasticity. *Science, 225,* 1287-1294.

Cotman, C.W., Cummings, B.J., Whitson, J.S. (1991). The role of misdirected plasticity in plaque biogenesis and Alzheimer's disease pathology. In: Hefti F, Brachet B, Christen WY, editors. *Growth factors and Alzheimer's disease.* Berlin: Springer-Verlag, p 222-233..

Counts, S.E., Nadeem, M., Lad, S.P., Wuu, J., and Mufson, E.J. (2006). Differential expression of synaptic proteins in the frontal and temporal cortex of elderly subjects with mild cognitive impairment. *Journal of Neuropathology and Experimental Neurology, 65,* 592-601.

Cremer, H., Lange, R., Christoph, A., Plomann, M., Vopper, G., Roes, J., Brown, R., Baldwin, S., Kraemer, P., Scheff, S., Barthels, D., Rajewsky, K., and Wille, W. (1994). Inactivation of the N-CAM gene in mice results in size reduction of the olfactory bulb and deficits in spatial learning. *Nature, 367,* 455-459.

Cross, D.A., Alessi, D.R., Cohen, P., Andjelkovich, M., and Hemmings, B.A. (1995). Inhibition of glycogen synthase kinase-3 by insulin mediated by protein kinase B. *Nature, 378,* 785-789.

Dalmau, I., Finsen, B., Zimmer, J., Gonzalez, B., and Castellano, B. (1998). Development of microglia in the postnatal rat hippocampus. *Hippocampus, 8,* 458-474.

Dalva, M.B., Takasu, M.A., Lin, M.Z., Shamah, S.M., Hu, L., Gale, N.W., and Greenberg, M.E. (2000). EphB receptors interact with NMDA receptors and regulate excitatory synapse formation. *Cell, 103,* 945-956.

Davies, C.A., Mann, D.M., Sumpter, P.Q., and Yates, P.O. (1987). A quantitative morphometric analysis of the neuronal and synaptic content of the frontal and temporal cortex in patients with Alzheimer's disease. *Journal of Neurological Sciences, 78,* 151-164.

Day, M., Wang, Z., Ding, J., An. X., Ingham, C.A., Shering, A.F., Wokosin, D., Ilijic, E., Sun, Z., Sampson, A.R., Mugnaini, E., Deutch, A.Y., Sesack, S.R., Arbuthnott, G.W., and Surmeier, D.J. (2006). Selective elimination of glutamatergic synapses on striatopallidal neurons in Parkinson disease models. *Nature Neuroscience, 9,* 251-259.

Deak, M., Clifton, A.D., Lucocq, L.M., and Alessi, D.R. (1998). Mitogen- and stress-activated protein kinase-1 (MSK1) is directly activated by MAPK and SAPK2/p38, and may mediate activation of CREB. *The EMBO Journal, 17,* 4426-4441.

de Leon, M.J., McRae, T., Rusinek, H., Convit, A., De Santi, S., Tarshish, C., Golomb, J., Volkow, N., Daisley, K., Orentreich, N., and McEwen, B. (1997). Cortisol reduces hippocampal glucose metabolism in normal elderly, but not in Alzheimer's disease. *Journal of Clinical Endocrinology and Metabolism, 82,* 3251-3259.

DeKosky, S.T., Scheff, S.W., and Styren, S.D. (1996). Structural correlates of cognition in dementia: quantification and assessment of synapse change. *Neurodegeneration, 5,* 417-421.

De Sarno, P., Bijur, G.N., Zmijewska, A.A., Li, X., and Jope, R.S. (2006). In vivo regulation of GSK3 phosphorylation by cholinergic and NMDA receptors. *Neurobiology of Aging, 27,* 413-422.

De Strooper, B., and Annaert, W. *J.* (2000). Proteolytic processing and cell biological functions of the amyloid precursor protein. *Journal of Cell Science, 113,* 1857-1870.

Dietschy, J.M., and Turley, S.D. (2001). Cholesterol metabolism in the brain. *Current Opinion in Lipidology, 12,* 105-112.

Dodart, J.C., Bales, K.R., Gannon, K.S., Greene, S.J., DeMattos, R.B., Mathis, C., DeLong, C.A., Wu, S., Wu, X., Holtzman, D.M., and Paul, S.M. (2002). Immunization reverses memory deficits without reducing brain Aβ burden in Alzheimer's disease model. *Nature Neuroscience, 5,* 452-457.

Dodson, S.E., Gearing, M., Lippa, C.F., Montine, T.J., Levey, A.I., and Lah, J.J. (2006). LR11/SorLA expression is reduced in sporadic Alzheimer disease but not in familial Alzheimer disease. *Journal of Neuropathology and Experimental Neurology, 65,* 866-872.

Dhavan, R., and Tsai, L.H. (2001). A decade of CDK5. *Nature Reviews Molecular Cell Biology, 2,* 749-759.

Ehlers, M.D. (2000). Reinsertion or degradation of AMPA receptors determined by activity-dependent endocytic sorting. *Neuron, 28,* 511-525.

Einstein, G., Buranosky, R., and Crain, B.J. (1994). Dendritic pathology of granule cells in Alzheimer's disease is unrelated to neuritic plaques. *Journal of Neuroscience, 14,* 5077-5088.

Engel, T., Hernández, F., Avila, J., and Lucas, J.J. (2006). Full reversal of Alzheimer's disease-like phenotype in a mouse model with conditional overexpression of glycogen synthase kinase-3. *Journal of Neuroscience, 26,* 5083-5090.

English, J.D., and Sweatt, J.D. (1996). Activation p42 mitogen-activated protein kinase in hippocampal long term potentiation. *Journal of Biological Chemistry, 271,* 24329-24332.

Esposito, D., Patel, P., Stephens, R.M., Perez, P., Chao, M.V., Kaplan, D.R., and Hempstead, B.L. (2001). The cytoplasmic and transmembrane domains of the p75 and Trk A receptors regulate high affinity binding to nerve growth factor. *Journal of Biological Chemistry, 276,* 32687-32695.

Evans, R.M., Hui, S., Perkins, A., Lahiri D.K., Poirier, J., and Farlow, M.R. (2004). Cholesterol and ApoE genotype interact to influence Alzheimer disease progression. *Neurology, 62,* 1869-1871.

Fagot-Campagna, A. (2000). Emergence of type 2 diabetes mellitus in children: epidemiological evidence. *Journal of Pediatric Endocrinology and Metabolism, 13,* 1395-1402.

Ferrer, I., and Gullotta, F. (1990). Down's syndrome and Alzheimer's disease: dendritic spine counts in the hippocampus. *Acta Neuropathologica (Berlin), 79,* 680-685.

Fifkova, E. (1985) A possible mechanism of morphometric changes in dendritic spines induced by stimulation. *Cellular and Molecular Neurobiology, 5,* 47-63.

Fillit, H., Ding, W.H., Buee, L., Kalman, J., Altstiel, L., Lawlor, B., and Wolf-Klein, G. (1991). Elevated circulating tumor necrosis factor levels in Alzheimer's disease. *Neuroscience Letters, 129,* 318-320.

Fiske, B.K., and Brunjes, P.C. (2000). Microglial activation in the developing rat olfactory bulb. *Neuroscience, 96,* 807-815.

Flood, D.G., Buell, S.J., Defiore, C.H., Horwitz, G.J., and Coleman, P.D. (1985). Age-related dendritic growth in dentate gyrus of human brain is followed by regression in the 'oldest old'. *Brain Research, 345,* 366-368.

Flood, D., and Coleman, P.D. (1990). Hippocampal plasticity in normal aging and decreased plasticity in Alzheimer's disease. *Progress in Brain Research, 83,* 435-443.

Fontán-Lozano, A., Sáez-Cassanelli, J.L., Inda, M.C., de los Santos-Arteaga, M., Sierra-Dominguez, S.A., López-Lluch, G., Delgado-Garcia, J.M., and Carrión, A.M. (2007). Caloric restriction increases learning consolidation and facilitates synaptic plasticity through mechanisms dependent on NR2B subunits of the NMDA receptor. *Journal of Neuroscience, 27,* 10185-10195.

Frade, J.M., and Barde, Y.A. (1998). Nerve growth factor: two receptors, multiple functions. *BioEssays, 20,* 137-145.

Geddes, J.W., Monaghan, D.T., Cotman, C.W., Lott, I.T., Kim, R.C., and Chui, H.C. (1985). Plasticity of hippocampal circuitry in Alzheimer's disease. *Science, 230,* 1179-1181.

Gehler, S., Shaw, A., Sarmiere, P., Bamburg, J., and Letourneau, P. (2004). Brain-derived neurotrophic factor regulation of retinal growth cone filopodial dynamics is mediated through actin depolymerizing factor/cofilin. *Journal of Neuroscience, 24,* 10741-10749.

Georganopoulou, D.G., Chang, L., Nam, J.M., Thaxton, C.S., Mufson, E.J., Klein, W.L., and Mirkin, C.A. (2005). Nanoparticle-based detection in cerebrospinal fluid of a soluble pathogenic biomarker for Alzheimer's disease. *Proceedings of the National Academy of Sciences, USA 102,* 2273-2276.

Gerozissis, K. (2003). Brain insulin: regulation, mechanisms of action and functions. *Cellular and Molecular Neurobiology, 23,* 1-25.

Gonatas, N.K., Anderson, W., and Evangelista, I. (1967). The contribution of altered synapses in the senile plaque: an electron microscopic study in Alzheimer's dementia. *Journal of Neuropathology and Experimental Neurology, 26,* 25-39.

Gong, Y., Chang, L., Viola, K.L., Lacor, P.N., Lambert, M.P., Finch, C.F., Krafft, G.A., and Klein, W.L. (2003). Alzheimer's disease affected brain: presence of oligomeric Aβ ligands (ADDLs) suggests a molecular basis for reversible memory loss. *Proceedings of the National Academy of Sciences, USA 100,* 10417-10422.

Goodman, C.S. (1996). mechanisms and molecules that control growth cone guidance. *Annual Review of Neuroscience, 19,* 341-377.

Goshima, Y., Nakamura, F., Strittmatter, P., and Strittmatter, S.M. (1995). Collapsin-induced growth cone collapse mediated by an intracellular protein related to UNC-33. *Nature, 376,* 509-514.

Green, K.N., Martinez-Coria, H., Khashwji, H., Hall, E.B., Yurko-Mauro, K.A., Ellis, L., and LaFerla, F.M. (2007). Dietary docosahexaenoic acid and docosapentaenoic acid ameliorate amyloid-β and tau pathology via a mechanism involving presenilin 1 levels. *Journal of Neuroscience, 27,* 4385-4395.

Grimm, M.O.W., Grimm, H.S., and Hartmann, T. (2007). Amyloid beta as a regulator of lipid homeostasis. *Trends in Molecular Medicine, 13,* 337-344.

Grossman, A.W, Elisseou, N.M, McKinney, B.C., and Greenough, W.T (2006). Hippocampal pyramidal cells in adult *Fmr1* knockout mice exhibit an immature-appearing profile of dendritic spines. *Brain Research, 1084,* 158-164.

Guan, Z., Guistetto, M., Lomvardas, S, Kim, J.H., Miniaci, M.C., Schwartz, J.H., Thanos, D., and Kandel, E.R. (2002). Integration of long-term-memory-related synaptic plasticity involves bidirectional regulation of gene expression and chromatin structure. *Cell, 111,* 483-493.

Haass, C., and Selkoe, D.J. (2007). Soluble protein oligomers in neurodegeneration: lessons from the Alzheimer's amyloid β-peptide. *Nature Reviews Molecular Cell Biology, 8,* 101-112.

Haes, A.J., Chang, L., Klein, W.L., and Van Duyne, R.P. (2005). Detection of a biomarker for Alzheimer's disease from synthetic and clinical samples using a nanoscale optical biosensor. *Journal of the American Chemical Society, 127,* 2266-2271.

Hardy, J., and Selkoe, D.J. (2002). The amyloid hypothesis of Alzheimer's disease: progress and problems on the road to therapeutics. *Science, 297,* 353-356.

Harigaya, Y., Shoji, M., Shirao, T., and Hirai, S. (1996). Disappearance of actin-binding protein, drebrin, from hippocampal synapses in Alzheimer's disease. *Journal of Neuroscience Research, 43,* 87-92.

Harris, K.M., and Kater, S.B. (1994). Dendritic spines: cellular specializations imparting both stability and flexibility to synaptic function. *Annual Review of Neuroscience, 17,* 341-371.

Harris, M.I., Hadden, W.C., Knowler, W.C., and Bennett, P.H. (1987). Prevalence of diabetes and impaired glucose tolerance and plasma glucose levels in U.S. population aged 20-74 yr. *Diabetes, 36,* 523-534.

Hartikka, J., and Hefti, F. (1988). Development of septal cholinergic neurons in culture: plating dendity and glial cells modulate effects of NGF on survival, fiber growth, and expression of transmitter-specific enzymes. *Journal of Neuroscience, 8,* 2967-2985.

Hernãndez, F., Borrell, J., Guaza, C., Avila, J., and Lucas, J.J. (2002). Spatial learning deficits in transgenic mice that conditionally over-express GSK-3β in the brain but do not form tau filaments. *Journal of Neurochemistry, 83,* 1529-1533.

Holcomb, L.A., Gordon, M.N., Jantzen, P., Hsiao K., Duff, K., and Morgan, D. (1999). Behavioral changes in transgenic mice expressing both amyloid precursor protein and presenilin-1 mutations: lack of association with amyloid deposits. *Behavioral Genetics, 29,* 177-185.

Hongpaisan, J., and Alkon, D.L. (2007). A structural basis for enhancement of long-term associative memory in single dendritic spines regulated by PKC. *Proceedings of the National Academy of Sciences, USA 104,* 19571-19576.

Hooper, C., Markevich, V., Plattner, F., Killick, R., Schofield, E., Engel, T., Hernandez, F., Anderton, B., Rosenblum, K., Bliss, T., Cooke, S.F., Avila, J., Lucas, J.J., Giese, K.P., Stephenson, J., and Lovestone, S. (2007). Glycogen synthase kinase-3 inhibition is integral to long-term potentiation. *European Journal of Neuroscience, 25,* 81-86.

Horner, H.C., Packan, D.R., and Sapolsky, R.M. (1990). Glucocorticoids inhibit glucose transport in cultured hippocampal neurons and glia. *Neuroendocrinology, 52,* 57-64.

Hosoya, T., Takizawa, K., Nitta, K., and Hotta, Y. (1995). *glial cells missing*: a binary switch between neuronal and glial determination in Drosophila. *Cell, 82,* 1025-1036.

Hoyer, S., and Lannert, H. (1999). Inhibition of neuronal insulin receptor causes Alzheimer-like disturbances in oxidative/energy brain metabolism and in behaviour in adult rats. *Annals of the New York Academy of Sciences, 893,* 301-303.

Hsia, A.Y., Masliah, E., McConlogue, L., Yu, G.Q., Tatsuno, G., Hu, K., Kholodenko, D., Malenka, R.C., Nicoll, R.A., and Mucke, L. (1999) Plaque-dependent disruption of neural circuits in Alzheimer's disease mouse models. *Proceedings of the National Academy of Sciences, USA 96,* 3228-3233.

Huh, C.Y.L., Danik, M., Manseau, F., Trudeau, L.E., and Williams, S. (2008) Chronic exposure to nerve growth factor increases acetykcholine and glutamate release from cholinergic neurons of the rat medial septum and diagonal band of Broca via mechanisms mediated by $p75^{NTR}$. *Journal of Neuroscience, 28,* 1404-1409.

Ibáñez, C.F. (1994). Structure-function relationships in the neurotrophin family. *Journal of Neurobiology, 25,* 1349-1361.

Ihara, Y. (1988). Massive somatodendritic sprouting of cortical neurons in Alzheimer's disease. *Brain Research, 459,* 138-144.

Impey, S., Obrietan, K., and Storm, D.R. (1999). Making new connections: role of ERK/MAP kinase signaling in neuronal plasticity. *Neuron, 23,* 11-14.

Irwin, S.A, Patel, B., Idupulapati, M., Harris, J.B, Crisostomo, R.A, Larsen, B.P, Kooy, F., Willems, P.J, Cras, P., Kozlowski, P.B, Swain, R.A, Weiler, I.J., and Greenough, W.T. (2001). Abnormal dendritic spine characteristics in the temporal and visual cortices of patients with fragile-X syndrome: a quantitative examination. *American Journal of Medical Genetics, 98,* 161-167.

Jacobsen, J.S., Wu, C.C., Redwine, J.M., Comery, T.A., Arias, R., Bowlby, M., Martone, R., Morrison, J.H., Pangalos, M.N., Reinhart, P.H., and Bloom, F.E. (2006). Early-onset behavioral and synaptic deficits in a mouse model of Alzheimer's disease. *Proceedings of the National Academy of Sciences, USA, 103,* 5161-5166.

Jarrett, J.T. Berger, E.P., and Lansbury, P.T. Jr. (1993). The carboxy terminus of the β amyloid protein is critical for the seeding of amyloid formation: implications for the pathogenesis of Alzheimer's disease. *Biochemistry, 32,* 4693-4697.

Jarvik, G.P., Wijsman, E.M., Kukull, W.A., Schellenberg, G.D., Yu, C., and Larson, E.B. (1995). Interactions of aoplipoprotein E genotype, total cholesterol level, age, and sex in prediction of Alzheimer's disease: A case-control study. *Neurology, 45,* 1092-1096.

Jaworski, J., Spangler, S., Seeburg, D.P., Hoogenraad, C.C., and Sheng, M. (2005). Control of dendritic arborizsation by the phosphoinositide-3'-kinase-Akt mammalian target of rapamycin pathway. *Journal of Neuroscience, 25,* 11300-11312.

Jenuwein, T., and Allis, C.D. (2001). Translating the histone code. *Science, 293,* 1074-1080.

Jiang, H., Guo, W., Liang, X., and Rao, Y. (2005). Both the establishment and the maintenance of neuronal polarity require active mechanisms: critical roles of GSK-3β and its upstream regulators. *Cell, 120,* 123-135.

Johnson, E.J., and Schaefer, E.J. (2006). Potential role of dietary n-3 fatty acids in the prevention of dementia and macular degeneration. *American Journal of Clinical Nutrition, 83 (suppl),* 1494S-1498S.

Jones, B.W., Fetter, R.D., Tear, G. and Goodman, C.S. (1995). *glial cells missing*: a genetic switch that controls glial versus neuronal fate. *Cell, 82,* 1013-1023.

Jope, R.S., and Johnson, G.V. (2004). The glamour and gloom of glycogen synthase kinase-3. *Trends in Biochemical Sciences, 29,* 95-102.

Kalmijn, S., van Boxtel M.P., Ocke, M., Verschuren, W.M., Kromhout, D., and Launer, L.J. (2004). Dietary intake of fatty acids and fish in relation to cognitive performance at middle age. *Neurology, 62,* 275-280.

Kang, H., Welcher, A.A., Shelton, D., and Schuman, E.M. (1997). Neurotrophins and time: different roles for TrkB signaling in hippocampal long-term potentiation. *Neuron, 19,* 653-664.

Kanterewicz, B.I., Urban, N.N., McMahon, D.B.T., Norman, E.D., Giffen, L.J., Favata, M.F., Scherle, P.A., Trzăskos, J.M., Barrionuevo, G., and Klann, E. (2000). The extracellular signal-regulated kinase cascade is required for NMDA receptor-independent LTP in area CA1 but not area CA3 of the hippocampus. *Journal of Neuroscience, 20,* 3057-3066.

Kaplan, R.J., Greenwood, C.E., Winocur, G., and Wolever, T.M.S. (2000). Cognitive performance is associated with glucose regulation in healthy elderly persons and can be enhanced with glucose and dietary carbohydrates. *American Journal of Clinical Nutrition, 72,* 825-836.

Kayed, R., Head, E., Thompson, J.L., McIntire, T.M., Milton, S.C., Cotman, C.W., and Glabe, C.G. (2003). Common structure of soluble amyloid oligomers implies common mechanism of pathogenesis. *Science, 300,* 486-489.

Kennedy, M.J., and Ehlers, M.D. (2006). Organelles and trafficking machinery for postsynaptic plasticity. *Annual Review of Neuroscience, 29,* 325-362.

Kiselyov, V.V., Skladchikova, G., Hinsby, A.M., Jensen, P.H., Kulahin, N., Soroka, V., Pedersen, N., Tsetlin, V., Poulsen, F.M., Berezin, V., and Bock, E. (2003). Structural basis for a direct interaction between FGFR1 and NCAM and evidence for a regulatory role of ATP. *Structure, 11,* 691-701.

Klein, W.L. (2006). Synaptic targeting by Aβ oligomers (ADDLs) as a basis for memory loss in early Alzheimer's disease. *Alzheimer's and Dementia, 2,* 43-55.

Knobloch, M., Konietzko, U., Krebs, D.C., and Nitsch, R.M. (2007a). Intracellular Aβ and cognitive deficits precede β-amyloid deposition in transgenic arcAβ mice. *Neurobiology of Aging, 28,* 1297-1306.

Knobloch, M., Farinelli, M., Konietzko, U., Nitsch, R.M., and Mansuy, I.M. (2007b). Aβ oligomer-mediated long-term potentiation impairment involves protein phosphatase 1-dependent mechanisms. *Journal of Neuroscience, 27,* 7648-7653.

Kokaia, Z., Andsberg, G., Yan, Q., and Lindvall, O. (1998). Rapid alterations of BDNF protein levels in the rat brain after focal ischemia: evidence for increased synthesis and anterograde axonal transport. *Experimental Neurology, 154,* 289-301.

Kondo, T., Shirasawa, T., Itoyama, Y., and Mori, H. (1996). Embryonic genes expressed in Alzheimer's disease brains. *Neuroscience Letters, 209,* 157-160.

Korte, M., Carroll, P., Wolf, E., Brem, G., Thoenen, H. and Bonhoeffer, T. (1995). Hippocampal long-term potentiation is impaired in mice lacking brain-derived neurotrophic factor. *Proceedings of the National Academy of Sciences, USA 92,* 8856-8860.

Korzus, E., Rosenfeld, M.G., and Mayford, M. (2004). CBP histone acetyltransferase activity is a critical component of memory consolidation. *Neuron, 42,* 961-972.

Kotilinek, L.A., Bacskai, B., Westerman, M., Kawarabayashi, T., Younkin, L., Hyman, B.T., Younkin, S., and Ashe, K.H. (2002). Reversible memory loss in a mouse transgenic model of Alzheimer's disease. *Journal of Neuroscience, 22,* 6331-6335.

Koudinov, A.R., and Koudinova, N.V. (2001). Essential role for cholesterol in synaptic plasticity and neuronal degeneration. *The FASEB Journal, 15,* 1858-1860.

Kuwada, J.Y. (1986) Cell recognition by neuronal growth cones in a simple vertrebrate embryo. *Science, 233,* 740-746.

Lacor, P.N., Buniel, M.C., Chang, L., Fernandez, S.J., Gong, Y., Viola, K.L., Lambert, M.P., Velasco, P.T., Bigio, E.H., Finch, C.E., Krafft, G.A., and Klein, W.L. (2004). Synaptic targeting by Alzheimer's-related amyloid β oligomers. *Journal of Neuroscience, 24,* 10191-10200.

Lacor, P.N., Buniel, M.C., Furlow, P.W., Clemente, A.S., Velasco, P.T., Wood, M., Viola, K.L., and Klein, W.L. (2007). Aβ oligomer-induced aberrations in synapse composition, shape, and density provide a molecular basis for loss of connectivity in Alzheimer's disease. *Journal of Neuroscience, 27,* 796-807.

Lambert, M.P., Barlow, A.K., Chromy, B.A., Edwards, C., Freed, R., Liosatos, M., Morgan, T.E., Rozovsky, I., Trommer, B., Viola, K.L., Wals, P., Zhang, C., Finch, C.E., Krafft, G.A., and Klein, W.L. (1998). Diffusible, nonfibrillar ligands derived from $A\beta_{1\text{-}42}$ are potent central nervous system toxins. *Proceedings of the National Academy of Sciences, USA 95,* 6448-6453.

Lanz, T.A., Carter, D.B., and Merchant, K.M. (2003). Dendritic spine loss in the hippocampus of young PDAPP and Tg2576 mice and its prevention by the ApoE2 genotype. *Neurobiology of Disease, 13,* 246-253.

Larson, J., Lynch, G., Games, D., and Seubert, P. (1999). Alterations in synaptic transmission and long-term potentiation in hippocampal slices from young and aged PDAPP mice. *Brain Research, 840,* 23-35.

Lassmann, H., Fischer, P., and Jellinger, K. (1993). Synaptic pathology of Alzheimer's disease. *Annals of the New York Academy of Sciences, 695,* 59-64.

Lauterborn, J.C., Rex, C.S., Kramár, E., Chen, L.Y., Pandyarajan, V., Lynch, G., and Gall, C.M. (2007). Brain-derived neurotrophic factor rescues synaptic plasticity in a mouse model of fragile X syndrome. *Journal of Neuroscience, 27,* 10685-10694.

Lee, C.C., Huang, C.C., Wu, M.Y., and Hsu, K.S. (2005). Insulin stimulates postsynaptic density-95 protein translation via the phosphoinositide 3-kinase-Akt-mammalian target of rapamycin signaling pathway. *Journal of Biological Chemistry, 280,* 18543-18550.

Levenson, J.M., O'Riordan, K.J., Brown, K.D., Trinh, M.A., Molfese, D.L., and Sweatt, J.D. (2004). Regulation of histone acetylation during memory formation in the hippocampus. *Journal of Biological Chemistry, 279,* 40545-40559.

Levi-Montalcini, R. (1987). The nerve growth factor 35 years later. *Science, 237,* 1154-1162.

Li, H.S., Xu, X.Z.S., and Montell, C. (1999). Activation of a TRPC3-dependent cation current through the neurotrophin BDNF. *Neuron, 24,* 261-273.

Li, R., Yang, L., Lindholm, K., Konishi, Y., Yue, X., Hampel, H., Zhang, D. and Shen, Y. (2004). Tumor necrosis factor death receptor signaling cascade is required for amyloid-β protein-induced neuron death. *Journal of Neuroscience, 24,* 1760-1771.

Lim, G.P., Calon, F., Morihara, T., Yang, F., Teter, B., Ubeda, O., Salem, N. Jr., Frautschy, S.A. and Cole, G.M. (2005). A diet enriched with omega-3 fatty acid docosahexaenoic acid reduces amyloid burden in an aged Alzheimer mouse model. *Journal of Neuroscience, 25,* 3032-3040.

Lin, C.H., Yeh, S.H., Lin, C.H., Lu, K.T., Leu, T.H., Chang, W.C., and Gean, P.W. (2001). A role for the PI-3 kinase signaling pathway in fear conditioning and synaptic plasticity in the amygdala. *Neuron, 31,* 841-851.

Lin, T.N., Kim, G.M., Chen, J.J., Cheung, W.M., He, Y.Y., and Hsu, C.Y. (2003). Differential regulation of thrombospondin-1 and thrombospondin-2 after focal cerebral ischemia/reperfusion. *Stroke, 34,* 177-186.

Lindvall, O., and Kokaia, Z. (2006). Stem cells for the treatment of neurological disorders. *Nature, 441,* 1094-1096.

Liu, J., and Kipreos, E.T. (2000). Evolution of cyclin-dependent kinases (CDKs) and CDK-activating kinases (CAKs): differential conservation of CAKs in yeast and metazoa. *Molecular Biology and Evolution, 17,* 1061-1074.

Liu, S.J., Zhang, A.H., Li, H.L., Wang, Q., Deng, H.M., Netzer, W.J., Xu, H., and Wang, J.Z. (2003). Overactivation of glycogen synthase kinase-3 by inhibition of phosphatidylinositol-3 kinase and protein kinase C leads to hyperphosphorylation of tau and impairment of spatial memory. *Journal of Neurochemistry, 87,* 1333-1344.

Liuzzi, F.J., and Lasek, R.J. (1987). Astrocytes block axonal regeneration in mammals by activating the physiological stop pathway. *Science, 237,* 642-645.

Lu, B. (2003). BDNF and activity-dependent synaptic modulation. *Learning and Memory, 10,* 86-98.

Lu, B., Pang, P.T., Woo, N.H. (2005). The yin and yang of neurotrophin action. *Nature Reviews Neuroscience, 6,* 603-614.

Lue, L.F., Kou, Y.M., Roher, A.E., Brachova, I., Shen, Y., Sue, I., Beach, T., Kurth, J.H., Rydel, R.E., and Rogers, J. (1999). Soluble amyloid beta peptide concentration as a predictor of synaptic change in Alzheimer's disease. *American Journal of Pathology, 155,* 853-862.

Lupien, S.J., de Leon, M.J., de Santi, S., Convit, A., Tarshish, C., Nair, N.P.V., Thakur, M., McEwen, B.S., Hauger, R.L., and Meaney, M.J. (1998). Cortisol levels during human aging predict hippocampal atrophy and memory deficits. *Nature Neuroscience, 1,* 69-73.

Lüscher, C., Xia, H., Beattie, E.C., Carroll, R.C., von Zastrow, M., Malenka, R.C., and Nicoll, R.A. (1999). Role of AMPA receptor cycling in synaptic transmission and plasticity. *Neuron, 24,* 649-658.

Lüscher, C., and Frerking, M. (2001). Restless AMPA receptors: implications for synaptic transmission and plasticity. *Trends in Neuroscience, 24,* 665-670.

Luthi, A., Schwyzer, L., Mateos, J.M., Gähwiler, B.H., and McKinney, R.A. (2001). NMDA receptor activation limits the number of synaptic connections during hippocampal development. *Nature Neuroscience, 4,* 1102-1107.

Lynch, G., Kramar, E.A., Rex, C.S., Jia, Y., Chappas, D., Gall, C.M., and Simmons, D.A. (2007). Brain-derived neurotrophic factor restores synaptic plasticity in a knock-in mouse model of Huntington's disease. *Journal of Neuroscience, 27,* 4424-4434.

Ma, Q.L., Teter, B., Ubeda, O.J., Morihara, T., Dhoot, D., Nyby, M.D., Tuck, M.L., Frautschy, S.A., and Cole, G.M. (2007). Omega-3 fatty acid docosahexaenoic acid increases SorLA/LR11, a sorting protein with reduced expression in sporadic Alzheimer's disease (AD): relevance to AD prevention. *Journal of Neuroscience, 27,* 14299-14307.

Magariños, A.M., and McEwen, B.S. (2000). Experimental diabetes in rats causes hippocampal dendritic and synaptic reorganization and increased glucocorticoid reactivity to stress. *Proceedings of the National Academy of Sciences, USA 97,* 11056-11061.

Mahley, R., and Huang, Y. (1999). Apolipoprotein E: from atherosclerosis to Alzheimer's disease and beyond. *Current Opinion in Lipidology, 10,* 207-217.

Mahley, R.W., and Rall, S.C. Jr. (2000). Aoplipoprotein E: far more than a lipid transport protein. *Annual Review of Genomics and Human Genetics, 1,* 507-537.

Malenka, R.C., and Nicoll, R.A. (1997). Silent synapses speal up. *Neuron 19,* 473-476.

Martin, K.C., Baraad, M., and Kandel, E.R. (2000). Local protein synthesis and its role in synapse-specific plasticity. *Current Opinion in Neurobiology, 10,* 587-592.

Masliah, E., Mallory, M., Hansen, L., Alford, M., Albright, T., DeTeresa, R., Terry, R., Baudier, J., and Saitoh T. (1991). Patterns of aberrant sprouting in Alzheimer's disease. *Neuron, 6,* 729-739.

Masliah, E., Mallory, M., Alford, M., Ge, N., and Mucke, L. (1995). Abnormal synaptic regeneration in hAPP695 transgenic and ApoE knockout mice. In: Iqbal K, Mortimer J, Winblad B, Wisniewski HM, editors. *Research advances in Alzheimer's disease and related disorders.* Chichester: Wiley, pp 405-414.

Masliah, E. (1998). Mechanisms of synaptic pathology in Alzheimer's disease. *Journal of Neural Transmission, 53,* 147-158.

Matus, A. (2005). Growth of dendritic spines: a continuing story. *Current Opinion in Neurobiology, 15,* 67-72.

Matynia, A., Kushner, S.A., and Silva, A.J. (2002). Genetic approaches to molecular and cellular cognition: a focus on LTP and learning and memory. *Annual Review of Genetics, 36,* 687-720.

McAllister, A.K., Katz, L.C.,and Lo, D.C. (1999). Neurotrophins and synaptic plasticity. *Annual Review of Neuroscience, 22,* 295-318.

McKee, A.C., Kowall, N.W., and Kosik, K.S. (1989). Microtubular reorganization and dendritic growth response in Alzheimer's disease. *Annals of Neurology, 26,* 652-659.

McKinney, R.A., Capogna, M., Dürr, R., Gähwiler, B.H., and Thompson, S.M. (1999). Miniature synaptic events maintain dendritic spines via AMPA receptor activation. *Nature Neuroscience, 2,* 44-49.

McNeill, T.H., Brown, S.A., Rafols, J.A., and Shoulson, I. (1988). Atrophy of medium spiny I striatal dendrites in advanced Parkinson's disease. *Brain Research, 455,* 148-152.

Meyer, M.R. (1998). APOE genotype predicts when-not whether-one is predisposed to develop Alzheimer disease. *Nature Genetics, 19,* 321-322.

Mesulam, M.M. (1999). Neuroplasticity failure in Alzheimer's disease: bridging the gap between plaques and tangles. *Neuron, 24,* 521-529.

Mesulam, M.M. (2000). A plasticity-based theory of the pathogenesis of Alzheimer's disease. *Annals of the New York Academy of Sciences, 924,* 42-52.

Mishizen-Eberz, A.J., Rissman, R.A., Carter, T.L., Ikonomovic, M.D., Wolfe, B.B., and Armstrong, D.M. (2004). Biochemical and molecular studies of NMDA receptor subunits NR1/2A/2B in hippocampal subregions throughout progression of Alzheimer's disease pathology. *Neurobiology of Disease, 15,* 80-92.

Mizuno, M., Yamada, K., Takei, N., Tran, M.H., He, J., Nakajima, A., Nawa, H., and Nabeshima, T. (2003). Phosphatidylinositol 3-kinase: a molecule mediating BDNF-dependent spatial memory formation. *Molecular Psychiatry, 8,* 217-224.

Mokin, M., Lindahl, J.S., and Keifer, J. (2006). Immediate-early gene-encoded protein Arc is associated with synaptic delivery of GluR4-containing AMPA receptors during in vitro classical conditioning. *Journal of Neurophysiology, 95,* 215-224.

Möller, J.C., Klein, M.A., Haas, S., Jones, L.L., Kreutzberg, G.W., and Raivich, G. (1996). Regulation of thrombospondin in the regenerating mouse facial motor nucleus. *Glia, 17,* 121-132.

Moolman, D.L., Vitolo, O.V., Vonsattel, J.P.G., and Shelanski, M.L. (2004) Dendrite and dendritic spine alterations in Alzheimer models. *Journal of Neurocytology, 33,* 377-387.

Mong, J.A., Glaser, E., and McCarthy, M.M. (1999). Gonadal steroids promote glial differentiation and alter neuronal morphology in the developing hypothalamus in a regionally specific manner. *Journal of Neuroscience, 19,* 1464-1472.

Morita, A., Yamashita, N., Sasaki, Y., Uchida, Y., Nakajima, O., Nakamura, F., Yagi, T., Taniguchi, M., Usui, H., Katoh-Semba, R., Takei, K., and Goshima, Y. (2006). Regulation of dendritic branching and spine maturation by semaphorin3A-Fyn signaling. *Journal of Neuroscience, 26,* 2971-2980.

Morris, R.G.M., and Davis, M. (1994). The role of NMDA receptors in learning and memory. In: Collingridge, G.L., Watkins, J.C. editors. *The NMDA receptor.* Oxford: Oxford University Press, pp 340-375.

Morris, M.C., Evans, D.A., Bienias, J.L., Tangney, C.C., Bennett, D.A., Wilson, R.S., Aggarwal, N., and Schneider, J. (2003). Conmsumption of fish and n-3 fatty acids and risk of incident Alzheimer disease. *Archives of Neurology, 60,* 940-946.

Morrison, J.H., and Hof, P.R. (1997). Life and death of neurons in the aging brain. *Science, 278,* 412-419.

Morrison, J.H., Hof, P.R., Campell, M.J., DeLima, A.D., Voigt, T., Bouras, C., Cox, K., and Young, W.G. (1990). Cellular pathology in Alzheimer's disease: implications for corticocortical disconnection and differential vulnerability. In: Rapoport, S.I., Petit, H., Leys, D., Christen, Y. editors. *Imaging, cerebral topography and Alzheimer's disease. Research and perspectives in Alzheimer's disease.* Berlin: Springer, pp 19-40.

Moser, M.B., Trommald, M., and Andersen, P. (1994). An increase in dendritic spine density on hippocampal CA1 pyramidal cells following spatial learning in adult rats suggests the formation of new synapses. *Proceedings of the National Academy of Sciences, USA 91,* 12673-12675.

Mucke, L., Masliah, E., Yu, G.Q., Mallory, M., Rockenstein, E.M., Tatsuno, G., Hu K., Kholodenko, D., Johnson-Wood, K., and McConlogue, L. (2000). High-level neuronal expression of $A\beta_{1-42}$ in wild-type human amyloid protein precursor transgenic mice: synaptotoxicity without plaque formation. *Journal of Neuroscience, 20,* 4050-4058.

Muddashetty, R.S., Kelić, S., Gross, C., Xu, M., and Bassell, G.J. (2007). Dysregulated metabotropic glutamate receptor-dependent translation of AMPA receptor and postsynaptic density-95 mRNAs at synapses in a mouse model of fragile X syndrome. *Journal of Neuroscience, 27,* 5338-5348.

Muñoz-Cueto, J.A., Garcia-Segura, L.M., and Ruiz-Marcos, A. (1991). Regional sex differences in spine density along the apical shaft of visual cortex pyramids during postnatal development. *Brain Research, 540,* 41-47.

Murphy, D.D., and Segal, M. (1996). Regulation of dendritic spine density in cultured rat hippocampal neurons by steroid hormones. *Journal of Neuroscience, 16,* 4059-4068.

Murk, J.L.A.N., Humbel, B.M., Ziese, U., Griffith, J.M., Posthuma, G., Slot, J.W., Koster, A.J., Verkleij, A.J., Geuze, H.J., and Kleijmeer, M.J. (2003). Endosomal compartmentalization in three dimensions: implications for membrane fusion. *Proceedings of the National Academy of Sciences, USA 100,* 13332-13337.

Nakamura, F., Kalb, R.G., and Strittmatter, S.M. (2000). Molecular basis of semaphorin-mediated axon guidance. *Journal of Neurobiology, 44,* 219-229.

Neely, M.D., Schmidt, D.E., and Deutch, A.Y. (2007). Cortical regulation of dopamine-depletion-induced dendritic spine loss in striatal medium spiny neurons. *Neuroscience, 149,* 457-464.

Neiiendam, J.L., Køhler, L.B., Christensen, C., Li, S., Pedersen, M.V., Ditlevsen, D.K., Kornum, M.K., Kiselyov, V.V., Berezin, V., and Bock, E. (2004). An NCAM-derived FGF-receptor agonist, the FGL-peptide, induces neurite outgrowth and neuronal survival in primary rat neurons. *Journal of Neurochemistry, 91,* 920-935.

Nelson, T.J., and Alkon, D.L. (2005). Insulin and cholesterol pathways in neuronal function, memory and neurodegeneration. *Biochemical Society Transactions, 33,* 1033-1036.

Nimmrich, V., Grimm, C., Draguhn, A., Barghorn, S., Lehmann, A., Shoemaker, H., Hillen, H., Gross, G., Ebert, U., and Bruehl, C. (2008). Amyloid β oligomers ($A\beta_{1\text{-}42}$ globulomer) suppress spontaneous synaptic activity by inhibition of P/Q-type calcium currents. *Journal of Neuroscience, 28,* 788-797.

Offe, K., Dodson, S.E., Shoemaker, J.T., Fritz, J.J., Gearing, M., Levey, A.I., and Lah, J.J. (2006). The lipoprotein receptor LR11 regulates amyloid β production and amyloid precursor protein traffic in endosomal compartments. *Journal of Neuroscience, 26,* 1596-1603.

Oksman, M., Iivonen, H., Hogyes, E., Amtul, Z., Penke, B., Leenders, I., Broersen, L., Lütjohann, D., Hartmann, T., and Tanila, H. (2006). Impact od different saturated fatty acid, polyunsaturated fatty acid and cholesterol containing diets on beta-amyloid accumulation in APP/PS1 transgenic mice. *Neurobiology of Disease, 23,* 563-572.

Oliveira, Jr. A.A., and Hodges, H.M. (2005). Alzheimer's disease and neural transplantation as prospective cell therapy. *Current Alzheimer Research, 2,* 79-95.

Opazo, P., Watabe, A.M., Grant, S.G.N., and O'Dell, T.J. (2003). Phosphatidylinositol 3-kinase regulates the induction of long-term potentiation through extracellular signal-related kinase-independent mechanisms. *Journal of Neuroscience, 23,* 3679-3688.

Oostra, B.A., and Hoogeveen, A.T. (1997). Animal model for fragile X syndrome. *Annals of Medicine, 29,* 563-567.

Ott, A., Stolk, R.P., Hofman, A., van Harskamp, F., Grobbee, D.E., and Breteler, M.M.B. (1996). Association of diabetes mellitus and dementia: The Rotterdam Study. *Diabetologia, 39,* 1392-1397.

Ozdinler, P., and Erzurumlu, R. (2001). Regulation of neurotrophin-induced axonal responses via Rho GTPases. *Journal of Comparative Neurology, 438,* 377-387.

Pakic, P. (1990). Principles of neural cell migration. *Experientia, 46,* 882-891.

Park, M., Salgado, J.M., Ostroff, L., Helton, T.D., Robinson, C.G., Harris, K.M., and Ehlers, M.D. (2006). Plasticity-induced growth of dendritic spines by exocytic trafficking from recycling endosomes. *Neuron, 52,* 817-830.

Patterson, S.L., Abel, T., Deuel, T.A., Martin, K.C., Rose, J.C., and Kandel, E.R. (1996). Recombinant BDNF rescues deficits in basal synaptic transmission and hippocampal LTP in BDNF knockout mice. *Neuron, 16,* 1137-1145.

Peineau, S., Taghibiglou, C., Bradley, C., Wong, T.P., Liu, L., Lu, J., Lo, E., Wu, D., Saule, E., Bouschet, T., Matthews, P., Isaac, J.T.R., Bortolotto, Z.A., Wang, Y.T., and Collingridge, G.L. (2007). LTP inhibits LTD in the hippocampus via regulation of GSK3β. *Neuron, 53,* 703-717.

Perry, R.T., Collins, J.S., Wiener, H., Acton, R., and Go, R.C. (2001). The role of TNF and its receptors in Alzheimer's disease. *Neurobiology of Aging 22,* 873-883.

Peters, A., Palay, S.L., and Webster, H.F. (1991). The Fine Structure of the Nervous System: The Neurons and Supporting Cells. Oxford: Oxford University Press.

Pfrieger, F.W., and Barres, B.A. (1995). What the fly's glia tell the fly's brain. *Cell, 83,* 671-674.

Pfrieger, F.W., and Barres, B.A. (1996). New views on synapse-glia interactions. *Current Opinion in Neurobiology, 6,* 615-621.

Pfrieger, F.W., and Barres, B.A. (1997). Synaptic efficacy enhanced by glial cells in vitro. *Science, 277,* 1684-1687.

Pierre, K., and Pellerin, L. (2005). Monocarboxylate transporters in the central nervous system: distribution, regulation and function. *Journal of Neurochemistry, 94,* 1-14.

Pihlajamäki, J., Gylling, H., Miettinen, T.A., and Laakso, M. (2004). Insulin resistance is associated with increased cholesterol synthesis and decreased cholesterol absorption in normoglycemic men. *Journal of Lipid Research, 45,* 507-512.

Plum, L., Schubert, M., and Bruning, J.C. (2005). The role of insulin receptor signaling in the brain. *Trends in Endocrinology and Metabolism, 16,* 59-65.

Pomeroy, S.L., and Purves, D. (1988). Neuron/glia relationships observed over intervals of several months in living mice. *Journal of Cell Biology, 107,* 1167-1175.

Poo, M.M. (2001). Neurotrophins as synaptic modulators. *Nature Review Neuroscience, 2,* 24-32.

Popov, V.I., Medvedev, N.I., Kraev, I.V., Gabbott, P.L., Davies, H.A., Lynch, M., Cowley, T.R., Berezin, V., Bock, E., and Stewart, M.G. (2008). A cell adhesion molecule mimetic, FGL peptide, induces alterations in synapse and dendritic spine structure in the dentate gyrus of aged rats: a three-dimensional ultrastructural study. *European Journal of Neuroscience, 27,* 301-314.

Raber, J., Wong, D., Buttini, M., Orth, M., Bellosta, S., Pitas, R.E., Mahley, R.W., and Mucke, L. (1998). Isoform-specific effects of human apolipoprotein E on brain function revealed in *ApoE* knockout mice: increased susceptibility of females. *Proceedings of the National Academy of Sciences, USA 95,* 10914-10919.

Rage, F., Lee, B.J., Ma, Y.J., and Ojeda, S.R. (1997). Estradiol enhances prostaglandin E2 receptor gene expression in luteinizing hormone-releasing hormone (LHRH) neurons and facilitates the LHRH response to PGE2 by activating a glia-to-neuron signaling pathway. *Journal of Neuroscience, 17,* 9145-9156.

Ramos, E.M., Lin, M.-T., Larson, E.B., Maezawa, I., Tseng, L.-H., Edwards, K.L., Schellenberg, G.D., Hansen, J.A., Kukull, W.A., and Jin, L.-W. (2006) Tumor necrosis factor α and interleukin 10 promoter region polymorphisms and risk of late-onset Alzheimer disease. *Archives of Neurology, 63,* 1165-1169.

Raper, J.A. (2000). Semaphorins and their receptors in vertebrates and invertebrates. *Current Opinions in Neurobiology, 10,* 88-94.

Rapoport, S.I. (1999). In vivo PET imaging and postmortem studies suggest potentially reversible and irreversible stages of brain metabolic failure in Alzheimer's disease. *European Archives of Psychiatry and Clinical Neuroscience 249 (Supplement),* 46-55.

Reichardt, L.F. (2006). Neurotrophin-regulated signalling pathways. *Philosophical Transactions of the Royal Society, B, 361,* 1545-1564.

Reisberg, B., Doody, R., Stöffler, A., Schmitt, F., Ferris, S., and Möbius H.J., for the Memantine Study Group. (2003). Memantine in moderate-to-severe Alzheimer's disease. *New England Journal of Medicine, 348,* 1333-1341.

Rex, C.S., Lauterborn, J.C., Lin, C.Y., Kramár, E.A., Rogers, G.A., Gall, C.M., and Lynch, G. (2006). Restoration of long-term potentiation in middle-aged hippocampus after induction of brain-derived neurotrophic factor. *Journal of Neurophysiology 96,* 677-685.

Rex, C.S., Lin, C.Y., Kramár, E.A., Chen, L.Y., Gall, C.M., and Lynch, G. (2007). Brain-derived neurotrophic factor promotes long-term potentiation-related cytoskeletal changes in adult hippocampus. *Journal of Neuroscience, 27,* 3017-3029.

Richardson, J.T. (1990). Cognitive function in diabetes mellitus. *Neuroscience and Biobehavioral Reviews, 14,* 385-388.

Rodriguez-Tebar, A., Dechant, G., and Barde, Y.A. (1990). Binding of brain-derived neurotrophic factor to the nerve growth factor receptor. *Neuron, 4,* 487-492.

Rogaeva, E., Meng, Y., Lee, J.H., Gu, Y., Kawarai, T., Zou, F., Katayama, T., Baldwin, C.T., Cheng, R., Hasegawa, H., Chen, F., Shibata, N., Kathryn Lunetta, L., Pardossi-Piquard, R., Bohm, C., Wakutani, Y., Cupples, L.A., Cuenco, K.T., Green, R.C., Pinessi, L., Rainero, I., Sorbi, S., Bruni, A., Duara, R., Friedland, R.P., Inzelberg, R., Hampe, W., Bujo, H., Song, Y.Q., Andersen, O.M., Willnow, T.E., Graff-Radford, N., Petersen, R.C., Dickson, D., Der, S.D., Fraser, P.E., Schmitt-Ulms, G., Younkin, S., Mayeux, R., Farrer, L.A., and St George-Hyslop, P. (2007). The neuronal sortilin-related receptor SORL1 is genetically associated with Alzheimer disease. *Nature Genetics, 39,* 168-177.

Roses, A.D., Saunders, A.M., Alberts, M.A., Strittmatter, W.J., Schmechel, D., Gorder, E., and Pericak-Vance, M.A. (1995). Apolipoprotein E E4 allele and risk of dementia. *Journal of the American Medical Association, 273,* 374-375.

Ross, F.M., Allan, S.M., Rothwell, N.J., and Verkhratsky, A. (2003). A dual role for interleukin-1 in LTP in mouse hippocampal slices. *Journal of Neuroimmunology, 144,* 61-67.

Rowan, M.J., Klyubin, I., Wang, Q., Hu, N.W., and Anwyl, R. (2007). Synaptic memory mechanisms: Alzheimer's disease amyloid β-peptide-induced dysfunction. *Biochemical Society Transactions, 35,* 1219-1223.

Rudelli, R., Brown, W., Wisniewski, K., Jenkins, E., Laure-Kamionowska, M., Connell, F., and Wisniewski, H. (1985). Adult fragile X syndrome. Clinico-neuropathologic findings. *Acta Neuropathologica, 67,* 289-295.

Ruggero, D. and Sonenberg, N. (2005). The Akt of translational control. *Oncogene, 24,* 7426-7434.

Saffell, J.L., Williams, E.J. Mason, I.J., Walsh, F.S. and Doherty, P. (1997). Expression of a dominant negative FGF receptor inhibits axonal growth and FGF receptor phosphorylation stimulated by CAMs. *Neuron, 18,* 231-242.

Sakamoto, H., Mezaki, Y., Shikimi, H., Ukena, K. and Tsutsui, K. (2003). Dendritic growth and spine formation in response to estrogen in the developing Purkinje cell. *Endocrinology, 144,* 4466-4477.

Salehi, A., Delcroix, J.-D. and Mobley, W.C. (2003). Traffic at the intersection of neurotrophic factor signaling and neurodegeneration. *Trends in Neuroscience, 26,* 73-80.

Sanchez-Heras, E., Howell, F.V., Williams, G. and Doherty, P. (2006). The fibroblast growth factor receptor acid box is essential for interactions with N-cadherin and all of the major isoforms of neural cell adhesion molecule. *Journal of Biological Chemistry, 281,* 35208-35216.

Sasaki, K., Tooyama, I., Li, A.J., Oomura, Y. and Kimura, H. (1999). Effects of an acidic fibroblast growth factor fragment analog on learning and memory and on medial septum cholinergic neurons in senescence-accelerated mice. *Neuroscience, 92,* 1287-1294.

Satoh, Y., Endo, S., Ikeda, T., Yamada, K., Ito, M., Kuroki, M., Hiramoto, T., Imamura, O., Kobayashi, Y., Watanabe, Y., Itohara, S., and Takishima, K. (2007). Extracellular signal-regulated kinase 2 (ERK2) knockdown mice show deficits in long-term memory; ERK2 has a specific function in learning and memory. *Journal of Neuroscience, 27,* 10765-10776.

Savitt, J.M., Dawson, V.L., and Dawson, T.M. (2006). Diagnosis and treatment of Parkinson disease: molecules to medicine. *Journal of Clinical Investigation, 116,* 1744-1754.

Scarpini, E., Scheltens, P., and Feldman, H. (2003). Treatment of Alzheimer's disease; current status and new perspectives. *Lancet Neurology, 2,* 539-547.

Schachner, M. (1997). Neural recognition molecules and synaptic plasticity. *Current Opinion in Cell Biology, 9,* 627-634.

Schaeffer, H.J., and Weber, M.J. (1999). Mitogen-activated protein kinases: specific messages from ubiquitous messengers. *Molecular and Cellular Biology, 19,* 2435-2444.

Scheff, S.W., DeKosky, S.T., and Price, D.A. (1990). Quantitative assessment of cortical synaptic density in Alzheimer's disease. *Neurobiology of Aging, 11,* 29-37.

Scheff, S.W., and Price, D.A. (2003). Synaptic pathology in Alzheimer's disease: a review of ultrastructural studies. *Neurobiology of Aging,24,* 1029-1046.

Scheibel, A.B. (1983). Dendritic changes. In: Reisberg B, editor. *Alzheimer's disease.* New York: The Free Press, pp 69-73.

Scott, S.A. (1993). Dendritic atrophy and remodeling of amygdaloid neurons in Alzheimer's disease. *Dementia, 4,* 264-272.

Segal, M. (2005). Dendritic spines and long-term plasticity. *Nature Reviews Neuroscience, 6,* 277-284.

Segal, R.A., and Greenberg, M.E. (1996). Intracellular signaling pathways activated by neurotrophic factors. *Annual Review of Neuroscience, 19,* 463-489.

Selcher, J.C., Nekrasova, T., Paylor, R., Landreth, G.E., and Sweatt, J.D. (2001). Mice lacking the ERK1 isoform of MAP kinase are unimpaired in emotional learning. *Learning and Memory, 8,* 11-19.

Selkoe, D.J. (2002).Alzheimer's disease is a synaptic failure. *Science, 298,* 789-791.

Selkoe, D.J., and Schenk, D. (2003).Alzheimer's disease: molecular understanding predicts amyloid-based therapeutics. *Annual Review of Pharmacology and Toxicology, 43,* 545-584.

Shelton, S.B., and Johnson, G.V. (2004). Cyclin-dependent kinase-5 in neurodegeneration. *Journal of Neurochemistry, 88,* 1313-1326.

Shen, J., Bronson, R.T., Chen, D.F., Xia, W., Selkoe, D.J., and Tonegawa, S. (1997). Skeletal and CNS defects in Presenilin-1-deficient mice. *Cell, 89,* 629-639.

Sheng, M., and Lee, S.H. (2001).AMPA receptor trafficking and the control of synaptic transmission. *Cell, 105,* 825-828.

Sherrington, R., Rogaev, E.I., Liang, Y., Rogaeva, E.A., Levesque, G., Ikeda, M., Chi, H., Lin, C., Li, G., Holman, K., Tsuda, T., Mar, L., Foncin, J.-F., Bruni, A.C., Montesi, M.P., Sorbi, S., Rainero, I., Pinessi, L., Nee, L., Chumakov, I., Pollen, D., Brookes, A.,

Sanseau, P., Pollinsky, R.J., Wasco, W., Da Silva, H.A.R., Haines, J.L., Pericak-Vance, M.A., Tanzi, R.E., Roses, A.D., and Fraser, P.E. (1995). Cloning of a gene bearing missense mutations in early-onset familial Alzheimer's disease. *Nature, 375,* 754-760.

Shi, S.H., Hayashi, Y., Petralia, R.S., Zaman, S.H., Wenthold, R.J., Svoboda, K., and Malinow, R. (1999). Rapid spine delivery and redistribution of AMPA receptors after synaptic NMDA receptor activation. *Science, 284,* 1811-1816.

Shim, K.S., and Lubec, G. (2002). Drebdin, a dendritic spine protein, is manifold decreased in brains of patients with Alzheimer's disease and Down's syndrome. *Neuroscience Letters, 324,* 209-212.

Shimokata, H., Muller, D.C., Fleg, J.L., Sorkin, J., Ziemba, A.W. and Andres, R. (1991). Age as independent determinant of glucose tolerance. *Diabetes, 40,* 44-51.

Silver, J., Lorenz, S.E., Wahlsten, D., and Coughlin, J. (1982). Axonal guidance during development of the great cerebral commissures: descriptive and experimental studies, in vivo, on the role of preformed glial pathways. *Journal of Comparative Neurology, 210,* 10-29.

Small, D.H. (2004). Mechanisms of synaptic homeostasis in Alzheimer's disease. *Current Alzheimer Research, 1,* 27-32.

Snyder, E.M., Nong, Y., Almeida, C.G., Paul, S., Moran, T., Choi, E.Y., Nairn, A.C., Salter, M.W., Lombroso, P.J., Gouras, G.K., and Greengard, P. (2005). Regulation of NMDA receptor trafficking by amyloid-β. *Nature Neuroscience, 8,* 1051-1058.

Sofroniew, M.V., Howe, C.L., and Mobley, W.C. (2001). Nerve growth factor signaling, neuroprotection, and neural repair. *Annual Reviews of Neuroscience, 24,* 1217-1281.

Spires, T.L., Meyer-Luehmann, M., Stern, E.A., McLean, P.J., Skoch, J., Nguyen, P.T., Bacskai, B.J., and Hyman, B.T. (2005). Dendritic spine abnormalities in amyloid precursor protein transgenic mice demonstrated by gene transfer and intravital nultiphoton microscopy. *Journal of Neuroscience, 25,* 7278-7287.

Standridge, J.B. (2006). Vicious cycles within the neuropathophysiologic mechanisms of Alzheimer's disease. *Current Alzheimer's Research, 3,* 95-108.

Stellwagen, D. and Malenka, R.C. (2006). Synaptic scaling mediated by glial TNF-α. *Nature, 440,* 1054-1059.

Stevens, B., Allen, N.J., Vazquez, L.E., Howell, G.R., Christopherson, K.S., Nouri, N., Micheva, K.D., Mehalow, A.K., Huberman, A.D., Stafford, B., Sher, A., Litke, A.M., Lambris, J.D., Smith, S.J., John, S.W.M., and Barres, B.A. (2007). The classical complement cascade mediates CNS synapse elimination. *Cell, 131,* 1164-1178.

Stewart, R., and Liolitsa, D. (1999). Type 2 diabetes mellitus, cognitive impairment and dementia. *Diabetic Medicine, 16.* 93-112.

Strachan, M.W.J., Deary, I.J., Ewing, F.M.E., and Frier, B.M. (2002). Recovery of cognitive function and mood after severe hypoglycaemia in adults with insulin-treated diabetes. *Diabetes Care, 23,* 305-312.

Styren, S.D., Bowser, R., and Dekosky, S.T. (1999). Expression of fetal ALZ-50 reactive clone 1 (FAC1) in dendate gyrus following entorhinal cortex lesion. *Journal of Comparative Neurology, 386,* 555-561.

Su, J.H., Cummings, B.J., and Cotman, C.W. (1993). Identification and distribution of axonal dystrophic neurites in Alzheimer's disease. *Brain Research, 625,* 228-237.

Su, J.H., Deng, G.M., and Cotman, C.W. (1997). Neuronal DNA damage precedes tangle formation and is associated with up-regulation of nitrotyrosine in Alzheimer's disease brain. *Brain Research, 774,* 193-199.

Sweatt, J.D. (2004). Mitogen-activated protein kinases in synaptic plasticity and memory. *Current Opinion in Neurobiology, 14,* 311-317.

Sze, C.I., Troncoso, J.C., Kawas, C., Mouton, P., Price, D.L., and Martin, L.J. (1997). Loss of the presynaptic vesicle protein synaptophysin in hippocampus correlates with cognitive decline in Alzheimer disease. *Journal of Neuropathology and Experimental Neurology, 56,* 933-944.

Sze, C.-I., Bi, H., Kleinschmidt-DeMasters, B.K., Filley, C.M., and Martin, L.J. (2001). N-Methyl-D-aspartate receptor subunit proteins and their phosphorylation status are altered selectively in Alzheimer's disease. *Journal of Neurological Sciences, 182,* 151-159.

Tan, Z.S., Beiser, A.S., Vasan, R.S., Roubenoff, R., Dinarello, C.A., Harris, T.B., Benjamin, E.J., Au, R., Kiel, D.P., Wolf, P.A., and Seshadri, S. (2007). Inflammatory markers and the risk of Alzheimer disease; the Framingham Study. *Neurology, 68,* 1902-1908.

Terry, R.D., Masliah, E., Salmon, D.P., Butters, N., DeTeresa, R., Hill, R., Hansen, L.A., and Katzman, R. (1991). Physical basis of cognitive alterations in Alzheimer's disease: synapse loss is the major correlate of cognitive impairment. *Annals of Neurology, 30,* 572-580.

Terry, R.D., Masliah, E., Hansen, L.A. (1994). Structural basis of the cognitive alterations in Alzheimer's disease. In: Terry, R.D., Katzman, R., Bick, K. editors. *Alzheimer's disease.* New York, USA: Raven Press, pp 179-196.

Teter, B. (2000). Apolipoprotein E isotype-specific effects in neurodegeneration. *Alzheimer's Reports, 3,* 199-212.

Teter, B., and Ashford, W. (2002). Neuroplasticity in Alzheimer's disease. *Journal of Neuroscience Research, 70,* 402-437.

Thomas, G.M., and Huganir, R.L. (2004). MAPK cascade signaling and synaptic plasticity. *Nature Reviews Neuroscience, 5,* 173-183.

Tobinick, E., Gross, H., Weinberger, A., and Cohen, H. (2006). TNF-alpha modulation for treatment of Alzheimer's disease; a 6-month pilot study. *Medscape General Medicine, 8,* 25.

Tobinick, E.L., and Gross, H. (2008). Rapid cognitive improvement in Alzheimer's disease following perispinal etanercept administration. *Journal of Neuroinflammation,* in press.

Todd, P., and Malter, J. (2002). Fragile X mental retardation protein in plasticity and disease. *Journal of Neuroscience Research, 70,* 623-630.

Tong, L., Thornton, P.L., Balazs, R., and Cotman, C.W. (2001). β-Amyloid-(1-42) impairs activity-dependent cAMP-response element-binding protein signaling in neurons at concentrations in which cell survival is not compromised. *Journal of Biological Chemistry, 276,* 17301-17306.

Tsacopoulos, M., and Magistretti, P.J. (1996). Metabolic coupling between glia and neurons. *Journal of Neuroscience, 16,* 877-885.

Tsankova, N.M., Kumar, A., and Nestler, E.J. (2004). Histone modifications at gene promoter regions in rat hippocampus after acute and chronic electroconvulsive seizures. *Journal of Neuroscience, 24,* 5603-5610.

Turrigiano, G.G., and Nelson, S.B. (2004). Homeostatic plasticity in the developing nervous system. *Nature Reviews Neuroscience, 5,* 97-107.

Tuszynski, M.H., Thal, L., Pay, M., Salmon, D.P., U, H.S., Bakay, R., Patel, P., Blesch, A., Vahlsing, H.L., Ho, G., Tong, G., Potkin, S.G., Fallon, J., Hansen, L., Mufson, E.J., Kordower, J.H., Gall, C., and Connor, J. (2005). A phase 1 clinical trial of nerve growth factor gene therapy for Alzheimer disease. *Nature Medicine, 11,* 551-555.

Tyler, W.J., Alonso, M., Bramham, C.R., and Pozzo-Miller, L.D. (2002). From acquisition to consolidation: on the role of brain-derived neurotrophic factor signaling in hippocampal-dependent learning. *Learning and Memory, 9,* 224-237.

Uemura, K., Kuzuya, A., Shimozono, Y., Aoyagi, N., Ando, K., Shimohama, S., and Kinoshita, A. (2007). GSK3β activity modifies the localization and function of Presenilin 1. *Journal of Biological Chemistry, 282,* 15823-15832.

Ullian, E.M., Sapperstein, S.K., Christopherson, K.S., and Barres, B.A. (2001). Control of synapse number by glia. *Science, 291,* 657-661.

Unverzagt, F.W., Gao, S., Baiyewu, O., Ogunniyi, A.O., Gureje, O., Perkins, A., Emsley, C.L., Dickens, J., Evans, R., Musick, B., Hakk, K.S., Hui, S.L., and Hendrie, H.C. (2001). Prevalence of cognitive impairment: Data from the Indianapolis Study of Health and Aging. *Neurology, 57,* 1655-1662.

Vanhanen, M.,Koivisto, K., Karjalainen, L., Helkala, E.L., Laakso, M., Soininen, H., and Riekkinen, P., Sr. (1997). Risk for non-insulin-dependent diabetes in the normoglycaemic elderly is associated with impaired cognitive function. *NeuroReport, 8* 1527-1530.

Venero, C., Herrero, A.I., Touyarot, K., Cambon, K., López-Fernández, M.A., Berezin, V., Bock, E., and Sandi, C. (2006). Hippocampal up-regulation of NCAM expression and polysialylation plays a key role on spatial memory. *European Journal of Neuroscience, 23,* 1585-1595.

Vora, N., Jovin, T., and Kondziolka, D. (2006). Cell transplantation for ischemic stroke. *Neurodegenerative Diseases, 3,* 101-105.

Walsh, F.S., and Dohery, P. (1997). Neural cell adhesion molecules on the immunoglobulin superfamily: role in axonal growth and guidance. *Annual Review of cell and Developmental Biology,13,* 425-456.

Wang, L.H., and Strittmatter, S.M. (1996). A family of rat CRMP genes is differentially expressed in the nervous system. *Journal of Neuroscience, 16,* 6197-6207.

Wang, H.-W., Pasternak, J.F., Kuo, H., Ristic, H., Lambert, M.P., Chromy, B., Viola, K.L., Klein, W.L., Stine, W.B., Krafft, G.A., and Trommer, B.L. (2002). Soluble oligomers of β amyloid (1-42) inhibit long-term potentiation but not long-term depression in rat dentate gyrus. *Brain Research, 924,* 133-140.

Wang, Q., Liu, L., Pei, L., Ju, W., Ahmadian, G., Lu, J., Wang, Y., Liu, F., Wang, Y.T. (2003). Control of synaptic strength, a novel function of Akt. *Neuron, 38,* 915-928.

Wang, Q., Wu, J., Rowan, M.J., and Anwyl, B. (2005). β-amyloid inhibition of long-term potentiation is mediated via tumor necrosis factor. *European Journal of Neuroscience, 22,* 2827-2832.

Weiler, I.J., Spangler, C.C., Klintsova, A.Y., Grossman, A.W., Kim, S.H., Bertaina-Anglade, V., Khaliq, H., de Vries, F.E., Lambers, F.A.E., Hatia, F., Base, C.K., and Greenough, W.T. (2004). Fragile X mental retardation protein is necessary for neurotransmitter-activated protein translation at synapses. *Proceedings of the National Academy of Sciences, USA, 101,* 17504-17509.

Williams, E.J., Furness, J., Walsh, F.S., and Doherty, P. (1994). Activation of the FGF receptor underlies neurite outgrowth stimulated by L1, N-CAM, and N-cadherin. *Neuron, 13,* 583-594.

Williams, E.J., Willams, G., Howell, F.V., Skaper, S.D., Walsh, F.S., and Doherty, P. (2001). Identification of an N-cadherin motif that can interact with the fibroblast growth factor receptor and is required for axonal growth. *J. Biol. Chem*, 276, 43879-43886.

Wilson, C.J., and Groves, P.M. (1980). Fine structure and synaptic connections of the common spiny neuron of the rat neostriatum: a study employing intracellular inject of horseradish peroxidase. *Journal of Comaprative Neurology, 194,* 599-615.

Winson, J. (1978). Loss of hippocampal theta rhythm results in spatial memory deficit in the rat. *Science, 201,* 160-163.

Wong, P.C., Zheng, H., Chen, H., Becher, M.W., Sirinathsinghji, D.J., Trumbauer, M.E., Chen, H.Y., Price, D.L., Van der Ploeg, L.H., and Sisodia, S.S. (1997). Presenilin 1 is required for Notch 1 and DII1 expression in the paraxial mesoderm. *Nature, 387,* 288-292.

Woodgett, J.R. (1990). Molecular cloning and expression of glycogen synthase kinase-3/factor A. *The EMBO Journal, 9,* 2431-2438.

Woolley, C.S., and McEwen, B.S. (1992). Estradiol mediates fluctuation in hippocampal synapse density during the estrous cycle in the adult rat. *Journal of Neuroscience, 12,* 2549-2554.

Woolley, C.S., and McEwen, B.S. (1993). Roles of estradiol and progesterone in regulation of hippocampal dendritic spine density during the estrous cycle in the adult rat. *Journal of Comparative Neurology, 336,* 293-306.

Woolley, C.S., and McEwen, B.S. (1994). Estradiol regulates hippocampal dendritic ine density via an N-methyl-D-aspartate receptor-dependent mechanism. *Journal of Neuroscience, 14,* 7680-7687.

Wyss-Coray, T. (2006). Inflammation in Alzheimer disease: driving force, bystander of beneficial response? *Nature Medicine, 12,* 1005-1015.

Xu, P.T., Gilbert, J.R., Qiu, H.L., Rothrock-Christian T., Settles, D.L., and Roses, A.D. (1998). Regionally specific neuronal expression of human APOE gene in transgenic mice. *Neuroscience Letters, 246,* 65-68.

Yamasaki, T.R., Blurton-Jones, M., Morrissette, D.A., Kitazawa, M., Oddo, S., and LaFerla, F.M. (2007). Neural stem cells improve memory in an inducible mouse model of neuronal loss. *Journal of Neuroscience, 27,* 11925-11933.

Yao, Z.X., and Papadopoulos, V. (2002). Function of β-amyloid in cholesterol transport: a lead to neurotoxicity. *The FASEB Journal, 16,* 1677-1679.

Yamashita, N., Morita, A., Uchida, Y., Nakamura, F., Usui, H., Ohshima, T., Taniguchi, M., Honnorat, J., Thomasset, N., Takei, K., Takahashi, T., Kolattukudy, P., and Goshima, Y., (2007). Regulation of spine development by semaphorin3A through cyclin-dependent kinase 5 phosphorylation of collapsin response mediator protein 1. *Journal of Neuroscience, 27,* 12546-12554.

Yoshimura, S., Takagi, Y., Harada, J., Teramoto, T., Thomas, S.S., Waeber, C., Bakowska, J.C., Breakefield, X.O., and Moskowitz, M.A. (2001). FGF-2 regulation of neurogenesis in adult hippocampus after brain injury. *Proceedings of the National Academy of Sciences, USA, 98,* 5874-5879.

Zaja-Milatovic, S., Milatovic, D., Schantz, A.M., Zhang, J., Montine, K.S., Samii, A., Deutch, A.Y., and Montine, T.J. (2005). Dendritic degeneration in neostriatal medium spiny neurons in Parkinson disease. *Neurology, 64,* 545-547.

Zalfa, F., Giorgi, M., Primerano, B., Moro, A., Di Penta, A., Reis, S., Oostra, B., and Bagni, C. (2003). The fragile X syndrome protein FMRP associates with *BC1* RNA and regulates the translation of specific mRNAs at synapses. *Cell, 112,* 317-327.

Zhao, W.Q., and Alkon, D.L. (2001). Role of insulin and insulin receptor in learning and memory. *Molecular and Cellular Endocrinology, 177,* 125-134.

Zheng, X., Rivabene, R., Cavallari, C., Napolitano, M., Avella, M., Bravo, E., and Botham, K.M. (2002). The effects of chylomicron remnants enriched in n-3 or n-6 polyunsaturated fatty acids on the transcription of genes regulating their uptake and metabolism by the liver: influence of cellular oxidative state. *Free Radical Biology and Medicine, 32,* 1123-1131.

Zhu, L.Q., Wang, S.H., Liu, D., Yin, Y.Y., Tian, Q., Wang, X.C., Wang, Q., Chen, J.G., and Wang, J.Z. (2007). Activation of glycogen synthase kinase-3 inhibits long-term potentiation with synapse-associated impairments. *Journal of Neuroscience,27,* 12211-12220.

Zhu, S.Q., Kum, W., Ho, S.K.S., Young, J.D., and Cockram, C.S. (1990). Structure-function relationships of insulin receptor interactions in cultured mouse astrocytes. *Brain Research, 529,* 329-332.

Zigova, T., Pencea, V., Wiegand, S.J., and Luskin, M.B. (1998). Intraventricular administration of BDNF increases the number of newly generated neurons in the adult olfactory bulb. *Molecular and Cellular Neuroscience, 11,* 234-245.

In: Synaptic Plasticity: New Research
Editors: Tim F. Kaiser and Felix J. Peters

ISBN: 978-1-60456-732-8

Chapter 2

MOLECULAR MECHANISMS OF LEARNING AND MEMORY BASED ON RESEARCH ON CA2+/CALMODULIN-DEPENDENT PROTEIN KINASE II

Takashi Yamauchi [*] ***and Hiroko Sugiura***
Department of Neuropharmacology, Tokyo Metropolitan Institute for Neurosciences

ABSTRACT

In the central nervous system (CNS), changes in the efficiency of synaptic transmission are important for a number of aspects of neural function. Much has been learned about the activity-dependent synaptic modifications, namely synaptic plasticity, that are thought to underlie memory storage, but these modifications are largely unknown at the molecular level.It is important to find and characterize the "memory molecules", and "memory apparatus or memory forming apparatus" in the brain. One of the best candidates for a molecular component of the memory apparatus is Ca^{2+}/calmodulin-dependent protein kinase II (CaMKII). The postsynaptic density (PSD) is also a good candidate for a body of the memory apparatus.

CaMKII is one of the most prominent protein kinases, and plays a multifunctional role in many intracellular events. CaMKII activity is regulated by autophosphorylation. It is present in essentially every tissue but most concentrated in the brain. Neuronal CaMKII is present in both presynapses and postsynapses, and is also the major component of the PSD. The PSD serves as a general organizer of the postsynaptic signal transduction machinery, which links regulatory molecules to their targets. Dysfunction of CaMKII may relate to neuronal disorders.

This review covers the molecular basis of learning and memory taking into consideration research on CaMKII, a major component of neurons.

* Address: Musashidai 2-6, Fuchu-City, Tokyo 183-8526, Japan. Email: yamauchi@tmin.ac.jp

List of Abbreviations

AD, Alzheimer's disease
AMPA, α-amino-3-hydroxy-5-methylisoxazole-4-propionic acid
Arc, Activity-regulated cytoskeleton-associated protein
BDNF, brain-derived neurotrophic factor
CaMKII, Ca^{2+}/calmodulin-dependent protein kinase II
CBP, CREB-binding protein
CDK, cyclin-dependent protein kinase
CNS, central nervous system
CPEB, Cytoplasmic polyadenylation element-binding protein
CREB, cAMP response element-binding protein
GABA, γ-aminobutyric acid
IP_3, inositol 1,4,5-trisphosphate
IRS p58/53, Insulin-receptor tyrosine kinase 58/53 kDa substrate
LTD, long-term depression
LTP, long-term potentiation
MAP, microtubule-associated protein
mGluR, metabotropic glutamate receptor
NFT, neurofibrillary tangle
NGF, nerve growth factor
NMDA, N-methyl-D-aspartate
nNOS, neuronal nitric oxide synthase
NT(s), neurotrophin(s)
PD, Parkinson's disease
PDZ, PSD-95/Disc-large/ZO-1
PHF, paired helical filament
PKA , Protein kinase A
PKC, protein kinase C
PP1, protein phosphatase 1
PSD, Post-synaptic density
SAP, synapse-associated protein
SynGAP, synaptic GTPase activating protein
TH, tyrosine hydroxylase
TPH, tryptophan hydroxylase
TNF, tumor necrosis factor
UTR, untranslated region

Introduction

In the central nervous system (CNS), the synapse is a specialized junctional complex by which axons and dendrites emerging from different neurons intercommunicate. Synaptic plasticity has a central role in learning and memory, and is defined as an activity-dependent change in synaptic transmission. Transient modifications of synapses have been associated with short-term memory and more lasting changes have been associated with long-term memory in the mature neuron. To understand these modifications at the molecular level, it is important to find and characterize the"memory molecules" and "memory apparatus or memory forming apparatus"in the brain. Synaptic plasticity depends on proper regulation of synaptic proteins, many of which can be rapidly regulated by phosphorylation/dephosphorylation. These synaptic phosphoproteins play a role in regulating both pre- and post-synaptic functions.

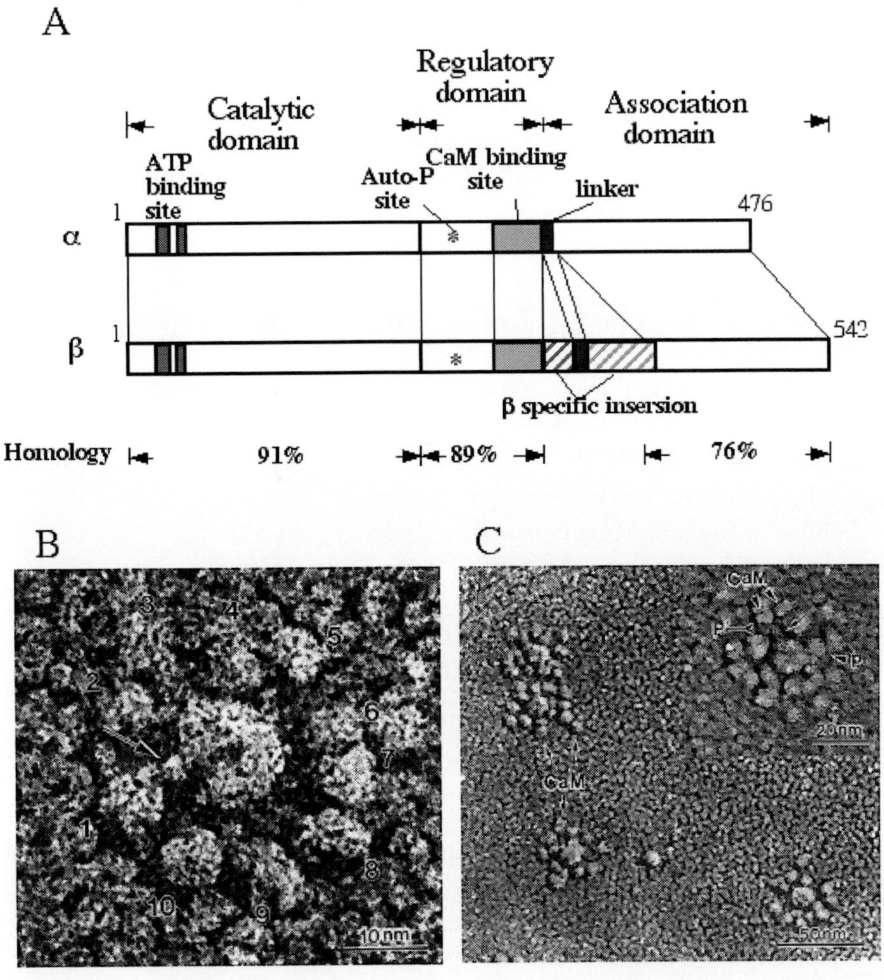

Figure 1. Structure of CaMKII (Kanaseki, et al. 1991). *A*, domain structure of α and β CaMKII. CaMKII is composed of three distinct functional domains, catalytic, regulatory, and association domains.The two isoforms are highly conserved. *B*, a high magnification electron micrograph of α CaMKII having 10 peripheral particles. An *arrow* indicates the linker, which is a thin projection linking peripheral and central particles. *C*, binding of α CaMKII with calmodulin. Calmodulin molecules (CaM) associated with the peripheral particles (P) from the outside. (*inset*) Two molecules of calmodulin are observed covering a peripheral particle (P').

Ca^{2+}/calmodulin–dependent protein kinase II (CaMKII), a multifunctional Ser/Thr kinase activated by Ca^{2+} and calmodulin, is an evolutionally conserved protein. Ca^{2+} is a universal second messenger in eukaryotic cells. Cells typically maintain an intracellular Ca^{2+} level of 10^{-7} M, which is 10^{4} times lower the level outside cells. The intracellular Ca^{2+} level rapidly increases up to 10^{-4} M derived from extracellular and intracellular sources in response to extra cellular stimuli. The predominant intracellular receptor of Ca^{2+} is calmodulin, a EF-hand family Ca^{2+}-binding protein and highly conserved Ca^{2+} sensor. Ca^{2+} plays an essential role in the basic operation of neurons through synaptic communication.

CaMKII is highly concentrated in the nervous system, and is specifically expressed during the most active period in the formation of the synaptic network. CaMKII is one of the major proteins in the postsynaptic density (PSD), which is an integral part of the postsynaptic signaling machinery. This kinase has an extremely broad substrate specificity and phosphorylates various kinds of proteins in the brain. Neuronal CaMKII is now recognized as a critical mediator of neuronal plasticity that links transiently triggered Ca^{2+} signals to persistent changes in neuronal physiology. It regulates important neuronal functions, such as neurotransmitter synthesis, neurotransmitter release, modulation of ion channel activity, cellular transport, cell morphology and neurite extension, synaptic plasticity, learning and memory, and gene expression. Because of these diverse functions, dysfunction of CaMKII may cause neurological disorders.

The key role of CaMKII in synaptic plasticity and behavior makes it important to understand its ability to achieve precise modulation of neuronal function. The basic molecular mechanisms of CaMKII's functions, including in learning and memory, lie in its interactions with and phosphorylation of putative modulatory targets. CaMKII is one of the best candidates for a molecular component of the memory apparatus.

We will review the literature, with special focus on studies of the action of CaMKII in the synapse, including both presynaptic terminals and postsynaptic regions. We also discuss that dysfunction of CaMKII may cause neurological disorders. Several other reviews on CaMKII provide additional perspectives for the interested reader (Hudmon & Schulman, 2002; Lisman et al., 2002; Griffith et al., 2003; Colbran & Brown, 2004; Yamauchi, 2005).

(1) What is CaMKII

In the nearly 30 years since its discovery, CaMKII has been of major interest in the region of brain science. There may be many new readers, however, who are not familiar with CaMKII. We briefly describe the historical background and summarize the characteristics of CaMKII. CaMKII was first identified in 1980 by gel filtration of Ca^{2+}/calmodulin-dependent protein kinases of rat brain by researchers monitoring the activation of tryptophan hydroxylase and the phosphorylation of endogenous proteins in the brain (Yamauchi & Fujisawa, 1980). It was the second peak eluted from a sizing column used to fractionate Ca^{2+}/calmodulin-dependent protein kinases from rat brain cytosol. The same kinase was independently reported as calmodulin-dependent protein kinese that phosphorylates site II of protein I (later named synapsin I) as a substrate (Kennedy & Greengard, 1981). Later, several groups identified and purified the same kinase from various tissues and species (see review; Hudmon & Schulamn, 2002; Yamauchi, 2005).

Table 1. Characteristics of CaMKII

*CaMKII is a serine/threonine protein kinase activated by Ca^{2+} and calmodulin.
*CaMKII is one of the most abundant protein kinases in the mammalian brain, and constitutes up to 2% of total protein in the hippocampus, a memory center.
*CaMKII has broad substrate specificity and phosphorylates a broad array of brain proteins.
*CaMKII is activated in the presence of Ca^{2+} and calmodulin, and then it has the ability to autophosphorylate, a process that confers Ca^{2+} -independent activity upon the kinase and greatly increases its affinity for calmodulin.
*The Ca^{2+}-independent activity prolongs the Ca^{2+} action transiently increased in response to nerve stimuli.
*CaMKII phosphorylates serine and threonine residues of the major consensus sequence RXXS/T. CaMKII also phosphorylates serine and threonine residues of the sequence S/TXD, a completely different sequence from the major consensus site; S, serine; T, threonine; D, aspartic acid; X, any amino acid
*CaMKII is increased rapidly during the most active phase in the formation of synapses in the postnatal brain, and is maintained at a high level after synaptic maturation.
*CaMKII is the major component of the postsynaptic density (PSD), where it plays a key role in synaptic signaling.
*CaM kinase II is an evolutionally conserved protein.
*Mammalian CaMKII has four isoforms (α,β,γ, and δ), and α and β the two major isoforms, are expressed almost exclusively in the nervous system.
*CaMKII holoenzyme exists as a multimeric structure consisting of 8-10 subunits, with a molecular mass of 500-600 kDa.
*CaMKII has a shape resembling that of a flower with 8 or 10 petals.
*CaMKII is one of the best candidates for a memory molecule.

CaMKII is an evolutionally conserved protein. Vertebrate CaMKII evolved *via* duplication of a single ancestral CaMKII gene, resulting in four genes, α,β, γ,and δ, in higher vertebrates (Tombes et al., 2003). α and β CaMKII are the two major isoforms of the kinase expressed in the brain, and expressed almost exclusively in the nervous system. CaMKII is unique among protein kinases because of its oligomeric assembly with a holoenzyme architecture. The subunit of CaMKII shares a domain structure consisting of catalytic, regulatory, and association domains (Lin et al., 1987). The molecular conformation of CaMKII and its binding to calmodulin have been investigated by electron microscopy (Fig. 1) (Kanaseki et al., 1991).

Gear-shaped model of α CaMKII was also reported using three-dimensional electron microscopy (Kolodziej et al. 2000). Table 1 summarizes the characteristics of the CaMKII molecule.

(2) Molecular Properties of CaMKII as a Memory Molecule

The interest in CaMKII has been fueled by its fascinating regulatory properties, which are based on autophosphorylation, distribution, developmental change, and translocation. Based on these properties, CaMKII is recognized as a memory molecule.

2-1. Autophosphorylation: Activation and inactivation of the kinase activity

Autophosphorylation provides critical regulation of CaMKII, both activation and inactivation.

CaMKII is completely inactive in the absence of Ca^{2+} and calmodulin, since the autoinhibitory domain, present in the regulatory domain, blocks the active site of the kinase. The autoinhibitory domain is disrupted by the binding of calmodulin at its C-terminal end, which leads to de-inhibition of the kinase. The autoinhibitory domain can be further disrupted by autophosphorylation of a key threonine residue common to all isoforms (Thr286 and Thr287 of the α and β isoforms, respectively) (Fong et al., 1989; Hanson et al., 1989). This phosphorylation converts the kinase to a Ca^{2+}-independent enzyme. Autophosphorylation increases the affinity of the kinase for calmodulin several hundred fold by reducing the dissociation rate (Meyer et al., 1992). The Ca^{2+}-independent activity of the enzyme prolongs the Ca^{2+} action transiently increased in response to nerve stimuli, and is involved in long-term potentiation (LTP), a basic process of learning and memory. Thus, CaMKII is postulated to act as a "molecular switch" (Lisman, 1994).

Autophosphorylation of Thr305 and Thr306, inhibitory autophosphorylation sites, on α and β CaMKII, respectively, occurs after phosphorylation at Thr286 (α) or Thr287 (β) in a Ca^{2+}-independent manner (Colbran & Soderling, 1990). This is responsible for the loss of ability of CaMKII to bind Ca^{2+}/calmodulin, resulting in a reduction of the kinase activity and the association of CaMKII with PSD.

CaMKII activity is regulated bidirectionally, activation and inactivation, by the autophosphorylation.

2-2. Distribution: Spatial and temporal expression of CaMKII in the brain

2-2-1. Immunocytochemistry

Immunoreactivity to CaMKII is present in neurons throughout the brain. CaMKII composes up to 1% of total protein in the forebrain and 2% of that in the hippocampus (Erondu & Kennedy, 1985). The ratio of α to β isoforms is about 3 : 1 and 1 : 4 in the adult forebrain and cerebellum, respectively (McGuinness et al., 1985; Miller & Kennedy, 1985).

In the forebrain, α CaMKII is more homogeneously distributed through cellular layers II to V than β CaMKII (Ochiishi et al., 1994b). In the cerebellum, the α isoform is present selectively in Purukinje cells, and a majority of the β isoform distributes in granular cells and neurons in the cerebellar nuclei (Ichikawa et al., 1992). Regional differences of distribution between α and β CaMKII are also shown in the retina and brainstem of rats (Ochiishi et al., 1994a; 1998). The distribution of α CaMKII corresponds with that of choline acetyl transferase in the retina, suggesting that the kinase participates in the regulation of the cholinergic system, especially the "light OFF" system in the retina (Ochiishi et al., 1994a). A different distribution of α and β isoforms is found in spinal cord of rat and monkey (Terashima et al., 1994). α CaMKII occurs in both dorsal and ventral corticospinal tract fibers, and β CaMKII is distributed in the neuropil of the gray matter.

2-2-2. Subcellular distribution

The subcellular localization and compartmentalization of specific proteins generally play a significant role in the functioning of signal transduction. In brain tissue, α CaMKII is found in the cytosolic fraction and PSD. α CaMKII is one of the major proteins in the PSD (Kennedy et al., 1983; Goldenring et al., 1984; Kelly et al., 1984). In the hippocampus, β CaMKII is associated with actin filaments (Shen et al., 1998).

The different subcellular distribution of α and β isoforms is demonstrated using neuroblastoma cells overexpressing each isoform as a model system. α CaMKII is mainly distributed in the cytosolic fraction, whereas the β isoform is in the particulate fraction (Yamauchi et al., 1990). Deletion analysis reveals that the second part of the β-specific insertion and oligomeric form are important to the particulate distribution of β CaMKII (Urushihara & Yamauchi, 2001).

2-2-3. Dendritic distribution of mRNA

mRNA of α CaMKII is distributed in dendrites of the cerebral cortex (Burgin et al., 1990).The 3' untranslated region (UTR) of α CaMKII mRNA is important to the dendritic distribution of the kinase (Miller et al., 2002). mRNAs of some neuronal proteins, including microtubule associated protein 2 (MAP2), calmodulin, and activity-regulated cytoskeleton-associated protein (Arc), inositol 1,4,5-trisphosphate (IP3) receptor, and N-methyl-D-aspartate (NMDA) receptor 2B subunit, are also found in dendrites (Steward & Schuman, 2001). It is interest that proteins translated from these mRNA are a substrate or regulating protein of CaMKII. Dendritic distribution of mRNA is related to the activity-dependent local protein synthesis without transcription of mRNA, and the translation of dendritic mRNAs may be regulated by signaling events at synapses. Therefore, local protein production during long-term synaptic plasticity has focused attention on the mechanism involved (Steward, 1997; Steward & Schuman, 2001).

2-3. Development:Relation to synaptic network formation

The levels of α and β proteins of CaMKII depend on the stage of development. There are two developmentally regulated isoforms of the kinase in the rat forebrain with α : β ratios for 10-day and adult enzymes of 1 : 1 and 2.3 : 1, respectively (McGuinness et al., 1985; Miller et al., 1985). The concentration of α and β proteins varies markedly in brain regions with age in the postnatal period. In early postnatal brain, the concentration of these proteins is low, and increases 20-60 fold between day 10 and 30 dependent on the region, indicating that the kinase is specifically expressed during the most active period in the formation of the synaptic network (Sugiura & Yamauchi, 1992).The expression of many substrates of CaMKII is also regulated developmentally, with levels increasing from neonates to adults according to the increase in the amount of CaMKII (Sugiura & Yamauchi, 1994).

The expression of α and β CaMKII is carefully regulated at the level of transcription. The α and β CaMKII genes both have strong transcriptional activity in the 5'-flanking region, but have no sequence identity or similarity in this region (Donai et al. 2001; Mima et al., 2001). Zic2, a zinc finger transcription factor, and rLRP157, rat leucine-rich protein 157 kDa protein, have been identified as one of the promoter-binding and activating proteins of α and β CaMKII, respectively (Sakurada et al., 2005; Ochiai et al., 2007). Some other promoter-binding proteins are found in the nuclear extract of the brain and should be identified.

2-4. Translocation in subcellular distribution

Autophosphorylation-dependent reversible translocation of α CaMKII to the PSD is important to the signal transduction in postsynaptic cells as described in a later section (Section 5-2).

(3) Involvement of CaMKII in Plasticity and/or Learning and Memory in Animal and Cell Models

A large number of extracellular signals have been shown to regulate protein phosphorylation in the nervous system. Genetic approaches, including the use of various mutant mice, have provided a wealth of information on the role of CaMKII and cognition (Elgersma et al., 2004). Cell models are also useful because of their high reproducibility and ease of handling.

3-1. CaMKII null mutant mice

Neuronal CaMKII was first recognized as involved in learning and memory based on the report that transgenic mice lacking the α isoform are defective in LTP in the hippocampus and spatial learning (Silva et al., 1992). Follow-up studies were carried out using subsequent generations of these mutant mice in a novel inbred background. Although LTP at 60 min post-tetanus is clearly deficient in these α CaMKII null mutant mice compared with α CaMKII control animals, the mutants mice do show a significant level of LTP. The amount of LTP observed in α CaMKII mutants is normally distributed and does not correlate with age (Hinds et al. 1998). The experience-dependent plasticity of the barrel cortex is also prevented in adult mice that lack the gene encoding α CaMKII, indicating that α CaMKII is necessary either for the induction or for the expression of plasticity (Glazewski et al., 1996). However, seizure susceptibility is increased in α CaMKII null mutant mice (Burtler et al., 1995). Thus, interest has been directed torward the molecular mechanism of learning and memory through the action of this kinase.

In the cerebellum of the α CaMKII null mutant mouse, a long-term depression (LTD) protocol results in only transient depression and in robust potentiation in adults. This suggests that the function of α CaMKII in parallel fiber-Purkinje cell plasticity is opposite to its function at excitatory hippocampal and cortical synapses. α CaMKII null mutant mice also show impaired gain-increase adaptation of both the vestibular ocular reflex and optokinetic reflex (Hansel et al., 2006).

3-2. Overexpression of CaMKII in mice and rats

When α CaMKII was overexpressed in the rat hippocampus using an adeno-associated viral vector, the transgenic rat exhibited improved performance in a water maze task, but no change in locomotor activity and exploratory behavior in an open field task, indicating that α CaMKII plays a role in spatial or explicit memory storage (Poulsen et al., 2007).

Using targeted chemical-genetic engineering, an *in vivo* conditional protein knockout and/or manipulation technology was developed (Wang et al., 2003). The α CaMKII-F86G mutant kinase is created based on the specific interaction interface between a modified protein domain and sensitized inhibitors. The mutant enzyme accepts ATP normally, but has highly sensitive to a specific inhibitor. The transgenic mice show a significant elevation in both Ca^{2+}-dependent and Ca^{2+}-independent CaMKII activity. CaMKII overexpression alters frequency–plasticity responses in the hippocampal Schaffer-collateral pathway. This effect is blocked by the CaMKII inhibitor. A precise level of CaMKII reactivation is essential for the consolidation of long-term memories in the brain (Wang et al., 2003).

Similarly, the β CaMKII-F90G mutant was created by targeted chemical-genetic engineering to investigate the functional difference between α CaMKII and β CaMKII*in vivo* (Cho et al., 2007). Experiments with the transgenic mice showed that β CaMKII activity in the dentate gyrus selectively impairs LTP in the dentate perforant path. The mice had normal 1-day memories, but were severely impaired in 10-day contextual fear memory, indicating that the initial day is a critical time within the postlearning consolidation period and is highly sensitive to change in β CaMKII (Cho et al., 2007).

3-3. Transgenic mice with CaMKII mutated at autophosphorylation sites

Autophosphorylation of α CaMKII at Thr 286 converts the kinase to a Ca^{2+}-independent enzyme. This Thr (T) residue is mutated to Ala (A), resulting in a deficiency of autophosphorylation and activation, and to Asp (D), resulting in mimicking the autonomous activity of the kinase autophosphorylated at Thr286. (The letter in the parenthesis indicates the amino acid as one letter.) Ca^{2+}-independent activity induced by autophosphorylation of α CaMKII is essential for the induction and maintenance of LTP (Lisman et al., 2002). The requirement of α CaMKII autophosphorylation for neocortical LTP and experience–

dependent synaptic plasticity was demonstrated using mice carrying a point mutation of α CaMKII at Thr286 to Ala (T286A) (Giese et al., 1998). In α CaMKII T286A mutant mice, experience-dependent plasticity in the barrel cortex was prevented in adult and adolescent mice homozygous for the mutation, but was normal in heterozygotes and wild-type littermates (Glazewski et al., 2000). The spatial tuning of place fields of α CaMKII T268A mutant mice is initially similar to that of wild-type mice, but completely failed to show an experience-dependent increase over days (Cacucci et al., 2007). α CaMKII T268A mutant mice also show impairments in ocular dominance plasticity (Taha et al, 2002).

Several lines of transgenic mice have been generated to increase CaMKII activity levels, such as transgenic T286D mutants with autonomous CaMKII activity. The mutant mice expressing α CaMKII T268D exhibited normal LTP in response to stimulation at 100 Hz. However, at lower frequencies, in the range of 1-10 Hz, there was a systematic shift in the size and direction of the resulting synaptic change in the transgenic animals that favored LTD. The regulation of this frequency-response is dependent on Ca^{2+}-independent CaMKII activity (Mayford et al., 1995). When the transgene is expressed at high levels in the lateral amygdala and the striatum but not other forebrain structures, there is a deficit in fear conditioning, an implicit memory task, that also is reversible. Thus, the CaMKII signaling pathway is critical for both explicit and implicit memory storage, in a manner that is independent of its potential role in development (Mayford et al. 1996). Mice expressing low levels of the α CaMKII T268D transgene have facilitated low-frequency-induced LTP, whereas mice with high levels of transgene expression have a deficit in this form of plasticity. Behavioral impairments in fear-conditioned memory and visible water maze correlate with the level of α CaMKII T268D expression. Mice with high levels of α CaMKII T268D have reversible, compensatory changes in the expression of genes associated with inhibitory neurotransmission (Bejar et al. 2002). These results indicate that the level of CaMKII activity is important in the experience–dependent synaptic plasticity.

Mutation of Thr305, an inhibitory autophosphorylation site, to Asp (T305D) results in the kinase becoming inactive because of inhibition of the binding to calmodulin. Mutation of Thr305 to Val (T305V) results in the active form in the presence of Ca^{2+}. It was demonstrated that inhibitory autophosphorylation controls the association of CaMKII with the PSD, synaptic plasticity, and learning using α CaMKII T305D mutant mice, (Elgersma et al., 2002). Inhibitory autophosphorylation of CaMKII is also required for hippocampal metaplasticity at the lateral perforant path-dentate granule cell synapse. Metaplasticity is known as the higher-order form of plasticity. Metaplasticity was absent in knock-in mice expressing the α CaMKII TT305/306VA mutant that cannot undergo inhibitory phosphorylation, indicating that inhibitory autophosphorylation at Thr306/Thr306 is a key mechanism for metaplasticity (Zhang et al., 2005).

3-4. Transgenic mice with CaMKII mRNA mutated at 3' UTR

α CaMKII mRNA in dendrites and the local synthesis of new α CaMII protein are required for late-phase LTP (Miller et al., 2002). The dendritic localization signal of α CaMKII mRNA is present in the 3' UTR. The signal is disrupted by deletion of the 3' UTR. In this mutant mouse, the protein-coding region of α CaMKII is intact, but mRNA is restricted to the soma. Mutant mice show a dramatic reduction of α CaMKII in the PSD, a reduction in late-phase LTP, and impairments in spatial memory, associative fear conditioning, and object recognition memory. These results demonstrate that local translation is important for synaptic delivery of the kinase and that local translation contributes to synaptic and behavioral plasticity. The results are supported by the finding that the induction of LTP increased the amount of α CaMKII mRNA in synaptosomes isolated from the dentate gyrus (Hivak et al., 2003).

3-5. Neuronal cells

The involvement of CaMKII in the increase in the number of synaptic contacts was demonstrated in pyramidal neurons (Pratt et al., 2003). Postsynaptic expression of the activated CaMKII T286D mutant increased the strength of transmission between pairs of pyramidal neurons, through a modest increase in quantal amplitude and a larger increase in the number of synaptic contacts.

In the CA1 region in hippocampal slices, a CaMKII inhibitor strongly reduced synaptic transmission. The inhibition occured in both LTP and control pathway, but only partially recovered after removal of the inhibitor. These data support the notion that CaMKII is involved in controlling basal synaptic strength (Sanhueza et al., 2007).

In cultures of dissociated rat hippocampal neurons, depolarization-induced secretion of postsynaptic neurotrophin (NT) is elicited by Ca^{2+} influx and inhibited in the presence of CaMKII inhibitor, indicating a critical dependence on the activation of CaMKII (Kolarow et al., 2007). The mammalian neurotrophins nerve growth factor (NGF), brain derived neurotrophic factor (BDNF), NT-3, and NT-4 constitute a family of secreted neuronal growth factors. NTs are implicated in several forms of activity-dependent synaptic plasticity. Taken together, depolarization-induced postsynaptic NT secretion is elicited by Ca^{2+} influx and activation of CaMKII.

CaMKII regulates gene expression *via* phosphorylation of transcription factors, such as cAMP response element-binding protein (CREB) and NeuroD. Using neuroblstoma cells expressing CREB and CaMKII, phosphorylation of serine 142 in CREB by CaMKII was shown to lead to the dissociation of the CREB dimer without impeding DNA-binding capacity. Dimeric CREB is required to recruit the CREB-binding protein (CBP). These results suggest that CaMKII confers a dominant inhibitory effect on transcription by preventing dimerization of CREB, and this mechanism is responsible for the attenuation of gene expression (Wu & McMurray, 2001). The transcription factor NeuroD mediates neuronal activity-dependent dendritogenesis. The genetic knockdown of NeuroD in primary granule neurons of cerebellar profoundly impaired the generation and maintenance of dendrites while sparing the development of axons. CaMKII phosphorylates NeuroD in primary neurons, and thereby stimulates dendritic growth, indicating that CaMKII-NeuroD signaling pathway plays important roles in synaptic plasticity in the developing and mature brain (Gaudilliere, et al., 2004).

A cell culture model was developed by overexpressing the α and β isoforms of CaMKII in neuroblastoma cells (Goshima et al., 1993; 99 Nomura et al., 1997). Expression of the isoforms stimulates neurite outgrowth and growth cone motility in these cells. This stimulation is enhanced by the selective protein kinase C (PKC) inhibitor, suggesting that the proliferation and differentiation of neuronal cells are regulated by the activity of CaMKII and PKC (Nomura et al., 1997). Autophosphorylation of Thr268 of α CaMKII is essential for this kinase to exert cellular functions efficiently, as demonstrated using α CaMKII T268A or T268D mutants (Goshima et al., 1993; Sogawa et al., 2000). The β-specific insertion of β CaMKII is involved in the subcellular distribution of the kinase, and the subcellular distribution is important in neurite extention (Urushihara & Yamauchi, 2001).

3-6. Toward a better understanding of molecular mechanisms

Remarkable progress has been made in understanding the role of CaMKII in various types of synaptic plasticity and in learning and memory. CaMKII is activated during the induction of LTP and this activation is necessary and sufficient for LTP. CaMKII also increases synaptic strength. CaMKII is involved in LTP, LTD, hippocampus-dependent learning, such as special learning, ocular dominance plasticity, seizure susceptibility, cued and contextual conditioning, metaplasticity, and neurite extension. CaMKII is also involved in protein synthesis and gene expression. These results indicate that careful regulation of the kinase activity is required for the normal functioning of CaMKII.The key experiments have been replicated in several laboratories and using independent methods.

Interest has been directed toward the molecular mechanism of these processes through the action of this kinase. CaMKII's actions are related to the phosphorylation and/or interaction of specific proteins. To understand the modulatory targets, and the impact that CaMKII has on learning and memory at the cellular and systemic level, we describe the basic molecular mechanisms of phosphorylation and binding interactions in the next sections.

(4) Presynaptic Proteins Regulated By CaMKII

CaMKII is involved in the regulation of neurotransmitter synthesis, neurotransmitter secretion, and microtubule function in the presynapse. Although CaMKII targets various kinds of proteins, CaMKII substrates and interacting proteins in the presynaptic terminal are shown in Table 2.

4-1. Regulation of neurotransmitter synthesis

The nervous system makes use of two main classical substances for signaling: small-molecule transmitters and neuroactive peptides. Neurotransmitters are contained in vesicles, which release their contents *via* an exocytotic mechanism. Catecholamine and serotonin transmitters are synthesized from the essential amino acids tyrosine and tryptophan, respectively. The synthesis of catecholamines and serotonin is regulated by CaMKII through phosphorylation of the rate-limiting enzymes of their biosynthesis, tyrosine hydroxylase (TH) and tryptophan hydroxylase (TPH), respectively (Yamauchi, 2005). TH is phosphorylated by CaMKII at Ser-19 (Itagaki et al., 1999), and TPH, at Ser-58 and Ser-260 (Jiang et al., 2000).

The phosphorylated enzymes are then activated by activator protein. Thus, the activation occurs in two steps, and a new mechanism of enzyme regulation is proposed; first, phosphorylation of TH and TPH by CaMKII, and second, activation of the phosphorylated enzymes by the activator protein (Yamauchi & Fujisawa,1981; Yamauchi et al., 1981; Yamauchi, 2005). Currently, the activator protein is known to be the same protein as 14-3-3 protein, and to be a regulator of the signal transduction/phosphorylation mechanism. Since these monoamines are known to be involved in normal mental function or in some neurological diseases, CaMKII may play an important role in mental function.

Table 2. CaMKII substrates and interacting proteins, and their regulation by CaMKII in the presynapse

Protein	Effect
Substrate protein	
TH	Activation[1]
TPH	Activation[1]
Synapsin	Stimulation of neurotransmitter release[2]
Tau	Regulation of microtubule assembly-disassembly[3]
Synaptotagmin	Increase in the interaction of syntaxin and SNAP-25 with synaptotagmin[4]
Interacting protein	
Syntaxin I	Stimulation of exocytosis[5]

1, Yamauchi, 2005; 2, Benfenati et al., 1992; 3, Singh et al., 1996; 4, Verona, et al., 2000; 5, Ohyama et al., 2002.

4-2. Synaptic vesicle proteins

CaMKII phosphorylates synaptic vesicle proteins, such as synapsin I and synaptotagmin. Synapsin I is a synaptic vesicle-associated phosphoprotein that is involved in the modulation of neurotransmitter release.CaMKII phosphorylates synapsin I, causes synapsin I to dissociate from synaptic vesicles, and increases neurotransmitter release (Benfenati et al., 1992). Synaptotagmin is associated with CaMKII, resulting in stimulation of the formation of fusion complex (Verona et al., 2000).

4-3. Mobilization of synaptic vesicles

Microtubules are involved in the transport of synaptic vesicles to active sites for secretion. Microtubule proteins, including tubulin, high molecular weight microtubule-associated proteins (MAPs), and the low molecular weight MAP tau, are suitable substrates for CaMKII. Assembly –disassembly of microtubules is regulated by the phosphorylation of various MAPs. Among MAPs, tau is mainly localized in axon and presynapse terminals. Tau is phosphorylated by CaMKII and the phosphorylation results in a reduction of affinity for tubulin and disassembly of microtubules (Singh et al., 1996).Synaptic vesicles may be released from microtubule, resulting in the stimulation of their mobility.

In *Drosophila* motor neuron terminals, ryanodine receptor and CaMKII are essential for post-tetanic potentiation of neuropeptide secretion. Ryanodine receptor-activated CaMKII increases vesicle mobility and potentiates neuropeptide release (Shakiryanova et al., 2007).

4-4. Fusion of synaptic vesicles to plasma membrane and exocytosis

When an action potential reaches a presynaptic terminal, Ca^{2+} enters it. The rise in the intracellular Ca^{2+} concentration causes the vesicles to fuse with the presynaptic membrane and thereby release their neurotransmitter *via* an exocytotic mechanism.

Synaptotagmin is a putative Ca^{2+} sensor, and is considered crucial for the Ca^{2+} dependence of release. It is also considered a molecular mediator of synaptic plasticity. Synaptotagmin is endogenously phosphorylated in synaptic vesicles by CaMKII. Its phosphorylation increases on interaction with syntaxin and SNAP-25, and stimulates exocytosis (Verona et al., 2000).

The interaction of α CaMKII with syntaxin 1A was also demonstrated using isolated proteins from the rat brain (Ohyama et al., 2002). Syntaxin 1A is a key component of the exocytotic molecular machinery. The binding is Ca^{2+} and ATP-dependent. A CaMKII-syntaxin complex forms in the presynaptic terminal. Microinjection of the CaMKII-binding domain peptide of syntaxin specifically results in a decrease in the frequency of exocytosis in chromaffin cells and in neurons, causing interference with the endogenous CaMKII-syntaxin complex. The Ca^{2+}/ATP-dependent binding of CaMKII to syntaxin is an important step in the regulation of exocytosis.

(5) Postsynaptic Proteins Regulated By CaMKII

CaMKII is involved in the regulation of the cytoskeleton, neurite extension, receptor and channel activity, and signal transduction in the postsynapse. CaMKII substrates and interacting proteins in the postsynapse are shown in Table 3.

Table 3. CaMKII substrates and interacting proteins in the PSD fraction[1]

Class
Substrate protein
Receptor and channel proteins NMDA receptor NR1, 2A and 2B subunits, AMPA receptor GluR1 subunit, mGluR, GABA receptor A subunit, Kvl.4,
Receptor-clustering, scaffold, and adaptor proteins PSD-95, SAP-97, SAP-90, PSD-95-associated protein (SAPAP), Homer 1b, ras GTPase-activating protein, SynGAP b1 and c proteins
Motor protein Myosin IIB
Cytoskeletal protein and associated proteins Neurofilament H, M, and L proteins, α-Internexin, α-Tubulin, β-Tubulin, Clipin C
Enzymes Dynamin 1, Cyclic nucleotide phosphodiesterase, CaM kinase II α, and β subunits (autophosphorylation), nNOS,
Membrane protein Densin 180
Others CPEB, TOAD-64, TNF receptor-associated factor 3, IRS pS8/S3
Interacting protein Arc, F-actin, α actinin, myosin Va (brain myosin V), Cdk5 activator p35 and p39

1. Data is summarized based on references (Yoshimura, et al., 2000 & 2002; see reviews, Fink & Meyer, 2002; Griffith et al., 2003; Yamauchi, 2002 & 2005), with some additions.

5-1. Regulation of cytoskeleton: Dynamic processes and movement of organelles and structural changes

Microtubule proteins are suitable substrates for CaMKII. Phosphorylation of MAP2 leads to a reduction in affinity for tubulin, and induces microtubule disassembly (Yamauchi & Fujisawa, 1983). The microtubule network plays an important role in maintaining cellular morphology, in membrane interaction, in intracellular trafficking, and in establishing neurite outgrowth of differentiating neurons (Drubin & Nelson, 1996).

Actin filament–microtubule interaction is also important for cellular structure, and the interaction of actin filament with microtubules is regulated by phosphorylation-dephosphorylation of MAP2. Phosphorylation of MAP2 by CaMKII inhibits the actin filament cross-linking activity of MAP2, indicating that CaMKII regulates microtubule-microfilament interaction (Yamauchi & Fujiswa, 1988). CaMKII also interacts with the tail domain of myosin V, enriched in the PSD fraction. CaMKII is activated in a CaM-independent manner via its association with myosin V after translocation to the PSD (Costa et al., 1999). Myosin V may function for CaMKII to shuttle between the cytosol and PSD in dendritic spines along the actin filament network. Thus, CaMKII is involved in the dynamic processes and movement of organelles in the nerve cells.

Neurite extension and branching are important neuronal plasticity mechanisms that can lead to the addition of synaptic contacts in developing neurons and changes in the number of synapses in mature neurons. CaMKII regulates the movement, extension, and branching of filopodia and fine dendrites as well as the number of synapses in hippocampal neurons. Only β CaMKII, not α CaMKII, has this morphogenic activity (Fink et al., 2003). CaMKII is capable of bundling F-actin through a stoichiometric interaction (Shen et al., 1998). In organotypic slice cultures of the hippocampus, RNAi-mediated down-regulation of CaMKII leads to a reduction in the volume of dendritic spine heads that is mediated by F-actin dynamics. This activity was associated with β. CaMKII in a manner requiring its actin-binding and association domains, indicating that this feature of CaMKII is necessary for maintaining the dendritic spine structure (Okamoto et al., 2007).Thus, CaMKII serves as a central signaling molecule in structural changes during synaptic plasticity.

5-2. Regulation of PSD protein by CaMKII

5-2-1. Molecular constituents of PSD

Important mechanisms for synaptic regulation, including LTP and LTD, may be based on the PSD (see review; Kennedy, 1997; Kennedy, 2000; Yamauchi, 2002; Sheng & Hoogenraad, 2007). The PSD is a tiny, amorphous structure located on and beneath the post-synaptic membrane and is visible under the electron microscope as tight complexes of post-synaptic junctional proteins. It is a disc-shaped subcellular organelle about 50 nm thick and 100-900 nm in diameter apposed to postsynaptic membranes. Many attempts have been made to identify and characterize the molecular constituents of the PSD, but, not all constituents are known (Yamauchi, 2002). Recently, molecular constituents have been analyzed using an integrated liquid chromatography-based protein identification system, and results provide a catalogue of the major protein sets associated with the PSD (Yoshimura et al., 2004). Hundreds of different proteins have been identified in the PSD. The PSD contains various proteins involved in signal transduction, including receptors, ion channel proteins, protein kinases and phosphatases, G-protein and related proteins, scaffold proteins, and adaptor proteins. Structural proteins, including membrane proteins involved in cell adhesion and cell-cell-interaction, proteins involved in endocytosis, motor proteins, and cytoskeletal proteins are also abundant.Similar results were reported somewhat later (Yoshimura et al., 2004; Peng et al., 2004; Sheng & Hoogenraad, 2007).

CaMKII is one of the major proteins in the PSD of the cerebral cortex and hippocampus (Kennedy et al., 1983; Goldenring et al., 1984; Kelly et al., 1984). Quantitative immunoblotting combined with scanning transmission electroscopy for estimation of the PSD mass revealed the CaMKII content per single PSD to be 80 holoenzymes, corresponding to 6% of the total PSD mass (Chen et al., 2005).

Many proteins in the PSD are phosphorylated and regulated by various protein kinases.

The presence and organization of the signaling machinery varies among different synaptic types. This information is crucial because the complement of signaling complexes at a synapse determines how it interacts and encodes information.

5-2-2. Translocation of CaMKII to the PSD

Recent studies have led to a model of the molecular steps of CaMKII's translocation and activation that can explain its role in neuronal plasticity. Autophosphorylation-dependent reversible translocation of α CaMKII to the PSD was demonstrated using an isolated PSD and purified CaMKII (Strack et al., 1997; Yoshimura et al., 1997). The discovery may be the initial step in elucidating this structural process and understanding the mechanism by which CaMKII increases synaptic strength. When CaMKII is autophosphorylated in the presence of Ca^{2+} and calmodulin, the kinase associates with the PSD to form the PSD-CaMKII complex. CaMKII is recruited to the NMDA receptor NR2B subunit through the cytoplasmic carboxyl-terminal domain of the subunit. The CaMKII-NR2B complex maintains the kinase-activated state (Bayer et al., 2001). After high-potassium treatment, the accumulation of CaMKII on the cytoplasmic face is observed in cultured hippocampal neurons, concomitant with the thickening of postsynaptic densities (Dosemeci et al. 2001). At the PSD, CaMKII associates with the cyclin-dependent protein kinase 5 (CDK5) activators p35 and p39, and the association is increased by the activation of the glutamate receptor (Dhavan et al., 2002). CaMKII also binds to α actinin *via* p35/p39. Cross-talk between the cdk5 and CaMKII signal transduction pathways may contribute to synaptic plasticity. CaMKII also interacts with densin-180, forming ternary complex with α actinin at the PSD (Walikonis et al., 2001).

After its dephosphorylation by the actions of protein phosphatase 1(PP1), CaMKII is released from the PSD (Yoshimura et al., 1999). The level of CaMKII in the PSD can affect LTP and hippocampal-dependent learning. Thus, α CaMKII is a key player in the regulation of plasticity.

5-2-3. Phosphorylation and regulation of PSD proteins by CaMKII

CaMKII substrates and interacting proteins

CaMKII of the PSD-CaMKII complex is active and has Ca^{2+}-independent activity. It can phosphorylate a large number of PSD proteins in both the presence and absence of Ca^{2+}. Most substrates have been identified by proteomic analysis (Yoshimura et al., 2000; Yoshimura et al., 2002; Fink & Meyer, 2002; Yamauchi, 2002). Table 3 summarizes CaMKII substrates and interacting proteins in the PSD fraction. The substrates include receptor and ion channel proteins, scaffold and adaptor proteins, motor proteins, cytoskeletal proteins, enzymes, and membrane proteins. Potential substrates are various glutamate receptors, synaptic GTPase activating protein (SynGAP), and PSD-95/Disc-large/ZO-1 (PDZ) proteins including PSD-95 and SAP-97.The interacting proteins include sytoskeletal proteins, motor proteins, and regulatory protein of protein kinases.

Regulation of receptors and ion channels in the PSD

The PSD contains various types of glutamate receptors, including NMDA receptors, α-amino-3-hydroxy-5-methylisoxazole-4-propionic acid (AMPA) receptors, and metabotropic glutamate receptors (mGluR). These receptors are a substrate of CaMKII (Yoshimura et al.,

2002).Glutamate receptors are also phosphorylated by various kinds of protein kinases, including PKC, cAMP-dependent protein kinase (PKA), and fyn tyrosin kinase, and regulated by phosphorylation (Yamauchi, 2002). The AMPA receptor GluR1 subunit contains a single phosphorylation site, Ser831, that when phosphorylated by CaMKII, enhances channel function (Barria et al., 1997a). Biochemical studies have shown that receptor phosphorylation occurs during LTP, as its induction promotes the incorporation of 32P into the GluR1 subunit by CaMKII (Barria et al., 1997b). The phosphorylation of Ser831 alters the induction of LTP which would be expected to increase the AMPA channel's conductance, and this has been directly observed (Benke et al., 1998). In rat hippocampal neurons, LTP or increased activity of CaMKII induces delivery of tagged AMPA receptors into synapses (Hayashi et al., 2000). This effect is blocked by mutating a PDZ domain interaction site, indicating that trafficking of AMPA receptors to synapses by CaMKII requires the association between the AMPA receptor and a PDZ domain protein.

The NMDA receptor NR2B subunit is phosphorylated at Ser1303 by CaMKII (Omkumar et al., 1996). α CaMKII enhances the extent and/or rate of desensitization of NMDA-induced macroscopic currents in HEK293 cells co-expressing NR2B with the NR1 subunit, without significantly changing other current parameters.This suggests a mechanism for the Ca^{2+}-dependent negative-feedback regulation of NMDA receptors (Sessoms-Sikes et al., 2005). CaMKII also binds to the NMDA receptor NR2A subunit C-terminal domain with high affinity. PKC-dependent phosphorylation at Ser-1416 of the NR2A C-terminal tail decreases its affinity for α CaMKII, and promotes the dissociation of the α CaMKII-NR2A complex, indicating that binding of CaMKII to the PSD is affected by PKC (Gardoni et al., 2001a & 2001b).

Members of the *Shaker* Kv channel family are localized to pre- and postsynaptic components, and possible targets for phosphorylation by CaMKII. Kv1.4, a rapidly inactivating Kv channel, is demonstrated to be phosphorylated and inactivated by CaMKII (Roeper et al., 1997). CaMKII phosphorylates an amino-terminal residue, Ser123. This phosphate is dephosphorylated by calcineurin (phosphatase 2B).The Ca^{2+}-sensitive phosphorylation/dephosphorylation of Kv1.4 has profound functional consequences for the inactivation.

Regulation of PSD proteins phosphorylated by CaMKII

Many scaffold proteins, including PSD-95, are good substrates for CaMKII. CaMKII-dependent phosphorylation of PSD-95 causes dissociation of NR2A from PSD-95, suggesting that PSD-95 regulates the signaling transduction pathway downstream of the NMDA receptor (Gardoni et al. 2006). Synaptic trafficking of synapse-associated protein 97 (SAP-97) is modulated by CaMKII in cultured hippocampal neurons. Activation of CaMKII promotes the recruitment of SAP-97 into dendritic spines (Mauceri et al., 2004). SAP-97 is involved in the correct delivery and clustering of glutamate ionotropic receptors and K^+ channel proteins to the PSD. CaMKII-dependent phosphorylation of SAP-97-Ser-39 caused a redistribution of the AMPA receptor GluR1 subunit (Mauceri et al., 2004). SAP-97 also interacts Kv4.2, and phosphorylation of SAP-97 by CaMKII regulates the subcellular localization of Kv4.2 (Gardoni et al. 2007). Kv4.2 is the pore-forming α subunit of the A-type K^+ channel and critically involved in the regulation of dendritic excitability and plasticity. Kv4.2 is enriched in the PSD fraction and specifically interacts with SAP-97 *via* the PDZ domain of SAP-97.

Thus, CaMKII-dependent phosphorylation of SAP-97 regulates the association of SAP-97 with the PSD, providing a fine molecular mechanism responsible for the synaptic delivery of SAP-97-interacting proteins, such as GluR1 and Kv4.2.

SynGAP is a ras GTPase-activating protein detected only in the brain (Chen et al., 1998). It plays a crucial role in the early development of the brain and in the control of synaptic plasticity in the adult brain (Komiyama et al., 2002). SynGAP has many sites of phosphorylation by CaMKII, and is a good substrate of that kinase. Phosphorylation of synGAP by CaMKII increases its Ras GTPase-activating activity by 70–95% (Oh et al., 2004).

Neuronal nitric oxide synthase (nNOS) is phosphorylated by various protein kinases, such as CaM kinases, PKA, and PKC (Bredt et al., 1992). nNOS activity is stimulated by increases in Ca^{2+} due to NMDA-receptor activation. CaMKII directly phosphorylates nNOS at Ser-847, and the enzyme activity decreases 50-60% with suppression of CaM binding (Hayashi et al., 1999).

Arc protein and mRNA expression is strongly induced by synaptic activation which evokes LTP (Lyford et al., 1995). Arc may play a role in stabilizing activity-dependent changes in synaptic efficacy. Arc protein is concentrated in the PSD, and is increased after electroconvulsive treatment (Donai et al. 2003). In neuroblastoma cells expressing Arc and CaMKII, Arc potentiates the action of CaMKII for neurite extension, suggesting that Arc and CaMKII in the PSD play an important role in activity-induced synaptic modification (Donai et al. 2003).

Protein synthesis-dependent late-phase LTP (L-LTP) in the hippocampus requires the influx of Ca^{2+} through NMDA receptor to activate CaMKII. CaMKII stimulates protein synthesis in depolarized hippocampal neurons through phosphorylation of the mRNA translation factor cytoplasmic polyadenylation element-binding protein (CPEB), and this phosphorylation is rapidly reversed by PP1 (Atkins et al., 2005).

The regulation of many other PSD proteins by CaMKII is not well characterized, and further studies would be required to understand the synaptic plasticity.

(6) Neuronal Disorders Related to a Dysfunction of CaMKII

6-1. Alzheimer's disease

Alzheimer's disease (AD), a progressive neurodegerative disorder, is characterized by the formation of neurofibrillary tangles (NFTs) and amyloid plaques. The tangles are composed of straight and paired helical filaments (PHFs), with a major component being an aberrantly hyperphosphorylated form of the microtuble-associated protein tau, normally expressed in axons. Abnormal phosphorylation of tau is related to the formation of PHFs in the AD brain. A number of protein kinases can phosphorylate tau (Lovestone & Reynolds, 1997). About one-fourth of the phosphorylation sites as found in AD tau are phosphorylated by CaMKII, suggesting that the kinase is involved in the abnormal phosphorylation of tau in AD brain (Singh, et al. 1996; Yoshimura et al. 2003). Increased phosphorylation of tau alone does not induce cell death in neuroblastoma cells overexpressing tau. Some additional stimuli may be required to induce the cell death associated with abnormal phosphorylation of tau in AD (Yoshizaki, et al. 2004). The involvement of phosphorylation of tau in apoptosis resembling AD was demonstrated using a model comprising P19 cells stably expressing human tau441 (tau/P19 cells) (Tsukane & Yamauchi, 2006). CaMKII is involved in the apoptosis of P19 cells expressing tau during neural differentiation induced by retinoic acid treatment.If CaMKII had been abnormally activated, due to a breakdown of the normal regulatory mechanisms, it would be responsible for the phosphorylation of tau in the AD brain.

6-2. Angelman's mental retardation syndrome

Angelman's mental retardation syndrome is a disorder of human cognition characterized by severe mental retardation and epilepsy. The *Ube3a* gene is identified as the genetic locus for Angelman's syndrome (Albrecht, et al. 1997). The *Ube3a* gene encodes for an E6-AP ubiquitin ligase, an enzyme involved in protein degradation through the ubiquitin-associated proteosome-mediated pathway. The behavioral phenotype of mice with a maternal deficiency in *Ube3a* resembles Angelman's syndrome, manifesting motor dysfunction, inducible seizures, and context-dependent association learning deficits (Weeber, et al. 2003). LTP is also severely impaired in the mice. Animal models of Angelman's syndrome exhibit a significant increase in phosphorylation at Thr268 and Thr305, with no corresponding change in the total level of CaMKII. Phosphorylation at Thr305 reduces CaMKII activity and its affinity for the PSD. These observations confirm that the phosphorylation at Thr305 is involved in the inhibition of synaptic responses. Thus, misregulation of □ CaMKII function may cause the neurological symptoms in Angelman's syndrome. The misregulation is probably caused by the decreased protein phosphatase PP1/PP2 activity (Weeber, et al. 2003).

6-3. Parkinson's disease, schizophrenia and pain

Parkinson's disease (PD) involves the degeneration of dopamine-containing nigrostriatal neurons leading to the motor symptoms observed in this disorder. It is demonstrated that NMDA receptor NR1 subunit and PSD-95 protein levels are selectively reduced in the PSD of dopamine -denervated striata in experimental Parkinsonism. These effects are accompanied by an increase in striatal levels of α CaMKII autophosphorylation. Abnormal α CaMKII autophosphorylation plays a causal role in the alterations of striatal plasticity and motor behavior that follow dopamine denervation. Normalization of CaMKII activity may be an important underlying mechanism of the therapeutic action of L-DOPA in PD (Picconi et al., 2004).

In searching for genes dysregulated in neuronal disease, it has been reported that the mRNA level of CaMKII is significantly elevated in postmortem frontal cerebral cortex tissues from patients who had died with schizophrenia, bipolar disorder, or severe, suggesting that altered expression of CaMKII in the cerebral cortex contributes to these diseases (Novak et al. 2006).

Relationship between CaMKII and pain has also been investigated. In morphine-treated mice, the levels of α CaMKII mRNA and protein were robustly increased and the abundance of phosphorylated α CaMKII was increased in spinal cord tissue, suggesting that α CaMKII is involved in opioid tolerance or pain (Liang et al., 2004).

CONCLUDING REMARKS: MEMORY MOLECULES AND MEMORY APPARATUS

Recent developments in molecular biology, gene techniques, and cell biology have helped shed light on synaptic plasticity and learning and memory at the molecular level. An initial step may be studies of CaMKII in the nerve cells. Biochemical studies have demonstrated that CaMKII has unique properties, including extremely broad substrate specificity, self regulation, and translocation. Furthermore, genetic approaches using mice have provided a great deal of information about the important roles that CaMKII plays in various types of plasticity and learning and memory. The involvement of CaMKII in the regulation of signaling in both pre- and post-synapses is shown in Fig. 2.

The exocytotic machinery is present in the presynaptic terminal. The PSD in the postsynapse exhibit dramatic changes in structure and composition and the efficiency of signal transduction during development and in response to synaptic activity. Various targets of CaMKII have been identified (Table 2 and 3), and the association of some well characterized molecules regulated by CaMKII in the synapse is shown in Fig. 2B.

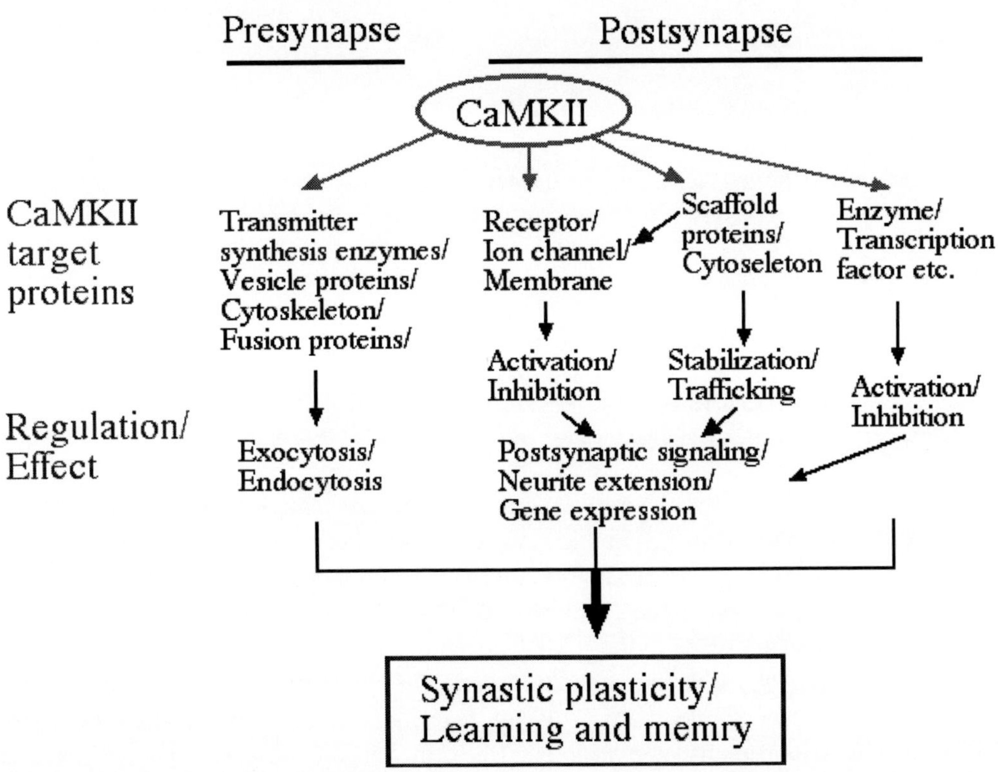

Figure 2. (Continued on the next page).

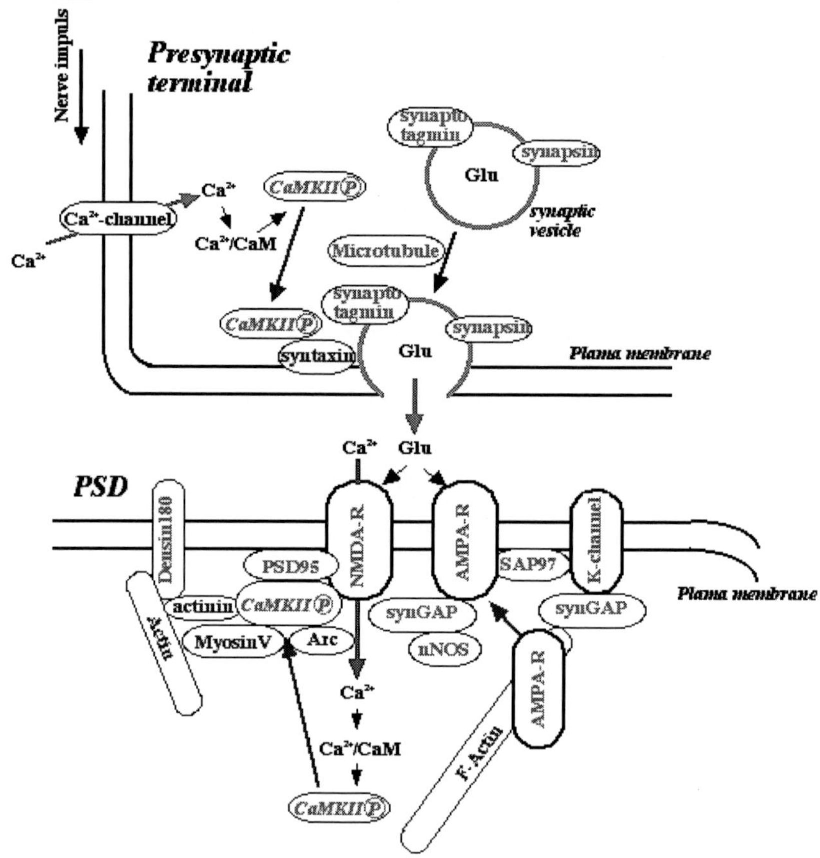

Figure 2. Schematic representation of regulation of CaMKII. *A*, Signal transduction of CaMKII.CaMKII has diverse functions in the nervous system based on the various categories of substrates and interacting proteins.Target molecules change *via* phosphorylation and/or association with CaMKII.Then, physiological reactions progress. *B*, Association of CaMKII and its target molecules well characterized in the presynaptic terminal and PSD of glutamatergic neurons. Although there are a great number of CaMKII targets, only well characterized molecules are shown. Note; In the nerve terminals of dopaminergic, noradrenergic, and serotonergic neurons, the rate-limiting enzymes of transmitter biosynthesis (TH and TPH) are phosphorylated by CaMKII, and neurotransmitter synthesis is increased (not shown).Red letter, CaMKII substrate; blue letter, CaMKII-interacting protein; blue arrow, phosphorylation-dependent translocation of CaMKII and AMPA receptor.

When a nerve impulse reaches the nerve terminals, local concentration of Ca^{2+} increases, and then CaKII phosphorylates synaptic vesicle proteins and microtubule proteins. Simultaneously, CaMKII is autophosphorylated at Thr286 and interacts with syntaxin in the plasma membrane, and then the neurotransmitter glutamate is released into the synaptic cleft by exocytosis. Glutamate binds to the AMPA receptor, and then the NMDA receptor is fully activated. Ca^{2+} enters postsynaptic cells through the NMDA receptor, binds calmodulin, and activates CaMKII. The activated CaMKII is autophosphorylated at Thr286 and translocated to the PSD, where it phosphorylates various PSD proteins. At the same time, the activated CaMKII also phosphorylates various proteins in postsynaptic cells. Arc potentiates CaMKII function. CaMKII also regulates gene expression and translation through the phosphorylation of transcription factors and translation factor, respectively. Phosphorylated proteins change their activity and regulate signaling pathways, and then new synapses are formed, resulting in a change of synaptic activity (Fig. 2).

The functional significance of the regulated change of many other substrates of CaMII needs to be investigated at the molecular level in the neural system. Furthermore, some neuronal diseases may be related to the disruption of synaptic activity *via* the impaired functioning of CaMKII. Many of CaMKII's targets are also phosphorylated by various protein kinases, including PKA, PKC, MAP kinase, and Src family tyrosine kinases, indicating that cross-talk of CaMKII signaling with other signaling systems is important to the synaptic plasticity. Taken together, CaMKII is one of the best candidates for a molecular component of the memory apparatus, and the PSD is a good candidate for the body of their apparatus.

REFERENCES

Albrecht, U., Sutcliffe, J. S., Cattanach, B. M., Beechey, C. V., Armstrong, D., Eichele, G., and Beaudet A. L. (1997). Imprinted expression of the murine Angelman syndrome gene, Ube3a, in hippocampal and Purkinje neurons. *Nature Genet*, 17, 75-78.

Atkins, C. M., Davare, M. A., Oh, M. C., Derkach, V., and Soderling, T. R. (2005). Bidirectional regulation of cytoplasmic polyadenylation element-binding protein phosphorylation by Ca^{2+}/calmodulin-dependent protein kinase II and protein phosphatase 1 during hippocampal long-term potentiation. *J. Neurosci*, 25, 5604-5610.

Barria, A., Derkach, V., and Soderling, T. (1997a). Identification of the Ca^{2+}/calmodulin-dependent protein kinase II regulatory phosphorylation site in the alpha-amino-3-hydroxyl-5-methyl-4-isoxazole-propionate-type glutamate receptor. *J. Boil. Chem*, 272, 32727-32730.

Barria, A., Muller, D., Derkach, V., Griffith, L. C., and Soderling, T. R. (1997b). Regulatory phosphorylation of AMPA-type glutamate receptors by CaM-KII during long-term potentiation. *Science,* 276, 2042-2045.

Bayer, K. U., Konlnck, P. D., Leonard, A. S., Hell, J. W., and Schulman, H. (2001). Interaction with the NMDA receptor locks CaMKII in an active conformation. *Nature,* 411, 801-805.

Bejar, R., Yasuda, R., Krugers, H., Hood, K., and Mayford, M. (2002). Transgenic calmodulin-dependent protein kinase II activation: dose-dependent effects on synaptic plasticity, learning, and memory. *J. Neurosci,*22, 5719-5726.

Benfenati, F., Valtorta, F., Rubenstein, J. L., Gorelick, F. S., Greengard, P., and Czernik, A. J. (1992). Synaptic vesicle-associated Ca^{2+}/calmodulin-dependent protein kinase II is a binding protein for synapsin I. *Nature,* 359, 417-420.

Benke, T. A., Luthi, A., Isaac, J. T. R., and Collingridge, G. L. (1998). Modulation of AMPA receptor unitary conductance by synaptic activity. *Nature,* 393, 793-797.

Bredt, D. S., Ferris, C. D., and Snyder, S. H. (1992). Nitric oxide synthase regulatory sites. Phosphorylation by cyclic AMP-dependent protein kinase, protein kinase C, and calcium/calmodulin-dependent protein kinase; Identification of flavin and calmodulin binding sites. *J. Biol. Chem*, 267, 10976-10981.

Burgin, K. E., Waxham, M. N., Rickling, S., Westgate, S. A., Mobley, W. C., and Kelly, P. T. (1990). In situ hybridization histochemistry of Ca^{2+}/calmodulin-dependent protein kinase in developing rat brain. *J. Neurosci*, 10, 1788-1798.

Butler, L. S., Silva, A. J., Abeliovich, A., Watanabe, Y., Tonegawa, S., and McNamara, J. O. (1995). Limbic epilepsy in transgenic mice carrying a Ca^{2+}/calmodulindependent kinase II alpha-subunit mutation. *Proc. Natl. Acad. Sci, U.S.A.* 92, 6852-6855.

Cacucci, F., Wills, T. J., Lever, C., Giese, K. P., and O'Keefe, J. (2007). Experience-dependent increase in CA1 place cell spatial information, but not spatial reproducibility, is dependent on the autophosphorylation of the alpha-isoform of the calcium/calmodulin-dependent protein kinase II. *J Neurosci,* 27, 7854-7859.

Chen, H.-J., Rojas-Soto, M., Oguni, A., and Kennedy, M. B. (1998). A synaptic Ras-GTPase activating protein (p135 SynGAP) inhibited by CaM kinase II. *Neuron,* 20, 895-904.

Chen, X., Vinade, L., Leapman, R.D., Petersen, J.D., Nakagawa, T., Phillips, T.M., Sheng, M., and Reese, T.S. (2005). Mass of the postsynaptic density and enumeration of three key molecules. *Proc. Natl. Acad. Sci, U.S.A.* 102, 11551–11556.

Cho, M. H., Cao, X., Wang, D., and Tsien, J. Z. (2007). Dentate gyrus-specific manipulation of beta-Ca^{2+}/calmodulin-dependent kinase II disrupts memory consolidation. *Proc. Natl. Acad. Sci. USA.* 104, 16317-16322.

Colbran, R. J., and Brown, A. M. (2004). Calcium/calmodulin-dependent protein kinase II and synaptic plasticity. *Curr. Opin. Neurobiol*, 14, 318-327.

Colbran, R. J., and Soderling, T. R. (1990). Calcium/calmodulin-independent autophosphorylation sites of calcium/calmodulin-dependent protein kinase II. Studies on the effect of phosphorylation of threonine 305/306 and serine 314 on calmodulin binding using synthetic peptides. *J. Biol. Chem*, 265, 11213-11219.

Costa, M.C., Mani, F., Santoro Jr.,W., Espreafico, E.M., and Larson, R.E., (1999). Brain myosin-V, a calmodulin-carrying myosin, binds to calmodulindependent protein kinase II and activates its kinase activity. *J. Biol. Chem*, 274, 15811–15819..

Dhavan, R., Greer, P. L., Morabito, M. A., Orlando, L. R., and Tsai, L. H. (2002). The cyclin-dependent kinase 5 activators p35 and p39 interact with the alpha-subunit of Ca^{2+}/calmodulin-dependent protein kinase II and alpha-actinin-1 in a calcium-dependent manner. *J. Neurosci*. 22, 7879-7891.

Donai, H., Morinaga, H., and Yamauchi, T. (2001). Genomic organization and neuronal cell type specific promoter activity of β isoform of Ca^{2+}/calmodulin-dependent protein kinase II of rat brain. *Mol. Brain Res*, 94, 35-47.

Donai, H., Sugiura, H., Ara, D., Yoshimura, Y., Yamagata, K., and Yamauchi, T. (2003). Interaction of Arc with CaM kinase II and stimulation of neurite extension by Arc in neuroblastoma cells expressing CaM kinase II. *Neurosci. Res*, 47, 399-408.

Dosemeci, A., Tao-Cheng, J. H., Vinade, L., Winters, C. A., Pozzo-Miller, L. and Reese, T. S. (2001). Glutamate-induced transient modification of the postsynaptic density. *Proc. Natl. Acad. Sci, USA,* 98, 10428-10432.

Drubin, D. G., and Nelson, W. J. (1996). Origins of cell polarity. *Cell*, 84, 335-344.

Elgersma, Y., Fedorov, N. B., Ikonen, S., Choi, E. S., Elgersma, M., Carvalho, O. M., Giese, K. P., and Silva, A. J. (2002). Inhibitory autophosphorylation of CaMKII controls PSD association, plasticity, and learning. *Neuron*, 36,493-505.

Elgersma, Y., Sweatt, J. D., and Giese, K. P. (2004). Mouse genetic approaches to investigating calcium/calmodulin-dependent protein kinase II function in plasticity and cognition. *J. Neurosci*, 24, 8410-8415.

Erondu, N. E., and Kennedy, M. B. (1985). Regional distribution of type II Ca^{2+}/calmodulin-dependent protein kinase in rat brain. *J. Neurosci*, 5, 3270-3277.

Fink, C. C., and Meyer, T. (2002). Molecular mechanisms of CaMKII activation in neuronal plasticity. *Curr. Opinion Neurobiol,* 12, 293–299.

Fink, C. C., Bayer, K. U., Myers, J. W., Ferrell, J. E. Jr., Schulman, H., and Meyer, T. (2003). Selective regulation of neurite extension and synapse formation by the beta but not the alpha isoform of CaMKII. *Neuron,* 39, 283-97.

Fong, Y. L., Taylor, W. L., Means, A. R., and Soderling, T. R. (1989).Studies of the regulatory mechanism of Ca^{2+}/calmodulin-dependent protein kinase II. Mutation of threonine 286 to alanine and aspartate. *J. Biol. Chem*, 264, 16759-16763.

Gardoni, F., Bellone, C., Cattabeni, F., and Luca, M. D. (2001a). Protein kinase C activation modulates α-calmodulin kinase II binding to NR2A subunit of N-methyl-D-aspartate receptor complex. *J. Biol. Chem*, 276, 7609-7613.

Gardoni, F., Schrama, L. H., Kamal, A., Gispen, W. H., Cattabeni, F., and Luca, M. D. (2001b).Hippocampal synaptic plasticity involves competition between Ca^{2+}/calmodulin-dependent protein kinase II and postsynaptic density 95 for binding to the NR2A subunit of the NMDA receptor. *J. Neurosci*, 21, 1501-1509.

Gardoni, F., Polli, F., Cattabeni, F., and Di Luca, M. (2006). Calcium-calmodulin-dependent protein kinase II phosphorylation modulates PSD-95 binding to NMDA receptors. *Eur. J. Neurosci.* 24, 2694-2704.

Gardoni, F., Mauceri, D., Marcello, E., Sala, C., DiLuca, M., and Jeromin, A. (2007). SAP-97 directs the localization of Kv4.2 to spines in hippocampal neurons: regulation by CaMKII. *J Biol Chem,* 282, 28691-28699.

Gaudilliere, B., Konishi, Y., de la Iglesia, N., Yao, G., and Bonni, A. (2004). A CaMKII-NeuroD signaling pathway specifies dendritic morphogenesis. *Neuron,* 41, 229-241.

Giese, K. P., Fedorov, N. B., Filipkowski, R. K. and Silva, A. J. (1998) Autophosphorylation at Thr286 of the calcium-calmodulin kinase II in LTP and learning. *Science,* 279,870-873.

Glazewski, S., Chen, C. M., Silva, A., and Fox, K. (1996) Requirement for alpha-CaMKII in experience-dependent plasticity of the barrel cortex. *Science*, 272, 421-423.

Glazewski, S., Giese, K. P., Silva, A., and Fox, K. (2000) The role of alpha-CaMKII autophosphorylation in neocortical experience-dependent plasticity. *Nature Neurosci*, 3, 911-918.

Goldenring, J. R., McGuire, J. S. Jr., and DeLorenzo, R. J. (1984). Identification of the major postsynaptic density protein as homologous with the major calmodulin-binding subunit of a calmodulin-dependent protein kinase. *J. Neurochem*, 42, 1077-1084.

Goshima, Y., Ohsako, S., and Yamauchi T. (1993). Overexpression of Ca^{2+}/calmodulin-dependent protein kinase II in Neuro 2a and NG108-15 neuroblastoma cell lines promotes neurite outgrowth and growth cone motility. *J. Neurosci*, 13, 559-567.

Griffith, L. C., Lu, C. S., and Sun, X. X. (2003). CaMKII, an enzyme on the move: regulation of temporospatial localization. *Mol. Interv*, 3, 386-403.

Hansel, C., de Jeu, M., Belmeguenai, A., Houtman, S. H., Buitendijk, G. H., Andreev, D., De Zeeuw, C. I., and Elgersma, Y. (2006). alphaCaMKII Is essential for cerebellar LTD and motor learning. *Neuron*, 51, 680-682.

Hanson, P. I., Kapiloff, M. S., Lou, L. L., Rosenfeld, M. G., and Schulman, H. (1989). Expression of a multifunctional Ca^{2+}/calmodulin-dependent protein kinase and mutational analysis of its autoregulation. *Neuron,* 3, 59-70.

Hayashi, Y., Nishio, M., Naito, Y., Yokokura, H., Nimura, Y., Hidaka, H., and Watanabe, Y. (1999). Regulation of neuronal nitric-oxide synthase by calmodulin kinases. *J. Biol. Chem*, 274, 20597-20602.

Hayashi, Y., Shi, S. H., Esteban, J. A., Piccini, A., Poncer, J. C., and Malinow, R. (2000). Driving AMPA receptors into synapses by LTP and CaMKII: Requirement for GluR1 and PDZ domain interaction. *Science.* 287, 2262-2267.

Hinds, H. L., Tonegawa, S., and Malinow, R. (1998). CA1 long-term potentiation is diminished but present in hippocampal slices from alpha-CaMKII mutant mice. *Learn Mem*, 5, 344-354

Hivak, B., Rokke, H., Bardsen, K., Davanger, S. and Bramham, C. R. (2003). Bursts of high-frequency stimulation trigger rapid delivery of pre-existing alpha-CaMKII mRNA to synapses: a mechanism in dendritic protein synthesis during long-term potentiation in adult awake rats. *Eur. J. Neurosci,*17, 2679-2689.

Hudmon, A., and Schulamn, H. (2002). Neuronal Ca^{2+}/calmodulin-dependent protein kinase II: the role of structure and autoregulation in cellular function. *Ann. Rev. Biochem*, 71, 473-510.

Ichikawa, T., Sekihara, S., Ohsako, S., Hirata, Y., and Yamauchi, T. (1992). Ca^{2+}/calmodulin-dependent protein kinase II in rat cerebellum; An immunohistochemical study with monoclonal antibodies specific to either α or β subunit. *J. Chem. Neuroanat.* 5, 383-390.

Itagaki, C., Isobe, T., Taoka, M., Natsume, T., Nomura, N., Horigome, T., Omata, S., Ichinose, H., Nagatsu, T., Greene, L. A., and Ichimura, T. (1999). Stimulus-coupled interaction of tyrosine hydroxylase with 14-3-3 proteins. *Biochemistry,* 38, 15673-15680.

Jiang, G. C., Yohrling, G. J., Schmitt, J. D., and Vrana, K. E. (2000). Identification of substrate orienting and phosphorylation sites within tryptophan hydroxylase using homology-based molecular modeling. *J. Mol. Biol*, 302, 1005-1017.

Kanaseki, T., Ikeuchi, Y., Sugiura, H., and Yamauchi, T. (1991).Structural feature of Ca^{2+}/calmodulin-dependent protein kinase II revealed by electron microscopy. *J. Cell Biol*, 115, 1049-1060.

Kelly, P. T., McGuinness, T. L., and Greengard, P. (1984). Evidence that the major postsynaptic density protein is a component of α Ca^{2+}/calmodulin-dependent protein kinase. *Proc. Natl. Acad. Sci, USA*, 81, 945-949.

Kennedy, M. B. (1997).The postsynaptic density at glutamatergic synapses. *Trends Neurosci*, 20, 264-268.

Kennedy, M. B. (2000). Signal-processing machines at the postsynaptic density. *Science,* 290, 750-754.

Kennedy, M. B., Bennett, M. K., and Erondu, N. E. (1983). Biochemical and immunochemical evidence that the "major postsynaptic density protein" is a subunit of a calmodulin-dependent protein kinase. *Proc. Natl. Acad. Sci, USA*, 80, 7357-7361.

Kennedy, M. B., and Greengard, P. (1981).Two calcium/calmodulin-dependent protein kinases, which are highly concentrated in brain, phosphorylate protein I at distinct sites. *Proc. Natl. Acad. Sci, USA*, 78, 1293-1297.

Kolarow, R., Brigadski, T., and Lessmann, V. (2007). Postsynaptic secretion of BDNF and NT-3 from hippocampal neurons depends on calcium calmodulin kinase II signaling and proceeds via delayed fusion pore opening. *J. Neurosci,* 27, 10350-10364.

Kolodziej, S. J., Hudmon, A., Waxham, M. N., and Stoops, J. K. (2000). Three-dimensional reconstructions of calcium/calmodulin-dependent (CaM) kinase IIalpha and truncated CaM kinase IIalpha reveal a unique organization for its structural core and functional domains. *J. Biol. Chem*, 275, 14354-14359.

Komiyama, N. H., Watabe, A. M., Carlisle, H. J., Porter, K., Charlesworth, P., Monti, J., Strathdee, D. J., O'Carroll, C. M., Martin, S. J., Morris, R. G., O'Dell, T. J., and Grant, S. G. (2002). SynGAP regulates ERK/MAPK signaling, synaptic plasticity, and learning in the complex with postsynaptic density 95 and NMDA receptor. *J. Neurosci,* 22, 9721–9732.

Liang, D., Li, X., and Clark, J. D. (2004) Increased expression of Ca^{2+}/calmodulin-dependent protein kinase II alpha during chronic morphine exposure. *Neuroscience,* 123, 769-775.

Lin, C. R., Kapiloff, M. S., Durgerian, S., Tatemoto,K., Russo, A. F., Hanson, P. I., Schulman, H., and Rosenfeld, M. G. (1987). Molecular cloning of a brain-specific calcium/calmodulin-dependent protein kinase. *Proc. Natl. Acad. Sci, USA*, 84, 5962-5966.

Lisman, J. (1994). The CaM kinase II hypothesis for the storage of synaptic memory. *Trends Neurosci*, 17, 406-412.

Lisman, J., Schulman, H., and Cline, H. (2002). The molecular basis of CaMKII function in synaptic and behavioural memory. *Nature Rev. Neurosci*, 3, 175-190.

Lovestone, S., and Reynolds, C. H. (1997). The phosphorylation of tau: a critical stage in neurodevelopment and neurodegenerative processes. *Neuroscience.* 78, 309-324.

Lyford, G. L., Yamagata, K., Kaufmann, W. E., Barnes, C. A., Sanders, L. K., Copeland, N. G., Gilbert, D. J., Jenkins, N. A., Lanahan, A.A., and Worley, P. F. (1995). Arc, a growth factor and activity-regulated gene, encodes a novel cytoskeleton-associated protein that is enriched in neuronal dendrites. *Neuron,* 14, 433-445.

Mauceri, D., Cattabeni, F., Di Luca, M., and Gardoni, F. (2004). Calcium/calmodulin-dependent protein kinase II phosphorylation drives synapse-associated protein 97 into spines. *J. Bio. Chem*, 279, 23813-23821.

Mayford, M., Bach, M. E., Huang, Y. Y., Wang, L., Hawkins, R. D., and Kandel, E. R. (1996). Control of memory formation through regulated expression of α CaMKII transgene. *Science,* 274,1678-1683.

Mayford, M., Wang, J., Kandel. E. R., and O'Dell, T. J. (1996). CaMKII regulates the frequency-response function of hippocampal synapses for the production of both LTD and LTP. *Cell*, 81, 891-904.

McGuinness, T. L., Lai, Y., and Greengard, P. (1985). Ca^{2+}/calmodulin-dependent protein kinase II. Isozymic forms from rat forebrain and cerebellum. *J. Biol. Chem*, 260, 1696-1704.

Meyer, T., Hanson, P. I., Stryer, L., and Schulman, H. (1992). Calmodulin trapping by calcium-calmodulin-dependent protein kinase. *Science,* 256, 1199-1202.

Miller, S., G., and Kennedy, M. B. (1985). Distinct forebrain and cerebellar isozymes of type II Ca^{2+}/calmodulin-dependent protein kinase associate differently with the postsynaptic density fraction. *J. Biol. Chem*, 260, 9039-9046.

Miller, S., Yasuda, M., Coats, J. K., Jones, Y., Martone, M. E., and Mayford, M. (2002). Disruption of dendritic translation of CaMKIIalpha impairs stabilization of synaptic plasticity and memory consolidation. *Neuron*, 36, 507-519.

Mima, K., Deguchi, S., and Yamauchi, T. (2001). Characterization of 5' flanking region of α isoform of rat Ca^{2+}/calmodulin-dependent protein kinase II gene and neuronal cell type specific promoter activity. *Neuosci. Lett*, 307, 117-121.

Nomura, T., Kumatoriya, K., Yoshimura, Y., and Yamauchi, T. (1997). Overexpression of α and β isoforms of Ca^{2+}/calmodulin-dependent protein kinase II in neuroblastoma cells ----- H-7 promotes neurite outgrowth. *Brain Res*, 766, 129-144.

Novak, G., Seeman, P., and Tallerico, T. (2006). Increased expression of calcium/calmodulin-dependent protein kinase IIbeta in frontal cortex in schizophrenia and depression. *Synapse,* 59, 61-68.

Ochiai, N., Masumoto, S., Sakagami, H., Yoshimura, Y., and Yamauchi, T. (2007). Rat leucine-rich protein binds and activates the promoter of the β isoform of Ca^{2+}/calmodulin-dependent protein kinase II gene. *Neurosci. Res*, 58, 67-76.

Ochiishi, T., Terashima, T., Sugiura, H., and Yamauchi, T. (1994a). Immunohistochmical localization of Ca^{2+}/calmodulin-dependent protein kinase II in the rat retina. *Brain Res*, 634, 257-265.

Ochiishi, T., Terashima, T., and Yamauchi, T. (1994b).Specific distribution of Ca^{2+}/calmodulin-dependent protein kinase II α and β isoforms in some structures of the rat forebrain. *Brain Res*, 659, 179-193.

Ochiishi, T., Terashima, T., and Yamauchi, T. (1998). Regional differences between the immunohistochemical distribution of Ca^{2+}/calmodulin-dependent protein kinase II α and β isoforms in the brainstem of the rat. *Brain Res*, 790, 129-140.

Oh, J. S., Manzerra, P., and Kennedy, M. B. (2004). Regulation of the neuron-specific Ras GTPase-activating protein, synGAP, by Ca^{2+}/calmodulin-dependent protein kinase II. *J. Biol. Chem,* 279, 17980-17988.

Ohyama, A., Hosaka, K., Komiya, Y., Akagawa, K., Yamauchi, E., Taniguchi, H., Sasagawa, N., Kumakura, K., Mochida,S., Yamauchi, T., and Igarashi, M. (2002). Regulation of exocytosis through Ca^{2+}/ATP-dependent binding of autophosphorylated Ca^{2+}/calmodulin-activated protein kinase II to syntaxin 1A . *J. Neurosci*, 22, 3342-3351.

Okamoto, K., Narayanan, R., Lee, S. H., Murata, K., and Hayashi, Y. (2007). The role of CaMKII as an F-actin-bundling protein crucial for maintenance of dendritic spine structure. *Proc. Natl. Acad. Sci, USA,*104, 6418-6423.

Omkumar, R. V., Kiely, M. J., Rosenstein, A. J., Min, K. T., and Kennedy, M. B. (1996). Identification of a phosphorylation site for calcium/calmodulindependent protein kinase II in the NR2B subunit of the N-methyl-D-aspartate receptor. *J. Biol. Chem*, 271, 31670-31678.

Peng, J., Kim, M. J., Cheng, D., Duong, D. M., Gygi, S. P., and Sheng, M. (2004). Semiquantitative proteomic analysis of rat forebrain postsynaptic density fractions by mass spectrometry. *J. Boil. Chem*, 279, 21003-21011.

Picconi, B., Gardoni, F., Centonze, D., Mauceri, D., Cenci, M. A., Bernardi, G., Calabresi, P., and Di Luca M. (2004). Abnormal Ca^{2+}-calmodulin-dependent protein kinase II function mediates synaptic and motor deficits in experimental parkinsonism. *J. Neurosci,* 24, 5283-5291.

Poulsen, D. J., Standing, D., Bullshields, K., Spencer, K., Micevych, P. E., and Babcock, A. M. (2007). Overexpression of hippocampal Ca^{2+}/calmodulin-dependent protein kinase II improves spatial memory. *J. Neurosci. Res,* 85, 735-739.

Pratt, K. G., Watt, A. J., Griffith, L. C., Nelson, S. B., and Turrigiano, G. G. (2003). Activity-dependent remodeling of presynaptic inputs by postsynaptic expression of activated CaMKII. *Neuron,* 39, 269-281.

Roeper, J., Lorra, C., and Pongs, O. (1997). Frequency-dependent inactivation of mammalian A-type K+ channel Kv1.4 regulated by Ca^{2+}/calmodulin-dependent protein kinase. *J. Neurosci*, 17, 3379-3391.

Sakurada, T., Mima, K., Kurisaki, A., Sugino, H., and Yamauchi, T. (2005). Neuronal cell type-specific promoter of the α CaM kinase II gene is activated by Zic2, a Zic family zinc finger protein, *Neurosci. Res*, 53, 323-330.

Sanhueza, M., McIntyre, C. C., and Lisman, J. E. (2007). Reversal of synaptic memory by Ca^{2+}/calmodulin-dependent protein kinase II inhibitor. *J. Neurosci,* 27, 5190-5199.

Sessoms-Sikes, S., Honse, Y., Lovinger, D. M., and Colbran, R. J. (2005). CaMKIIalpha enhances the desensitization of NR2B-containing NMDA receptors by an autophosphorylation-dependent mechanism. *Mol. Cell. Neurosci,* 29, 139-147.

Shakiryanova, D., Klose, M. K., Zhou, Y., Gu, T., Deitcher, D. L., Atwood, H. L., Hewes, R. S., and Levitan, E. S. (2007). Presynaptic ryanodine receptor-activated calmodulin kinase II increases vesicle mobility and potentiates neuropeptide release. *J. Neurosci*, 27, 7799-7806.

Sheng, M., and Hoogenraad, C. C. (2007).The postsynaptic architecture of excitatory synapses: a more quantitative view. *Annu. Rev. Biochem.* 76, 823-47.

Shen, K., Teruel, M. N., Subramanian, K., and Meyer, T. (1998). CaMKIIbeta functions as an F-actin targeting module that localizes CaMKIIalpha/beta heterooligomers to dendritic spines. *Neuron*, 21, 593-606.

Silva A. J., Paylor, R., Wehner, J. M., and Tonegawa, S. (1992). Impaired spatial learning in alpha-calcium-calmodulin kinase II mutant mice. *Science,* 257, 206-211.

Singh, T. J., Wang, J.-Z., Novak, M., Kontzekova, E., Grundke-Iqubal, I., and Iqubal, K. (1996).Calcium/calmodulin-dependent protein kinase II phosphorylates tau at Ser-262 but only partially inhibits its binding to microtubules. *FEBS Lett*, 387, 145-148.

Sogawa, Y., Yoshimura, Y., Otaka, A., and Yamauchi, T. (2000). Ca^{2+}-independent activity of Ca^{2+}/calmodulin-dependent protein kinase II involved in stimulation of neurite outgrowth in neuroblastoma cells. *Brain Res*, 881, 165-175.

Steward, O. (1997). mRNA localization in neurons: a multipurpose mechanism? *Neuron*, 18, 9-12.

Steward, O., and Schuman, E. M. (2001). Protein synthesis at synaptic sites on dendrites. *Annu. Rev. Neurosci*, 24, 299-325.

Strack, S., Choi, S., Lovinger, D. M. and Colbran, R. J. (1997). Translocation of autophosphorylated calcium/calmodulin-dependent protein kinase II to the postsynaptic density. *J. Biol. Chem*, 272, 13467-13470.

Sugiura, H. and Yamauchi, T. (1992). Developmental changes in the levels of Ca^{2+}/calmodulin-dependent protein kinase II α and β proteins in soluble and particulate fractions of the rat brain. *Brain Res*, 593, 97-104.

Sugiura, H. and Yamauchi, T. (1994). Developmental changes of protein substrates of Ca^{2+}/calmodulin-dependent protein kinase II in the rat forebrain. *Brain Res*, 659, 42-54.

Taha, S., Hanover, J. L., Silva, A. J., and Stryker, M. P. (2002). Autophosphorylation of alphaCaMKII is required for ocular dominance plasticity. *Neuron,* 36, 483-91.

Terashima, T., Ochiishi, T., and Yamauchi, T. (1994). Immunohistochemical detection of calcium/calmodulin-dependent protein kinase II in the spinal cord of the rat and monkey with special reference to the corticospinal tract. *J. Comp. Neurol*, 340, 469-479.

Tombes, R. M., Faison, M. O., and Turbeville, J. M. (2003). Organization and evolution of multifunctional Ca^{2+}/CaM-dependent protein kinase genes. *Gene.* 322, 17-31.

Tsukane, M., and Yamauchi, T. (2006). Increase in apoptosis with neural differentiation and shortening of the lifespan of P19 cells overexpressing tau. *Neurochem. Inter*, 48, 243-254.

Urushihara, M., and Yamauchi, T. (2001). Role of β isoform-specific insertions of Ca^{2+}/calmodulin-dependent protein kinase II. *Eur. J. Biochem*, 268, 4802-4808.

Verona, M., Zanotti, S., Schäfer, T., Racagni, G., and Popoli, M. (2000). Changes of synaptotagmin interaction with t-SNARE proteins in vitro after calcium/calmodulin-dependent phosphorylation. *J Neurochem,*74, 209-221.

Walikonis, R.S., Oguni, A., Khorosheva, E.M., Jeng, C.J., Asuncion, F.J., and Kennedy, M.B. (2001). Densin-180 forms a ternary complex with the α-subunit of Ca^{2+}/calmodulin-dependent protein kinase II and α-actinin. *J. Neurosci,* 21, 423–433.

Wang, H., Shimizu, E., Tang, Y. P., Cho, M., Kyin, M., Zuo, W., Robinson, D. A., Alaimo, P. J., Zhang, C., Morimoto, H., Zhuo, M., Feng, R., Shokat, K.M., and Tsien, J. Z. (2003). Inducible protein knockout reveals temporal requirement of CaMKII reactivation for memory consolidation in the brain. *Proc. Natl. Acad. Sci. USA.*100,

4287-4292.

Weeber, E. J., Jiang, Y. H., Elgersma, Y., Varga, A. W., Carraquillo, Y., Brown, S. E., Christian, J. M., Mirnikjoo, B., Silva, A., Beaudet, A. L. and Sweatt, J. D. (2003) Derangements of hippocampal calcium/calmodulin-dependent protein kinase II in a mouse model for Angelman mental retardation syndrome. *J. Neurosci*, 23, 2634-2644.

Wu, X. and McMurray, C. T. (2001). Calmodulin kinase II attenuation of gene transcription by preventing cAMP response element-binding protein (CREB) dimerization and binding of the CREB-binding protein. *J. Biol. Chem*, 276, 1735-1741.

Yamauchi, T. (2002). Molecular constituents and phosphorylation-dependent regulation of the post-synaptic density. *Mass Spectrometry Rev*, 21, 266-286.

Yamauchi, T. (2005). Neuronal Ca^{2+}/calmodulin-dependnet protein kinase II --- Discovery, progress in a quarter of a century, and perspective: Implication for learning and memory. *Biol. Pharm. Bull*, 28, 1342-1354.

Yamauchi, T., and Fujisawa, H. (1980). Evidence for three distinct forms of calmodulin-dependent protein kinases from rat brain. *FEBS Lett*, 116, 141-144.

Yamauchi, T. and Fujisawa, H. (1981).Tyrosine 3-monooxygenase is phosphorylated by Ca^{2+}-,calmodulin-dependent protein kinase, followed by activation by activator protein. *Biochem. Biophys. Res. Commun,* 100, 807-813.

Yamauchi, T., Nakata, H., and Fujisawa, H. (1981). A new activator protein that activates tryptophan 5-monoooxygenase and tyrosine 3-monooxygenase in the presence of Ca^{2+}-,calmodulin-dependent protein kinase, Purification and characterization. *J. Biol. Chem*, 256, 5404-5409.

Yamauchi, T., and Fujisawa, H. (1983). Disassembly of microtubules by the action of calmodulin-dependent protein kinase (Kinase II) which occurs only in the brain tissues. *Biochem. Biophys. Res. Commun*, 110, 287-291.

Yamauchi, T., and Fujisawa, H. (1988). Regulation of the interaction of actin filaments with microtubule-associated protein 2 by calmodulin-dependent protein kinase II. *Biochim. Biophys. Acta* 968, 77-85.

Yamauchi, T., Sekihara, S., and Ohsako, S. (1990). Subcellular distribution of α and β subunit proteins of Ca^{2+}/calmodulin-dependent protein kinase II expressed in Chinese hamster ovary cells. *FEBS Lett*. 266, 55-58.

Yoshimura, Y., and Yamauchi, T. (1997). Phosphorylation-dependent reversible association of Ca^{2+}/calmodulin-dependent protein kinase II with the postsynaptic densities. *J. Biol. Chem*, 272, 26354-26359.

Yoshimura, Y., Sogawa, Y., and Yamauchi T. (1999). Protein phosphatase 1 is involved in the dissociation of Ca^{2+}/calmodulin-dependent protein kinase II from postsynaptic densities. *FEBS Lett*, 446, 239-242.

Yoshimura, Y., Aoi, C., and Yamauchi, T. (2000). Investigation of protein substrates of Ca^{2+}/calmodulin-dependent protein kinase II translocated to the postsynaptic density. *Mol. Brain Res*, 81, 118-128.

Yoshimura, Y., Shinkawa, T., Taoka, M., Kobayashi, K., Isobe, T., and Yamauchi, T. (2002). Identification of protein substrates of Ca^{2+}/calmodulin-dependent protein kinase II in the postsynaptic density by protein sequencing and mass spectrometry. *Biochem. Biophys. Res. Commun,* 290, 948-954.

Yoshimura, Y., Ichinose, T., and Yamauchi, T. (2003). Phosphorylation of tau protein to sites found in Alzheimer's disease brain is catalyzed by Ca^{2+}/calmodulin-dependent protein kinase II as demonstrated tandem Mass Spectrometry, *Neurosci. Lett*, 353, 185-188.

Yoshimura, Y., Yamauchi, Y., Shinkawa, T., Taoka, M., Donai, T., Takahashi, N., Isobe, T., and Yamauchi, T. (2004). Molecular constituents of the postsynaptic density fraction revealed by proteomic analysis using multidimensional liquid chromatography-tandem mass spectrometry. *J. Neurochem*, 88, 759-768.

Yoshizaki, C., Tsukane, M., and Yamauchi, T. (2004). Overexpression of tau leads to the stimulation of neurite outgrowth, the activation of caspase 3 activity, and accumulation and phosphorylation of tau in neuroblastoma cells on cAMP treatment, *Neurosci. Res*, 49, 363-371.

Zhang, L., Kirschstein, T., Sommersberg, B., Merkens, M., Manahan-Vaughan, D., Elgersma, Y., Beck, H. (2005). Hippocampal synaptic metaplasticity requires inhibitory autophosphorylation of Ca^{2+}/calmodulin-dependent kinase II. *J. Neurosci*, 25, 7697-707.

In: Synaptic Plasticity: New Research
Editors: Tim F. Kaiser and Felix J. Peters
ISBN: 978-1-60456-732-8

Chapter 3

SYNAPTIC PLASTICITY: EMERGING ROLE FOR THE ENDOCANNABINOID SYSTEM

***Balapal S. Basavarajappa*[1,2,3,*] *and Ottavio Arancio*[4]**

[1] Division of Analytical Psychopharmacology, New York State Psychiatric Institute
[2] Nathan Kline Institute for Psychiatric Research,
Orangeburg, Orangeburg, New York 10962, USA
[3] Department of Psychiatry
[4] Department of Pathology, Taub Institute for Research on Alzheimer's Disease and the Aging Brain, College of Physicians and Surgeons, Columbia University, New York, New York 10032, USA

1. SUMMARY

Changes in synaptic strength are thought to be crucial to experience-dependent modifications of neural function. The diversity of mechanisms underlying these changes is far greater than previously expected. In the last few years, a new class of use-dependent synaptic plasticity that requires endocannabinoid signaling system has been identified in several brain regions. The endocannabinoid signaling system is composed of the cannabinoid receptors; their endogenous ligands, the endocannabinoids; the enzymes that produce and inactivate the endocannabinoids; and the endocannabinoid transporters. Endogenous cannabinoids (endocannabinoids) (ECs) are lipid mediators that activate these same cannabinoid receptors. Elegant work from several laboratories over the past 6 years has established that ECs are produced on demand in activity-dependent manners and released from postsynaptic neurons. The released ECs travel backward across the synapse, activate presynaptic CB1 receptors, and modulate presynaptic functions. Retrograde EC signaling is crucial for certain forms of short-term and long-term synaptic plasticity at excitatory or inhibitory synapses in many brain

* Nathan Kline Institute for Psychiatric Research 140 Old Orangeburg Rd, Orangeburg, NY-10962, Tel: 845-398-3234 or 5454 Fax: 845-398-5451 E-mail: Basavaraj@nki.rfmh.org

regions, and thereby contributes to various aspects of brain function including learning and memory. Thus, the EC system is emerging as a major player in synaptic plasticity. In this review, the authors describe molecular mechanisms of the endocannabinoid-mediated synaptic modulation and its possible physiological significance.

Keywords: endocannabinoids, CNS, synaptic plasticity, CB1 receptors, retrograde signaling, short-term plasticity, long-term plasticity

2. Introduction

The earliest anthropological evidence of Cannabis use comes from the oldest known Neolithic culture in China where it was used in the production of hemp for ropes and textiles, and also for its psychotropic effects [106] and have been used across various cultures for centuries [16].

The major psychoactive constituent of Cannabis sativa (such as marijuana, hashish and bhang) is Δ^9-tetrahydrocannabinol (Δ^9-THC, dronabinol), which is mainly responsible for the pharmacological effects of the Cannabis plant [58, 97]. Currently Δ^9-THC and its analogs are used for the treatment of nausea and vomiting induced by radiotherapy or chemotherapy, and wasting syndrome in AIDS patients. Cannabinoids are also useful for the treatment of pain, aspasticity, glaucoma and other disorders [210]. However, the clinical usefulness of Δ^9-THC and its anlogs is greatly hampered by their profound effects on mental state. These include euphoric or rewarding properties [131], impairement of attention, working memory [85] and excutive function [69]. These behavioural effcts are consistent with the findings that Δ^9-THC and its analogs (cannabinoids) have widespread actions upon neuronal function in the central nervous system (CNS).

In recent years, cannabinoid research received a tremendos attention from various researchers due to the breakthrough and discovery of the receptors that bind Δ^9-THC (Cannabinoid receptors) and thier endogenous ligands, endocannabinoids (ECs) in animal tissues. This emerging body of research has revealed multiple ways in which the endocannabinoid system functions to regulate synaptic neurotransmission in various brain areas[118, 156, 212]. Growing research has provided vital functions for EC signaling in molecular pathways that underlie both short and long lasting alterations in synaptic strength [2]. Infact, the critical involvement of ECs in some mechanisms of synaptic plasticity may change the current thinking of cellular models of learning and memory. These models may be pivotal in understanding and providing potential treatment for the rewarding and amnestic actions of drugs of abuse including cannabinoids and alcohol.

2.1 Cannabinoid receptors

Cannabinoids have two specific G-protein-coupled heptahelical receptor subtypes, which have been cloned. These are named CB1 and CB2. Evidence for a third type of G-protein-coupled cannabinoid receptor ("CB3" or "Anandamide receptor") in brain and in endothelial tissues is mounting [28, 60, 104, 207]. However, the cloning, expression and characterization of CB3 is yet to come. cDNA sequences encoding CB1- or CB2-like receptors have been reported for the rat [139], human [72, 151], mouse [1, 41], cow (Wessner, GeneBank submission, 1997), cat [71] (GeneBank submission, 1997), puffer fish [214], leech [183], zebra finch [181], and newt [182]. Although significant progress has been achieved into many aspects of the biology of the endocannabinoid system, and our knowledge of cannabinoid genomics and proteomics is increasing, the regulation of cannabinoid receptor genes is poorly understood.

The CB1 receptor is mainly expressed in the brain and spinal cord and thus is often referred to as the "brain cannabinoid receptor". The CB2 receptor is sometimes referred to as the "peripheral cannabinoid receptor" because initial studies suggested that CB2 receptors were predominantly present in immune cells in the periphery [67, 151]. Recent studies suggested that CB2 cannabinoid receptors are functionally expressed in neurons in the brain [66, 78, 92, 161, 199]. CB1 receptors are among the most abundant G-protein-coupled receptors in the brain, their densities being similar to the levels of γ-aminobutyric acid (GABA)- and glutamate-gated ion channels [91]. CB1 receptors have been shown to be localized presynaptically on GABAergic interneurons and glutamatergic neurons [83, 84, 107, 108] and is believed to mediate most of the effects described in this chapter. This would be consistent with the proposed role of endocannabinoid compounds in modulating neurotransmission.

(a) The signal transduction mechanism of cannabinoid receptors

Activation of a cannabinoid receptor promotes its interaction with G proteins, resulting in guanosine diphosphate/guanosine triphosphate exchange and subsequent dissociation of the α and βγ subunits. These subunits regulate the activity of multiple effector proteins to bring about biological functions (Fig. 1). CB1 is coupled with G_i or G_o proteins. CB1 receptors differ from many other GPCR proteins in being constitutively active, as they are precoupled with G-proteins in the absence of exogenously added agonists [149]. Among its cellular actions are inhibitions of

adenylate cyclase activity [44, 99, 163], inhibition of N- type voltage-gated channels [39, 125, 155, 162], inhibition of N-type, P/Q-type calcium channels and D-type potassium channels [98, 99], activation of A-type and inwardly rectifying potassium channels [148] and inhibition of synaptic transmission [68, 98]. Based on these findings, it has been suggested that CB1 receptors play a role in regulation of neurotransmitter release [68, 98].

In addition, one of the most interesting research areas is the regulation of neuritogenesis, axonal growth and synaptogenesis by CB1 receptors. The molecular mechanism involved in this process is not yet clear. The CB1 receptor activates MAPK pathway [209]. In some cells, CB1 receptor-mediated activation of MAPK was mediated through the PI3 kinase pathway [27, 209]. AEA, CP,55, 940 and WIN 55,212-2 increased phosphorylation of FAK+ 6,7, a neural isoform of FAK, in hippocampal slices and in cultured neurons [54]. CB1 receptor activation stimulate phosphorylation of the Tyr-397 residue of FAK in the hippocampus, which is crucial for FAK activation [55] and increase phosphorylation of p130-Cas, a protein associated with FAK in the hippocampus. CB1 receptor-stimulated FAK-autophosphorylation was shown to be upstream of the Src family kinases [55]. These new downstream effectors of CB1 receptors are quite likely play a role in some forms of synaptic plasticity through gene regulation, but needs further investigation.

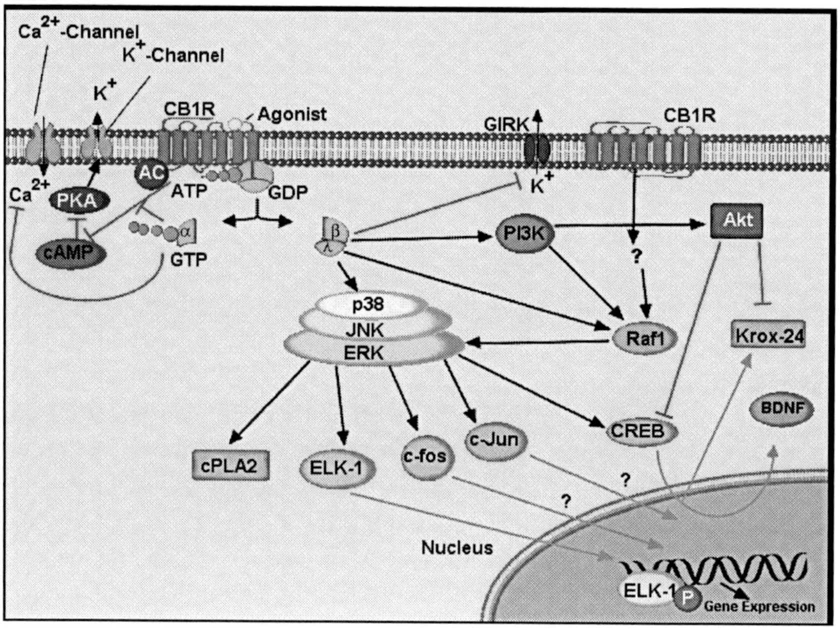

Figure 1. Schematic summary of CB1 receptor signaling. CB1 receptors are 7-transmembrane domain, G-protein-coupled proteins located in the cell membrane. The Ca2+ channels inhibited by CB1 receptors include N-, P/Q- and L-type channels. Actions on Ca2+ channels and adenylyl cyclase (AC) are thought to be mediated by the α subunits of the G-protein, and those on GIRK and PI3K by the βγ subunits. Inhibition of AC and the subsequent decrease in cAMP decreases activation of cAMP-dependent protein kinase A (PKA), which leads to decreased phosphorylation of the K+ channels. Stimulatory effects are shown by a (→) sign and inhibitory effects by a (⊥) sign

2.2 Endocannabinoids

The ECs are lipid signaling molecules that bind to and activate cannabinoid receptors. These lipid compounds are formed from phospholipids precursors [17, 19, 20, 33, 61, 142] within cells throughout the body, and are released from these cells on demand in a nonvasicular manner to act in a paracrine fashion [17, 19, 20, 61, 76, 142].

Beginning in 1992, the first endogenous cannabinoid was identified as anandamide (AEA, arachidonylethanolamide). It was named from the Sanskrit ananda, "internal bliss,'' making reference to its chemical structure (the amide of arachidonic acid and ethanolamine) [57]. Subsequently, another endogenous cannabinoid receptor ligand, 2-arachidonylglycerol (2-AG) was discovered and characterized [141, 187]. The third ether-type EC, 2-arachidonylglycerol ether (noladin ether), was isolated from the CNS and shown to display pharmacological properties similar to AEA [88]. The fourth type of EC, virodhamine, in contrast to the previously described endocannabinoids, is a partial agonist with in vivo antagonist activity at the CB1 receptor [168]. The fifth type of EC, N-arachidonyl-dopamine (NADA), not only binds to CB1 receptor but also stimulates vanilloid receptors (VR1) [101]. It should be noted that except AEA and 2-AG, to date, there is little evidence about the physiological actions of these compounds.

AEA is believed to be made from N-arachidonyl phosphatidylethanolamine (N-ArPE), which is believed to originate from the transfer of arachidonic acid (AA) from the sn-1 position of 1,2-sn-di-arachidonylphosphatidylcholine to phosphatidylethanolamine, catalyzed by a calcium-dependent N-acyltransferase (NAT) (Fig. 2).

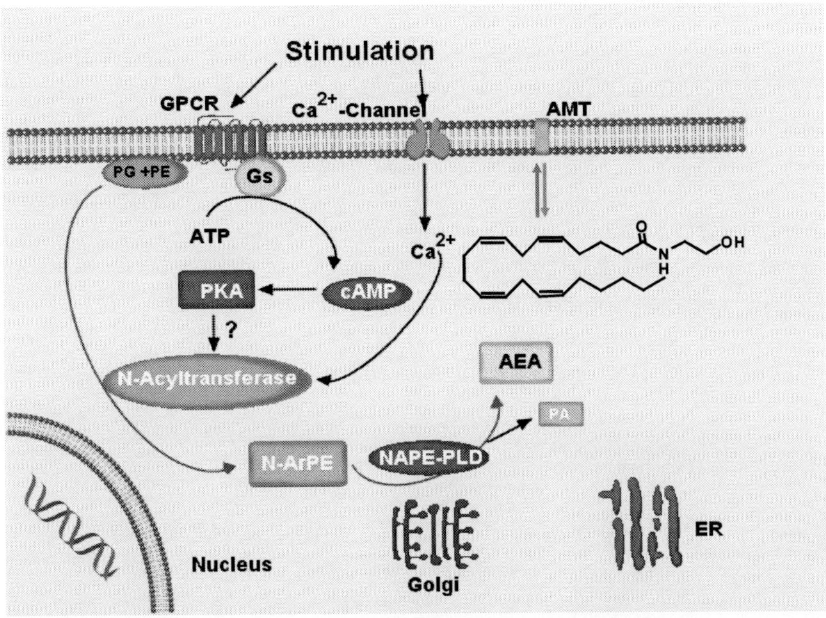

Figure 2. The potential pathways of anandamide biosynthesis. Stimulation of adenylate cyclase and cAMP-dependent protein kinase potentiate the N-acyltransferase (Ca2+-dependent transacylase, CDTA). A fatty arachidonic acid chain is transferred by CDTA from the sn-1 position of phospholipids to the primary amine of phosphatidylethanolamine, in a Ca2+-dependent manner, forming an N-arachidonyl phosphatidylethanolamine (N-ArPE). This N-ArPE intermediate is then hydrolyzed by a phospholipase D (PLD)-like enzyme to yield the anandamide (AEA). Once synthesized, AEA can transported to the outside of the cell through a process that has not yet been well characterized. AMT, anandamide membrane transporter

N-ArPE is then cleaved by a N-acyl phosphatidylethanolamine (NAPE)-specific phospholipase D (PLD) [61, 153, 176], which releases AEA and phosphatidic acid. It is not clear whether the NAT or the NAPE-PLD controls the rate-limiting step of AEA synthesis [59, 86, 186]. AEA biosynthesis was unaffected in NAPE-PLD knockout mice suggesting the involvement of other enzymes [120]. Another pathway which involves the conversion of NAPE into 2-lysol-NAPEs via the action of secretory PLA_2 has also been reported. 2-Lysol-NAPEs are then converted into N-acyl-ethanolamides, including AEA, via a selective lyso phospholipase D (lyso-PLD) [190]. A recent study proposed the existence in mouse brain and RAW264.7 macrophages of a parallel pathway through which AEA is generated from NAPE by a two-step process involving the PLC-catalyzed cleavage of NAPE to yield pAEA, which is subsequently dephosphorylated by protein tyrosine phosphatases (PTPN22) [121]. Notably, there is a strong evidence for calcium dependence in both of these synthesis steps, which may underlie the requirement for postsynaptic Ca^{2+} in certain forms of synaptic plasticity (see below). As a putative neuromodulator, AEA that is released into the synaptic cleft is expected to be rapidly inactivated. In general, two mechanisms are known that could remove endocannabinoids from the synaptic cleft to ensure rapid signal inactivation: re-uptake or enzymatic degradation. AEA is inactivated by reuptake [22, 24] via uncharacterized membrane transport molecule, the 'AEA membrane transporter' (AMT) [20, 22, 23, 75, 93, 94, 124], and subsequent intracellular enzymatic degradation. AEA is metabolized to arachidonic acid and ethanolamine via the action of the fatty acid amide hydrolase (FAAH), and this activity plays a significant role in the rapid clearance of AEA from extracellular compartments [56, 77]. In addition to hydrolysis by FAAH, AEA is metabolized by COX-2, LOX and cytochrome P450. COX-2 has been shown to metabolize AEA in to PGE_2-ethanolamide (PGE2-EA) [173]. 12- and 15-LOX, nonheme iron-containing enzymes convert AEA into 12- and 15-hydroxy-AEA (12- and 15-HAEA) in vitro, respectively [115, 124]. Cytochrome P450 also metabolizes AEA into several polar lipids [32]. Recently, in the absence of FAAH, exogenously injected AEA has been shown to be converted into o-phosphorylcholine (PC)-AEA in the brain and spinal cord. The choline-specific phosphodiesterase (NPP6) was found to convert PC-NAE into NAE [150]. Further research is required to elucidate the exact mechanism and enzymes involved in this pathway of AEA metabolism.

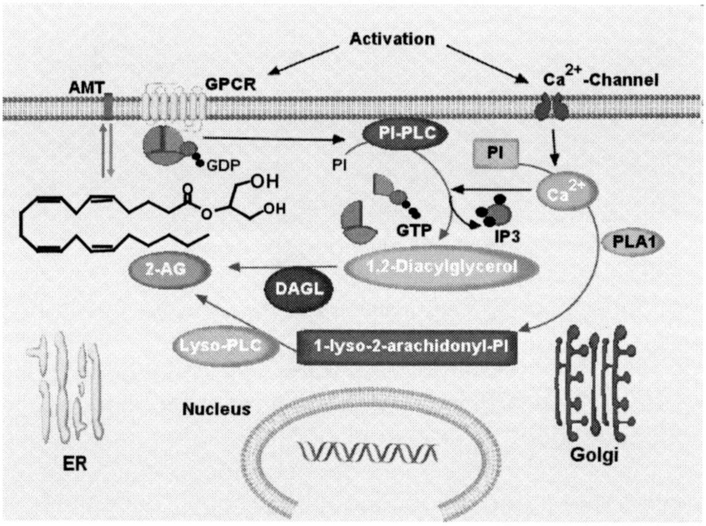

Figure 3. The potential pathways of 2-arachidonylglycerol biosynthesis. Intracellular Ca2+ initiates 2-AG biosynthesis by inducing the formation of diacylglycerol (DAG) in the membrane by stimulating the phosphatidyl-inositol-phospholipase C (PI-PLC) pathway. 2-AG is the product of DAG-lipase (DAGL) acting on DAG. The second pathway involves hydrolysis of PI by phospholipase A1 (PLA1) and hydrolysis of the resultant lyso-PI by a specific lyso-PLC. Once synthesized, 2-AG can transported to the outside of the cell through a process that has not yet been characterized. AMT, anandamide membrane transporter

The second widely recognized endogenous CB1 agonist is 2-arachidonylglycerol (2-AG) was characterized soon after the discovery of AEA [141, 187]. 2-AG has been characterized as a unique molecular species of monoacylglycerol isolated from both the canine gut [141] and the rat brain [188], where it presumably functions as an endogenous cannabinoid receptor ligand. 2-AG biosynthesis occurs by two possible routes in neurons, which are illustrated in

Figure 3 and also in recent review [14]. Phospholipase C (PLC)-mediated hydrolysis of membrane phospholipids may produce diacylglycerol (DAG), which may be subsequently converted to 2-AG by diacylglycerol lipase (DAGL) activity [169, 187]. The formation of DAG also involves the hydrolysis of phosphatidic acid through Mg^{2+} and Ca^{2+}-dependent PA phsophohydrolase activity [25, 36]. Alternatively, phospholipase A1 (PLA1) may generate a lysophospholipid, which may be hydrolyzed to 2-AG by lyso-PLC activity [187]. Under certain conditions, 2-AG can also be synthesized through the conversion of 2-arachidonyl lysophosphatidic acid (LPA) by phosphatase to yield 2-AG [152]. Molecular characterization of these potential pathways remains to be accomplished. 2-AG, like AEA, is found in a variety of tissues throughout the body and brain, and appears to be released from cells in response to certain stimuli. 2-AG activates the CB1 receptor with greater efficacy than does AEA. 2-AG is inactivated by reuptake [22, 24] via uncharacterized membrane transport molecule, the 'AEA membrane transporter' (AMT) [20, 22, 23, 75, 93, 94, 124], and subsequent intracellular enzymatic degradation [53, 56, 61] by monoacylglycerol (MAGL) lipase (Fig. 6), like other monoacylglycerols [114]. Similarly, 2-AG is metabolized by MAGL lipase from porcine brain cytosol and particulate fractions [80]. Interestingly, MAGL is expressed in presynaptic terminals [64, 81], suggesting it has a role in terminating EC signaling at presynaptic neurons [185]. 2-AG is metabolized to 2-arachidonyl LPA through the action of monoacyl glycerol kinase(s). 2-Arachidonyl LPA is then converted into 1-steroyl-2-arachidonyl PA [178]. 1-steroyl-2-arachidonyl PA is further utilized in the "PI cycle" or is used in the de novo synthesis of PC and PE. Furthermore, 2-AG is metabolized by enzymatic oxygenation of 2-AG by COX-2 into PGH2 glycerol esters. The biological activity and the role of oxygenated 2-AG are yet to be determined.

2.3 Synaptic Plasticity

Changes in the strength and number of synaptic connections between neurons are believed to be one of the major mechanisms underlying learning and memory and mediating other physiological functions of the CNS. This phenomenon is called synaptic plasticity. This characteristic is present both during brain development and in the adult life. In its most general form, the synaptic plasticity and memory hypothesis states that "activity-dependent synaptic plasticity is induced at appropriate synapses during memory formation and is both necessary and sufficient for the information storage underlying the type of memory mediated by the brain area in which that plasticity is observed." Several key molecules are involved in normal synaptic formation [5-7, 38, 47, 109, 126, 132-134, 154], but their interactions are not well understood. There are various forms of synaptic plasticity differing with respect to their persistence over time and their underlying induction and expression mechanisms. Table 1 gives an overview of different mechanisms, their time scales and synaptic location.

2.3.1 Short-term synaptic plasticity

Synaptic transmission is subject to a wide range of short-term changes in synaptic strength, termed short-term synaptic plasticity. Short-term synaptic plasticity enables neurons to not just relay but rather, to actively transform their inputs to produce a patterned output. The differences in short term synaptic plasticity among neurons, and in particular the differences between excitatory and inhibitory neurons, are important for information processing and self-regulation of neural networks. Synaptic efficacy is dynamic. For instance, when closely spaced action potentials reach a presynaptic terminal, the synapse does not transmit them identically to a postsynaptic neuron. This form of synaptic plasticity, termed short-term plasticity, is diverse. At facilitating synapses, the postsynaptic responses to later spikes in repetitive presynaptic firing are larger than that to the first one, whereas at depressing synapses, they are smaller. Whether a synapse is facilitating or depressing depends upon the type of synapse. Hippocampal mossy fibre- CA3 synapses and climbing fiber-Purkinje cell synapses are typically facilitating, whereas parallel fiber- Purkinje cell synapses display depression. However, the biophysical mechanisms underlying short-term plasticity are multiple and complex, and therefore in many types of synapses, including hippocampal Schaffer collateral-CA1 synapses, these two forms of plasticity, i.e., facilitation and depression, often coexist, resulting in complicated profiles of short-term plasticity.

Table 1. Activity dependent synaptic mechanisms, a rough estimate of their decay constants and an indication of whether they are depending on pre- or postsynaptic activity or both are given [123, 212]

Mechanism	Duration	Synaptic Location
Short-term Plasticity		
Paired-pulse facilitation (PPF)	100 ms	Pre
Augmentation	10 s	Pre
Post-tetanic potentiation (PTP)	1 min	Pre
Depolarization-induced suppression of inhibition (DSI)	50 –75 ms	Pre
Depolarization-induced suppression of excitation (DSE)	50 –75 ms	Pre
Paired pulse depression (PPD)	100 ms	Pre
Depletion	10s	Pre
Long-term plasticity	15 min	Post
Short-term Potentiation (STP)	> 30 min	Pre and Post
Long-term Potentiation (LTP)	>30 min	Pre and Post
Long-term depression (LTD)		

Short-term synaptic enhancement has been most thoroughly characterized at invertebrate synapses and at the neuromuscular junction in vertebrates [8, 129]. High-frequency stimulus trains enhance release both during and after stimulation. Based upon differences in time course and pharmacology, this enhancement is separated into four components: post tetanic potentiation (PTP), augmentation, facilitation component F2, and facilitation component Fl, with time constants of decay of 30-90 set, 5-10 set, 200-500 msec, and 20-l00 msec, respectively. Quanta1 analysis indicates that these forms of enhancement are presynaptic in origin. Short-term memory involves modifications of preexisting proteins and transient strengthening of preexisting synaptic connections.

(A) ECs-Mediated Short-Term Plasticity

The discovery of ECs such as AEA and 2-AG and the widespread localization of CB1 receptors in the brain have stimulated considerable excitement over the previously unrecognized cannabinoid system and questions about the function of this ubiquitous network in the nervous system. There is now overwhelming evidence that AEA and 2-AG interact with CB1 receptors and share some of the biological properties of other cannabinoids, but with significant differences. These significant differential effects involve other non-CB1 receptors and/or postulated CB3 receptors as described. In recent years, the functions of ECs at the synaptic and network levels have been elucidated.

In 2001, three groups independently revealed that ECs are released when neuronal cells (postsynaptic neurons and possibly presynaptic terminals as well) are activated. They travel in a retrograde direction and transiently (<1 min) suppress presynaptic neurotransmitter release by activating CB1 receptor-mediated inhibition of voltage-gated Ca^{2+} channels [118, 156, 212]. Such a negative feedback mechanism should be effective in calming stimulated neurons after excitation. Since then, dozens of papers have been published that have confirmed the role of ECs as a retrograde messenger in various regions of the brain. It is now established that EC release can be induced by four stimulation protocol, namely, postsynaptic depolarization, activation of postsynaptic Gq-coupled receptors, combined Gq-coupled activation and depolarization, and repetitive synaptic activation. In the following section, we address the mechanisms of EC release by each of the four stimulation protocols.

(a) Depolarization-induced EC release

A number of recent studies have demonstrated that a well-known form of short-term plasticity at hippocampal GABAergic synapses, called depolarization-induced suppression of inhibition (DSI), is in fact mediated by the retrograde actions of endocannabinoids released in response to depolarization of the postsynaptic cells. Despite the widespread interest and potential physiological importance of DSI, many questions regarding the physiological relevance of DSI remain. Brief activation of CA1 pyramidal cells in the hippocampus [2, 3, 159, 165-167] or Purkinje cells in the cerebellum [122, 204-206] (Fig. 4) is known to cause a reduction in the amplitude of GABAergic inhibitory postsynaptic currents (IPSCs). The DSI is initiated postsynaptically by the voltage-dependent influx of Ca^{2+} into the soma and dendrites of the neuron, but is expressed presynaptically through inhibition of transmitter release from axon terminals of GABA interneurons. This suggests that a chemical messenger generated during depolarization of the pyramidal neurons must travel backwards across the synapse to induce DSI. DSI has been observed in both excitatory and inhibitory neurons in hippocampal cell culture [158], in CA3 pyramidal cells [146], in dentate gyrus granule cells [2], and in neocortical pyramidal cells [218].

The retrograde messenger in DSI remained unknown until recent investigations by Wilson and Nicoll [211-213] and by Ohno-Shosaku et al. [156] indicated that in hippocampal cells the messenger was likely to be an EC. Shortly thereafter, cerebellar DSI was also reported to be mediated by an EC [62, 117, 216]. Furthermore, it was reported that CB1 receptor agonists selectively reduced IPSCs in both the hippocampus [83, 95, 108] and cerebellum [194]. There is strong evidence that this retrograde signaling process involves an EC. (a) CB1 receptor antagonists selectively blocked DSI whereas agonists enhanced it [156, 212]. (b) DSI is absent in CB1 receptor knockout mice [211, 216]. (c) The GABA

4.A

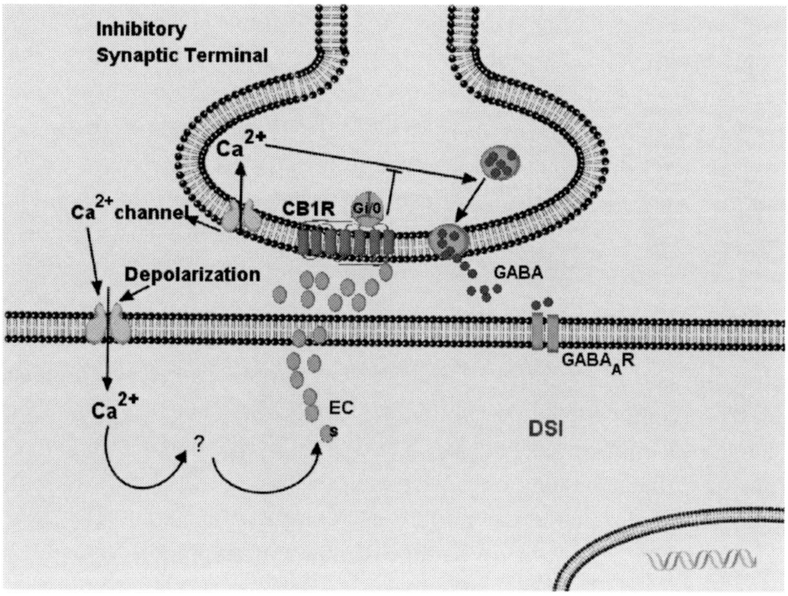

4.B

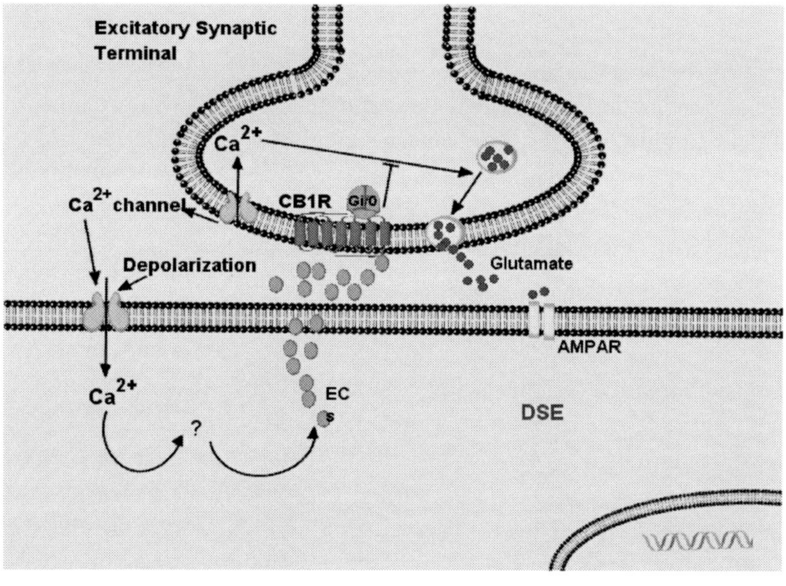

Figure 4. Schematic diagram to illustrate the mechanism of depolarization-induced suppression of inhibition (DSI) and depolarization-induced suppression of excitation (DSE). Depolarization of a postsynaptic neuron leads to Ca2+ influx through voltage-gated Ca2+ channels. Elevation of intracellular Ca2+ concentration triggers biosynthesis of endocannabinoids. Endocannabinoids are then released from postsynaptic neurons, activate CB1 receptors at presynaptic neuron, and suppress GABA (DSI) (A) or glutamate (DSE) (B) release by inhibiting Ca2+ channels [95, 100, 177]. GluR, Glutamate receptors.

interneurons that are implicated in DSI express high levels of CB1 receptors, which are localized to their axon terminals [108]. (d) Neuronal activity and Ca^{2+} entry stimulate the synthesis of 2-AG in hippocampal neurons and AEA and 2-AG in other neuronal cells [17, 19, 20]. Recently, DSI mediated by 2-AG was shown in the mouse substantia nigra pars reticulate and rat cerebellum [192]. It remains to be established that EC-mediated DSI is present in other brain regions such as the ventromedial medulla [203], amygdala [108], and striatum [191], in which exogenously applied CB1 receptor agonists are known to suppress IPSCs. These reports convincingly established that ECs are important mediators of short-term plasticity.

The neurons in the hippocampus and cerebellum use ECs to carry out a signaling process that is analogous in mechanism but opposite in sign to DSI, called depolarization-induced suppression of excitation (DSE). Like DSI, DSE is induced by neuronal depolarization; it consists of a transient depression in neurotransmitter release, and it requires a retrograde endocannabinoid messenger. But unlike DSI, DSE targets glutamatergic rather than GABA axon terminals and therefore it reduces the excitatory input to the affected cell [2, 164]. DSE is mimicked and blocked by agonists and antagonists of CB1 receptors respectively [118, 127] and it is absent in the CB1 receptor knockout mouse [160]. CB1 receptor agonists suppress EPSCs in other areas of the brain, evidently through presynaptic actions. For instance, similar DSE was reported in the ventral tegamental area (VTA) as a Ca^{2+}-dependent phenomenon, blocked by both CB1 receptor antagonists AM281 and SR141716A (rimonabant), and enhanced by WIN55212-2 [144]. Importantly, DSE was partially blocked by the D_2 DA antagonist eticlopride and enhanced by the D_2 DA agonist quinpirole without changing the presynaptic cannabinoid activity [144]. These observations indicate that activation of D_2 DA receptors in the VTA significantly enhances the depolarization-induced release of ECs, which are responsible for the inhibition of glutamate transmission in the VTA [144]. The synchronous release of mEPSCs in Sr^{2+}-substituted extracellular solution was found to be reduced by ECs in the prefrontal cortex and striatum [9, 73]. Recently, it was shown that 2-AG is the retrograde messenger for train-induced suppression of excitation at the VTA-DA synapses [143]. It remains to be demonstrated whether or not DSE is present in the striatum [73], substantia nigra [193], periaqueductal gray [202], and spinal cord [147].

(b) Receptor-Driven EC release

Another form of EC-mediated short-term plasticity, which is driven by receptor activation was first discovered in the cerebellum [127]. Metabotropic glutamate receptors (mGluRs) are G-protein-coupled receptors distributed throughout the CNS that modulate multiple CNS functions, including neuronal excitability [4, 49] and neurotransmitter release [37]. Recent data from several investigators have begun to uncover an entirely novel signaling mechanism for mGluRs, namely the production and subsequent release of ECs.

Some of the effects (short- and long-term forms of synaptic plasticity) previously attributed directly to mGluR activation are in fact indirectly mediated by signaling through the EC system [65]. Recent studies suggest that mGluR/EC signaling is a widespread feature of neuronal circuitry [65], given the widespread expression of postsynaptic group I mGluRs throughout the CNS and a similar extensive expression of CB1 receptors. Activation of group I mGluRs can cause the release of ECs in the cerebellum [127] and hippocampus [200].

5.A

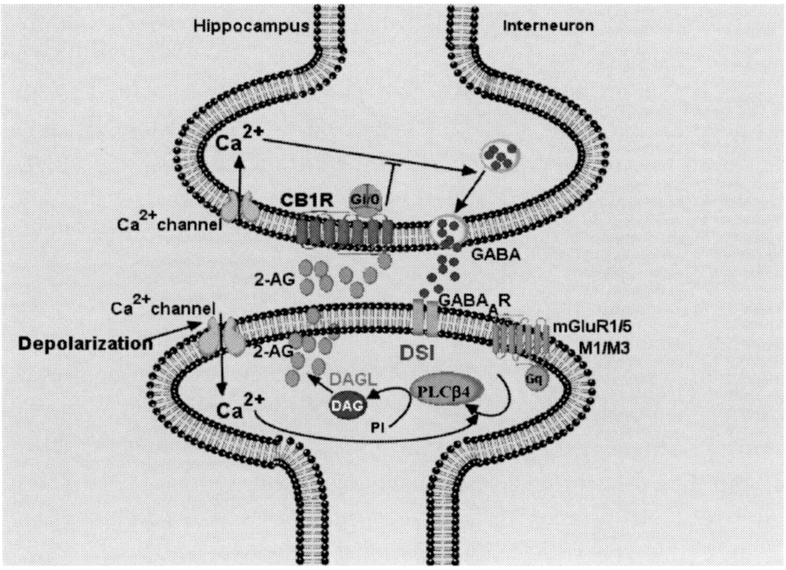

5.B

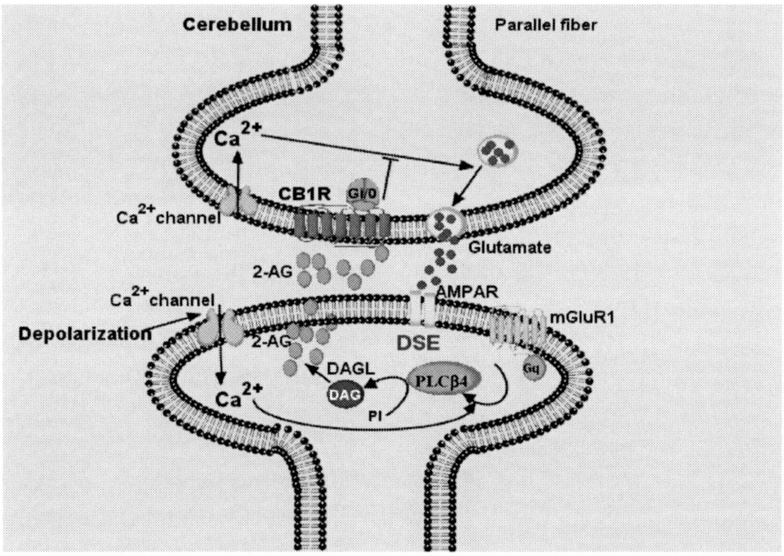

Figure 5. Scheme illustrating the potential mechanisms of receptor-driven endocannabinoid release and Ca2+-assisted receptor-driven endocannabinoid release. A, In the hippocampus, activation of GluR1/5 or M1/M3 muscarinic receptors stimulates PLCβ1-DAGL cascade and induces the formation of 2-AG. As a retrograde messenger, 2-AG activates CB1 receptors at presynaptic neuron and suppresses the GABA release. B, In the cerebellum, activation of mGluR1 receptors in Purkinje cells stimulates LCβ4 by inducing the formation of diacylglycerol (DAG). DAG-lipase (DAGL) converts DAG to 2-AG. 2-AG activates presynaptic CB1 receptors on parallel fibers and suppresses the glutamate release. These signaling pathways (A and B) are facilitated by depolarization-induced Ca2+elevation because of the Ca2+dependency of PLCβ1/4 (Ca2+-assisted receptor-driven endocannabinoid release). PLC, phospholipase C

Synaptic depression in the cerebellum has been observed at glutamatergic synapses. A similar mechanism operates in the hippocampus. As in the cerebellum, activation of postsynaptic group I mGluRs depresses neurotransmitter release through EC-mediated retrograde activation of presynaptic CB1 receptors. In contrast to the cerebellum, however, synaptic depression in the hippocampus has been observed at GABAergic rather than at glutamatergic synapses.

In addition to group I mGluRs, other types of Gq-coupled receptors also induce EC release. Muscarinic acetylcholine receptors, which are coupled to Gq protein[70], induced transient suppression of inhibitory synaptic transmission is mediated through release of ECs in the hippocampus [111]. In the dorsal raphe nucleus, orexin receptor, another Gq/11-coupled receptor, was found to drive EC release [82].

It should be noted here that EC release driven by these Gq-coupled receptors is dependent on tissue specific PLCβ isoenzymes (PLCβ1-4). In the hippocampus, activation of Gq-coupled receptors, such as mGluR1/5 and M1/M3 muscarinic receptors, stimulates PLCβ1 and induces the production and release of 2-AG through DAGL activity (Fig 5A). 2-AG then activates presynaptic CB1 receptors and suppresses the GABA release [89]. Activation of I mGluRs stimulates PLCβ4 in cerebellar purkinje cells and yields DAG, which is then converted to 2-AG by DAGL (Fig 5B). Then, 2-AG is released from the postsynaptic neuron, activates presynaptic CB1 receptors, and suppresses the glutamate release [128].

(c) Ca2+-Assisted Receptor-Driven EC release

This is another form of EC-mediated short-term plasticity. It is driven by two distinct stimuli, Gq-coupled receptor activation and Ca^{2+} elevation, which facilitate PLCβ dependent and independent pathways respectively. It was noted that simultaneous elevation of Ca^{2+} and activation of either group I mGluR or muscarinic receptors, the amount of ECs released was several times higher than the simple sum of the amounts released by individual stimuli applied separately [157, 160]. This is partly due to Ca^{2+} dependency of PLCβ [89, 128] and this effect was completely eliminated in PLCβ knockout mice[89]. This mode of EC release seems physiologically important, because mild Ca^{2+} elevation and mild receptor activation, both of which are subthreshold for inducing EC release when applied alone, can effectively induce EC release when applied conjointly. In this Ca^{2+} -assisted receptor driven EC release, PLCβ detects the coincidence of Ca^{2+} elevation reflecting postsynaptic activity and the receptor activation reflecting presynaptic activity. In this regard, PLCβ and the EC signal can work as a coincidence detector and a coincidence signal, respectively, for activity-dependent synaptic plasticity.

(d) Synaptically Triggered EC Release

EC release during short-term plasticity could be induced experimentally by the aforementioned three stimulation protocols. Under physiological conditions, the EC signaling should be triggered by synaptic activities. It is important to understand the kind of synaptic activity and the type of pathway could facilitate physiological relevant EC release. There are several studies that examined EC release during synaptic activity. In the cerebellum, brief bursts of PF stimulation (for example,50–100 Hz, 10 pulses) induced EC release from PCs and suppressed the transmitter release from PF terminals [30, 128]. This type of synaptic suppression was dependent on both mGluR1 activation and postsynaptic Ca^{2+} elevation [128].

When PF stimulation was combined with CF stimulation (100 Hz, 5 pulses), only two to five pulses to PFs were enough to induce EC release [29]. This associative short-term plasticity induced by coactivation of PF and CF synapses was also dependent on both mGluR1 activation and postsynaptic Ca^{2+} elevation. In VTA dopamine neurons, brief-burst stimulation (5 Hz, 10 pulses) of excitatory inputs from the prefrontal cortex induced EC-mediated suppression of the excitatory transmission, which was sensitive to both mGluR1 antagonist and the blockade of postsynaptic Ca^{2+} elevation [144]. All these observations indicate the significance of Ca^{2+}-assisted receptor-mediated pathway for synaptically triggered EC release. In addition, the other two pathways, namely, the depolarization induced pathway being mediated by Ca^{2+} elevation alone [29] and the receptor-driven pathway being triggered by Gq-coupled receptor activation alone [127], can also be involved in the synaptically triggered EC release. Besides the temporal pattern, the spatial pattern of synaptic activation is also important for EC signaling in the cerebellum. Although spatially dispersed synapse activation failed to induce retrograde EC signaling, activation of nearby synapses induced retrograde inhibition of PF-PC synapses, because of activation of mGluRs by glutamate spillover from nearby active synapses [135].

(B) CB1-Dependent Suppression of Transmitter Release: Presynaptic Mechanisms

EC release during short-term plasticity activates presynaptic CB1 receptors and suppresses transmitter release reversibly. Several studies addressed the issue of how activation of CB1 receptors affect transmitter release [2]. Three mechanisms have been suggested for the CB1-mediated suppression of transmitter release, which include inhibition of voltage-gated Ca^{2+} channels, activation of K^{+} channels, and inhibition of release machinery. First, the possibility of Ca^{2+} channel inhibition has been most intensively studied and well supported by many lines of evidence. CB1 receptors are pertussis-sensitive G-protein-coupled receptors, and their activation inhibits L-type, N-type, and Q-type Ca^{2+} channels [39, 40, 125, 162, 195]. The studies using Ca^{2+}-channel blockers and K^{+}-channel blockers suggested that the cannabinoid-mediated suppression was caused by inhibition of presynaptic Ca^{2+} channels rather than activation of K^{+} channels in the hippocampus and cerebellum [31, 95]. Second, the possibility of K^{+}-channel activation has also been suggested [51, 52, 63]. It is thought that activation of K^{+} channels changes the action potential wave form and indirectly suppresses the Ca^{2+} influx into presynaptic terminals. Third, inhibition of the release machinery has also been suggested to contribute to CB1-mediated suppression of transmitter release [194, 215]. In some cells, it appears that the CB1 receptor could reduce GABA release from at least some nerve terminals through a mechanism that is independent of N-P/Q-type Ca^{2+} channels [73, 194, 200, 202], perhaps by direct action on the transmitter release machinery. In cerebellar PCs, CB1 activation had no effect on basal miniature postsynaptic events but selectively suppressed miniature postsynaptic events enhanced by Ca^{2+} elevation in presynaptic terminals [215]. Thus, CB1 activation appears to regulate processes of spontaneous transmitter release by acting downstream of Ca^{2+} entry into presynaptic terminals.

2.3.2 Long-term synaptic plasticity

In addition to short-term plasticity, central synapses often show long-term plasticity that is they are capable of increasing or decreasing their efficacy of transmission in response to brief repetitive synaptic activation and thereafter maintaining the changed efficacy for a long time. LTP, the long lasting enhancement of synaptic transmission first reported by Bliss and Lomo [26] over 30 years ago, has been the focus of an enormous amount of investigation. The temporal pattern of synaptic stimulation determines whether synaptic efficacy is strengthened (long-term potentiation, LTP) or weakened (long-term depression, LTD). LTP represents long-lasting 'memory' at the sub-neuronal level and is widely believed to underlie learning and memory at the behavioral level. Since it's discovery in the perforant path of the hippocampal formation, the great majority of the work related to LTP has been through electrophysiological investigations. During this time, evidence for a number mechanisms for the induction and expression of this functionality have been reported including increased glutamate release (pre-synaptic mechanism,) and activation of previously silent synapses [102]. Long-term memory involves altered gene expression, protein synthesis and the growth of new and stronger synaptic connections within existing circuits. Intracellular signaling pathways convert short-lasting stimulus events to persistent changes in synaptic strength.

(A) Regulation of long-term synaptic plasticity by ECs

As in EC-mediated short-term plasticity, all the studies to date suggest that EC-mediated long-term plasticity takes the form of depression of neurotransmission in various brain regions. It was observed that long-term depression (LTD) was absent in CB1 receptor knockout mice, reduced or eliminated by CB1 receptor blockade, and enhanced by CB1 receptor activation in various brain regions, indicating the involvement of EC signaling [74]. Soon after this publication, similar EC mediated LTD was reported at both excitatory (LTDe) and inhibitory (LTDi) neurotransmission in various brain regions [42, 136, 170]. Another form of EC-mediated LTDe was described in the visual cortex [179]. All these forms of EC-mediated LTD expressed presynaptically as persistent decrease in neurotransmitter release. By contrast, cerebellar LTD, which is well known to be expressed postsynaptically, was reported to require EC signaling [174]. In the following sections, we describe these different LTD's and also discuss the functional significance of the EC signaling in various neuronal functions.

(B) Evidence for EC retrograde messengers in long-term synaptic plasticity

(a) Dorsal Striatum

In 1997, it was demonstrated that high frequency stimulation (for example, 100 Hz, 1 s) of corticostriatal glutamatergic afferents in medium spiny neurons of the dorsal striatum was known to induce LTD of the excitatory input. This striatal LTDe was suggested to be expressed as long-lasting suppression of glutamate release through the elevation of postsynaptic Ca^{2+}, implying the involvement of a retrograde signal [34, 45, 46]. It should be noted here the critical role of postsynaptic intracellular Ca^{2+} in the formation of ECs, because there are strong evidences that AEA synthesis is stimulated by Ca^{2+} signaling [61, 68]. Moreover, striatal medium spiny neurons grown in culture had been shown to synthesize and release AEA, in a Ca^{2+}-dependent manner, in response to depolarizing stimuli[61]. Furthermore, striatal LTD is dependent on activation of D2 (as well as D1) dopamine receptors. Accordingly, depolarization and D2 receptor activation led to an increased detection of AEA measured in the dorsal striatum of rats in vivo, and that these effects were additive [76]. Based on these discoveries, it was expected that ECs might work as retrograde messengers in LTDe induction. It was found that LTDe was blocked by CB1 antagonist and was absent in CB1-knockout mice, and suggesting that striatal LTDe was mediated by ECs [74]. Further, postsynaptic loading with AEA transporter inhibitors prevented striatal LTDe, suggesting the requirement of transporter-mediated release of AEA for LTDe induction [172]. Dopamine also modulated striatal EC release and LTDe induction in medium-spiny neurons [116]. All these observations suggest that EC can act as a retrograde messenger in striatal LTDe. The dorsal striatum is an important brain area for motor control and habit learning. Because the striatum receives excitatory inputs from the cortex and thalamus, synaptic plasticity of excitatory synapses in this area is thought to be crucial for such striatum-related functions. The retrograde EC signaling might play a role in the striatal functions through the contribution to LTDe. As for the molecular identity of EC for EC mediated -LTD, AEA and 2-AG appear to function in different brain regions. Although it is less clear how LTD-inducing synaptic activity leads to production of AEA in the striatum, recent data suggest that AEA mediate LTDe in the striatum [74, 172].

(b) Nucleus Accumbens

As in the striatum, EC-LTDe was observed in the nucleus accumbens (NAc)[170]. NAc-LTDe was induced by prolonged, moderate frequency stimulation (10min at 13Hz) of prelimbic cortical glutamatergic synapses. As in the striatal LTDe, NAc-LTDe was prevented by CB1 receptor antagonists, enhanced by CB1 receptor agonists, and absent in CB1 receptor knockout mice, indicating the involvement of EC signaling [170]. Importantly, once NAc LTD was induced, the antagonist did not affect it, demonstrating that the LTD was not maintained by a continual release of ECs, but rather represented a persistent effect of transient CB1 receptor activation. The EC that mediated LTD was evidently released as a retrograde messenger, because LTD was prevented by chelating postsynaptic Ca^{2+} (with 20mM BAPTA) in the recorded cell [170]. NAc-LTDe required both activation of mGluR5 and Ca^{2+} release from intracellular stores. Interestingly, in vivo exposure to Δ^9-THC blocked NAc-LTDe, which was explained by a functional tolerance of CB1 receptors [96, 138]. Because NAc is crucial for behaviors related to motivation and reward, these results suggest that NAc- LTDe might be related to addiction behavior. Synaptically triggered EC release in VTA dopaminergic neurons was mainly driven by group I mGluR activation, was blocked by inhibition of DAGL [143] suggesting the participation of 2-AG as a retrograde messenger in NAc-LTDe.

(c) Hippocampus

It has been shown that CB1 receptor activation inhibits both LTP and LTD induction in the hippocampus [184, 189]. EC-LTDi was also observed in the hippocampus [42]. Two trains of high-frequency stimulation (100 Hz, 100 pulses) or theta burst stimulation in the stratum radiatum of the CA1 region caused LTD at GABAergic inhibitory synapses. This hippocampal LTDi was presynaptically expressed, blocked by CB1 antagonist [42] and eliminated in CB1 knockout mice [43], suggesting the involvement of EC signaling. LTDi was prevented by pharmacological blockade of mGluR1/5, PLC, and DAGL, but not by postsynaptic loading of the Ca^{2+} chelator BAPTA, suggesting that the generation of EC through the mGluR1/5-PLCβ-DAGL pathway is required for LTDi induction. By examining the effects of CB1 antagonist at different time periods before, during, and after LTDi, the induction of LTDi was shown to require continuous activation of CB1 for 5 to 10 minutes.

High frequency (two brief 100Hz trains) stimulation of Schaffer collaterals releases glutamate, which activates postsynaptic mGluR1/5, leading to the production of 2-AG through the PLCβ-DAGL pathway. 2- AG is then released, activates presynaptic CB1 on nearby GABAergic interneurons, and causes long-term suppression of GABA release, if CB1 activation continues for several minutes [42]. Further, the expression of LTDi facilitated subsequent induction of LTP at excitatory synapses [42, 217]. Enhancement of LTP likely results from mechanisms similar to those previously implicated in priming of LTP during EC-mediated DSI and LTDi [35, 43]. Facilitation of LTP induction by mGluR activation was also observed in a previous study [145], and similar EC actions may underlie this enhancement. It is likely that mGluR5 and CB1 blockade prevent stimulus-primed LTP by interfering with EC signaling during low frequency stimulation. However, application of SR141716 after low frequency stimulation (LFS) but during theta burst stimulation (TBS) does not abolish the LFS facilitation of LTP. Thus, CB1 activation is not directly involved in LTP induction. Because EC signaling is blocked when the CB1 antagonist is present during TBS, no DSI would take place during LTP induction, and thus LFS-enhanced DSI could not contribute to LTP enhancement [42, 217]. Up-regulation of retrograde EC signaling and LTDi contribute to long-lasting enhancement of glutamatergic transmission through inhibition of GABAergic transmission [217]. These processes might thus contribute to EC enhancement of learning and memory. Therefore, the EC signaling could significantly contribute to the memory formation through the induction of local metaplasticity. LTP elicited by moderate stimulations (20 or 50 pulses) was facilitated in slices treated with a CB1 antagonist, whereas LTP elicited with robust stimulations (100 or 200 pulses) was unchanged by CB1 blockade. LTP elicited with TBS also was facilitated with CB1 blockade, revealing a tonic inhibitory influence of ECs on the hippocampal LTP induction. Conversely, inhibition of cyclooxygenase-2 (COX-2) prevented LTP elicited with TBS. Inhibition of COX-1 or other routes of EC degradation did not affect LTP. These observations suggest that COX-2 regulates the formation of ECs that negatively regulate LTP [180]. Possible involvement of the EC system in extinction processes has been suggested in a behavioral study [201]. Performance of CB1-knockout mice was evaluated in the Morris water maze test, a standard task for examination of hippocampus-dependent spatial memory in rodents. CB1-knockout mice exhibited a deficit in learning a new platform location during the reversal text suggesting that the EC signaling plays a key role in facilitating extinction processes [201]. In contrast, CB1-knockout mice exhibited normal acquisition and extinction of trace eyeblink conditioning that is known to be dependent on the hippocampus [113]. Animals treated with a low dose of SR intrahippocampally enhanced learning and memory without effecting the procedural learning [171]. It remains to be investigated the extent to which EC-LTDi contributes to extinction processes of hippocampus-dependent learning. All these observations support the notion that spatial learning may activate ECs and stimulate CB1 receptors in hippocampus. Although the molecular identity of the retrograde signal involved in DSI/DSE is not fully determined, two studies have suggested that 2-AG mediates DSI. DSI in CA1 pyramidal cells was not affected by FAAH inhibition but was prolonged by inhibition of COX-2, which can degrade both 2-AG and AEA [110]. Because FAAH inhibition was shown to facilitate the effect of exogenously applied AEA, the negative effect of FAAH inhibition on DSI suggests that AEA does not play a dominant role in DSI. The inhibitors of MAGL (URB754 and URB602) increased 2- AG levels and prolonged DSI in CA1 pyramidal cells, suggesting the involvement of 2-AG [130]. However, third study suggests that DSI was not affected by application of inhibitors of PLC and DAGL [42] and suggest that the involvement of AEA in DSI. Further studies are required to determine the enzymes for the EC production and the related signaling molecule involved in hippocampal EC mediated LTD.

(d) Amygdala

EC mediated LTD has been found at GABAergic inhibitory synapses within the basolateral nucleus of the amygdala (BLA) [137]. This LTD of inhibitory inputs (LTD_i) is induced by low-frequency (1 Hz, 100 pulses) stimulation, and PPF evidence indicates that expression of this form of plasticity involves a presynaptic decrease in neurotransmitter release and required CB1 activation. A further study reported that induction of LTDi was dependent on mGluR1 activation but not on postsynaptic Ca^{2+} influx [10]. Pharmacological experiments with inhibitors of PLC and DAGL suggested that AEA rather than 2-AG was involved in LTDi. Consistent with this idea, LTDi was enhanced in mice lacking the FAAH enzyme [10]. Although it is not clear how mGluR1 activation causes AEA production, the authors suggested that adenylyl-cyclase and protein kinase A might be involved. The amygdala is crucial for acquisition and storage of fear memory [119] and presumably also for its extinction. CB1 knockout mice showed strongly impaired short-term and long-term extinction in auditory fear-conditioning tests, with unaffected memory acquisition and consolidation. Treatment of wild-type mice with CB1 receptor antagonist mimicked the phenotype of CB1 knockout mice, suggesting that CB1 is required at the moment of fear memory extinction [136]. Although, the mechanism needs to be elucidated, these studies suggest that EC signaling is important for the induction, but not the expression, phase of LTD. EC mediated LTDi in the amygdala may underlie this process. It is less clear how LTD-inducing synaptic activity leads to production of ECs and the identity of the EC involved in EC mediated LTD in the amygdala needs to be investigated.

(e) Cortex

CB1 receptors are present on glutamatergic terminals in the prefrontal cortex [90], and activation of the CB1 receptor by agonists suppresses glutamate EPSCs in layer V slices of rat cortex, evidently by acting at a presynaptic site [9]. Cannabinoids facilitates LTD, at expense of LTP in slices of rodent prefrontal cortex [9, 13]. Conversely, blockade of CB1 receptors with the antagonist SR141716A led to an increased likelihood of observing LTP, although LTD was not entirely absent. Therefore, the EC system may serve to promote LTD in layer V neurons of the PFC, without being absolutely required for the LTD. It remains to be determined whether natural balance between LTD and LTP in the PFC is regulated by ECs and CB1 receptors. In corticostriatal slice cultures, mGluR5 activation induced 2-AG formation through the PLC-DAGL cascade [105]and remains to be determined the extent to which 2-AG acts as a retrograde messenger in cortex LTD.

(f) Neocortex

Neocortical synapses exhibit spike-timing-dependent plasticity, which is induced by pre- and postsynaptic firings with a certain pre-to-post timing [50]. When presynaptic firing repeatedly precedes postsynaptic firing by 0 to 20 ms, LTP is usually induced. By contrast, when presynaptic firing follows postsynaptic firing with a delay up to 100 ms, LTD is induced. This timing-dependent LTD at glutamatergic synapses (LTDe) in visual cortical layer 5 pyramidal neuron, was expressed presynaptically and was dependent on activation of CB1 receptors [179]. Importantly, it requires coincident activation of presynaptic CB1 and NMDA receptors. Studies have suggested that the spike timing-dependent plasticity can provide a fundamental mechanism, by which neural networks can perform computational functions, such as causality detection and sequence learning [50]. The EC signaling might contribute to these neural functions through mediating timing-dependent LTDe in the neocortex.

(g) Cerebellum

Although several forms of EC-LTD described above are all expressed presynaptically, postsynaptically expressed EC-LTD was reported in the cerebellum [174]. It is well accepted that cerebellar LTD at PF to PC synapses is a cellular basis for certain forms of discrete motor learning [103]. This LTD is induced at PF-PC excitatory synapses by conjunctive stimulation of PFs and CFs. The induction of LTDe was blocked by a CB1 antagonist and abolished in CB1-knockout mice suggesting the EC requirement for cerebellar LTDe. Postsynaptic loading of DAGL inhibitors also blocked cerebellar LTDe, suggesting the involvement of 2-AG. Because cerebellar LTDe is known to be expressed postsynaptically [103], presynaptic CB1 activation should eventually bring the message to postsynaptic neurons. Inhibition of nitric oxide (NO) synthesis prevented LTD induction even in the presence of a CB1 agonist suggesting that NO may work as an anterograde messenger [174]. The classical eyeblink conditioning, a well-known form of cerebellum-dependent discrete motor learning, was severely impaired in CB1- knockout mice, and was blocked by the CB1 antagonist SR141716A suggesting the involvement of EC-signaling in motor learning [112]. Interestingly, extinction of conditioned eyeblink response was not affected by SR141716A. These observations suggest that the EC signaling plays an important role in cerebellar LTDe and contributes to acquisition of cerebellum-dependent discrete motor learning. Cerebellar DSE was resistant to DAGL inhibitors [174]. Because PLC and DAGL are key enzymes for 2- AG production, suggesting the participation of alternative pathways independent of PLC/DAGL (Sugiura and others 2006) for the synthesis of 2-AG. Although the molecular identity of the retrograde signal involved in DSI/DSE is not fully determined, studies have suggested that 2-AG mediates DSI in cerebellum. The studies on cerebellar PCs of PLCβ4-knockout mice [128] demonstrated that the EC release driven by group I mGluRs or muscarinic receptors was abolished in these PLCβ-knockout neurons. Synaptically triggered EC release in cerebellar PCs [128, 174] was mainly driven by group I mGluR activation, and was blocked by inhibition of DAGL. Moreover, biochemical measurements of 2-AG indicate that driving mGluR1-PLCβ4 cascade induces 2-AG production [128].

These early investigations are just beginning to address the effects of ECs on the neurophysiology of the brain, and further studies are necessary before the roles of ECs in short- and long-term plasticity are fully elucidated. Further studies are also required to determine the enzymes for the EC production and the related signaling molecule involved in EC mediated- short- and long-term plasticity.

2.4 Therapeutic opportunity

Even though the detailed pathophysiology of the EC system is not yet fully understood, there is already overwhelming evidence indicating that a pharmacological modulation of the endogenous cannabinoid system could provide new tools for a number of disease states, including drug addiction. Recent evidence suggests that the blockade of CB1 receptors with SR141617A (Fig. 6) might be beneficial to alleviate motor inhibition typical of Parkinson's disease (PD) [79]. In addition to SR, several specific EC transport inhibitors, FAAH and MAGL inhibitors which regulate brain EC levels might have a therapeutic value in the protection against Aβ-induced neurodegeneration [197] and memory deficit in rodents [140].

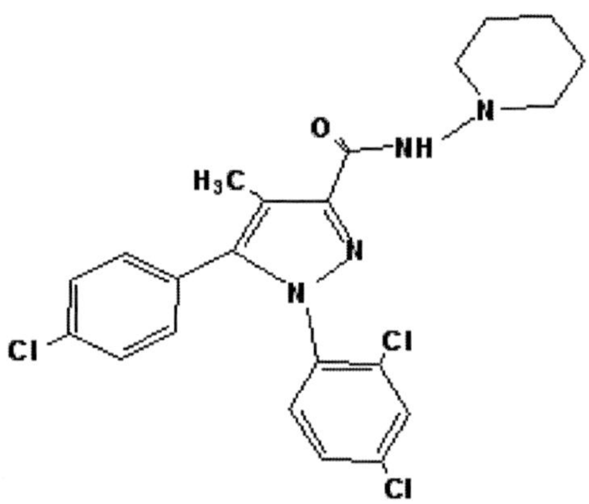

SR141716A

Figure 6. Molecular structure of CB1 receptor-selective antagonist/inverse agonist, rimonabant. SR141716A is a highly potent and selective CB1 receptor ligand that readily prevents and reverses CB1 mediated effects both in vitro and in vivo [98]

The CB1 receptor antagonist SR has progressed furthest and is in late phase III trials for the treatment of obesity and as an aid for smoking cessation [48, 198]. An NIAAA clinical study of the efficacy of SR to reduce voluntary alcohol drinking is in phase I trials. Pending the results of the clinical trials, SR could become an important addition to the limited arsenal of effective treatments for alcoholism. During disease or drug abuse, including alcohol abuse[15], there are changes in EC levels in various regions of the brain [12, 18, 175, 208]. Therefore, drugs or agents which regulate the level of ECs by inhibiting their metabolism (FAAH inhibitors such as URB597) or uptake (AM404) or synthesis (orlistat) could locally target sites while limiting the effects on uninvolved cognitive areas, and would thus be expected to have a higher therapeutic value [21, 87]. EC interactions with the dopamine system have been offered as a possible mechanism for some of the therapeutic potential of cannabinoid-based drugs in alcoholism.

3. Conclusion

In this chapter, we focused on the roles of ECs as retrograde modulators of short-term and long-term forms of synaptic plasticity. It is now widely accepted that ECs are released from postsynaptic neurons in an activity-dependent manner and induce transient or persistent suppression of transmitter release. These EC- mediated forms of synaptic plasticity are observed in various brain regions including the striatum, hippocampus, cortex, neocortex, amygdale, NAc, and cerebellum. Because CB1 is widely distributed in the CNS, it is expected that the EC signaling may be involved in synaptic plasticity throughout the CNS and contribute to various aspects of brain functions. In addition to the roles as retrograde messengers at synapses, ECs have other important functions that are discussed elsewhere. For example, ECs are reported to control the excitability of neocortical GABAergic interneurons in an autocrine manner [11]. ECs also play an important role in neuroprotection [196]. As reviewed in this chapter, recent studies have greatly expanded our knowledge of the EC system in the CNS. The development in EC research is also very important from a clinical point of view, because the EC system has been expected to provide potential targets not only for the treatment of habit forming behaviors but also neurological disorders.

4. Acknowledgements

The authors acknowledge support in part by grants from the National Institutes of Health (NIH AA11031 and NS049442), and the New York State Psychiatric Institute (BSB).

5. References

[1] Abood, M.E., Ditto, K.E., Noel, M.A., Showalter, V.M., Tao, Q. (1997). Isolation and expression of a mouse CB1 cannabinoid receptor gene. Comparison of binding properties with those of native CB1 receptors in mouse brain and N18TG2 neuroblastoma cells. *Biochem Pharmacol*, 53, 207-214.

[2] Alger, B.E. (2002). Retrograde signaling in the regulation of synaptic transmission: focus on endocannabinoids. *Progress in Neurobiology*, 68, 247-286.

[3] Alger, B.E., Pitler, T.A., Wagner, J.J., Martin, L.A, .Morishita, W., Kirov, S.A., Lenz, R.A. (1996). Retrograde signalling in depolarization-induced suppression of inhibition in rat hippocampal CA1 cells. *J Physiol*, 496, 197-209.

[4] Anwyl, R. (1999). Metabotropic glutamate receptors: electrophysiological properties and role in plasticity. *Brain Res Brain Res Rev*, 29, 83-120.

[5] Arancio, O., Kandel, E.R., Hawkins, R.D. (1995). Activity-dependent long-term enhancement of transmitter release by presynaptic 3',5'-cyclic GMP in cultured hippocampal neurons. *Nature*, 376, 74-80.

[6] Arancio, O., Kiebler, M., Lee, C.J., Lev-Ram, V., Tsien, R.Y., Kandel, E.R., Hawkins, R.D. (1996). Nitric oxide acts directly in the presynaptic neuron to produce long-term potentiation in cultured hippocampal neurons. *Cell*, 87, 1025-1035.

[7] Arancio, O., Lev-Ram, V., Tsien, R.Y., Kandel, E.R., Hawkins, R.D. (1996). Nitric oxide acts as a retrograde messenger during long-term potentiation in cultured hippocampal neurons. *J Physiol Paris*, 90, 321-322.

[8] Atwood, H.L., Wojtowicz, J.M. (1986). Short-term and long-term plasticity and physiological differentiation of crustacean motor synapses. *Int Rev Neurobiol*, 28, 275-362.

[9] Auclair, N., Otani, S., Soubrie, P., Crepel, F. (2000). Cannabinoids modulate synaptic strength and plasticity at glutamatergic synapses of rat prefrontal cortex pyramidal neurons. *J Neurophysiol*, 83, 3287-3293.

[10] Azad, S.C., Monory, K., Marsicano, G., Cravatt, B.F., Lutz, B., Zieglgansberger, W., Rammes, G. (2004). Circuitry for associative plasticity in the amygdala involves endocannabinoid signaling. *J Neurosci*, 24, 9953-9961.

[11] Bacci, A., Huguenard, J.R., Prince, D.A. (2004). Long-lasting self-inhibition of neocortical interneurons mediated by endocannabinoids. *Nature*, 431, 312-316.

[12] Baker, D., Pryce, G., Croxford, J.L., Brown, P., Pertwee, R.G., Makriyannis, A., Khanolkar, A., Layward, L., Fezza, F., Bisogno, T., Di Marzo, V. (2001). Endocannabinoids control spasticity in a multiple sclerosis model. *FASEB J*, 15, 300-302.

[13] Barbara, J.G., Auclair, N., Roisin, M.P., Otani, S., Valjent, E., Caboche, J., Soubrie, P., Crepel, F. (2003). Direct and indirect interactions between cannabinoid CB1 receptor and group II metabotropic glutamate receptor signalling in layer V pyramidal neurons from the rat prefrontal cortex. *Eur J Neurosci*, 17, 981-990.

[14] Basavarajappa, B.S. (2007). Critical Enzymes Involved in Endocannabinoid Metabolism. *Protein and Peptide letters*, 14, 237-246.

[15] Basavarajappa, B.S. (2007). The endocannabinoid signaling system: a potential target for next-generation therapeutics for alcoholism. *Mini-Reviews in Medicinal Chemistry*, 7, 769-779.

[16] Basavarajappa, B.S. (2007). Neuropharmacology of the endocannabinoid signaling system-Molecular mechanisms, biological actions and synaptic plasticity. *Current Neuropharmacology*, 5, 81-97.

[17] Basavarajappa, B.S., Hungund, B.L. (1999). Chronic Ethanol Increases the Cannabinoid Receptor Agonist, Anandamide and its Precursor N-Arachidonyl phosphatidyl ethanolamine in SK-N-SH Cells. *J. Neurochem*, 72, 522-528.

[18] Basavarajappa, B.S., Hungund, B.L. (2002). Neuromodulatory role of the endocannabinoid signaling system in alcoholism: an overview. *Prostaglandins Leukot Essent Fatty Acids*, 66, 287-299.

[19] Basavarajappa, B.S., Saito, M., Cooper, T.B., Hungund, B.L. (2000). Stimulation of cannabinoid receptor agonist 2-arachidonylglycerol by chronic ethanol and its modulation by specific neuromodulators in cerebellar granule neurons. *Biochemica Biophysica Acta*, 1535, 78-86.

[20] Basavarajappa, B.S., Saito, M., Cooper, T.B., Hungund, B.L. (2003). Chronic ethanol inhibits the anandamide transport and increases extracellular anandamide levels in cerebellar granule neurons. *Eur J Pharmacol*, 466, 73-83.

[21] Basavarajappa, B.S., Yalamanchili, R., Cravatt, B.F., Cooper, T.B., Hungund, B.L. (2006). Increased ethanol consumption and preference and decreased ethanol sensitivity in female FAAH knockout mice. *Neuropharmacology*, 50, 834-844.

[22] Beltramo, M., Piomelli, D. (2000). Carrier-mediated transport and enzymatic hydrolysis of the endogenous cannabinoid 2-arachidonylglycerol. *NeuroReport*, 11, 1231-1235.

[23] Beltramo, M., Stella, N., Calignano, A., Lin, S.Y., Makriyannis, A., Piomelli, D. (1997). Functional role of high-affinity anandamide transport, as revealed by selective inhibition. *Science*, 277, 1094-1097.

[24] Bisogno, T., MacCarrone, M., De Petrocellis, L., Jarrahian, A., Finazzi-Agro, A., Hillard, C., Di Marzo, V. (2001). The uptake by cells of 2-arachidonoylglycerol, an endogenous agonist of cannabinoid receptors. *Eur J Biochem*, 268, 1982-1989.

[25] Bisogno, T., Melck, D., De Petrocellis, L., Di Marzo, V. (1999). Phosphatidic acid as the biosynthetic precursor of the endocannabinoid 2-arachidonoylglycerol in intact mouse neuroblastoma cells stimulated with ionomycin. *Journal of Neurochemistry*, 72, 2113-2119.

[26] Bliss, T.V., Gardner-Medwin, A.R. (1973). Long-lasting potentiation of synaptic transmission in the dentate area of the unanaestetized rabbit following stimulation of the perforant path. *J Physiol*, 232, 357-374.

[27] Bouaboula, M., Poinot-Chazel, C., Bourrie, B., Canat, X., Calandra, B., Rinaldi-Carmona, M., Le Fur, G., Casellas, P. (1995). Activation of mitogen-activated protein kinases by stimulation of the central cannabinoid receptor CB1. *Biochem J*, 312, 637-641.

[28] Breivogel, C.S., Griffin, G., Di Marzo, V., Martin, B.R. (2001). Evidence for a new G protein-coupled cannabinoid receptor in mouse brain. *Mol Pharmacol*, 60, 155-163.

[29] Brenowitz, S.D., Regehr, W.G. (2005). Associative short-term synaptic plasticity mediated by endocannabinoids. *Neuron*, 45, 419-431.

[30] Brown, S.P., Brenowitz, S.D., Regehr, W.G. (2003). Brief presynaptic bursts evoke synapse-specific retrograde inhibition mediated by endogenous cannabinoids. *Nat Neurosci*, 6, 1048-1057.

[31] Brown, S.P., Safo, P.K., Regehr, W.G. (2004). Endocannabinoids inhibit transmission at granule cell to Purkinje cell synapses by modulating three types of presynaptic calcium channels. *J Neurosci*, 24, 5623-5631.

[32] Burstein, S.H., Rossetti, R.G., Yagen, B., Zurier, R.B. (2000). Oxidative metabolism of anandamide. *Prostaglandins Other Lipid Mediat*, 61, 29-41.

[33] Cadas, H., di Tomaso, E., Piomelli, D. (1997). Occurrence and biosynthesis of endogenous cannabinoid precursor, N-arachidonoyl phosphatidylethanolamine, in rat brain. *J. Neurosci*, 17, 1226-1242.

[34] Calabresi, P., Maj, R., Pisani, A., Mercuri, N.B., Bernardi, G. (1992). Long-term synaptic depression in the striatum: physiological and pharmacological characterization. *J Neurosci*, 12, 4224-4233.

[35] Carlson, G., Wang, Y., Alger, B.E. (2002). Endocannabinoids facilitate the induction of LTP in the hippocampus. *Nat Neurosci*, 5, 723-724.

[36] Carrier, E.J., Kearn, C.S., Barkmeier, A.J., Breese, N.M., Yang, W.Nithipatikom, K.Pfister, S.L., Campbell, W.B., Hillard, C.J. (2004). Cultured rat microglial cells synthesize the endocannabinoid 2-arachidonylglycerol, which increases proliferation via a CB2 receptor-dependent mechanism. *Mol Pharmacol*, 65, 999-1007.

[37] Cartmell, J., Schoepp, D.D. (2000). Regulation of neurotransmitter release by metabotropic glutamate receptors. *J Neurochem*, 75, 889-907.

[38] Castillo, P.E., Schoch, S., Schmitz, F., Sudhof, T.C., Malenka, R.C. (2002). RIM1alpha is required for presynaptic long-term potentiation. *Nature*, 415, 327-330.
[39] Caulfield, M.P., Brown, D.A. (1992). Cannabinoid receptor agonists inhibit Ca current in NG108-15 neuroblastoma cells via a pertussis toxin-sensitive mechanism. *Br J Pharmacol*, 106, 231-232.
[40] Caulfield, M.P., Robbins, J., Brown, D.A. (1992). Neurotransmitters inhibit the omega-conotoxin-sensitive component of Ca current in neuroblastoma x glioma hybrid (NG 108-15) cells, not the nifedipine-sensitive component. *Pflugers Arch*, 420, 486-492.
[41] Chakrabarti, A., Onaivi, E.S., Chaudhuri, G. (1995). Cloning and sequencing of a cDNA encoding the mouse brain-type cannabinoid receptor protein. *DNA Seq*, 6, 385-388.
[42] Chevaleyre, V., Castillo, P.E. (2003). Heterosynaptic LTD of hippocampal GABAergic synapses: a novel role of endocannabinoids in regulating excitability. *Neuron*, 38, 461-472.
[43] Chevaleyre, V., Castillo, P.E. (2004). Endocannabinoid-mediated metaplasticity in the hippocampus. *Neuron*, 43, 871-881.
[44] Childers, S.R., Sexton, T., Roy, M.B. (1994). Effects of anandamide on cannabinoid receptors in rat brain membranes. *Biochem. Pharmacol*, 47, 711-715.
[45] Choi, S., Lovinger, D.M. (1997). Decreased frequency but not amplitude of quantal synaptic responses associated with expression of corticostriatal long-term depression. *J Neurosci*, 17, 8613-8620.
[46] Choi, S., Lovinger, D.M. (1997). Decreased probability of neurotransmitter release underlies striatal long-term depression and postnatal development of corticostriatal synapses. *Proc Natl Acad Sci U S A*, 94, 2665-2670.
[47] Citri, A., Malenka, R.C. (2008). Synaptic plasticity: multiple forms, functions, and mechanisms. *Neuropsychopharmacology*, 33, 18-41.
[48] Cleland, J.G., Ghosh, J., Freemantle, N., Kaye, G.C., Nasir, M., Clark, A.L., Coletta, A.P. (2004). Clinical trials update and cumulative meta-analyses from the American College of Cardiology: WATCH, SCD-HeFT, DINAMIT, CASINO, INSPIRE, STRATUS-US, RIO-Lipids and cardiac resynchronisation therapy in heart failure. *Eur J Heart Fail*, 6, 501-508.
[49] Conn, P.J., Pin, J.P. (1997). Pharmacology and functions of metabotropic glutamate receptors. *Annu Rev Pharmacol Toxicol*, 37, 205-237.
[50] Dan, Y., Poo, M.M. (2004). Spike timing-dependent plasticity of neural circuits. *Neuron*, 44, 23-30.
[51] Daniel, H., Crepel, F. (2001). Control of Ca(2+) influx by cannabinoid and metabotropic glutamate receptors in rat cerebellar cortex requires K(+) channels. *J Physiol*, 537, 793-800.
[52] Daniel, H., Rancillac, A., Crepel, F. (2004). Mechanisms underlying cannabinoid inhibition of presynaptic Ca2+ influx at parallel fibre synapses of the rat cerebellum. *J Physiol*, 557, 159-174.
[53] Day, T.A., Rakhshan, F., Deutsch, D.G., Barker, E.L. (2001). Role of fatty acid amide hydrolase in the transport of the endogenous cannabinoid anandamide. *Mol Pharmacol*, 59, 1369-1375.

[54] Derkinderen, P., Toutant, M., Burgaya, F., Le Bert, M., Siciliano, J.C., de Franciscis, V., Gelman, M., Girault, J.A. (1996). Regulation of a neuronal form of focal adhesion kinase by anandamide. *Science*, 273, 1719-1722.

[55] Derkinderen, P., Toutant, M., Kadare, G., Ledent, C., Parmentier, M., Girault, J.A. (2001). Dual role of Fyn in the regulation of FAK+6,7 by cannabinoids in hippocampus. *J Biol Chem*, 276, 38289-38296.

[56] Deutsch, D.G., Glaser, S.T., Howell, J.M., Kunz, J.S., Puffenbarger, R.A., Hillard, C.J., Abumrad, N. (2001). The cellular uptake of anandamide is coupled to its breakdown by fatty-acid amide hydrolase. *J Biol Chem*, 276, 6967-6973.

[57] Devane, W.A., Hanus, L., Breuer, A., Pertwee, R.G., Stevenson, L.A., Griffin, G., Gibson, D., Mandelbaum, A., Etinger, A., Mechoulam, R. (1992). Isolation and structure of a brain constituent that binds to the cannabinoid receptor. *Science*, 258, 1946-1949.

[58] Dewey, W.L. (1986). Cannabinoid pharmacology. *Pharmacol Rev*, 38, 151-178.

[59] Di Marzo, V. (1998). 'Endocannabinoids' and other fatty acid derivatives with cannabimimetic properties: biochemistry and possible. *Biochim Biophys Acta*, 1392, 153-175.

[60] Di Marzo, V., Breivogel, C.S., Tao, Q., Bridgen, D.T., Razdan, R.K., Zimmer, A.M., Zimmer, A., Martin, B.R. (2000). Levels, metabolism, and pharmacological activity of anandamide in CB(1) cannabinoid receptor knockout mice: evidence for non-CB(1), non-CB(2) receptor-mediated actions of anandamide in mouse brain. *J Neurochem*, 75, 2434-2444.

[61] Di Marzo, V., Fontana, A., Cadas, H., Schinelli, S., Cimino, G., Schwartz, J.C., Piomelli, D. (1994). Formation and inactivation of endogenous cannabinoid anandamide in central neurons. *Nature*, 372, 686-691.

[62] Diana, M.A., Levenes, C., Mackie, K., Marty, A. (2002). Short-term retrograde inhibition of GABAergic synaptic currents in rat Purkinje cells is mediated by endogenous cannabinoids. *J Neurosci*, 22, 200-208.

[63] Diana, M.A., Marty, A. (2003). Characterization of depolarization-induced suppression of inhibition using paired interneuron--Purkinje cell recordings. *J Neurosci*, 23, 5906-5918.

[64] Dinh, T.P., Carpenter, D., Leslie, F., M.Freund, T.F., Katona, I., Sensi, S.L., Kathuria, S., Piomelli, D. (2002). Brain monoglyceride lipase participating in endocannabinoid inactivation. *Proc Natl Acad Sci U S A*, 99, 10819-10824.

[65] Doherty, J., Dingledine, R. (2003). Functional interactions between cannabinoid and metabotropic glutamate receptors in the central nervous system. *Curr Opin Pharmacol*, 3, 46-53.

[66] Ellert-Miklaszewska, A., Grajkowska, W., Gabrusiewicz, K., Kaminska, B., Konarska, L. (2007). Distinctive pattern of cannabinoid receptor type II (CB2) expression in adult and pediatric brain tumors. *Brain Res*, 1137, 161-9.

[67] Facci, L., Dal Toso, R., Romanello, S., Buriani, A., Skaper, S.D., Leon, A. (1995). Mast cells express a peripheral cannabinoid receptor with differential sensitivity to anandamide and palmitoylethanolamide. *Proc Natl Acad Sci U S A*, 92, 3376-3380.

[68] Freund, T.F., Katona, I., Piomelli, D. (2003). Role of endogenous cannabinoids in synaptic signaling. *Physiol Rev*, 83, 1017-1066.

[69] Fried, P., Watkinson, B., James, D., Gray, R. (2002). Current and former marijuana use: preliminary findings of a longitudinal study of effects on IQ in young adults. *Cmaj*, 166, 887-891.

[70] Fukudome, Y., Ohno-Shosaku, T., Matsui, M., Omori, Y., Fukaya, M., Tsubokawa, H., Taketo, M.M., Watanabe, M., Manabe, T., Kano, M. (2004). Two distinct classes of muscarinic action on hippocampal inhibitory synapses: M2-mediated direct suppression and M1/M3-mediated indirect suppression through endocannabinoid signalling. *Eur J Neurosci*, 19, 2682-2692.

[71] Gebremedhin, D., Lange, A.R., Campbell, W.B., Hillard, C.J., Harder, D.R. (1999). Cannabinoid CB1 receptor of cat cerebral arterial muscle functions to inhibit L-type Ca2+ channel current. *Am J Physiol*, 276, H2085-2093.

[72] Gerard, C.M., Mollereau, C., Vassart, G., Parmentier, M. (1991). Molecular cloning of a human cannabinoid receptor which is also expressed in testis. *Biochem J*, 279, 129-134.

[73] Gerdeman, G., Lovinger, D.M. (2001). CB1 cannabinoid receptor inhibits synaptic release of glutamate in rat dorsolateral striatum. *J Neurophysiol*, 85, 468-471.

[74] Gerdeman, G.L., Ronesi, J., Lovinger, D.M. (2002). Postsynaptic endocannabinoid release is critical to long-term depression in the striatum. *Nat Neurosci*, 5, 446-451.

[75] Giuffrida, A., Beltramo, M., Piomelli, D. (2001). Mechanisms of endocannabinoid inactivation: biochemistry and pharmacology. *J Pharmacol Exp Ther*, 298, 7-14.

[76] Giuffrida, A., Parsons, L.H., Kerr, T.M., Rodriguez de Fonseca, F., Navarro, M., Piomelli, D. (1999). Dopamine activation of endogenous cannabinoid signaling in dorsal striatum. *Nat Neurosci*, 2, 358-363.

[77] Glaser, S.T., Abumrad, N.A., Fatade, F., Kaczocha, M., Studholme, K.M., Deutsch, D.G. (2003). Evidence against the presence of an anandamide transporter. *Proc Natl Acad Sci U S A*, 100, 4269-4274.

[78] Gong, J.P., Onaivi, E.S., Ishiguro, H., Liu, Q.R., Tagliaferro, P.A., Brusco, A., Uhl, G.R. (2006). Cannabinoid CB2 receptors: immunohistochemical localization in rat brain. *Brain Res*, 1071, 10-23.

[79] Gonzalez, S., Scorticati, C., Garcia-Arencibia, M., de Miguel, R., Ramos, J.A., Fernandez-Ruiz, J. (2006). Effects of rimonabant, a selective cannabinoid CB1 receptor antagonist, in a rat model of Parkinson's disease. *Brain Res*, 1073-1074, 209-219.

[80] Goparaju, S.K., Ueda, N., Yamaguchi, H., Yamamoto, S. (1998). Anandamide amidohydrolase reacting with 2-arachidonoylglycerol, another cannabinoid receptor ligand. *FEBS Lett*, 422, 69-73.

[81] Gulyas, A.I., Cravatt, B.F., Bracey, M.H., Dinh, T.P., Piomelli, D., Boscia, F., Freund, T.F. (2004). Segregation of two endocannabinoid-hydrolyzing enzymes into pre- and postsynaptic compartments in the rat hippocampus, cerebellum and amygdala. *Eur J Neurosci*, 20, 441-458.

[82] Haj-Dahmane, S., Shen, R.Y. (2005). The wake-promoting peptide orexin-B inhibits glutamatergic transmission to dorsal raphe nucleus serotonin neurons through retrograde endocannabinoid signaling. *J Neurosci*, 25, 896-905.

[83] Hajos, N., Katona, I., Naiem, S.S., MacKie, K., Ledent, C., Mody, I., Freund, T.F. (2000). Cannabinoids inhibit hippocampal GABAergic transmission and network oscillations. *Eur J Neurosci*, 12, 3239-3249.

[84] Hajos, N., Ledent, C., Freund, T.F. (2001). Novel cannabinoid-sensitive receptor mediates inhibition of glutamatergic synaptic transmission in the hippocampus. *Neuroscience*, 106, 1-4.

[85] Hampson, R.E., Deadwyler, S.A. (1999). Cannabinoids, hippocampal function and memory. *Life Sci*, 65, 715-723.

[86] Hansen, H.H., Hansen, S.H., Schousboe, A., Hansen, H.S. (2000). Determination of the phospholipid precursor of anandamide and other N-acylethanolamine phospholipids before and after sodium azide-induced toxicity in cultured neocortical neurons. *J Neurochem*, 75, 861-871.

[87] Hansson, A.C., Bermudez-Silva, F.J., Malinen, H., Hyytia, P., Sanchez-Vera, I., Rimondini, R., Rodriguez de Fonseca, F., Kunos, G., Sommer, W.H., Heilig, M. (2006). Genetic Impairment of Frontocortical Endocannabinoid Degradation and High Alcohol Preference. *Neuropsychopharmacology*.

[88] Hanus, L., Abu-Lafi, S., Fride, E., Breuer, A., Vogel, Z., Shalev, D.E., Kustanovich, I., Mechoulam, R. (2001). 2-arachidonyl glyceryl ether, an endogenous agonist of the cannabinoid CB1 receptor. *Proc Natl Acad Sci U S A*, 98, 3662-3665.

[89] Hashimotodani, Y., Ohno-Shosaku, T., Tsubokawa, H., Ogata, H., Emoto, K., Maejima, T., Araishi, K., Shin, H.-S., Kano, M. (2005). Phospholipase C[beta] Serves as a Coincidence Detector through Its Ca2+ Dependency for Triggering Retrograde Endocannabinoid Signal. *Neuron*, 45, 257-268.

[90] Herkenham, M.A.B. L., Little, M.D., Johnson, M.R., Melvin, L.S., de Costa, B.R., Rice, K.C. (1990). Cannabinoid receptor localization in brain. *Proc. Natl. Acad. Sci. USA*, 87, 1932-1936.

[91] Herkenham, M., Lynn, A.B., Johnson, M.R., Melvin, L.S., de Cost, B.R., Rice, K.C. (1991). Characterization and localization of cannabinoid receptors in rat brain: a quantitative in vitro autoradiographic study. *J Neurosci*, 16, 8057-8066.

[92] Hill, E.L., Gallopin, T., Ferezou, I., Cauli, B., Rossier, J., Schweitzer, P., Lambolez, B. (2007). Functional CB1 receptors are broadly expressed in neocortical GABAergic and glutamatergic neurons. *J Neurophysiol*.

[93] Hillard, C.J, .Edgemond, W.S., Jarrahian, A., Campbell, W.B. (1997). Accumulation of N-arachidonoylethanolamine (anandamide) into cerebellar granule cells occurs via facilitated diffusion. *J Neurochem*, 69, 631-638.

[94] Hillard, C.J., Jarrahian, A. (2000). The movement of N-arachidonoylethanolamine (anandamide) across cellular membranes. *Chem Phys Lipids*, 108, 123-134.

[95] Hoffman, A.F., Lupica, C.R. (2000). Mechanisms of cannabinoid inhibition of GABA(A) synaptic transmission in the hippocampus. *J Neurosci*, 20, 2470-2479.

[96] Hoffman, A.F., Oz, M., Caulder, T., Lupica, C.R. (2003). Functional tolerance and blockade of long-term depression at synapses in the nucleus accumbens after chronic cannabinoid exposure. *J Neurosci*, 23, 4815-4820.

[97] Hollister, L.E. (1986). Health aspects of cannabis. *Pharmacol Rev*, 38, 1-20.

[98] Howlett, A.C., Barth, F., Bonner, T.I., Cabral, G., Casellas, P., Devane, W.A., Felder, C.C., Herkenham, M., Mackie, K., Martin, B.R., Mechoulam, R., Pertwee, R.G. (2002). International Union of Pharmacology. XXVII. Classification of cannabinoid receptors. *Pharmacol Rev*, 54, 161-202.

[99] Howlett, A.C., Mukhopadhyay, S. (2000). Cellular signal transduction by anandamide and 2-arachidonoylglycerol. *Chem Phys Lipids*, 108, 53-70.

[100] Huang, C.C., Lo, S.W., Hsu, K.S. (2001). Presynaptic mechanisms underlying cannabinoid inhibition of excitatory synaptic transmission in rat striatal neurons. *J Physiol*, 532 (Pt3), 731-748.

[101] Huang, S.M., Bisogno, T., Trevisani, M., Al-Hayani, A., De Petrocellis, L., Fezza, F., Tognetto, M., Petros, T.J., Krey, J.F., Chu, C.J., Miller, J.D., Davies, S.N., Geppetti, P., Walker, J.M., Di Marzo, V. (2002). An endogenous capsaicin-like substance with high potency at recombinant and native vanilloid VR1 receptors. *Proc Natl Acad Sci U S A*, 99, 8400-8405.

[102] Isaac, J.T., Nicoll, R.A., Malenka, R.C. (1995). Evidence for silent synapses: implications for the expression of LTP. *Neuron*, 15, 427-434.

[103] Ito, M. (2001). Cerebellar long-term depression: characterization, signal transduction, and functional roles. *Physiol Rev*, 81, 1143-1195.

[104] Jarai, Z., Wagner, J.A., Varga, K., Lake, K.D., Compton, D.R., Martin, B.R., Zimmer, A.M., Bonner, T.I., Buckley, N.E., Mezey, E., Razdan, R.K., Zimmer, A., Kunos, G. (1999). Cannabinoid-induced mesenteric vasodilation through an endothelial site distinct from CB1 or CB2 receptors. *Proc Natl Acad Sci U S A*, 96, 14136-14141.

[105] Jung, K.M., Mangieri, R., Stapleton, C., Kim, J., Fegley, D., Wallace, M., Mackie, K., Piomelli, D. (2005). Stimulation of endocannabinoid formation in brain slice cultures through activation of group I metabotropic glutamate receptors. *Mol Pharmacol*, 68, 1196-1202.

[106] Kabelik, J., Krejci, Z., Santavy, F. (1960). Cannabis as a Medicant. *Bull. Narc*, 12, 5-23.

[107] Katona, I., Rancz, E.A., Acsady, L., Ledent, C., Mackie, K., Hajos, N., Freund, T.F. (2001). Distribution of CB1 cannabinoid receptors in the amygdala and their role in the control of GABAergic transmission. *J Neurosci*, 21, 9506-9518.

[108] [108]Katona, I., Sperlagh, B., Sik, A., Kafalvi, A., Vizi, E.S., Mackie, K., Freund, T.F. (1999). Presynaptically located CB1 cannabinoid receptors regulate GABA release from axon terminals of specific hippocampal interneurons. *J Neurosci*, 19, 4544-4558.

[109] Kauer, J.A., Malenka, R.C. (2006). LTP, AMPA receptors trading places. *Nat Neurosci*, 9, 593-594.

[110] Kim, J., Alger, B.E. (2004). Inhibition of cyclooxygenase-2 potentiates retrograde endocannabinoid effects in hippocampus. *Nat Neurosci*, 7, 697-698.

[111] Kim, J., Isokawa, M., Ledent, C., Alger, B.E. (2002). Activation of muscarinic acetylcholine receptors enhances the release of endogenous cannabinoids in the hippocampus. *J Neurosci*, 22, 10182-10191.

[112] Kishimoto, Y., Kano, M. (2006). Endogenous cannabinoid signaling through the CB1 receptor is essential for cerebellum-dependent discrete motor learning. *J Neurosci*, 26, 8829-8837.

[113] Kishimoto, Y., Nakazawa, K., Tonegawa, S., Kirino, Y., Kano, M. (2006). Hippocampal CA3 NMDA receptors are crucial for adaptive timing of trace eyeblink conditioned response. *J Neurosci*, 26, 1562-1570.

[114] Konrad, R.J., Major, C.D., Wolf, B.A. (1994). Diacylglycerol hydrolysis to arachidonic acid is necessary for insulin secretion from isolated pancreatic islets: sequential actions of diacylglycerol and monoacylglycerol lipases. *Biochemistry*, 33, 13284-13294.

[115] Kozak, K.R., Crews, B.C., Morrow, J.D., Wang, L.H., Ma, Y.H., Weinander, R.Jakobsson, P.J., Marnett, L.J. (2002). Metabolism of the endocannabinoids, 2-

arachidonylglycerol and anandamide, into prostaglandin, thromboxane, and prostacyclin glycerol esters and ethanolamides. *J Biol Chem*, 277, 44877-44885.

[116] Kreitzer, A.C., Malenka, R.C. (2005). Dopamine modulation of state-dependent endocannabinoid release and long-term depression in the striatum. *J Neurosci*, 25, 10537-10545.

[117] Kreitzer, A.C., Regehr, W.G. (2001). Cerebellar depolarization-induced suppression of inhibition is mediated by endogenous cannabinoids. *J Neurosci*, 21, RC174.

[118] Kreitzer, A.C., Regehr, W.G. (2001). Retrograde inhibition of presynaptic calcium influx by endogenous cannabinoids at excitatory synapses onto Purkinje cells. *Neuron*, 29, 717-727.

[119] LeDoux, J.E. (2000). Emotion circuits in the brain. *Annu Rev Neurosci*, 23, 155-184.

[120] Leung, D., Saghatelian, A., Simon, G.M., Cravatt, B.F. (2006). Inactivation of N-acyl phosphatidylethanolamine phospholipase D reveals multiple mechanisms for the biosynthesis of endocannabinoids. *Biochemistry*, 45, 4720-4726.

[121] Liu, J., Wang, L., Harvey-White, J., Osei-Hyiaman, D., Razdan, R., Gong, Q., Chan, A.C., Zhou, Z., Huang, B.X., Kim, H.Y., Kunos, G. (2006). A biosynthetic pathway for anandamide. *Proc Natl Acad Sci U S A*, 103, 13345-13350.

[122] Llano, I., Leresche, N., Marty, A. (1991). Calcium entry increases the sensitivity of cerebellar Purkinje cells to applied GABA and decreases inhibitory synaptic currents. *Neuron*, 6, 565-574.

[123] Maass, W., Bishop, C.M. (1999). Pulsed Neural Networks. MIT Press.

[124] Maccarrone, M., van der Stelt, M., Rossi, A., Veldink, G.A., Vliegenthart, J.F., Agro, A.F. (1998). Anandamide hydrolysis by human cells in culture and brain. *J Biol Chem*, 273, 32332-32339.

[125] Mackie, K., Hille, B. (1992). Cannabinoids inhibit N-type calcium channels in neuroblastoma-glioma cells. *Proc Natl Acad Sci U S A*, 89, 3825-3829.

[126] Madison, D.V., Malenka, R.C., Nicoll, R.A. (1991). Mechanisms underlying long-term potentiation of synaptic transmission. *Annu Rev Neurosci*, 14, 379-397.

[127] Maejima, T., Ohno-Shosaku, T., Kano, M. (2001). Endogenous cannabinoid as a retrograde messenger from depolarized postsynaptic neurons to presynaptic terminals. *Neurosci Res*, 40, 205-210.

[128] Maejima, T., Oka, S., Hashimotodani, Y., Ohno-Shosaku, T., Aiba, A., Wu, D., Waku, K., Sugiura, T., Kano, M. (2005). Synaptically Driven Endocannabinoid Release Requires Ca2+-Assisted Metabotropic Glutamate Receptor Subtype 1 to Phospholipase C {beta}4 Signaling Cascade in the Cerebellum. pp. 6826-6835.

[129] Magleby, K.L. (1987). Short-term changes in synaptic efficacy. In: Edelman, G.M.G. W.E, Cowan, W.M, Ed, In: Synaptic function. New York, Wiley. pp. 21-56.

[130] Makara, J.K., Mor, M., Fegley, D., Szabo, S.I., Kathuria, S., Astarita, G., Duranti, A., Tontini, A., Tarzia, G., Rivara, S., Freund, T.F., Piomelli, D. (2005). Selective inhibition of 2-AG hydrolysis enhances endocannabinoid signaling in hippocampus. *Nat Neurosci*, 8, 1139-1141.

[131] Maldonado, R., Rodriguez de Fonseca, F. (2002). Cannabinoid addiction: behavioral models and neural correlates. *J Neurosci*, 22, 3326-3331.

[132] Malenka, R.C. (1991). The role of postsynaptic calcium in the induction of long-term potentiation. *Mol Neurobiol*, 5, 289-295.

[133] Malenka, R.C. (2003). The long-term potential of LTP. *Nat Rev Neurosci*, 4, 923-926.

[134] Malenka, R.C., Bear, M.F. (2004). LTP and LTD: an embarrassment of riches. *Neuron*, 44, 5-21.

[135] Marcaggi, P., Attwell, D. (2005). Endocannabinoid signaling depends on the spatial pattern of synapse activation. *Nat Neurosci*, 8, 776-781.

[136] Marsicano, G., Wotjak, C.T., Azad, S.C., Bisogno, T., Rammes, G., Cascio, M.G., Hermann, H., Tang, J., Hofmann, C., Zieglgansberger, W., Di Marzo, V., Lutz, B. (2002). The endogenous cannabinoid system controls extinction of aversive memories. *Nature*, 418, 530-534.

[137] Marsicano, G., Wotjak, C.T., Azad, S.C., Bisogno, T., Rammes, G., Cascio, M.G., Hermann, H., Tang, J., Hofmann, C., Zieglgansberger, W., Di Marzo, V., Lutz, B. (2002). The endogenous cannabinoid system controls extinction of aversive memories. *Nature*, 418, 530-534.

[138] Mato, S., Chevaleyre, V., Robbe, D., Pazos, A., Castillo, P.E., Manzoni, O.J. (2004). A single in-vivo exposure to delta 9THC blocks endocannabinoid-mediated synaptic plasticity. *Nat Neurosci*, 7, 585-586.

[139] Matsuda, L.A., Bonner, T.I., Lolait, S.J. (1993). Localization of cannabinoid receptor mRNA in rat brain. *J Comp Neurol*, 327, 535-550.

[140] Mazzola, C., Micale, V., Drago, F. (2003). Amnesia induced by beta-amyloid fragments is counteracted by cannabinoid CB1 receptor blockade. *Eur J Pharmacol*, 477, 219-225.

[141] Mechoulam, R., Ben-Shabat, S., Hanus, L., Ligumsky, M., Kaminski, N.E., Schatz, A.R., Gopher, A., Almog, S., Martin, B.R., Compton, D.R., Pertwee, R.G., Griffin, G.Bayewitch, M., Barg, J., Vogel, Z. (1995). Identification of an endogenous 2-monoglyceride, present in canine gut, that binds to cannabinoid receptors. *Biochem Pharmacol*, 50, 83-90.

[142] Mechoulam, R., Fride, E., Di Marzo, V. (1998). Endocannabinoids. *Eur J Pharmacol*, 359, 1-18.

[143] Melis, M., Perra, S., Muntoni, A.L., Pillolla, G., Lutz, B., Marsicano, G., Di Marzo, V., Gessa, G.L., Pistis, M. (2004). Prefrontal cortex stimulation induces 2-arachidonoyl-glycerol-mediated suppression of excitation in dopamine neurons. *J Neurosci*, 24, 10707-10715.

[144] Melis, M., Pistis, M., Perra, S., Muntoni, A.L., Pillolla, G., Gessa, G.L. (2004). Endocannabinoids Mediate Presynaptic Inhibition of Glutamatergic Transmission in Rat Ventral Tegmental Area Dopamine Neurons through Activation of CB1 Receptors. *J. Neurosci*, 24, 53-62.

[145] Miura, M., Watanabe, M., Offermanns, S., Simon, M.I., Kano, M. (2002). Group I metabotropic glutamate receptor signaling via Galpha q/Galpha 11 secures the induction of long-term potentiation in the hippocampal area CA1. *J Neurosci*, 22, 8379-8390.

[146] Morishita, W., Alger, B.E. (2000). Differential effects of the group II mGluR agonist, DCG-IV, on depolarization-induced suppression of inhibition in hippocampal CA1 and CA3 neurons. *Hippocampus*, 10, 261-268.

[147] Morisset, V., Urban, L. (2001). Cannabinoid-induced presynaptic inhibition of glutamatergic EPSCs in substantia gelatinosa neurons of the rat spinal cord. *J Neurophysiol*, 86, 40-48.

[148] Mu, J., Zhuang, S.Y., Kirby, M.T., Hampson, R.E., Deadwyler, S.A. (1999). Cannabinoid receptors differentially modulate potassium A and D currents in hippocampal neurons in culture. *J. Pharmacol. Exp. Ther*, 291, 893-902.

[149] Mukhopadhyay, S., McIntosh, H.H., Houston, D.B., Howlett, A.C. (2000). The CB(1) cannabinoid receptor juxtamembrane C-terminal peptide confers activation to specific G proteins in brain. *Mol Pharmacol*, 57, 162-170.

[150] Mulder, A.M., Cravatt, B.F. (2006). Endocannabinoid Metabolism in the Absence of Fatty Acid Amide Hydrolase (FAAH): Discovery of Phosphorylcholine Derivatives of N-Acyl Ethanolamines. *Biochemistry*, 45, 11267-11277.

[151] Munro, S., Thomas, K.L., Abu-Shaar, M. (1993). Molecular characterization of a peripheral receptor for cannabinoids. *Nature*, 365, 61-65.

[152] Nakane, S., Oka, S., Arai, S., Waku, K., Ishima, Y., Tokumura, A., Sugiura, T. (2002). 2-Arachidonoyl-sn-glycero-3-phosphate, an arachidonic acid-containing lysophosphatidic acid: occurrence and rapid enzymatic conversion to 2-arachidonoyl-sn-glycerol, a cannabinoid receptor ligand, in rat brain. *Arch Biochem Biophys*, 402, 51-58.

[153] Natarajan, V., Reddy, P.V., Schmid, P.C., Schmid, H.H. (1981). On the biosynthesis and metabolism of N-acylethanolamine phospholipids in infarcted dog heart. *Biochim Biophys Acta*, 664, 445-448.

[154] Nicoll, R.A., Kauer, J.A., Malenka, R.C. (1988). The current excitement in long-term potentiation. *Neuron*, 1, 97-103.

[155] Nogueron, M.I., Porgilsson, B., Schneider, W.E., Stucky, C.L., Hillard, C.J. (2001). Cannabinoid receptor agonists inhibit depolarization-induced calcium influx in cerebellar granule neurons. *J Neurochem*, 79, 371-381.

[156] Ohno-Shosaku, T., Maejima, T., Kano, M. (2001). Endogenous cannabinoids mediate retrograde signals from depolarized postsynaptic neurons to presynaptic terminal. *Neuron*, 29, 729-738.

[157] Ohno-Shosaku, T., Matsui, M., Fukudome, Y., Shosaku, J., Tsubokawa, H., Taketo, M.M., Manabe, T., Kano, M. (2003). Postsynaptic M1 and M3 receptors are responsible for the muscarinic enhancement of retrograde endocannabinoid signalling in the hippocampus. *Eur J Neurosci*, 18, 109-116.

[158] Ohno-Shosaku, T., Sawada, S., Kano, M. (2000). Heterosynaptic expression of depolarization-induced suppression of inhibition (DSI) in rat hippocampal cultures. *Neurosci Res*, 36, 67-71.

[159] Ohno-Shosaku, T., Sawada, S., Yamamoto, C. (1998). Properties of depolarization-induced suppression of inhibitory transmission in cultured rat hippocampal neurons. *Pflugers Arch*, 435, 273-279.

[160] Ohno-Shosaku, T., Tsubokawa, H., Mizushima, I., Yoneda, N., Zimmer, A., Kano, M. (2002). Presynaptic cannabinoid sensitivity is a major determinant of depolarization-induced retrograde suppression at hippocampal synapses. *J Neurosci*, 22, 3864-3872.

[161] Onaivi, E.S., Ishiguro, H., Gong, J.P., Patel, S., Perchuk, A., Meozzi, P.A., Myers, L., Mora, Z., Tagliaferro, P., Gardner, E., Brusco, A., Akinshola, B.E., Liu, Q.R., Hope, B., Iwasaki, S., Arinami, T., Teasenfitz, L., Uhl, G.R. (2006). Discovery of the presence and functional expression of cannabinoid CB2 receptors in brain. *Ann N Y Acad Sci*, 1074, 514-536.

[162] Pan, X., Ikeda, S.R., Lewis, D.L. (1996). Rat brain cannabinoid receptor modulates N-type Ca2+ channels in a neuronal expression system. *Mol Pharmacol*, 49, 707-714.

[163] Pinto, J.C., Potie, F., Rice, K.C., Boring, D., Johnson, M.R., Evans, D.M., Wilken, G.H., Cantrell, C.H., Howlett, A.C. (1994). Cannabinoid receptor binding and agonist activity of amides and esters of arachidonic acid. *Mol. Pharmacol*, 46, 516-522.

[164] Piomelli, D. (2003). The molecular logic of endocannabinoid signalling. *Nat Rev Neurosci*, 4, 873-884.

[165] Pitler, T.A., Alger, B.E. (1990). Activation of the pharmacologically defined M3 muscarinic receptor depolarizes hippocampal pyramidal cells. *Brain Res.*, *534*, 257-262.

[166] Pitler, T.A., Alger, B.E. (1992) Postsynaptic spike firing reduces synaptic GABAA responses in hippocampal pyramidal cells. *J Neurosci*, 12, 4122-4132.

[167] Pitler, T.A., Alger, B.E. (1994). Depolarization-induced suppression of GABAergic inhibition in rat hippocampal pyramidal cells: G protein involvement in a presynaptic mechanism. *Neuron*, 13, 1447-1455.

[168] Porter, A.C., Sauer, J.M., Knierman, M.D., Becker, G.W., Berna, M.J., Bao, J., Nomikos, G.G., Carter, P., Bymaster, F.P., Leese, A.B., Felder, C.C. (2002). Characterization of a novel endocannabinoid, virodhamine, with antagonist activity at the CB1 receptor. *J Pharmacol Exp Ther*, 301, 1020-1024.

[169] Prescott, S.M., Majerus, P.W. (1983). Characterization of 1,2-diacylglycerol hydrolysis in human platelets. Demonstration of an arachidonoyl-monoacylglycerol intermediate. *J Biol Chem*, 258, 764-769.

[170] Robbe, D., Kopf, M., Remaury, A., Bockaert, J., Manzoni, O.J. (2002). Endogenous cannabinoids mediate long-term synaptic depression in the nucleus accumbens. *Proc Natl Acad Sci U S A*, 99, 8384-8388.

[171] Robinson, L., McKillop-Smith, S., Ross, N.L., Pertwee, R.G., Hampson, R.E., Platt, B., Riedel, G. (2007). Hippocampal endocannabinoids inhibit spatial learning and limit spatial memory in rats. *Psychopharmacology (Berl)*.

[172] Ronesi, J., Gerdeman, G.L., Lovinger, D.M. (2004). Disruption of endocannabinoid release and striatal long-term depression by postsynaptic blockade of endocannabinoid membrane transport. *J Neurosci*, 24, 1673-1679.

[173] Ross, R.A., Craib, S.J., Stevenson, L.A., Pertwee, R.G., Henderson, A., Toole, J., Ellington, H.C. (2002). Pharmacological characterization of the anandamide cyclooxygenase metabolite: prostaglandin E2 ethanolamide. *J Pharmacol Exp Ther*, 301, 900-907.

[174] Safo, P.K., Regehr, W.G. (2005). Endocannabinoids control the induction of cerebellar LTD. *Neuron*, 48, 647-659.

[175] Schabitz, W.R., Giuffrida, A., Berger, C., Aschoff, A., Schwaninger, M., Schwab, S., Piomelli, D. (2002). Release of fatty acid amides in a patient with hemispheric stroke: a microdialysis study. *Stroke*, 33, 2112-2114.

[176] Schmid, P.C., Reddy, P.V., Natarajan, V., Schmid, H.H. (1983). Metabolism of N-acylethanolamine phospholipids by a mammalian phosphodiesterase of the phospholipase D type. *J Biol Chem*, 258, 9302-9306.

[177] Shen, M., Thayer, S.A. (1998). The cannabinoid agonist Win55,212-2 inhibits calcium channels by receptor-mediated and direct pathways in cultured rat hippocampal neurons. *Brain Res*, 783, 77-84.

[178] Simpson, C.M., Itabe, H., Reynolds, C.N., King, W.C., Glomset, J.A. (1991). Swiss 3T3 cells preferentially incorporate sn-2-arachidonoyl monoacylglycerol into sn-1-stearoyl-2-arachidonoyl phosphatidylinositol. *J Biol Chem*, 266, 15902-15909.

[179] Sjostrom, P.J., Turrigiano, G.G., Nelson, S.B. (2003). Neocortical LTD via coincident activation of presynaptic NMDA and cannabinoid receptors. *Neuron*, 39, 641-654.

[180] Slanina, K.A., Roberto, M., Schweitzer, P. (2005). Endocannabinoids restrict hippocampal long-term potentiation via CB1. *Neuropharmacology*, 49, 660-668.

[181] Soderstrom, K., Johnson, F. (2000). CB1 cannabinoid receptor expression in brain regions associated with zebra finch song control. *Brain Res*, 857, 151-157.

[182] Soderstrom, K., Johnson, F. (2000). CB1 cannabinoid receptor expression in brain regions associated with zebra finch song control. *Brain Res*, 857, 151-157.

[183] Stefano, G.B., Salzet, B., Salzet, M. (1997). Identification and characterization of the leech CNS cannabinoid receptor: coupling to nitric oxide release. *Brain Res*, 753, 219-224.

[184] Stella, N., Schweitzer, P., Piomelli, D. (1997). A second endogenous cannabinoid that modulates long-term potentiation. *Nature*, 388, 773-778.

[185] Straiker, A., Mackie, K. (2005). Depolarization-induced suppression of excitation in murine autaptic hippocampal neurones. *J Physiol*, 569, 501-517.

[186] Sugiura, T., Kobayashi, Y., Oka, S., Waku, K. (2002). Biosynthesis and degradation of anandamide and 2-arachidonoylglycerol and their possible physiological significance. *Prostaglandins Leukot Essent Fatty Acids*, 66, 173-192.

[187] Sugiura, T., Kondo, S., Sukagawa, A., Nakane, S., Shinoda, A., Itoh, K., Yamashita, A., Waku, K. (1995). 2-Arachidonoylglycerol: a possible endogenous cannabinoid receptor ligand in brain. *Biochem Biophys Res Commun*, 215, 89-97.

[188] Sugiura, T., Yoshinaga, N., Kondo, S., Waku, K., Ishima, Y. (2000). Generation of 2-arachidonoylglycerol, an endogenous cannabinoid receptor ligand, in picrotoxinin-administered rat brain. *Biochem Biophys Res Commun*, 271, 654-658.

[189] Sullivan, J.M. (2000). Cellular and molecular mechanisms underlying learning and memory impairments produced by cannabinoids. *Learn Mem*, 7, 132-139.

[190] Sun, Y.X., Tsuboi, K., Okamoto, Y., Tonai, T., Murakami, M., Kudo, I., Ueda, N. (2004). Biosynthesis of anandamide and N-palmitoylethanolamine by sequential actions of phospholipase A2 and lysophospholipase D. *Biochem J*, 380, 749-756.

[191] Szabo, B., Dorner, L., Pfreundtner, C., Norenberg, W., Starke, K. (1998). Inhibition of GABAergic inhibitory postsynaptic currents by cannabinoids in rat corpus striatum. *Neuroscience*, 85, 395-403.

[192] Szabo, B., Urbanski, M.J., Bisogno, T., Di Marzo, V., Mendiguren, A., Baer, W.U., Freiman, I. (2006). Depolarization-induced retrograde synaptic inhibition in the mouse cerebellar cortex is mediated by 2-arachidonoylglycerol. *J Physiol*, 577, 263-280.

[193] Szabo, B., Wallmichrath, I., Mathonia, P., Pfreundtner, C. (2000). Cannabinoids inhibit excitatory neurotransmission in the substantia nigra pars reticulata. *Neuroscience*, 97, 89-97.

[194] Takahashi, K.A., Linden, D.J. (2000). Cannabinoid receptor modulation of synapses received by cerebellar Purkinje cells. *J Neurophysiol*, 83, 1167-1180.

[195] Twitchell, W., Brown, S., Mackie, K. (1997). Cannabinoids inhibit N- and P/Q-type calcium channels in cultured rat hippocampal neurons. *J Neurophysiol*, 78, 43-50.

[196] Van der Stelt, M., Fox, S.H., Hill, M., Crossman, A.R., Petrosino, S., Di Marzo, V., Brotchie, J.M. (2005). A role for endocannabinoids in the generation of parkinsonism and levodopa-induced dyskinesia in MPTP-lesioned non-human primate models of Parkinson's disease. *Faseb J*, 19, 1140-1142.

[197] Van der Stelt, M., Mazzola, C., Esposito, G., Matias, I., Petrosino, S., De Filippis, D., Micale, V., Steardo, L., Drago, F., Iuvone, T., Di Marzo, V. (2006). Endocannabinoids and beta-amyloid-induced neurotoxicity in vivo: effect of pharmacological elevation of endocannabinoid levels. *Cell Mol Life Sci*, 63, 1410-1424.

[198] Van Gaal, L., F.Rissanen, A., M.Scheen, A.J., Ziegler, O., Rossner, S. (2005). Effects of the cannabinoid-1 receptor blocker rimonabant on weight reduction and cardiovascular risk factors in overweight patients: 1-year experience from the RIO-Europe study. *Lancet*, 365, 1389-1397.

[199] Van Sickle, M.D., Duncan, M., Kingsley, P.J., Mouihate, A., Urbani, P., Mackie, K., Stella, N., Makriyannis, A., Piomelli, D., Davison, J.S., Marnett, L.J., Di Marzo, V., Pittman, Q.J., Patel, K.D., Sharkey, K.A. (2005). Identification and functional characterization of brainstem cannabinoid CB2 receptors. *Science*, 310, 329-332.

[200] Varma, N., Carlson, G.C., Ledent, C., Alger, B.E. (2001). Metabotropic glutamate receptors drive the endocannabinoid system in hippocampus. *J Neurosci*, 21, RC188.

[201] Varvel, S.A., Lichtman, A.H. (2002) Evaluation of CB1 receptor knockout mice in the Morris water maze. *J Pharmacol Exp Ther*, *301*, 915-924.

[202] Vaughan, C.W., Connor, M., Bagley, E.E., Christie, M.J. (2000). Actions of cannabinoids on membrane properties and synaptic transmission in rat periaqueductal gray neurons in vitro. *Mol Pharmacol*, 57, 288-295.

[203] Vaughan, C.W., McGregor, I.S., Christie, M.J. (1999). Cannabinoid receptor activation inhibits GABAergic neurotransmission in rostral ventromedial medulla neurons in vitro. *Br J Pharmacol*, 127, 935-940.

[204] Vincent, P., Armstrong, C.M., Marty, A. (1992). Inhibitory synaptic currents in rat cerebellar Purkinje cells: modulation by postsynaptic depolarization. *J Physiol*, 456, 453-471.

[205] Vincent, P., Marty, A. (1993). Neighboring cerebellar Purkinje cells communicate via retrograde inhibition of common presynaptic interneurons. *Neuron*, 11, 885-893.

[206] Vincent, P., Marty, A. (1996). Fluctuations of inhibitory postsynaptic currents in Purkinje cells from rat cerebellar slices. *J Physiol*, 494 (Pt 1), 183-199.

[207] Wagner, J.A., Varga, K., Jarai, Z., Kunos, G. (1999). Mesenteric vasodilation mediated by endothelial anandamide receptors. *Hypertension*, 33, 429-434.

[208] Walker, J., M., Huang, S.M. (2002). Endocannabinoids in pain modulation. *Prostaglandins Leukot Essent Fatty Acids*, 66, 235-242.

[209] Wartmann, M., Campbell, D., Subramanian, A., Burstein, S.H., Davis, R.J. (1995). The MAP kinase signal transduction pathway is activated by the endogenous cannabinoid anandamide. *FEBS Lett*, 2-3, 133-136.

[210] Watson, S.J., Benson, J., A., Jr., Joy, J.E. (2000). Marijuana and medicine: assessing the science base: a summary of the 1999 Institute of Medicine report. *Arch Gen Psychiatry*, 57, 547-552.

[211] Wilson, R., I.Kunos, G., Nicoll, R.A. (2001). Presynaptic specificity of endocannabinoid signaling in the hippocampus. *Neuron*, 31, 453-462.

[212] Wilson, R.I., Nicoll, R.A. (2001). Endogenous cannabinoids mediate retrograde signalling at hippocampal synapses. *Nature*, 410, 588-592.

[213] Wilson, R.I., Nicoll, R.A. (2002). Endocannabinoid Signaling in the Brain. *Science*, 296, 678-682.

[214] Yamaguchi, F., Macrae, A.D., Brenner, S. (1996). Molecular cloning of two cannabinoid type 1-like receptor genes from the puffer fish Fugu rubripes. *Genomics*, 35, 603-605.

[215] Yamasaki, M., Hashimoto, K., Kano, M. (2006). Miniature synaptic events elicited by presynaptic Ca2+ rise are selectively suppressed by cannabinoid receptor activation in cerebellar Purkinje cells. *J Neurosci*, 26, 86-95.

[216] Yoshida, T., Hashimoto, K., Zimmer, A., Maejima, T., Araishi, K., Kano, M. (2002). The Cannabinoid CB1 Receptor Mediates Retrograde Signals for Depolarization-Induced Suppression of Inhibition in Cerebellar Purkinje Cells. *J Neurosci*, 22, 1690-1697.

[217] Zhu, P.J., Lovinger, D.M. (2007). Persistent synaptic activity produces long-lasting enhancement of endocannabinoid modulation and alters long-term synaptic plasticity. *J Neurophysiol*, 97, 4386-4389.

[218] Zilberter, Y. (2000). Dendritic release of glutamate suppresses synaptic inhibition of pyramidal neurons in rat neocortex. *J Physiol*, 528 (Pt 3), 489-496.

In: Synaptic Plasticity: New Research
Editors: Tim F. Kaiser and Felix J. Peters
ISBN: 978-1-60456-732-8

Chapter 4

THE PRESENCE OF PERFORATED SYNAPSES IN THE STRIATUM AFTER DOPAMINE DEPLETION: IS THIS A SIGN OF NEGATIVE BRAIN PASTICITY?

Maria Rosa Avila-Costa*[1]*, Ana Luisa Gutierrez-Valdez, Jose Luis Ordoñez-Librado, Verónica Anaya-Martínez, Laura Colin-Barenque, César Sánchez Vázquez del Mercado and Leonardo Reynoso-Erazo
Universidad Nacional Autonoma de Mexico, FES Iztacala, Dept. Neurociencias, Mexico

ABSTRACT

Synaptic plasticity is the process by which long-lasting changes take place at synaptic connections. The concept of plasticity can be applied to molecular as well as to environmental events. The phenomenon itself is complex and can involve many levels of organization. Some authors separate forms into adaptations that have positive or negative consequences for the animal. For example, if an organism, after a stroke, can recover to normal levels of performance, that adaptiveness could be considered an example of "positive plasticity". An excessive level of neuronal growth leading to spasticity or tonic paralysis, or an excessive release of neurotransmitters in response to injury, which could kill nerve cells, would have to be considered perhaps as a "negative or maladaptive" plasticity.

The striatum is the point of entry of information into the basal ganglia, and it has important roles in motor control and habit learning. The neocortex provides the major excitatory inputs to striatal medium spiny projection neurons. Morphological studies have demonstrated that the majority of these afferent terminals impinge on the head of the spines on the dendrites of these striatal neurons, whereas most dopaminergic afferent fibers coming from the substantia nigra make synapses on the necks of the same dendritic spines. This close anatomical localization of these two types of synapses suggests that dopamine released from the nigrostriatal afferent terminals may have modulatory effects on the excitatory signals generated from the cortex.

The importance of dopamine in normal striatal function is evidenced by the severe disruption of behavior observed in Parkinson's disease and after chemical lesions of nigral dopaminergic inputs to striatum. In recent years attention has been focused on perforated synapses considering their possible involvement in synaptic plasticity in the nervous system. It has been hypothesized that an increase in the number of synapses may represent a structural basis for the enduring expression of synaptic plasticity during some events that involve memory and learning; also it has been suggested that perforated synapses increase in number after some experimental situations. The aim of this chapter was to analyze whether the dopamine depletion produces changes in the synaptology of the corpus striatum of rats after the unilateral injection of 6-OHDA. The findings suggest that after the lesion, both contralateral and ipsilateral striata present a significant increment in the number of perforated synapses, suggesting brain plasticity that might be deleterious for the spines, because this type of synaptic contacts are excitatory, and in the absence of the modulatory effects of dopamine, the neuron could die by excitotoxic mechanisms. Thus, we can conclude that the presence of perforated synapses after striatal dopamine depletion might be a form of negative synaptic plasticity.

INTRODUCTION

Brain plasticity refers to the lifelong capacity for physical and functional brain change enjoyed by humans and other animals and is inherently bidirectional: through the same mechanisms and plasticity processes, brain function can either be strengthened or degraded, depending on the circumstances. During normal aging, individuals typically undergo physical, behavioral, and environmental changes that, in the aggregate, promote negative plastic changes that degrade brain function. These root causes of functional decline involve a complex interplay of physical brain deterioration, behavioral and environmental changes, and brain plasticity processes (Mahncke et al., 2006).

One of the greatest challenges in neuroscience is understanding how the nervous system acquires, stores, and utilizes information derived from the sensory world. With the establishment of the "neuron doctrine" by Cajal (1894), which stated that the nervous system is made up of discrete units (neurons), neuroscientists including Cajal proposed that modifications might occur in the interaction between neurons. They suggested that certain neuronal modifications might underlie developmental processes as well as processes underlying learning and memory (Chen and Tonegawa, 1997).

In 1949, Hebb proposed a well-defined rule of synaptic plasticity: Coincident activity in two connected neurons leads to strengthening of their connection. Hebb further postulated that associative learning could be based on this synaptic modification. Today we know that synaptic plasticity is expressed in many forms. Thus, Hebb's coincident rule can be applied only to some forms of synaptic plasticity. Yet the notion that neural activity leads to synaptic

[1] Laboratorio de Neuromorfología, UNAM FES Iztacala.Av. de los Barrios # 1 Los Reyes Iztacala. C.P. 54090

modifications remains central in our current understanding of activity-dependent development, learning, memory and brain damage (Chen and Tonegawa, 1997).

In 1973 it was discovered that brief tetanic stimulation produced a long lasting form of synaptic plasticity, long-term potentiation (LTP) that can last for hours or days in the mammalian hippocampus (Bliss and Lømo 1973). Just before that the involvement of the hippocampal formation in memory was established by clinical data indicating that lesions of this structure in humans produce anterograde amnesia (Milner 1966).

Throughout development and in adult life, the brain responds to experience by adjusting the strength of communication at individual synapses and by changing the physical pattern of synaptic connections between neurons. In this way, information can be stored by the nervous system in the form of altered structure and chemistry of synapses and/or by the formation of new synapses and the elimination of old ones. Neuronal plasticity is associated with critical physiological processes in the developing and adult brain.

Activity-dependent remodeling of synaptic efficacy and neuronal connectivity is a remarkable property of synaptic transmission and characteristic of plastic events in the nervous system. Neuronal plasticity involves, in part, changes in cell morphology. These changes have been observed as a consequence of a variety of experimental manipulations, including associative learning (Black et al., 1990; Federmeier et al., 1994; Kleim et al., 1994, 1997), environmental rearing conditions (Turner and Greenough, 1985; Volkmar and Greenough 1972), and increased synaptic "use" induced by direct electrical stimulation (Wojtowicz et al., 1989; Geinisman, 1993; Buchs and Muller 1996;), as well as in relation to the processes of normal development and aging (De Groot and Bierman 1983; Dyson and Jones 1984; Harris et al., 1992). Structural characteristics identified as "plastic," or susceptible to environmental and experiential influence, include size and shape of the postsynaptic spine head, length of the postsynaptic spine neck, length and thickness of the postsynaptic density (PSD), and changes in the number of presynaptic vesicles and presynaptic active zones (Liaw et al., 1999).

It has been demonstrated that synapses are constantly being formed, eliminated and/or reshaped. There is evidence that LTP of synaptic efficacy induces synaptic spine changes in the hippocampus (Engert and Bonhoeffer, 1999; Toni et al., 1999). It was also shown that synaptic structures undergo a conformational change after a treatment to induce olfactory memory formation in mice (Matsuoka et al., 1997).

Adaptive reorganization of neuronal connectivity, which allows the acquisition of new information, both during development and in the mature brain, is thus based upon the strengthening of existing, synapses, the formation of new synapses and the destabilization of previously established synaptic contacts. With the increasing need during evolution to organize brain structures of increasing complexity, these processes of dynamic stabilization and destabilization might become more and more important. At the same time, however, the delicate balance between stabilization and destabilization might also provide the basis for an increasing rate of failure. The effects of plasticity can, therefore, lead to either positive or negative changes. Thus, one can envisage of a spectrum of types of neuronal modifications that lead, at one end, to beneficial modifications as they may occur in learning and, at the other end, to detrimental effects as neurodegeneration and cell death (Caroni, 1998; McEachern and Shaw, 1999; Mattson and Furukawa, 1998).

An interesting finding of recent years is that synapses are extremely dynamic structures that may change not only their functioning with activity but also their morphology. The number of synapses in the nervous system change under the influence of a variety of normal physiological factors, including hormonal status (Kretz et al., 2004), activity (Devaud and Ferrus, 2003; Harris et al., 2003), or age (Gan et al., 2003; Rosenzweig and Barnes, 2003; Coggan et al., 2004). Also, cognitive deficits associated with aging or certain pathologies result from widespread synapse loss in brain neurons (Spires and Hyman, 2004). Synaptic loss is currently established as the best neurobiological correlate of the cognitive and motor deficits in neurodegenerative diseases (Honer, 2003; Scheff and Price, 2003), schizophrenia and mood disorders (Kolomeets et al., 2005). The changes that have been observed include alterations of the postsynaptic structure (Forno and Norville, 1979; Machado-Salas et al., 1989; Roberts and DiFiglia 1990; Ingham et al., 1991; Pickel et al., 1992; Avila-Costa et al., 1998; Fiala et al., 2002; Avila-Costa et al., 2004; Avila-Costa et al., 2005b and others), presynaptic ending edema (Ingham et al., 1991; Pickel et al., 1992; Avila-Costa et al., 2005b) an addition of postsynaptic receptors to the postsynaptic density (Lüscher et al., 2000; Zhu et al., 2000) and modifications of the pre and postsynaptic membranes –perforations— (Vrensen and Nunez, 1981; Sirevaag and Greenough, 1985; Geinisman et al., 1988; Calverley and Jones, 1987; Meshul and Casey, 1989; Geinisman et al., 1992; Toni et al., 2001 and others). The presence of the perforated synapses suggests an increase in activity of that synaptic terminal. However, despite the compelling evidence relating structural modification, the mechanisms by which perforated synapses contribute to synaptic plasticity remain unknown.

In this way, in our laboratory we investigated whether the dopamine depletion produces changes in the synaptology of the corpus striatum of rats after unilateral injection of 6-OHDA. In this chapter our focus is to describe briefly the characteristics of perforated synapses, synaptic organization of the corpus striatum, structure which plays an important role in Parkinson's disease, and to analyze the synaptic changes after dopamine depletion, focusing mainly in the formation of perforated synapses.

Perforated Synapses

A synapse is an intercellular junction defined ultrastructurally as a postsynaptic electron density (PSD) in direct opposition to a presynaptic profile associated with synaptic vesicles that is referred to as an active zone. The synaptic cleft is a tight intercellular junction that is resistant to biochemical disruption. The intervening space at the synapse is termed the synaptic cleft (10 to 20 nm wide) (figure 1).

The chemical synapse is by far the most common type of synapse in the central nervous systems of mammals. Because an axon terminal can form a synapse with any part of the surface of another neuron, synapses in which an axon forms the presynaptic component may be designated as being:

- axo-dendritic
- axo-somatic
- axo-axonal

Also, there are examples of synapses that occur between two dendrites (dendro-dendritic), between perikarya of two neurons (somato-somatic), and between perikarya and dendrites (somato-dendritic and dendro-somatic).

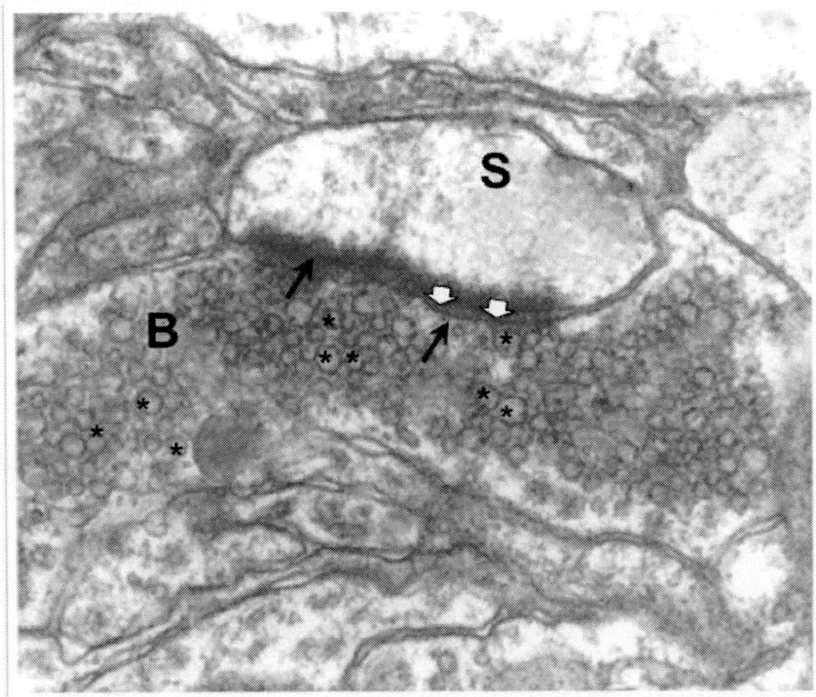

Figure 1. Electron micrograph of an axon terminal (B) that forms asymmetric synapse with a dendritic spine (S). This axon terminal contains spherical vesicles (*). Note the membrane asymmetry (arrows) called the postsynaptic electron density and the synaptic cleft (white arrowheads).

In the late 1950s Gray was the first to classify synapses on the basis of their junctional characteristics. He referred to those synapses with prominent postsynaptic densities as type 1, and described them as possessing a widened synaptic cleft, the separation between the faces of the presynaptic and postsynaptic membranes being 20 nm wide (Fig. 2A); Gray also found a different kind of synapse on the dendritic trunks and he referred to these as type 2 synapses. Such synapses have a narrower synaptic cleft, about 12 nm wide, and dense regions of the junction can be intermittent and have a less pronounced postsynaptic density than those of type 1 synapses (Fig. 2B). In a later evaluation of the synapses came to conclusion that type 1 and type 2 synapses represent the extremes of a morphological continuum, and he chose to refer them as asymmetric and symmetric synapses, on the basis of the disposition of the cytoplasmic density on each side of the junction. Frequently, asymmetric synapses contain round vesicles, and symmetric synapses contain both round and pleomorphic vesicles (Peters et al., 1991).

The stereotypical and most abundant type of synapse in the central nervous system is the asymmetric synapse occurring between an axon and a dendritic spine (Figure 2A).

The principal neurons of most brain regions are covered with small protrusions known as dendritic spines. Spines are extremely numerous on many kinds of dendrites; in fact they account for the majority of postsynaptic sites in the vertebrate brain. Dendritic spines typically are in excitatory synapses, and thus typically receive the neurotransmitter glutamate from their partner axon. Spines are found on the dendrites of most principal neurons in the brain, and are notably found in the pyramidal neurons of the cerebral cortex, the medium spiny neurons of the striatum, and the Purkinje cells of the cerebellum.

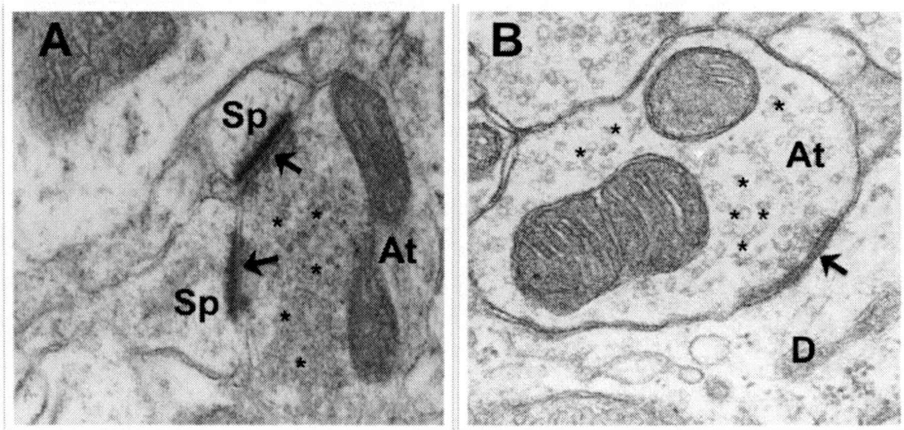

Figure 2. **A**. This picture shows an axon terminal (At) establishing an asymmetric synapse with two dendritic spines (Sp). The synaptic bouton contains spherical vesicles (*). The arrows show the postsynaptic electron densities. **B**. This electron micrograph shows an axon terminal (At) forming a symmetric synapse with a dendrite (D). This synaptic bouton contains pleomorphic synaptic vesicles (*). The arrow shows the postsynaptic electron density.

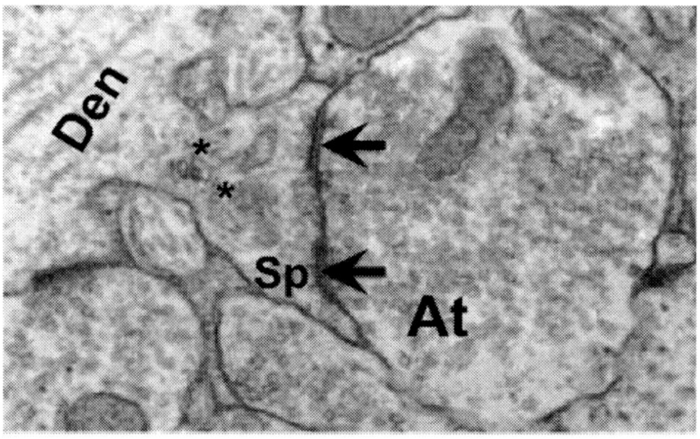

Figure 3. In this picture there is a spiny branchlet of a pyramidal cell dendrite (Den). The dendritic spine (Sp) form asymmetric synapses (arrows) with the axon terminal (At). Spine can be recognized by its spine apparatus (asterisks).

At ultrastructural level, spines can be distinguished from other dendritic elements in the neuropil by the presence of a characteristic spine apparatus (figure 3) composed of a calcium-binding protein, and it has been an important marker for spines in quantitative electron microscopic studies. Within cerebral cortex, for example, about 79% of all excitatory synapses are made onto spines and the rest directly onto dendrites, whereas 31% of all inhibitory synapses are made onto spines. A spine with an inhibitory synapse always carries an excitatory synapse as well (Beaulieu and Colonnier, 1989). Given the dominance of excitatory synapses, about 15% of all dendritic spines carry both excitatory and inhibitory synaptic profiles, as in the case of the striatum, structure that is the main target of this chapter.

One possible function of dendritic spines is the increase of the surface area of dendrites and thus the number of possible synapses per dendritic length. Furthermore, spines allow dendrites to reach multiple axons, minimizing the distances from one synapse to the next. In addition, the narrow spine neck restricts the diffusion of molecules into and out of the spine (Nimchimsky et al., 2002). This diffusional biochemical compartmentalization may help to retain molecules at the synapse, i.e. Ca^{2+} influx upon synaptic stimulation is limited to the stimulated spine and does not affect synapses on neighboring spines (Sabatini et al., 2001; Nimchimsky et al., 2002).

Spines may be isolated functional entities at times; calcium influx from NMDA receptors or calcium channels activated by weak synaptic inputs may cause an increase in calcium concentration within the spine (Yuste et al., 2000). This may lead to the activation of signaling cascades other than membrane potential changes. For instance, the length and shape of the spine neck, which determines how well the synaptic potentials that are generated within a spine will spread to the dendritic shaft, could conceivably vary with cytoskeletal rearrangements that are dependent on this calcium influx (Matus, 2000). It has been proposed that a moderate increase of cytoplasmic calcium concentration causes elongation of spines, whereas a very large increase of calcium concentration causes shrinkage and collapse of spines (Segal et al., 2005). The possible deleterious effects of high concentrations of Ca^{2+} produced by excitatory synaptic activity have suggested the hypothesis that "a major role of spines is to protect the parent dendrite from a rise of Ca^{2+} to levels that can be toxic to the cell" (Shepherd, 1996).

Although recent imaging studies have focused on spine formation and pruning, or on spine expansion and shrinkage, electron microscopy reconstruction studies have led to discoveries of other types of change in spines. These include changes in the length of the postsynaptic density at the spine head (Desmond and Levy, 1986), spine splitting (Edwards, 1995), the formation of perforated spines (Geinisman et al., 1987, 1988; 2001; Geinisman, 2000, and others) changes in spine curvature and the formation of multiple spine synapses (Toni et al., 1999). Some authors have attempted to provide a unified view that considers the different spine changes as subclasses of postsynaptic density enlargement (Harris et al., 2003).

Pathological changes in spines can be classified into two general categories, pathologies of distribution and pathologies of structure. Pathologies of distribution include dramatic increases and decreases in spine density, and widespread changes in morphology. Commonly observed morphological changes include an overall reduction in spine size or alteration in spine shape, dendritic beading with concomitant loss of spines, and sprouting of spines in abnormal locations. Pathologies of structure include all those changes observable in single spines, such as densification of the cytoplasm, hypertrophy of organelles or spine volume, and formation of aberrant synapse-like connections (Fiala et al., 2002).

The loss of spines upon deafferentation suggests that they are somehow maintained by their afferent input. Because spines bear glutamatergic synapses, one may reason that some aspect of glutamatergic neurotransmission acts as a signal to maintain the spine and that interference with normal synaptic activity may therefore affect spine shape or density

(Nimchinsky et al., 2002); moderately increased levels of excitatory synaptic activity can induce spine formation, but that excessive and unrestrained activation can cause excitotoxic loss of spines.

The majority of spines contain one continuous PSD, representing one synaptic contact. Nevertheless, the PSD of some spines appears interrupted and therefore perforated, and it was suggested that these perforated synapses represent an intermediate step during spine division and are thus involved in the process of synaptogenesis (Geinisman, 1993).

It has been proposed that some brain processes like learning and memory may elicit the conversion of some morphological subtypes of synapses into others (Chang and Greenough, 1984). The existence of distinct morphological subtypes of axospinous synapses is consistent with this idea and suggests a hypothetical model of synapse restructuring that may account for synaptic plasticity associated with the induction phase of LTP. According to this model, LTP induction initiates a sequence of structural synaptic modifications, which initiates with the enlargement of typical small-nonperforated synapses and their conversion into atypically large nonperforated ones. This is followed by the consecutive formation of perforated synapses that have initially a focal spine partition with a fenestrated post synaptic density, and finally a complete partition with a segmented post synaptic density. Synapses of the latter subtype have multiple transmission zones instead of only a single one, and an increase in their number after LTP induction, may result in an augmentation of synaptic transmission (Calverley and Jones, 1990).

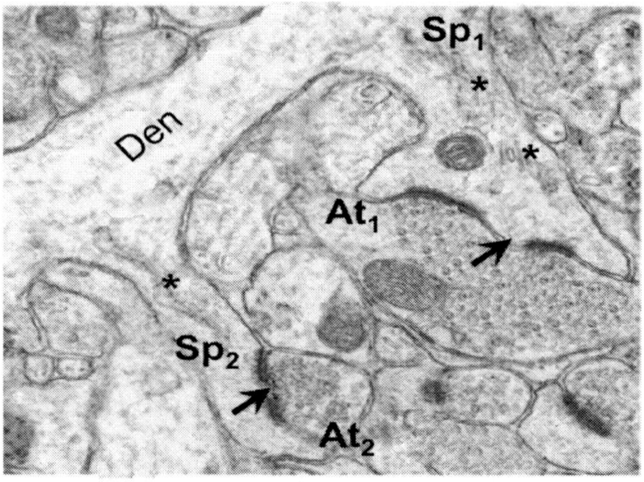

Figure 4. The typical perforated synapses can be distinguished with a rupture toward the presynaptic terminal membrane (arrow), and the presynaptic density is in association to the spine apparatus (*); Den: dendrite; Sp: spine; At: presynaptic button or axon terminal.

Ultrastructuraly, perforated synapses are characterized by a perforation (fenestration) extended through the paramembranous densities, from the presynaptic terminal across the cleft and into the postsynaptic process. This type of synapses has been reported to increase in number during development (Itarat and Jones, 1992) and under various experimental conditions such as complex environments (Sirevaag and Greenough, 1985), behavioral training (Vrensen and Nunez, 1981), repetitive electrical stimulation (Geinisman et al., 1988), and hormonal alterations (Hatton and Ellisman, 1982). It has also been suggested that a preserved complement of hippocampal perforated synapses is required for the maintenance of good spatial memory during aging (Geinisman, 2000).

Calverley and Jones (1987) classified the perforated synapses as follows:

- The site of the perforation projects into the presynaptic terminal.
- The active zone has one or more negatively curved components that are separated by a central region of the active zone that projects into the presynaptic terminal.
- The presynaptic density is in close association to the spine apparatus or an extension of it (see figure 4).

Synaptic Organization Of The Striatum

The striatum, a large subcortical nucleus, is an integral part of the basal ganglia, a group of interconnected structures involved in various aspects of the control of movement (Calabresi et al., 1997a; Chesselet and Delfs 1996; Marsden and Obeso 1994).

The basal ganglia are a group of nuclei involved in a variety of processes including motor, associative, cognitive and mnemonic functions. The dorsal division of the basal ganglia consists of the striatum (or caudate-putamen), the globus pallidus (GP, external segment of the globus pallidus in primates), entopeduncular nucleus (EP, internal segment of globus pallidus in primates, GPi), the subthalamic nucleus (STN) and the substantia nigra (SN), which is divided into two main parts, the dorsal pars compacta (SNc) in which the dopaminergic nigrostriatal neurons are located and the more ventral pars reticulata (SNr).

The most widely accepted views of basal ganglia function are based on observations of human afflicted with degenerative diseases that attack these structures. In all cases these diseases produce severe deficits of movement. In some, such as Parkinson's disease (PD), movements are more difficult to make, as if the body were somehow made rigid and resistive to changes in position. In others, such as Huntington´s disease, useless and unintended movements interfere with the execution of useful and intended ones. In general, these symptoms affect only voluntary movements, purposive movements, with reflexive movements being relatively unaffected. These clinical observations have led most investigators to view basal ganglia as components of a widespread system that is somehow involved in the generation of goal-directed voluntary movements, but in complex and subtle aspects of that process (Wilson, 1996).

The major input to the basal ganglia is derived from the cortex; virtually the whole cortex projects onto the basal ganglia in a highly topographical manner. The main point of entry of this cortical information to the basal ganglia is the striatum. The corticostriatal projection imparts functionality on to the striatum and consequently other divisions of the basal ganglia. In what is now considered the classic view of basal ganglia circuitry (Albin et al., 1989; DeLong, 1990; Smith et al., 1998), the functional organization is such that cortical information carried by the corticostriatal projection is processed within the striatum, integrated with the many other inputs to the basal ganglia (e.g. intralaminar thalamic nuclei, amygdala, hippocampus, dorsal raphe) which primarily innervate the striatum, and then the information is transmitted to the output nuclei of the basal ganglia, the EP and the SNr. The basal ganglia influence behavior by these output nuclei projecting to the ventral thalamus and then back to the cortex or by projecting to subcortical `premotor' regions (figure 5) (see Albin et al., 1989; DeLong, 1990; Bolam and Bennett, 1995; Gerfen and Wilson, 1996; Smith et al., 1998 for review).

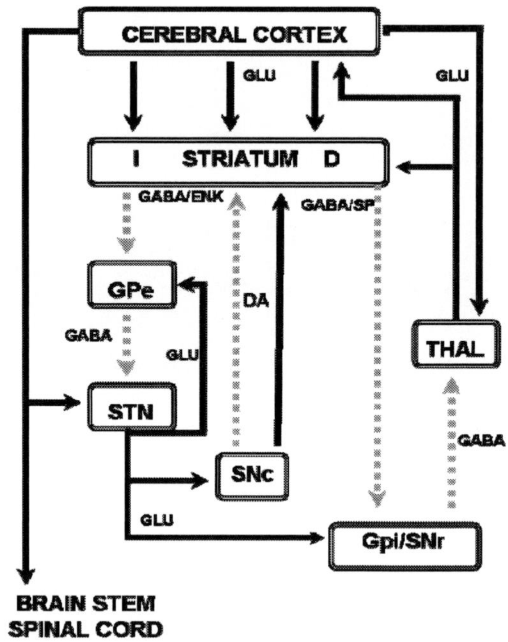

Figure 5. Basal ganglia motor circuit. Areas of the motor cortex project in a somatotopic pattern to the striatum, where they synapse through excitatory glutamatergic neurons onto the medium spiny striatal neurons. These striatal neurons use GABA as their primary neurotransmitter and substance P (SP) or enkephalin (Enk) as co-transmitters, and are organized into two pathways: the 'direct' (D) and the 'indirect' (I) pathway. The direct pathway connects the striatum to the internal segment of the globus pallidus (GPi) and the substantia nigra pars reticulata (SNr). The GPi and SNr are the output nuclei of the basal ganglia (GPi/SNr) and project to the brainstem and the thalamus and from the latter to the cortex. The influence of the GPi and SNr on the thalamus is inhibitory, whereas the thalamic projection to the cortex is excitatory. The indirect pathway also connects the striatum to the output nuclei of the basal ganglia but these fibres first pass through synaptic connections in the external segment of the globus pallidus (GPe) and then the subthalamic nucleus (STN). Output from the STN to the GPi/SNr is excitatory. Dopaminergic neurons (DA) of the SNc provide a massive feedback projection to the striatum and modulate the flow of cortical information. Excitatory projections are shown in black; inhibitory connections are shown in mottled gray lines.

The transmission of cortical information through the basal ganglia occurs through two routes, the `direct' and `indirect' pathways (Albin et al., 1989; DeLong, 1990). In the direct pathway corticostriatal information is transmitted directly from the striatum to the output nuclei (SNr/GPi). In the indirect pathway corticostriatal information is transmitted indirectly to the output nuclei via the complex network interconnecting the GPe and STN.

The great complexity of the circuits and the manner in which the basal ganglia accomplish their diverse functions is better explained through the analysis of a single neuronal cell type in the striatum: the medium sized spiny neuron (MSN) (figure 6). The striatum contains both, projection neurons and several populations of interneurons (Bolam and Bennett, 1995).

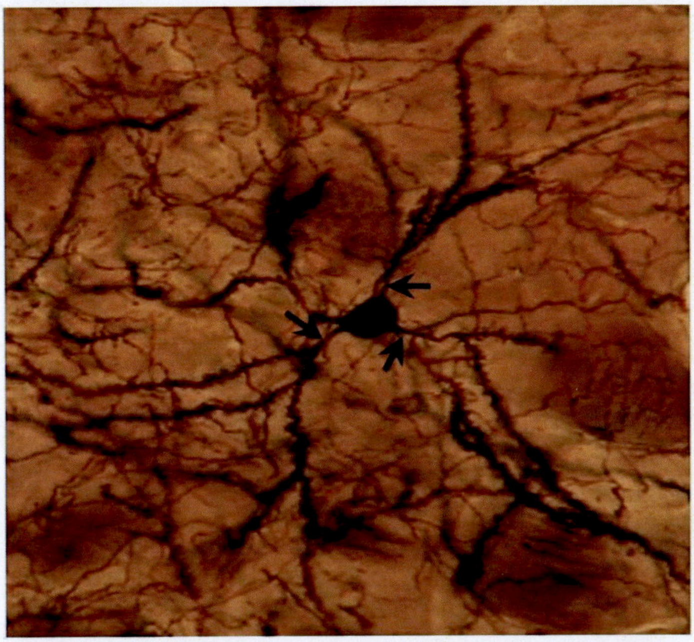

Figure 6. Light micrograph of a Golgi impregnated medium size spiny neuron in the rat striatum. Note the medium sized perikaryon (approximately 20 μm in diameter), the spine-free proximal dendrites (arrows) and the densely spiny secondary and higher order dendrites.

This neuron cell type, which constitutes over 90% of striatal neurons, is the major output neuron of the striatum. Combined ultrastructural and neuroanatomical methods have elucidated the organization of afferent connectivity to these neurons. The major physiologic function of striatal efferent activity appears to be inhibition of tonically active GABAergic neurons in the GP and SNr. Thus, the excitatory input from the cerebral cortex, whose afferents make asymmetric synapses with the spines of MSN, appears to drive the efferent activity of the striatum. Other extrinsic and intrinsic afferent synapses are situated in a position to regulate the effect of the corticostriatal excitatory input to the MSN. For example, dopaminergic afferents from the midbrain make mainly symmetric synapses with the spine necks and dendritic shafts of the MSN. These neurons themselves have local axon collaterals, which serve to link together local clusters of MSN. These local axon collaterals, which contain, either GABA, substance P or enkephalin, also make mainly symmetric synapses with the necks of spines or dendritic shafts of MSN. Other afferents with similar synaptic connections to these neurons arise from cholinergic or somatostatinergic striatal interneurons. Additionally, the patterns of extrinsic and intrinsic afferents to MSN and their extrinsic projections are related to the organization of MSN into two mosaically organized macroscopic compartments, the striatal patches and matrix (Gerfen, 1988). Figure 7 summarizes the synaptic organization of the medium spiny neuron.

Of particular importance, as we mentioned above, is the input from the dopaminergic terminals derived from the SNc, which degenerate in PD. These terminals form symmetric synaptic contacts mainly with the necks of dendritic spines of MSN (Bouyer et al., 1984; Freund et al., 1984; Smith et al., 1994). The head of spines that receive the dopaminergic input invariably receive glutamatergic input from terminals forming asymmetric synapses (Freund et al., 1984), which are generally derived from the cortex (Bouyer et al., 1984; Smith et al., 1994) (see Fig. 8). This anatomical arrangement is ideally suited for the dopamine released from the nigrostriatal terminal, which is likely to act on dopamine receptors localized both within the synapse and at extrasynaptic sites (Yung et al., 1996), to very selectively modulate the response to the excitatory input at the head of the spine. Other inputs to spiny neurons are the cholinergic, which exhibit a similar anatomical organization (Izzo and Bolam, 1988) and GABAergic terminals also observed in contact with the necks of spines (Bolam and Bennett, 1995).

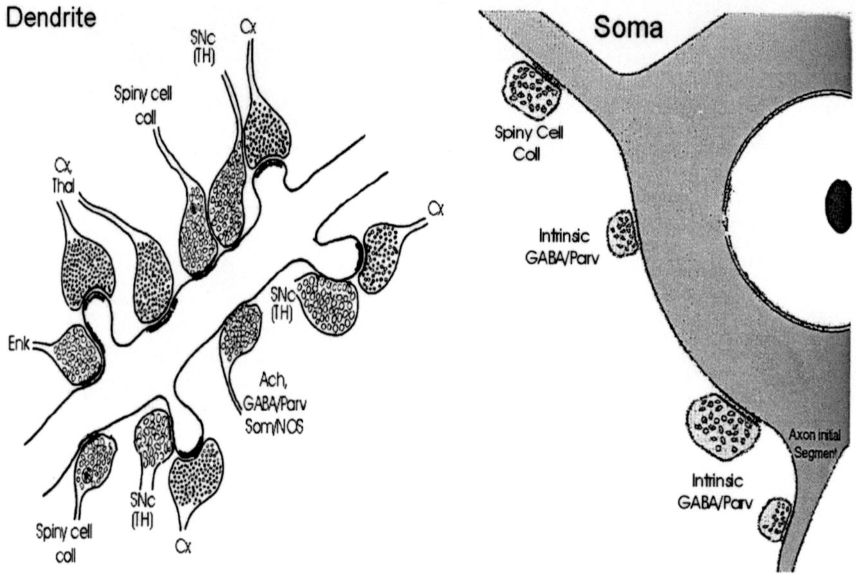

Figure 7. The major synaptic types of the striatal spiny neuron. The distal spiny dendrites receive inputs with round synaptic vesicles, which form asymmetrical contacts primarily on the dendritic spines, but occasionally on the shafts of the dendrites. These arise mostly from afferent fibers from the cerebral cortex (Cx) and thalamus (Thal), which contact the head of the spines. Spiny cell collaterals, TH-staining axons from substantia nigra compacta (SNc), and intrinsic intrastriatal connections (from aspiny cholinergic neurons) form symmetrical contacts with pleomorphic and flattened vesicles on the stalks of dendritic spines, on the proximal part of the spine heads, and on dendritic shafts. The inputs to the soma or to the proximal surface of the spiny projection neurons are from interneurons and collateral arborizations of the spiny neurons. They form symmetrical synapses with pleomorphic or flattened synaptic vesicles at very low density on the aspiny initial portion of the dendrites, the soma and axon initial segment (Modified from Gerfen, 1988 and Wilson, 1996).

For many years, much of the work devoted to the striatum has focused on the dopaminergic nigrostriatal input (Björklund and Lindvall 1984). This interest has been sustained by the realization, in the early 1960s, that loss of dopaminergic neurons in the pars compacta is the hallmark of PD (Bernheimer et al., 1973). As a result, many studies have focused on the development and plasticity of the nigrostriatal pathway (Murrin and Ferrer 1984; Voom et al., 1988; Weihmuller and Bruno 1989; Zigmond and Striker 1989).

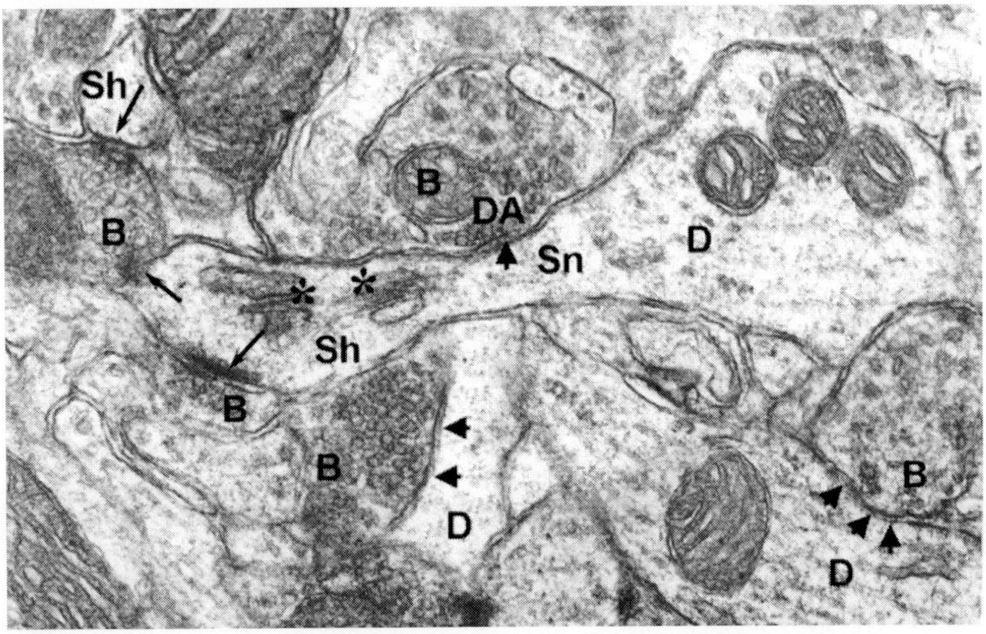

Figure 8. Electron micrograph from the striatum neuropil. At the center of the micrograph lies a typical dendritic spine, which contains an evident spine apparatus (*) receiving three synaptic contacts: two asymmetric, probably glutamatergic (arrows) on the head of the spine (Sh) and one symmetric (arrow head), probably dopaminergic (DA) with the neck of the spine (Sn). Along the micrograph it can be distinguish various synaptic contacts between presynaptic buttons (B) establishing asymmetric contacts (arrow) with the head of a dendritic spine (Sh) and two more symmetric (arrow heads) with dendrites (D).

There have been relatively few studies on ultrastructural changes within the striatum following dopamine (DA) deafferentation. Ingham et al. (1991) first reported that the size of enkephalin-immunoreactive terminals and length of the synaptic specialization was larger up to 13 months post-lesion. They later reported that there was also an increase in the length of the synaptic specialization associated with asymmetric synapses (Ingham et al., 1993). This later observation would suggest changes in striatal glutamate synapses.

Although this anatomical configuration suggests that DA has a direct modulatory effect on cortical signaling (Arbuthnott et al., 1998), the role of DA in presynaptic modification of corticostriatal afferents has been controversial because of the extraordinary complexity of MSN innervation (Akopian and Walsh, 2002) and the challenges inherent in using postsynaptic recordings to determine alterations in presynaptic activity (Van der Kloot, 1991; Sulzer and Pothos, 2000; Reynolds and Wickens, 2002). Electron microscopy (Fisher et al., 1994; Sesack et al., 1994; Wang and Pickel, 2002) and electrophysiology (Calabresi et al., 1993; O'Donnell and Grace, 1994; Hsu et al., 1995; Flores-Hernandez et al., 1997; Cepeda et al., 2001; Tang et al., 2001; West and Grace, 2002; Bamford et al., 2004) studies, however, have supported the concept that DA directly regulates glutamate release from corticostriatal terminals by stimulating D2 receptors located on a subpopulation of cortical afferents, providing a mechanism for dampening critical cortical signals (Bamford et al., 2004). Tang et al., (2001) suggest that the major role for DA and D2 receptors in striatum is to limit the efficacy of striatal glutamatergic synaptic inputs to MSN.

The dopaminergic lose in the striatal spiny neurons is followed by a cascade of events that ultimately changes its structure and the activity of basal ganglia circuits, resulting in the development of PD symptomatology. The specific mechanisms leading to the spiny neurons morphological changes are not well understood, but may involve glutamate hyperactivity (Ingham et al., 1998).

The etiology of PD is still not fully understood, but animal models, human post-mortem material and genetic analyses have provided important clues.

Chemical neurotoxins have been widely used in creating several animal models of human neurodegenerative diseases in order to assess the neurochemical, physiological and behavioral effects of lesioning specific neuronal populations. The catecholamine-specific neurotoxin 6-hydroxydopamine (6-OHDA) has been widely used to destroy dopamine-containing cells in the SNc and produces an animal model of PD (Dauer and Przedborski, 2003; Schober, 2004).

In recent years attention has been focused on perforated synapses considering their possible involvement in synaptic plasticity in the nervous system. It has been hypothesized that an increase in the number of synapses may represent a structural basis for the enduring expression of synaptic plasticity during some events that involve memory and learning; also it has been suggested that perforated synapses increase in number after some experimental situations. Thus the aim of this study was to analyze whether the DA depletion produces changes in the synaptology of the corpus striatum of rats after the unilateral injection of 6-OHDA.

METHODS

The experiments were carried out in 70 male Wistar rats weighing 190 ± 10 g at the beginning of the study. The animals were housed in a controlled environment with a 12-h light/dark cycle and free access to food pellets and water.

Surgical and Drug Treatment Procedures

The rats were anesthetized with sodium pentobarbitone (35 mg/Kg i.p.) and placed in a stereotaxic apparatus. The rats were injected with 4 μl of a saline solution containing 8 μg of 6-OHDA (Sigma Chemical, Co.) (n = 35) and 0.2 mg of ascorbic acid into the right medial forebrain bundle and sham lesion was made with the vehicle (n = 35). The injections were given over a 4-min period with a Hamilton syringe attached to a glass micropipette with a tip diameter of 20–50 μm. The stereotaxic coordinates were as follows: AP = –4mm anterior of the ear bar; L = 1.4 mm lateral of bregma; V = –7.7 mm vertical of dura (according to Paxinos & Watson, 1986). After recovery from the anaesthesia the animals were returned to their home cages with free access to food and water, in a cyclical 12-h light-dark environment.

Apomorphine (Sigma Chemical, USA; 0.25 mg/Kg i.p.) induced rotational behavior was tested two days after lesioning (Ungerstedt, 1968). Only those animals exhibiting more than 200 complete turns in a 30' period were included in the study. 3, 4, 10, 20, 30, 60 and 120 days after lesioning under i.p. sodium pentobarbitone anaesthesia, and via the aorta, all animals were perfused with saline solution (0.9%), followed by a fixative solution containing 2% glutaraldehyde and 2% paraformaldehyde in 0.1 M phosphate buffer.

Ultrastructural Analysis

The brains were carefully removed and placed in the same fixative solution during one hour. Using a dissection microscope, we took small fragments from the dorsomedial quadrant of the right and left striatum and the right and left SN for its ultrastructural study in a JEOL 100 X II electron microscope (Japan).

Striatal ultrastructural analysis was performed in 50 randomly selected synaptic endings per striatum. In each synaptic button we observed all its membrane and organelles features, and we measured (see Fig. 9):

- The diameters of the presynaptic button using two axes, which were perpendicular one to each other and intersected at the center of the synaptic terminal; the diameter was measured directly from the electron microscope screen with a grid placed inside the eyepiece (Avila-Costa et al., 2005b).
- The number of dendritic spines or dendrites as postsynaptic targets.
- The number of perforated synapses (Avila-Costa et al., 2005a).

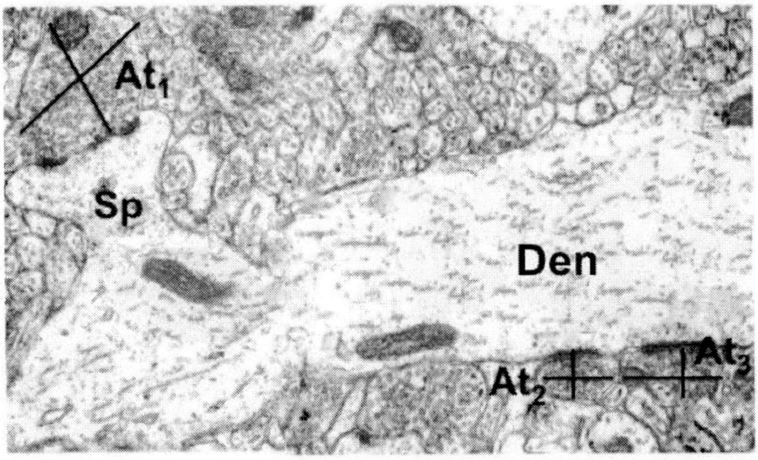

Figure 9. Synaptic ending (At_1) showing the two axes measured, establishing a perforated synaptic contact with a dendritic spine (Sp). At_2 and At_3 also showing the two axes measured and establishing synaptic contacts with a dendritic shaft (Den).

Synapses were defined by the presence of a clear postsynaptic density facing at least three presynaptic vesicles. Perforated synapses were identified on micrographs of serial sections and were defined by the presence of a discontinuity in the postsynaptic density (Geinisman et al., 1987). To minimize subjectivity, classification was carried out blind by at least two experimenters and if distinction was unclear, the synapse was not included in the quantification.

Statistical analysis

The unpaired Student's t and Kruskal-Walis tests were used to detect significant differences between sham lesioned group with 6-OHDA lesioned striatum; and the paired Student's t test to detect differences between ipsi and contralateral striatum ($p<0.05$).

RESULTS

Diameters of synaptic endings

Sham lesioned rats did not show any differences between both striata, nor alterations at the different stages after the surgery (figures 10 and 11-1).

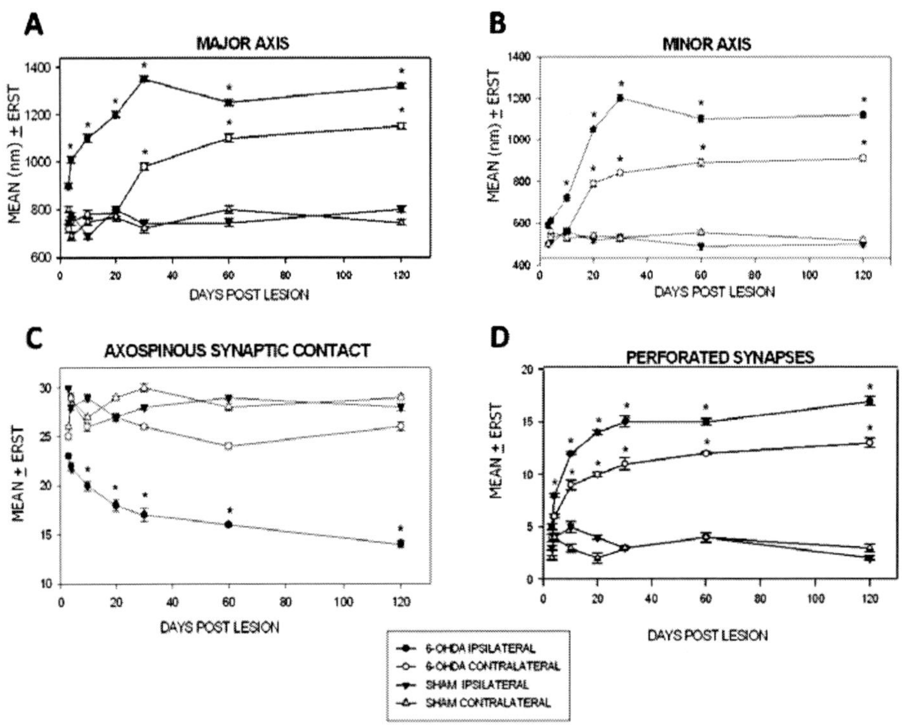

Figure 10. A-B: Time course of changes for synaptic ending diameter (major (A) and minor (B) axes) in ipsi and contralateral striatum following 6-OHDA and sham lesions. * $P < 0.001$. C: Mean of the total number of synaptic endings establishing synapses with a dendritic spine. * $P < 0.001$. D: Mean of the total number of perforated synapses in ipsi and contralateral striatum following 6-OHDA and sham lesions. * $P < 0.001$

In 6-OHDA lesioned rats we observed a statistically significant increase in the diameter of the synaptic ending in both axes; in the ipsilateral striatum this increase was evident since the 3rd day after the lesion and reached to the maximum at day 30th (figure 10-A and B, and figure 12-2). The contralateral striatum of 6-OHDA lesioned rats disclosed an increase in the diameter at day 20-30 after the lesion; the increment persisted until the 120th day (figures 10-A and B, and 11-3).

Postsynaptic target

As it is shown in figures 10-C and 11, the contralateral striatum presents similar values to those found in the sham operated group, being the axospinous synaptic contact the most common. In contrast, in the ipsilateral striatum, the axodendritic contacts prevailed.

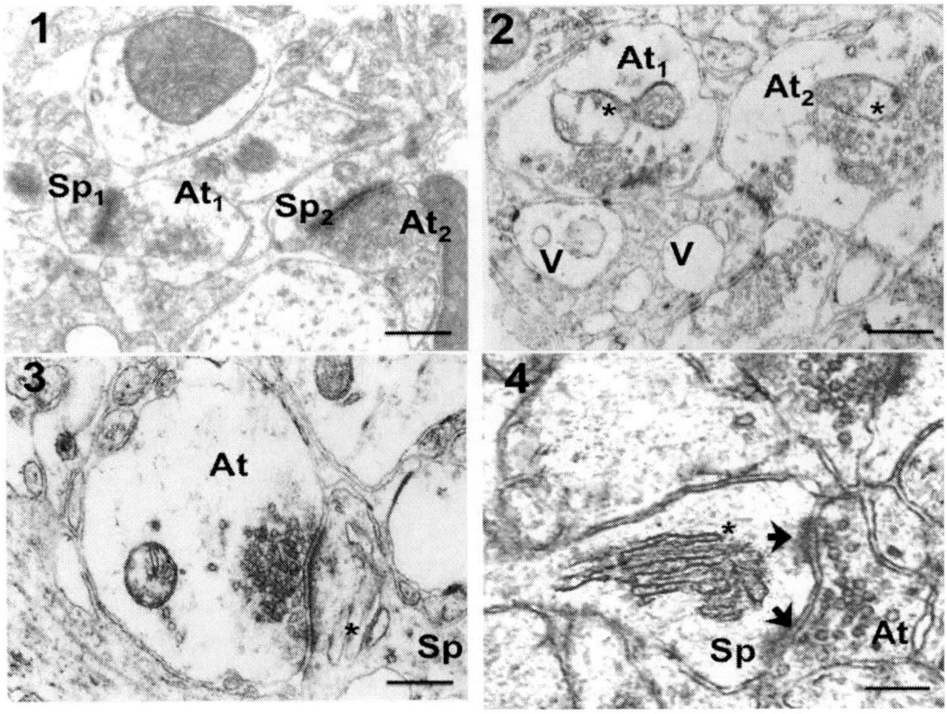

Figure 11. Electron micrographs from the striatum neuropil of the sham lesioned group (1); 6-ohda lesioned ipsilateral striatum (2); 6-ohda contralateral striatum (3); 6-ohda lesioned ipsilateral striatum (4). 1, In sham group, the mean size of the synaptic buttons (At_1, At_2) was 750 X 500 nm and the predominant postsynaptic target was the dendritic spines (Sp_1, Sp_2), it can be observe that the neuropil is well preserved 40,000 X. 2, This image corresponds to ipsilateral striatum neuropil and shows two swollen synaptic buttons (At_1, At_2) and some vacuoles (V) within a dendrite; note the edematous mitochondrion (*) 40,000 X. 3, This image demonstrates an edematous presynaptic ending (At) of the contralateral striatum establishing a synaptic contact with a dendritic spine (Sp) with dilated spine apparatus (*) 40,000 X. 4, An increase in the presence of perforated synaptic contacts was notorious in both striata of lesioned animals (arrows). (At) Synaptic button; (Sp) dendritic spine; (*) spine apparatus. 40,000X. Bar: 0.25μm

Perforated synapses

The ipsilateral lesioned striatum exhibits a prominent increase in perforated synaptic contacts from the 4th to the 120th day. Similar changes were distinguished in the contralateral striatum from the 60th day after the lesion (figures 10D and 11-4). In contrast, the sham lesioned striatum displayed a continuous discrete number of perforated synaptic contacts (figure 10D).

The ultrastructural analysis of the ipsilateral and contralateral striatum neuropil throughout the different stages of evolution after 6-OHDA lesion of the SNc of rats revealed that this neurotoxin rapidly induces an important, and time dependent derangement of the ipsilateral striatum neuropil, characterized by synaptic ending edema, alterations in the postsynaptic target, and changes in the number of perforated synaptic contacts.

The contralateral striatum also exhibited statistically significant alterations in almost all of the criteria evaluated in this study, however, not as dramatic as those observed in the ipsilateral striatum.

Diameters of synaptic endings

The present analysis confirms previous observations referring to the fact that the dopamine depletion of the nigrostriatal pathway induces cell alterations between 48-72 hrs after the lesion (Zuch et al., 2000) and causes an increment in the size of the presynaptic profile (Ingham et al., 1991; Pickel et al., 1992). We assume that this swelling is due to an inherent degenerative process caused by 6-OHDA lesion; it seems that this nigrostriatal denervation triggers a widely distributed edematous response in almost all striatum synaptic endings. These observations are also confirmed with the analysis of the caudate nucleus neuropil of PD patients (Machado-Salas et al., 1989; Zaja-Milatovic et al., 2005).

Postsynaptic target

It is known from previous ultrastructural studies that spines of medium-sized spiny neurons receive mainly axospinous synaptic contacts (Bolam et al., 2000; Solis et al., 2007). In accordance with other authors (Ingham et al., 1991; Pickel et al., 1992), we found that the proportion of axospinous synapses was significantly reduced in the ipsilateral striatum of the 6-OHDA lesioned rats in all postlesion intervals. These findings are also confirmed by the observations reported in PD patients (McNeill et al., 1988; Machado-Salas et al., 1989; Zaja-Milatovic et al., 2005), where the synaptic contacts were predominantly of the axodendritic type. It is established that the dopaminergic input to the striatum originates in the SNc. Therefore, 6-OHDA lesion of the nigrostriatal pathway provokes a decrement of dopaminergic axons and there upon of the dopaminergic buttons establishing synaptic contact with the spines of the MSN of the striatum. The strongly lateralized effect of loss of the axospinous synaptic contacts is explained in terms of the predominant ipsilateral projection of the SN fibers (Yung et al., 1996). Ingham et al. (1998) suggest that the loss of spines may be a random process. This would imply that dopamine subserves a neurotrophic function and could play a role in the maintenance of spines (Arbuthnott et al., 2000). Indeed, the dopamine-containing cells have been shown to contain neurotrophins of various classes, including BDNF and NT3 (Seroogy et al., 1994) and it may be the release of these factors, rather than dopamine, that is important for spine survival.

Alterations in the contralateral striatum

We found degenerative changes in the contralateral striatum after 20-30 days of lesioning; the changes consist in synaptic ending edema and increment in perforated synaptic contacts. Yang et al., (2007) argue that changes that occur in the ipsilateral SNc affect the contralateral side because his electrophysiological data have shown that the SNc from the contralateral brain side influences nigrostriatal dopamine cell activity. Moreover, Fass and Butcher (1981) and Emsley et al., (2001) have reported that nigrostriatal projection is primarily ipsilateral, but also comprises a small contralateral component. Thus, this could explain in part the contralateral alterations we found in our experiment. However, further studies are necessary to explain the relationship between both striata. It is important to stand out that special attention should be paid to the interpretations formulated about the studies using this experimental model of Parkinson's disease, since unilateral 6-OHDA induces severe modifications in the contralateral non-lesioned striatum, at least 20-30 days after 6-OHDA lesion, since some investigators preferentially use contralateral striatum as control structure to compare against the lesioned side. However, between 3-20 days after dopamine depletion, the neuropil is well preserved, comparable to sham-lesioned group, thus it could serve as control structure.

PERFORATED SYNAPSES

Of particular interest is the presence of perforated synapses due to their supposed participation in synaptic plasticity. Our data reveal a great number of perforated synapses after the 6-OHDA lesion in both striatum nuclei in comparison to the control group.

Since the late 1970s an increasing number of studies has appeared in the literature, supporting the idea that perforated synapses are involved as intermediate structures in synaptic plasticity in mechanisms of learning and memory (Calverley and Jones, 1990; Itarat and Jones, 1992) and it has been reported that they increase in some experimental conditions such as complex environment (Sirevaag and Greenough, 1985), repetitive electrical stimulation (Geinisman et al., 1992) and behavioral training (Geinisman et al., 2001). It has also been suggested that a preserved complement of hippocampal perforated synapses is required for the maintenance of good spatial memory during aging (Geinisman et al., 1991).

Some experimental data in rats and in non-human primates suggest that this type of synapses correspond mainly to glutamatergic corticostriatal afferents to medium spiny GABAergic neurons (Smith and Bolam, 1990; Meshul et al., 1994). Thus, our data would therefore suggest that the reduced nigrostriatal dopaminergic transmission occurring in 6-OHDA model results in an increase in glutamate-mediated corticostriatal synaptic transmission. Such hyperactivity accords with the increased concentration and release of glutamate in the rat striatum following striatal dopaminergic denervation (Lindefors and

Ungerstedt, 1990) or a blockade of striatal dopamine receptors by neuroleptics (Meshul et al., 1994).

In this way, Meshul et al. (2000) found that after one month following unilateral ablation of the rat frontal cortex, removing corticostriatal input, or the injection of the neurotoxin 6-OHDA, into the SNc, removing nigrostriatal input or a combined ipsilateral cortical and 6-OHDA lesion (CTX/6-OHDA) a significant increase in all three lesion groups in the mean percentage of asymmetrical synapses associated with a perforated postsynaptic density. They suggest that following a CTX and/or 6-OHDA lesions, there is an increase in striatal glutamatergic function. The large increase in the percentage of multiple synaptic boutons in the combined lesion group suggests that dopamine or other factors released by the dopamine terminals assist in regulating synapse formation. The same authors (Meshul et al., 1999) reported that unilateral lesion of the rat nigrostriatal pathway with the neurotoxin 6-OHDA, results in a time-dependent change in striatal glutamatergic function. One month following the lesion, there is an increase in the extracellular level of striatal glutamate, as determined by *in vivo* microdialysis. In addition, there is an increase in the mean percentage of striatal asymmetrical nerve terminals associated with a perforated, or discontinuous, postsynaptic density, a finding similar to that reported by Ingham et al. (1998). An increase in this particular type of asymmetrical synaptic contact suggests an increase in activity of that synaptic terminal (Greenough et al., 1978).

Increases in such synapses have been reported to be associated with increased neuronal activity, as observed after the induction of long-term potentiation, hippocampal kindling, and increases in neuronal input to the visual cortex (Geinisman et al., 1988; Geinisman et al., 1991; Greenough et al., 1978; Meshul et al., 1994). Of interest is that the change in glutamate synapses following a 6-OHDA lesion is primarily associated with alterations of the ipsilateral corticostriatal pathway.

As we mentioned above, interactions between glutamate and dopamine occur both presynaptically and postsynaptically within the striatum. These neurotransmitters act at particular receptors on the pre and postsynaptic membranes. Striatal neurons, and nerve terminals immediately afferent to them, contain both ionotropic (AMPA/kainate and N-methyl-D-aspartate, NMDA, type) and metabotropic (mGluR family) glutamate receptors, and D1-like (D1, D5 subtype) and D2-like (D2, D3 and D4 subtype) dopamine receptors. The precise anatomical location and the degree of receptor subtype colocalisation on pre and postsynaptic membranes are issues that remain particularly controversial (Gerfen et al., 1990; Tarazi and Baldessarini, 1999). There are evidences that largely support a reciprocal regulation of dopamine and glutamate release in the striatum, through NMDA receptor-mediated augmentation and D2-like receptor-mediated reduction of neurotransmitter release (Reynolds and Wickens, 2002).

A major form of interaction between glutamate and dopamine that occurs postsynaptically at the level of individual spiny projection neurons is the modulation of membrane excitability. This affects the probability that a spiny projection neuron will fire action potentials in response to an excitatory event (Cepeda et al., 2001), thus dopamine is seen as a modulator of corticostriatal synaptic transmission. It has been demonstrated that DA depletion also appears to increase the excitability of MSN by diminishing the capacity of these neurons to modulate intracellular calcium (Ca^{2+}) levels (Day et al., 2006).

Moreover, previous studies have demonstrated that a pathological form of synaptic plasticity in the striatum related to supersensitivity of NMDA receptors could cause the development of atypical motor patterns leading to dyskinesias (Chase et al., 2000, 2004). Thus, as the number of activated NMDA channels increases, a higher amount of Ca^{2+} will enter the cell. The resulting rapid increase in Ca^{2+} concentration in the neuron induces the storage of this ion in the mitochondria, which further compromises energy supply. In fact, Ca^{2+} overload of mitochondria inhibits ATP synthesis (Miller et al., 1989). The latter event irreversibly blocks the respiratory chain leading to activation of phospholipases, excitotoxicity and neuronal death (Turski and Turski, 1993).

In this way, Neely et al., (2007) demonstrate that removal of the cortex after lesioning the striatal dopamine innervation completely prevented the spine loss. Their findings are thus similar to *in vivo* studies where prolonged blockade of excitatory transmission led to increased spine density (Rocha and Sur, 1995), and to observations made by Kirov et al. (2004), who found that blocking excitatory transmission in acute slices from adult rats results in an increase in spine density in CA1 pyramidal neurons. Moreover, preliminary studies in 6-OHDA lesioned rats show that blockade of the NMDA subset of glutamate receptors normalize both the D1 system downregulation and the D2 system upregulation (Chase et al., 1994). In this context, antiglutamatergic drugs may be of interest in PD. Yet, before such therapy can be envisaged, the exact nature of the receptors for excitatory amino acids involved in corticostriatal neurotransmission has to be analyzed in order to develop specific therapeutic agents without adverse side effects.

The perforated synapses are particularly interesting for several reasons. They have large PSD and thus probably also more receptors (Desmond and Weinberg, 1998). These morphological changes could be directly related to the increase in synaptic strength, because the process of membrane expansion that characterizes synapses with segmented PSD includes an enlargement of the PSD area and thus probably also insertion of new receptors in the synaptic membrane (Lüscher et al., 2000). Furthermore, the formation of segmented, fully partitioned PSD may result in the creation of two independent release sites, with their own release probabilities (Geinisman, 1993; Edwards, 1995). This suggests that perforated synapses may release more glutamate, which could trigger other biochemical changes that are important in the induction of excitatory potentials, and possibly excitotoxicity and more cell damage.

Calabresi et al. (1997b) demonstrated that D2Rs play a key role in mechanisms underlying the direction of long-term changes in synaptic efficacy in the striatum. These authors also show that an imbalance between D2R and NMDA receptor activity induces altered synaptic plasticity at corticostriatal synapses. This abnormal synaptic plasticity might cause the movement disorders observed in PD. Thus, we consider that the increase in the number of perforated synapses in the denervated striatum might be a sign of negative synaptic plasticity, since this type of synapses seems to induce more glutamate release, excitotoxicity and neuronal death. Cell death results in appearance of focal dendritic and axon terminals swellings or disappearance of dendritic spines, as we found here. There is also strong evidence that swelling and spine loss are caused by activation of excitatory amino acid receptors (Smart and Halpain, 2000). Furthermore, swelling appears to be a potentially very damaging process, disrupting the membrane continuity. It is very interesting in this respect that the phenomenon may in fact occur on dendrites, spines, as well as presynaptic terminals, being therefore not structure specific.

In conclusion, selective synaptic changes in shape and function are possibly signs of excitotoxic injury, and observed in diverse neurological diseases and neurodegenerative disorders. Elucidating mechanisms that mediate the synaptic alterations under pathological conditions may be of fundamental importance to understanding mechanisms of neuronal injury.

Despite of many new findings there are still various questions to be answered and further experiments to be done. The mechanisms of synaptic plasticity are still not completely clear —the role of retrograde messengers, details in the molecular cascades leading to gene expression and new protein synthesis or to growth of new synapses, finding the more accurate causal connection between plasticity and various forms of learning, memory and cell damage. The use of regulated and anatomically restricted genetic modification, combined with morphologic analysis, should provide a powerful set of tools for elucidating synaptic plasticity mechanisms.

References

Akopian, G., Walsh, J.P. (2002). Corticostriatal paired-pulse potentiation produced by voltage-dependent activation of NMDA receptors and L-type Ca(2+) channels. *J Neurophysiol*, 87, 157-165.

Albin, R.L., Young, A.B., Penney, J.B. (1989). The functional anatomy of basal ganglia disorders. *Trends Neurosci*, 12, 366-375.

Arbuthnott, G.W., Ingham,C.A., Wickens, J.R. (1998). Modulation by dopamine of rat corticostriatal input. *Adv Pharmacol*, 42, 733-736.

Arbuthnott, G. W., Ingham, C. A., Wickens, J. R. (2000). Dopamine and synaptic plasticity in the neostriatum. *J Anat*, 196, 587–596.

Avila-Costa, M.R., Colín-Barenque, L., Espinosa-Villanueva, J., Machado-Salas, J. (1998). Degeneración del neuropilo del núcleo caudado en la enfermedad de Parkinson y en el modelo experimental provocado con 6-OHDA: análisis ultraestructural comparativo. *Patología*, 36, 297-301.

Avila-Costa, M.R., Montiel-Flores, E., Colin-Barenque, L., Ordoñez, J.L., Gutierrez, A.L., Niño-Cabrera, H.G., Mussali-Galante, P., Fortoul, T.I. (2004). Nigrostriatal modifications after vanadium (V205) inhalation. An immunocytochemical and cytological approach. *Neurochem. Res*, 7, 1357-1362.

Avila-Costa, M.R., Colín-Barenque, L., Aley-Medina, P., Gutiérrez Valdez, A.L., Ordóñez Librado, J.L., Flores Martínez, E., and Fortoul, T.I. (2005a). Bilateral increase of perforated synapses after unilateral dopamine depletion. *Intern. J. Neuroscience*,115,79-86.

Avila-Costa, M.R., Colín-Barenque, L., Montiel-Flores, E., Aley-Medina, P., Gutiérrez Valdez, A.L., Ordóñez-Librado, J.L., Flores Martínez, E., Anaya Martínez, V., Mussali-Galante, P., and Fortoul, T.I. (2005b). Bromocriptine Treatment in a Murine Parkinson's Model. Ultrastructural Evaluation after Dopaminergic Deafferentation. *Int. J. of Neuroscience*, 115 (6), 851-859.

Bamford, N.S., Zhang, H., Schmitz, Y., Wu, N.P., Cepeda, C., Levine, M.S., Schmauss, C., Zakharenko, S.S., Zablow, L., Sulzer, D. (2004). Heterosynaptic dopamine neurotransmission selects sets of corticostriatal terminals. *Neuron,* 42, 653-663.

Beaulieu, C., Colonnier, M. (1989). Number and size of neurons and synapses in the motor cortex of cats raised in different environmental complexities. *J Comp Neurol*, 289,178-181.

Bemheimer, H., Birkmayer, W., Honykiewicz, 0., Jellinger, K., Seitelberger, F. (1973). Brain dopamine and the syndromes of Parkinson and Huntington. *j. Neurol. Sci,* 20, 415-455.

Björklund, A., Lindvall, 0. (1984). Dopamine-containing systems in the CNS. *Handbook of Chemical Neuroanatomy,* Vol. 2,*Classical Transmitters in the CNS, Part* I, A. Bjorklund, and T. Hokfelt, eds., pp. 55-122. Amsterdam, Elsevier.

Black, J. E., Isaacs, K. R., Anderson, B. J., Alcantara, A. A., and Greenough, W. T. (1990). Learning causes synaptogenesis, whereas motor activity causes angiogenesis, in cerebellar cortex of adult rats. *Proc. Natl. Acad. Sci, USA,* 87, 5568-72.

Bliss, T.V.P., Lømo, T. (1973). Long-lasting potentiation of synaptic transmission in the dentate area of the anaesthetized rabbit following stimulation of the perforant path. *J. Physiol*, 232, 331– 56.

Bolam, J., Bennett, D. (1995). Microcircuitry of the neostriatum: molecular and Cellular Mechanisms of Neostriatal Function. In *Molecular and Cellular Mechanisms of Neostriatal Function,* M. A. Arian, D. J. Surmeier, eds., pp. 1-20. Austin, TX, R. G. Landes.

Bolam, J.P., Hanley, J.J., Booth, P.A.C., Bevan, M.D. (2000). Synaptic organisation of the basal ganglia. *J. Anat*, 196, 527-542.

Bouyer, J.J., Park, D.H., Joh, T.H., Pickel, V.M (1984). Chemical and structural analysis of the relation between cortical inputs and tyrosine hydroxylase-containing terminals in rat neostriatum. *Brain Res*, 302, 267-275.

Buchs, P.A., Muller, D. (1996). Induction of long-term potentiation is associated with major ultrastructural changes of activated synapses. *Proc. Natl. Acad. Sci, USA,* 93, 8040-8045.

Cajal, S.R. (1894). La fine structure des centre nerveux. *Proc. R. Soc*, London B 55, 444– 68.

Calabresi P, Mercuri NB, Sancesario G, Bernardi G (1993) Electrophysiology of dopamine-denervated striatal neurons. Implications for Parkinson's disease. *Brain*, 116, 433-452.

Calabresi, P., De Murtas, M., and Bernardi, G. (1997a). The neostriatum beyond the motor function:experimental and clinical evidence. *Neuroscience, 78,* 39-60.

Calabresi, P., Saiardi, A., Pisani, A., Baik, J.H., Centonze, D., Mercuri, N.B., Bernardi, G., Borrelli, E. (1997b). Abnormal synaptic plasticity in the striatum of mice lacking dopamine D2 receptors. *J. Neurosci*, 17, 4536–78.

Calverley, R.K.S., Jones, D.G.A. (1987). Serial-section study of perforated synapses in rat neocortex. *Cell Tiss Res*, 247, 565–572.

Calverley, R.K.S., Jones, D.G. (1990). Contributions of dendritic spines and perforated synapses to synaptic plasticity. *Brain Res. Rev*, 15, 215– 49.

Caroni, P. (1998). Neuro-regeneration: plasticity for repair and adaptation. *Essays Biochem*, 33, 53–64.

Cepeda, C., Ariano, M.A., Calvert, C.R., Flores-Hernandez, J., Chandler, S.H., Leavitt, B.R., Hayden, M.R., Levine, M.S. (2001). NMDA receptor function in mouse models of Huntington disease. *J Neurosci Res*, 66, 525-539.

Chase, T.N., Engber, T.M., Mouradian, M.M. (1994). Glutamatergic influences and motor complications in Parkinson's disease. *New trends Clin Neuropharmacol*, 3, 18.

Chase, T.N., Oh, J.D. (2000). Striatal mechanisms and pathogenesis of parkinsonian signs and motor complications. *Ann Neurol*, 47, S122–S9.

Chase, T.N. (2004). Striatal plasticity and extrapyramidal motor dysfunction. *Parkinsonism Relat Disord*, 10, 305–13.

Chang, F.L.F., Greenough, W.T. (1984). Transient and enduring morphological correlates of synaptic activity and efficacy change in the rat hippocampal slice. *Brain Res*, 309, 35-46.

Chen, C., Tonegawa, S. (1997). Molecular genetic analysis of synaptic plasticity, activity-dependent neural development, learning, and memory in the mammalian brain. *Ann Rev Neurosci*, 20, 157-184.

Chesselet, M.F., Delfs, J.M. (1996). Basal ganglia and movement disorders: an update. *Trends Neurosci,* 19, 417-422.

Coggan, J.S., Grutzendler, J., Bishop, D.L., Cook, M.R., Gan, W., Heym, J., Lichtman, J.W. (2004). Age-associated synapse elimination in mouse parasympathetic ganglia. *J. Neurobiol*, 60, 214 –226.

Dauer, W., Przedborski, S. (2003). Parkinson's disease: mechanisms and models. *Neuron*, 11, 889-909.

Day, M., Wang, Z., Ding, J., An, X., Ingham, C.A., Shering, A.F., Wokosin, D., Ilijic, E., Sun, Z., Sampson, A.R., Mugnaini, E., Deutch, A.Y., Sesack, S.R., Arbuthnott, G.W., Surmeier, D.J. (2006). Selective elimination of glutamatergic synapses on striatopallidal neurons in Parkinson disease models. *Nat Neurosci,* 9, 251–259.

De Groot, D.M., Bierman, E. P. (1983). The complex-shaped "perforated" synapse, a problem in quantitative stereology of the brain. *J. Microsc,* 131, 355-60.

Delong, M.R. (1990). Primate models of movement disorders of basal ganglia origin. *Trends in Neuroscience*, 13, 281-285.

Desmond, N.L., Levy, W.B. (1986). Changes in the postsynaptic density with long-term potentiation in the dentate gyrus. *J. Comp. Neurol,* 253, 476–482

Desmond, N.L., Weinberg, R.J. (1998). Enhanced expression of AMPA receptor protein at perforated axospinous synapses. *NeuroReport*, 9, 857–860.

Devaud, J.M., Ferrus, A. (2003). Molecular genetics of activity-dependent structural changes at the synapse. *J. Neurogenet*, 17, 271–293.

Dyson, S.E., Jones, D.G. (1984). Synaptic remodeling during development and maturation: junction differentiation and splitting as a mechanism for modifying connectivity. *Brain Res,* 315, 125-37.

Edwards, F.A. (1995) Anatomy and electrophysiology of fast central synapses lead to a structural model for long-term potentiation. *Physiol. Rev*, 75, 759–787.

Emsley, J.G., Lu, X., Hagg, T. (2001). Retrograde Tracing Techniques Influence Reported Death Rates of Adult Rat Nigrostriatal Neurons. *Exp Neurol*, 168, 425-433.

Engert, F., Bonhoeffer, T. (1999). Dendritic spine changes associated with hippocampal long-term synaptic plasticity. *Nature*, 399, 66–70.

Fass, B., Butcher, L.L. (1981). Evidence for a crossed nigrostriatal pathway in rats. *Neursci Lett*, 22, 109-113.

Federmeier, K., Kleim, J. A., Anderson, B. J., and Greenough, W. T. (1994). Formation of double synapses in the cerebellar cortex of the rat following motor learning. *Soc. Neurosci. Abstr,* 20, 1435.

Fiala, J. C., Spacek, J., Harris, M. (2002). Dendritic Spine Pathology: Cause or Consequence of Neurological Disorders? *Brain Res. Rev*, 39, 29–54.

Fisher, R.S., Levine, M.S., Sibley, D.R., Ariano, M.A. (1994). D2 dopamine receptor protein location: Golgi impregnation-gold toned and ultrastructural analysis of the rat neostriatum. *J Neurosci Res*, 38, 551-564.

Flores-Hernandez, J., Galarraga, E., Bargas, J. (1997). Dopamine selects glutamatergic inputs to neostriatal neurons. *Synapse*, 25, 185-195.

Forno, L.S., Norville, R.L. (1979). Ultrastructure of the neostriatum Huntington's and Parkinson's disease. *Advances in Neurology*, 23, 123- 135.

Freund, T.F., Powell, J., Smith, A.D. (1984). Tyrosine hydroxylase-immunoreactive boutons in synaptic contact with identified striatonigral neurons, with particular reference to dendritic spines. *Neuroscience*, 13, 1189-1215.

Gan, W.B., Kwon, E., Feng, G., Sanes, J.R., Lichtman, J.W. (2003). Synaptic dynamism measured over minutes to months: age-dependent decline in an autonomic ganglion. *Nat. Neurosci,* 6, 956 –960.

Geinisman, Y., Morrell, F., de Toledo-Morrell, L. (1987). Axospinous synapses with segmented postsynaptic densities: A morphologically distinct synaptic subtype contributing to the number of profiles of "perforated" synapses visualized in random sections. *Brain Research*, 423, 179–188.

Geinisman, Y., Morrell, F., de Toledo-Morrell, L. (1988). Remodeling of synaptic architecture during hippocampal "kindling." *Proc. Natl. Acad. Sci*, USA 85, 3260–3264.

Geinisman, Y., de Toledo-Morrell, L., Morrell, F. (1991). Induction of long-term potentiation is associated with an increase in the number of axospinous synapses with segmented postsynaptic densities. *Brain Res*, 566, 77–88.

Geinisman, Y., Morrell, F., de Toledo Morrell, L. (1992). Increase in the number of axospinous synapses with segmented postsynaptic densities following hippocampal kindling. *Brain Res*, 569, 341 347.

Geinisman, Y. (1993). Perforated axospinous synapses with multiple, completely partitioned transmission zones: probable structural intermediates in synaptic plasticity. *Hippocampus,* 3, 417-434.

Geinisman, Y. (2000). Structural synaptic modifications associated with hippocampal LTP and behavioral learning. *Cereb Cortex*, 10, 952–962.

Geinisman, Y., Berry, R. W., Disterhoft, J. F., Power, J. M., Van der Zee, E.A. (2001). Associative learning elicits the formation of multiple-synapse boutons. *J. Neurosci*, 21, 5568–5573.

Gerfen, C.R. (1988). Synaptic Organization of the Striatum. *J. Elec. Micros. Thech*, 10, 265-281.

Gerfen, C.R., Engber, T. M., Mahan, L. C., Susel, Z., Chase, T. N., Monsma, F.J., Sibley, D.R. (1990). D1 and D2 dopamine receptor-regulated gene expression of striatonigral and striatopallidal neurons. *Science*, 250, 1429–1432.

Gerfen, C.R., Wilson, C.J. (1996). In Björklund A, Hökfelt T, Swanson L (eds.) *The Basal Ganglia*. Handbook of Chemical Neuroanatomy, Integrated Systems of the CNS, Part III, (pp. 369-466). Amsterdam: Elsevier Science.

Greenough, W. T., West, R., DeVoogd, T. J. (1978). Subsynaptic plate perforations: Changes with age and experience in the rat. *Science*, 202, 1096–1098.

Harris, K.M., Jensen, F.E., Tsao, B. (1992). Three-dimensional structure of dendritic spines and synapses in rat hippocampus (CA1) at postnatal day 15 and adult ages: Implications for the maturation of synaptic physiology and long-term potentiation. *J. Neurosci*, 12, 2685-2705.

Harris, K.M., Fiala, J.C., Ostroff, L. (2003). Structural changes at dendritic spine synapses during long-term potentiation. *Philos. Trans. R. Soc. Lond. B. Biol. Sci*, 358, 745–748.

Hatton, J.D., Ellisman, M.H. (1982). A restructuring of hypothalamic synapses is associated with motherhood. *J. Neurosci*, 2, 704 707.

Hebb, D.O. (1949). *The Organization of Behavior*. New York, USA: Wiley.

Honer, W.G. (2003). Pathology of presynaptic proteins in Alzheimer's disease: more than simple loss of terminals. *Neurobiol. Aging*, 24, 1047–1062.

Hsu, K.S., Huang, C.C., Yang, C.H., Gean, P.W (1995). Presynaptic D2 dopaminergic receptors mediate inhibition of excitatory synaptic transmission in rat neostriatum. *Brain Res*, 690, 264-268.

Ingham, C.A., Hood, S.H., Arbuthnott, G.W. (1991). A light and electron microscopical study of enkephalin-immunoreactive structures in the rat neostriatum after removal of the nigrostriatal dopaminergic pathway. *Neuroscience*, 42, 715-730.

Ingham,C.A., Hood, S.H., VanMaldengen, B., Weenink, A., Arbuthnot, G.W. (1993). Morphological changes in the rat neostriatum after unilateral 6-hydroxydopamine injection into the nigrostriatal pathway. *Exp. Brain Res*, 93, 17-27.

Ingham, C.A., Hood, S.H., Arbuthnott, G.W. (1998). Plasticity of synapses in the rat neostriatum after unilateral lesion of the nigrostriatal dopaminergic pathway. *J. Neurosci*, 18, 4732-4743.

Itarat, W., Jones, D.G. (1992). Perforated synapses are present during synaptogenesis in rat neocortex. *Synapse*, 11, 279–286.

Izzo, P.N., Bolam, J.P. (1988). Cholinergic synaptic input to different parts of spiny striatonigral neurons in the rat. *J. Comparative Neurol*, 269, 219-234.

Kirov, S.A., Goddard,C.A., Harris, K.M. (2004). Age-dependence in the homeostatic upregulation of hippocampal dendritic spine number during blocked synaptic transmission. *Neuropharmacology,* 47, 640–648.

Kleim, J. A., Napper, R. M. A., Swain, R. A., Armstrong, K. E., Jones, T. A., Greenough, W. T. (1994). Selective synaptic plasticity in the cerebellar cortex of the rat following complex motor learning. *Soc. Neurosci. Abstr*, 20, 1435.

Kleim, J. A., Vij, K., Ballard, D. H., and Greenough, W. T. (1997). Learning-dependent synaptic modifications in the cerebellar cortex of the adult rat persist for at least 4 weeks. *J. Neurosci*, 17, 717-721.

Kolomeets, N.S., Orlovskaya, D.D., Rachmanova, V.I., Uranova, N.A. (2005). Ultrastructural alterations in hippocampal mossy fiber synapses in schizophrenia: a postmortem morphometric study. *Synapse*, 57, 47–55.

Kretz, O., Fester, L., Wehrenberg, U., Zhou, L., Brauckmann, S., Zhao, S., Prange-Kiel, J., Naumann, T., Jarry, H., Frotscher, M., Rune, G.M. (2004). Hippocampal synapses depend on hippocampal estrogen synthesis. *J. Neurosci*, 24, 5913–5921.

Liaw, J.S., Xie, X., Ghaffari, T., Baudry, M., Chauvet, G.A., and Berger, T. W. (1999). *Role of Synaptic Geometry in the Dynamics and Efficacy of Synaptic Transmission*. In: Advances in Synaptic Plasticity. M. Baudry, J. L. Davis and R. F. Thompson (Eds). The MIT Press, NY. PP. 103-153.

Lindefors, N., Ungerstedt, U. (1990). Bilateral regulation of glutamate tissue and extracellular levels in caudate-putamen by midbrain dopamine neurons. *Neurosci Lett,* 115, 248–252.

Lüscher, C., Nicoll, R.A., Malenka, R.C., Muller, D. (2000). Synaptic plasticity and dynamic modulation of the postsynaptic membrane. *Nat. Neurosci*, 3, 545–550.

Machado-Salas, J.P., Ibarra, O., Martínez-Fong, D., Cornejo, A., Aceves, J., Kuri, J. (1989). Degenerative ultrastructural changes observed in the neuropil of caudate nuclei from Parkinson's disease patients. *Stereotactic. Functional Neurosurgery*, 54+55, 297-305.

Mahncke, H.W., Bronstone, A., Merzenich, M.M. (2006). Brain Plasticity and Functional Losses in the Aged: Scientific Bases for a Novel Intervention. *Prog Brain Res*, 157, 81-109.

Marsden, C. D., and Obeso, J. A. (1994). The functions of the basal ganglia and the paradox of stereotaxic surgery in Parkinson's disease. *Brain,* 117, 877-897.

Mattson, M.P., Furukawa, K. (1998). Signaling events regulating the neurodevelopmental triad. Glutamate and secreted forms of β-amyloid precursor protein as examples. *Persp. devl Neurobiol*, 5, 337–352.

Matsuoka, M., Kaba, H., Mori, Y., Ichikawa, M. (1997). Synaptic plasticity in olfactory memory formation in female mice. Learning and Memory. *Neuroreport,* 8, 2501-2504.

Matus, A. (2000). Actin-based plasticity in dendritic spines. *Science*, 290,754–758.

McEachern, J.C., Shaw, C.A. (1999). The plasticity–pathology continuum: defining a role for the LTP phenomenon. *J. Neurosci. Res*, 58, 42–61.

McNeill, T.H., Brownn, S.A., Rafols, J.A., Shoulson, I. (1988).Atrophy of medium spiny I striatal dendrites in advanced Parkinson's disease. *Brain Res*, 455,148-152.

Meshul, C.K., Casey, D.E. (1989). Regional, reversible ultrastructural changes in rat brain with chronic neuroleptic treatment. *Brain Res,* 489, 338 –346.

Meshul, C. K., Stallbaumer, R. K., Taylor, B., Janowsky, A. (1994). Haloperidol-induced synaptic changes in striatum are associated with glutamate synapses. *Brain Res*, 648, 181–195.

Meshul, C. K., Emre, N., Nakamura, C. M., Allen, C., Donohue, M. K., Buckman, J. F. (1999). Time-dependent changes in striatal glutamate synapses following a 6-hydroxydopamine lesion. *Neuroscience,* 88, 1–16.

Meshul, C. K., Cogen, J. P., Cheng, H.W., Moore, C., Krentz, L., and McNeill, T. H. (2000). Alterations in Rat Striatal Glutamate Synapses Following a Lesion of the Cortico- and/or Nigrostriatal Pathway. *Exp Neurol*, 165, 191–206.

Miller, R.J., Murphy, S.N., Glaum, S.R. (1989). Neuronal calcium channels and their regulation by excitatory amino acids. *Ann New York Acad Sci*, 568, 149-158.

Milner, B. (1966). *Amnesia following operation on the temporal lobes*. In Amnesia: Clinical, Psychological and Medicolegal Aspects, ed. CWM Whitty, OL Zangwill, pp. 109– 133. London, UK: Butterworths.

Murrin, C., Ferrer, J.R. (1984). Ontogeny of the rat striatum: correspondence of dopamine terminals, opiate receptors and acetylcholinesterase. *Neurosci. Lett,* 47, 155-160.

Neely, M. D., Schmidt, D. E., Deutch, A.Y. (2007). Cortical regulation of dopamine depletion-induced dendritic spine loss in striatal medium spiny neurons. *Neuroscience*, 149, 457–464.

Nimchinsky, E.A., Sabatini, B.L., Svoboda, K. (2002). Structure and function of dendritic spines. *Annu. Rev. Physiol*, 64, 313-353.

O'Donnell, P., Grace, A.A. (1994). Tonic D2-mediated attenuation of cortical excitation in nucleus accumbens neurons recorded in vitro. *Brain Res*, 634, 105-112.

Paxinos, G., and Watson, C. (1986). *The rat brain in Stereotaxic Coordinates* (2nd ed.). New York, USA: Academic Press.

Peters, A., Palay, S., Webster, H. (1991). *Synapses. In: The fine Structure of the nervous system*. 3rd edition. Oxford University Press, New York,USA.

Pickel, V.M., Johnson, E., Carson, M., Chan, J. (1992). Ultrastructure of spared dopamine terminals in caudate-putamen nuclei of adult rats neonatally treated with intranigral 6-hydroxidopamine. *Developmental Brain Research*, 70, 75-86.

Reynolds, J.N.J., Wickens, J. (2002). Dopamine-dependent plasticity of corticostriatal synapses. *Neural Networks*, 15, 507-521.

Roberts, R., DiFiglia, M. (1990). Evidence for synaptic proliferation, reorganization, and growth in the exitotoxic lesioned adult rat caudate nucleus. *Exp Neurol*, 107, 1-10.

Rocha, M., Sur, M. (1995). Rapid acquisition of dendritic spines by visual thalamic neurons after blockade of N-methyl-D-aspartate receptors. *Proc Natl Acad Sci*, U S A 92, 8026–8030.

Rosenzweig, E.S., Barnes, C.A. (2003). Impact of aging on hippocampal function: plasticity, network dynamics, and cognition. *Prog. Neurobiol*, 69, 143–179.

Sabatini, B.L., Maravall, M., Svoboda, K. (2001). Ca2+ signaling in dendritic spines. *Curr Opin Neurobiol*, 11, 349-356.

Scheff, S.W., Price, D.A. (2003). Synaptic pathology in Alzheimer's disease: a review of ultrastructural studies. *Neurobiol. Aging*, 24, 1029 –1046.

Schober, A. (2004).Classic toxin-induced animal models of Parkinson's disease: 6-OHDA and MPTP. *Cell Tissue Res*, 318, 215-224.

Segal, M. (2005). Dendritic spines and long-term plasticity. Nat Rev Neurosci 6, 277-284.

Seroogy, K.B., Lundgren, K.H., Tran,T.M.D., Guthrie, K.M., Isackson, P.J., Gall, C.M. (1994). Dopaminergic neurons in rat ventral midbrain express brain-derived neurotrophic factor and neurotrophin-3 mRNAs. *J. Comp. Neurol*, 342, 321-334.

Sesack, S.R., Aoki, C., Pickel, V.M. (1994). Ultrastructural localization of D2 receptor-like immunoreactivity in midbrain dopamine neurons and their striatal targets. *J Neurosci*, 14, 88-106.

Shepherd, G.M. (1996). The dendritic spine: A multifunctional integrative unit. *J Neurophysiol,* 75, 2197-2210.

Sirevaag, A.M., Greenough, W.T. (1985). Differential rearing effects on rat visual cortex synapses. II. Synaptic morphometry. *Dev. Brain Res*, 19, 215 226.

Smart, F.M., Halpain, S. (2000). Regulation of dendritic spine stability. *Hippocampus*, 10, 542–554.

Smith, A.D., Bolam, J.P. (1990). The neuronal network of the basal ganglia as revealed by the study of synaptic connections of identified neurones. *Trends Neurosci*, 13, 259-265.

Smith, Y., Bennett, B.D., Bolam, J.P., Parent, A., Sadikot, A.F. (1994). Synaptic relationships between dopaminergic afferents and cortical or thalamic input in the sensorimotor territory of the striatum in monkey. *J Comp Neurol*, 344, 1-19.

Smith, Y., Bevan, M.D., Shink, E., Bolam, J.P. (1998). Microcircuitry of the direct and indirect pathways of the basal ganglia. *Neuroscience,* 86, 353-387.

Solis, O., Limón, D.I., Flores-Hernández, J., Flores, G. (2007). Alterations in dendritic morphology of the prefrontal cortical and striatum neurons in the unilateral 6-OHDA-rat model of Parkinson's disease. *Synapse*, 61, 450 – 458.

Spires, T.L., Hyman, B.T. (2004). Neuronal structure is altered by amyloid plaques. *Rev Neurosci,* 15, 267–278.

Sulzer, D., Pothos, E.N. (2000). Regulation of quantal size by presynaptic mechanisms. *Rev Neurosci*, 11, 159-212.

Tang, K., Low, M.J., Grandy, D.K., Lovinger, D.M. (2001). Dopamine-dependent synaptic plasticity in striatum during in vivo development. *Proc Natl Acad Sci*, USA 98, 1255-1260.

Tarazi, F.I., Baldessarini, R.J. (1999). Regional localization of dopamine and ionotropic glutamate receptor subtypes in striatolimbic brain regions. *J Neurosci Res*, 55, 401–410.

Toni, N., Buchs, P.A., Nikonenko, I., Bron, C.R., Muller, D. (1999). LTP promotes formation of multiple spine synapses between a single axon terminal and a dendrite. *Nature*, 402, 421-425.

Toni, N., Buchs, P.A., Nikonenko, I., Povilaitite, P., Parisi, L., and Muller, D. (2001). Remodeling of Synaptic Membranes after Induction of Long-Term Potentiation. *J. Neurosci*, 21, 6245–6251.

Turner, A.M., Greenough, W.T. (1985). Differential rearing effects on rat visual cortex synapses. I. Synaptic and neuronal density and synapses per neuron. *Brain Res*, 329, 195-203.

Turski, L., Turski, W.A. (1993). Towards an understanding of the role of glutamate in neurodegenerative disorders: energy metabolism and neuropathology. *Experientia*, 49, 1064-1072.

Ungerstedt, U. (1968). 6-Hydroxydopamine induced degeneration of central monoaminergic neurons. *Eur J Pharmacol*, 5, 107–110.

Van der Kloot, W. (1991). The regulation of quantal size. *Prog Neurobiol*, 36, 93-130.

Volkmar, F. R., Greenough, W. T. (1972). Rearing complexity affects branching of dendrites in the visual cortex of the rat. *Science,* 176, 1145-7.

Voom, P., Kalsbeek, A., Jorritsma-Byham, B., Groenewegen, H.J. (1988). The pre- and postnatal development of the dopaminergic cell groups in the ventral mesencephalon and the dopaminergic innervation of the striatum of the rat. *Neuroscience,* 25, 857-887.

Vrensen, G., Nunez, J. (1981). Changes in size and shape of synaptic connections after visual training: an ultrastructural approach of synaptic plasticity. *Brain Res*, 218, 79 97.

Wang, H., Pickel, V.M. (2002). Dopamine D2 receptors are present in prefrontal cortical afferents and their targets in patches of the rat caudateputamen nucleus. *J Comp Neurol*, 442, 392-404.

Weihmuller, F. B., Bruno, J.P. (1989). Age-dependent plasticity in the dopaminergic control of sensorimotor development. *Behay. Brain Res,* 35, 95-109.

West, A.R., Grace, A.A. (2002). Opposite influences of endogenous dopamine D1 and D2 receptor activation on activity states and electrophysiological properties of striatal neurons: studies combining in vivo intracellular recordings and reverse microdialysis. *J Neurosci*, 22, 294-304.

Wilson, C.J. (1996). *Basal Ganglia. In Gordon M. Shepherd* (Ed.). The synaptic Organization of the Brain (pp. 329-352). New York, USA: Oxford University Press.

Wojtowicz, J. M., Marin, L., and Atwood, H. L (1989). Synaptic restructuring during long-term facilitation at the crayfish neuromuscular junction. *Can. J. Physiol. Pharmacol*, 67, 167-71.

Yang, J., Sadler, T.R., Givrad, T.K., Maarek, J.M.I., Holschneider, D.P. (2007). Changes in brain functional activation during resting and locomotor states after unilateral nigrostriatal damage in rats. *Neuroimage*, 36, 755–773.

Yung, K.K.L., Smith, A.D., Levey, A.I., Bolam, J.P. (1996). Synaptic connections between spiny neurons of the direct and indirect pathways in the neostriatum of the rat: evidence from dopamine receptor and neuropeptide immunostaining. *Eur. J. Neurosci*, 8, 861-869.

Yuste, R., Majewska, A., Hotlhoff, K. (2000). From form to function: calcium compartmentalization in dendritic spines. *Nat. Neurosci*, 3, 653– 59.

Zaja-Milatovic, S., Milatovic, D., Schantz, A.M., Zhang, J., Montine, K. S., Samii,A., Deutch, A.Y., Montine, T. J. (2005). Dendritic degeneration in neostriatal medium spiny neurons in Parkinson disease. *Neurol,* 64, 545–547.

Zhu, J.J., Esteban, J.A., Hayashi,Y., Malinow, R. (2000). Postnatal synaptic potentiation: delivery of GluR4-containing AMPA receptors by spontaneous activity. *Nat. Neurosci*, 3, 1098–1106.

Zuch, C.L., Nordstroem, V.K., Briedrick, L.A., Hoernig, G.R., Granholm, A.C., Bickford, P.C. (2000). Time course of degenerative alterations in nigral dopaminergic neurons following a 6-hydroxydopamine lesion. *J Comp Neurol*, 427, 440-54.

Zigmond, M.J., Striker, E.M. (1989). Animal models of parkinsoninsm using selective neurotoxins: clinical and basic implications. *Int. Rev. Neurobiol,* 31, 1-79.

In: Synaptic Plasticity: New Research
Editors: Tim F. Kaiser and Felix J. Peters

ISBN: 978-1-60456-732-8

Chapter 5

SYNAPTIC PLASTICITY AND MOTOR LEARNING IN THE CEREBELLUM

Shun Tsuruno and Tomoo Hirano
Department of Biophysics, Kyoto University, Japan

ABSTRACT

The cerebellum plays a key role in motor learning. Since Marr and Albus proposed the perceptron model of cerebellar cortex, extensive study has been performed to clarify the mechanism of motor learning. The cerebellar long-term depression (LTD) is a type of synaptic plasticity occurring at the parallel fiber – Purkinje cell synapses, which was predicted by Albus and has been regarded as a cellular basis of motor learning. Not only its involvement in motor learning but also its regulation mechanisms at a molecular level have been clarified. On the other hand, other forms of synaptic plasticity have been reported in the cerebellum. Long-tem potentiation (LTP) and LTD occur at both excitatory and inhibitory synapses in the cortex and also in the cerebellar nuclei. Their molecular mechanisms and implication in motor learning have also been studied.

In this article, we begin by reviewing researches on the regulatory molecular mechanisms of the cerebellar LTD. Then, we turn to other forms of synaptic plasticity. Finally, we summarize the involvement of cerebellar synaptic plasticity in several motor learning tasks by reviewing studies on animals with surgical lesion, chemical inactivation or genetic manipulation of a specific region of the cerebellar circuit.

INTRODUCTION

The cerebellum is involved in motor control and motor learning. Recent progress in brain imaging techniques has revealed that the cerebellum is also involved in cognitive functions such as processing of language [1,2]. The cerebellum is composed of cortex and nuclei [3]. Five types of neurons, Purkinje cells, granule cells, Golgi cells, basket cells and stellate cells, are found in the cortex. The main inputs into the cerebellar cortex are mossy fibers and climbing fibers (Figure 1).

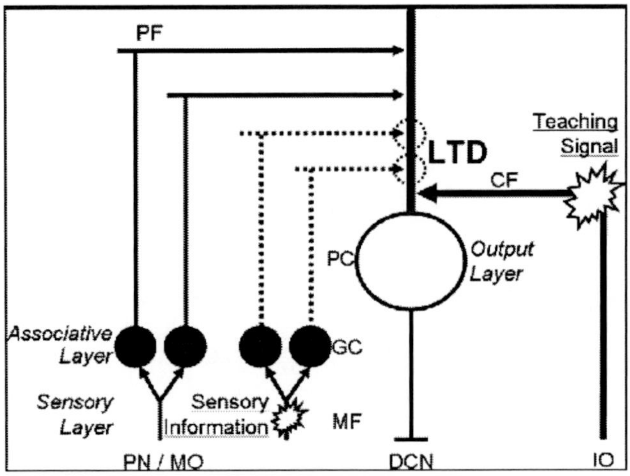

Figure 1. Main neural circuits of the cerebellar cortex. Sensory information is transmitted to the cerebellar cortex through mossy fibers (MF). They are regarded as elements of the sensory layer in a three-layered perceptron. Mossy fibers project to granule cells (GC), corresponding to elements of the associative layer in the perceptron. Granule cells project to a Purkinje cell (PC), corresponding to elements of the output layer. A climbing fiber (CF) relays the teaching signal to a Purkinje cell. LTD occurs at the synapses between parallel fibers (PF) and a Purkinje cell, when the synaptic activity is followed by the climbing fiber activity. CF: climbing fiber, DCN: deep cerebellar nuclei, GC: granule cell, IO: inferior olivary nuclei, MF: mossy fiber, MO: medulla oblongata, PC: Purkinje cell, PF: parallel fiber, PN: pontine nuclei.

On the other hand, the output from the cortex is confined to axons of Purkinje cells, which form GABAergic inhibitory synapses on neurons in the deep cerebellar nuclei or in the vestibular nuclei. The cerebellar cortex has three layers – the molecular, Purkinje and granular layer. The outermost molecular layer contains two types of inhibitory interneurons, basket and stellate cells, dendrites of Purkinje cells and axons of granule cells called parallel fibers. Parallel fibers run laterally to the body axis, and perpendicularly to the flat dendrites of Purkinje cells. Beneath the molecular layer is the Purkinje layer, where cell bodies of Purkinje cells spread over in a single layer. The innermost granular layer contains cell bodies of granule and Golgi cells. Climbing fibers originate from neurons in the inferior olivary nuclei located in the ventral side of brainstem. A mature Purkinje cell receives synaptic inputs from only one climbing fiber, which forms as many as 300 glutamatergic synapses and provides a strong excitatory effect inducing a characteristic action potential called complex spike [3]. Mossy fibers arise from neurons in the pontine nuclei or in the medulla oblongata. They form excitatory synapses on granule cells. An axon of a granule cell goes up to the molecular layer, where it bifurcates into a parallel fiber. A parallel fiber forms excitatory glutamatergic synapses on Purkinje cells. Each of parallel fiber – Purkinje cell synapse is weak, but a single Purkinje cell has more than 100 thousand parallel fiber synapses. Parallel fibers also form synapses on basket, stellate and Golgi cells. Both basket and stellate cells form inhibitory

GABAergic synapses on Purkinje cells, whereas Golgi cells inhibit activity of granule cells in a feedback manner.

Around 1970, Marr and Albus proposed that the neural circuit in the cerebellar cortex can be regarded as a three-layered perceptron [4,5]. A perceptron is a type of network system that learns to distinguish input patterns. A three-layered perceptron consists of the sensory, associative and output layers. Elements in the sensory layer send signals to elements in the associative layer, and they in turn send signals to elements in the output layer. Information processing in a perceptron is transformed by the teaching signal which tells whether the output pattern of perceptron is appropriate or not. The efficacy of information transmission between elements of the associative and the output layers is weakened if the output is inappropriate, and strengthened if appropriate. Marr and Albus regarded mossy fibers as elements in the sensory layer, granule cells as those in the associative layer and Purkinje cells as those in the output layer (Figure 1). They thought that climbing fibers provide teaching signals. Albus considered that climbing fibers code an error signal which is sent when the output is inappropriate. It depresses the efficacy of synaptic transmission between parallel fibers (granule cells) and a Purkinje cell, which occurred just before the arrival of error signal. In the early 1980's, Masao Ito and his colleagues showed that conjunctive stimulation of parallel fibers and a climbing fiber leads to long-term depression (LTD) of the information transmission at the parallel fiber – Purkinje cell synapses [6].

The deep cerebellar nuclei (DCN) consist of the dentate, emboliform, globose and fastigial nuclei. Neurons in DCN receive excitatory synaptic inputs from mossy and climbing fibers, and inhibitory synaptic inputs from Purkinje cells. Some DCN neurons project to premotor and motor areas of the cerebral cortex through the thalamus. Different functional roles are assigned to the distinct regions of DCN. Some neurons in the vestibular nuclei also receive synaptic inputs from Purkinje cells in the flocculus or in the ventral paraflocculus of cerebellar cortex. Therefore, the cerebellar cortex participates in the neural computation through modulation of outputs from DCN and vestibular nuclei.

In this chapter, we will first review the molecular mechanisms of LTD induction at parallel fiber – Purkinje cell synapses. Then, we will introduce other forms of synaptic plasticity in the cerebellum, and explain their implication in motor learning.

1. Long-Term Depression

The cerebellar LTD occurs at the parallel fiber – Purkinje cell synapses, when a Purkinje cell receives concurrent synaptic inputs from parallel fibers and a climbing fiber [6-8]. It lasts for more than 24 hours [9]. Both parallel and climbing fibers release glutamate as the neurotransmitter. It is known that N-methyl-D-aspartate (NMDA) type of ionotropic glutamate receptor plays an important role in the induction of synaptic plasticity in the hippocampus [10]. However, the expression level of NMDA receptor is very low in mature Purkinje cells [11,12]. Thus, implication of NMDA receptor in the cerebellar LTD is unlikely. Major glutamate receptors on Purkinje cells are α-amino-3-hidroxy-5-methylisoxazolpropionic acid (AMPA) type ionotropic glutamate receptor and type I metabotropic glutamate receptor, mGluR1. The δ2 subunit of glutamate receptor is also localized at the postsynaptic membrane of parallel fiber – Purkinje cell synapses, although it does not seem to work as an ion-conducting channel [13,14].

Since a climbing fiber forms numerous synapses on a Purkinje cell, a single action potential can induce a strong postsynaptic depolarization through activation of AMPA receptor, leading to large Ca^{2+} influx through voltage-gated Ca^{2+} channel, which is abundantly expressed in dendrites of Purkinje cells [15] (Figure 2).

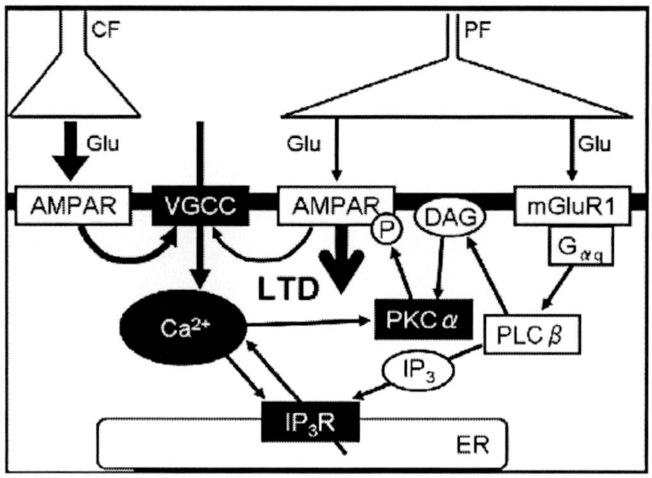

Figure 2. The main molecular signaling pathways involved in induction of the cerebellar LTD. The candidates of coincidence detectors are shown in white characters. AMPAR: AMPA receptor, CF: climbing fiber, DAG: diacylglycerol, ER: endoplasmic reticulum, $G_{\alpha q}$: Gq protein α subunit, Glu: glutamate, IP_3R: IP_3 receptor, mGluR1, metabotropic type I glutamate receptor, PF: parallel fiber, PKCα: protein kinase Cα, PLCβ: phospholipase Cβ, VGCC: voltage-gated Ca^{2+} channel.

The increase in the intracellular Ca^{2+} concentration is necessary for the induction of LTD. Glutamate released from a parallel fiber activates AMPA receptor and mGluR1. mGluR1 activates phospholipase Cβ (PLCβ) through $G_{\alpha q}$. PLCβ produces inositol-1,4,5-triphosphate (IP_3) and diacylglycerol (DAG) from phosphatidylinositol biphosphate (PIP_2) in the plasma membrane (Figure 2). IP_3 is released to the cytoplasm, where it binds to IP_3 receptors on the membrane of endoplasmic reticulum and induces Ca^{2+} release from the endoplasmic reticulum to the cytoplasm. Thus, both the Ca^{2+} influx through voltage-gated Ca^{2+} channel and the Ca^{2+} release from the intracellular store cooperatively increase the intracellular Ca^{2+} concentration. DAG produced by mGluR1/PLCβ pathway activates protein kinase C (PKC) together with Ca^{2+} [16]. PKC phosphorylates the PSD-95/DlgA/zo-1 (PDZ) domain binding motif in the C-terminus of GluR2 subunit of AMPA receptor [17]. LTD induction depends on the activity of PKCα but not of PKCγ, another subtype of PKC abundantly expressed in Purkinje cells [18]. This specificity is ascribed to the PDZ-binding motif found in PKCα, but not in PKCγ. In the basal condition, AMPA receptors are accumulated in the postsynaptic membrane and bind to glutamate receptor interacting protein (GRIP) [19]. After phosphorylation of GluR2 by PKCα, AMPA receptor is released from GRIP and binds to protein interacting with C-kinase-1 (PICK1) [17]. The binding to PICK1 is thought to lead to endocytosis of the receptor. Thus, AMPA receptor on the postsynaptic membrane is reduced in the number [20,21]. This is a current prevailing scheme of the molecular induction mechanism of cerebellar LTD [22].

One important feature of LTD induction is its requirement for concurrent synaptic inputs from two pathways, parallel fibers and a climbing fiber. A protocol for LTD induction is pairing stimulation of parallel fibers and a climbing fiber at 1-4 Hz for 100-600 times. LTD is induced when each climbing fiber stimulation follows each parallel fiber stimulation with a delay of up to 250 ms [23,24]. This LTD induction condition is consistent with the Albus model, which suggests that an error signal coded as a climbing fiber input is fed back to a Purkinje cell, and depresses the parallel fiber – Purkinje cell synaptic transmission which has contributed to an inappropriate output.

There are four candidate molecules or ions playing a key role in the coincidence detection of two inputs. They are Ca^{2+}, voltage-gated Ca^{2+} channel, IP_3 receptor and PKC (Figure 2). Ca^{2+} enters the cytoplasm through two types of channels, voltage-gated Ca^{2+} channel on the plasma membrane and IP_3 receptor on the endoplasmic reticulum. Cytoplasmic Ca^{2+} concentration might reach the threshold for LTD induction only when the two types of channel open concurrently. The second candidate is voltage-gated Ca^{2+} channel. Paired activation of parallel fibers and a climbing fiber may cause local depolarization larger than that caused by each. The steep voltage-dependence of open probability of voltage-gated Ca^{2+} channel may contribute to the supralinear activation of Ca^{2+} channel near the parallel fiber – Purkinje cell synapses [24]. The third candidate is IP_3 receptor. IP_3 receptor is a type of Ca^{2+} channel localized not on the plasma membrane but on the membrane of endoplasmic reticulum, that is opened by binding to IP_3. It is known that their opening probability increases when the cytoplasmic Ca^{2+} concentration is increased [25]. Thus, coincident activation of parallel fibers and a climbing fiber induces a large increase in the intracellular Ca^{2+} concentration depending on the Ca^{2+} release from the endoplasmic reticulum [24]. This response exceeds the simple sum of each response. Computational simulation study supports a role of IP_3 receptor for the coincidence detection [26]. LTD is absent in a mutant mouse lacking endoplasmic reticulum in the postsynaptic spines of a PN, which might also support the role of IP_3 receptor [27]. The fourth candidate is PKCα. PKCα translocates from the cytoplasm to the plasma membrane by binding Ca^{2+}, and then becomes fully activated by binding DAG [16]. A climbing fiber input induces a large increase in the intracellular Ca^{2+} concentration, and parallel fiber inputs increase DAG in the plasma membrane [15]. In the hippocampus, concurrent activation of Ca^{2+} permeable NMDA receptors and mGluR induces synergistic activation of PKCγ [28]. This result suggests that PKCα integrates the Ca^{2+} signal and the mGluR signal, and may work as a coincidence detector for the LTD induction in a Purkinje cell. However, a live-imaging study of PKCα tagged with green fluorecent protein (GFP) reported that the activity of PKCα is not apparently prolonged by the coincident activation of Ca^{2+} channel and mGluR1 [29]. Considering the requirement for sequential inputs from parallel fibers and a climbing fiber in the LTD induction, IP_3 receptor may play a main role in the coincidence detection [26].

There are other molecules involved in the LTD induction such as mitogen-activated protein kinase (MAPK), phospholipase A_2 (PLA_2), nitric oxide (NO), protein kinase G (PKG), Ca^{2+}/calmodulin-dependent protein kinase II (CaMKII), protein phosphatase 2B (PP2B, calcineurin), PTPMEG, protein tyrosine kinases and GluRδ2 subunit [30-42]. NO is released from stellate cells activated by parallel fibers [43-45]. It diffuses into Purkinje cells and activates guanylyl cyclase, producing cyclic GMP (cGMP) [34,35,46,47]. cGMP activates PKG, which in turn phosphorylates G-substrate. Phosphorylated G-substrate suppresses protein phosphatases such as PP2A which counteracts kinases involved in the LTD induction [48]. LTD is induced not only at synapses which are active during induction, but also at nearby inactive synapses [49,50]. This heterosynaptic LTD is suggested to depend on diffusion of nitric oxide [51,52].

Although δ2 subunit does not form an ion-conducting channel, it is grouped as an ionotropic glutamate receptor according to its primary structure [53,54]. Extensive studies have been conducted on this molecule. It is specifically expressed on the postsynaptic membrane of parallel fiber – Purkinje cell synapses and is required for the LTD induction [13,42,53-56]. δ2 knockout mouse shows not only LTD impairment but also reduced number of parallel fiber synapses, motor incoordination and impaired motor learning [55,57-60]. Physiological ligand of δ2 has not been identified, although serine and glycine bind to δ2 [61,62]. LTD is also rescued in a δ2-null Purkinje cell by transfection of truncated δ2 subunit that contains highly-charged membrane-proximal motif in the cytoplasmic region but not by transfection of the mutant δ2 subunit without the charged motif [63]. δ2 subunit interacts with PICK1 through this charged motif, and this interaction is required for the LTD induction. Other studies demonstrated that the PDZ-binding motif in the C-terminus of δ2 subunit is also required for the LTD induction [64,65]. Thus, δ2 seems to regulate the LTD induction through the interaction with intracellular molecules, although the detail is enigmatic.

As described above, various molecules are involved in the LTD induction. However, it is not clear how their interaction is regulated in the complex intracellular signaling cascade. A computational simulation model of molecular signaling cascades involved in the LTD induction has been constructed in an attempt to clarify the role of each molecule [37,66].

Long-Term Potentiation and Other Forms of Synaptic Plasticity

Synaptic plasticity in the cerebellar cortex

Long-term potentiation (LTP) is induced at the parallel fiber – Purkinje cell synapses by repetitive stimulation of parallel fibers [8,67-71]. Two forms of LTP have been reported (Figure 3).

One is accompanied with the increased glutamate release from the presynaptic terminal, and the other with the increased postsynaptic glutamate responsiveness. The former is induced by the 2-8 Hz repetitive stimulation, and the latter by the 1 Hz stimulation. While the induction of presynaptic LTP depends on cyclic AMP (cAMP) in the presynaptic terminal, the induction of postsynaptic LTP depends on NO and moderate increase in the postsynaptic intracellular Ca^{2+} concentration [69-71]. It is suggested that the postsynaptic LTP reverses the cerebellar LTD by increasing the number of AMPA receptors on the postsynaptic membrane [72].

Long-term synaptic plasticity is also reported at the GABAergic inhibitory synapses between basket/stellate cells and a Purkinje cell. When a Purkinje cell is strongly depolarized, for example by repetitive climbing fiber inputs, the efficacy of synaptic transmission is potentiated for more than 30 minutes. [73]. This phenomenon is called rebound potentiation

(RP), and is accompanied with the enhancement of postsynaptic GABA response mediated by ionotropic $GABA_A$ receptors. Induction of RP depends on the postsynaptic CaMKII activity and structural alteration of $GABA_A$ receptor-associated protein (GABARAP), which binds to both $GABA_A$ receptor γ2 subunit and tubulin, the component of microtubule [74,75]. A unique property of RP is that its induction depends on the heterosynaptic excitatory inputs. Thus, RP induction does not depend on the activity of synapse undergoing potentiation. However, when GABA is released at an inhibitory synapse during postsynaptic depolarization, RP induction is suppressed at the synapse [76]. This suppression enables the synapse-specific regulation of RP. RP suppression is mediated by activation of the postsynaptic metabotropic $GABA_B$ receptors, which inhibits CaMKII through a signaling cascade involving $G_{i/o}$, adenylyl cyclase, cAMP, protein kinase A, dopamine- and cAMP-regulated phosphoprotein of 32kDa (DARPP-32) and PP1 [77]. RP is also suppressed by integrin, a cell adhesion molecule, through activation of c-Src [78]. RP induction is occluded in a δ2 knockout mouse through the enhanced climbing fiber activity *in vivo* [79]. LTD is also reported at the synapse between a basket/stellate cell and a Purkinje cell [80].

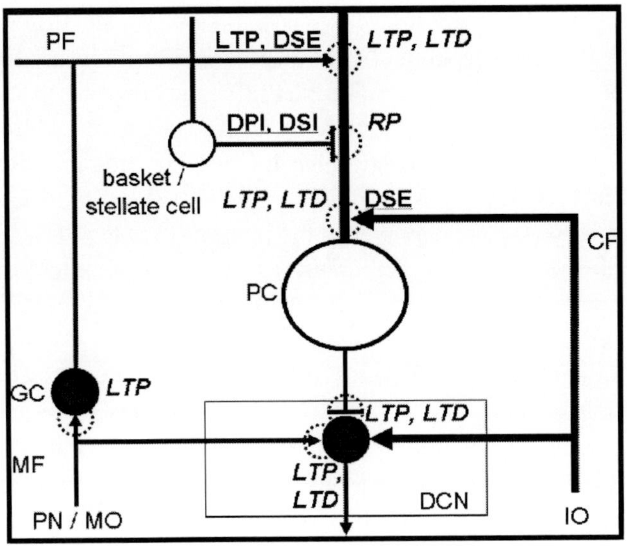

Figure 3. Various forms of synaptic plasticity in the cerebellum. Underlined words indicate the synaptic plasticity expressed presynaptically and ITALIC words indicate that expressed postsynaptically. Filled circles and arrows show somata and axons of excitatory neurons. Open circles and lines ended with bars indicate somata and axons of inhibitory neurons. Dpi: depolarization-induced potentiation of inhibition, dse: depolarization-induced suppression of excitation, dsi: depolarization-induced suppression of inhibition, ltd: long-term depression, ltp: long-term potentiation, rp: rebound potentiation. Cf: climbing fiber, dcn: deep cerebellar nuclei, gc: granule cell, io: inferior olivary nuclei, mf: mossy fiber, mo: medulla oblongata, pc: purkinje cell, pf: parallel fiber, pn: pontine nuclei.

LTP and LTD have also been reported at climbing fiber – Purkinje cell synapses [81,82]. In P14-26 rats, LTD is induced by repetitive stimulation of a climbing fiber, depending on the increase in postsynaptic intracellular Ca^{2+} and on the PKC activity [81]. Multiple climbing fibers innervate a Purkinje cell in a neonatal rat. The number of innervating climbing fibers decreases during development, resulting in the strong innervation by one climbing fiber by P20. In P6-9 rats, a Purkinje cell is innervated by one strong climbing fiber and several weak climbing fibers. Pairing depolarization of a Purkinje cell with activation of a strongly-innervating climbing fiber induces homosynaptic LTP, whereas that with activation of a weakly-innervating climbing fiber induces homosynaptic LTD [82]. LTP and LTD in P6-9 rats were suggested to be involved in the developmental reduction of number of innervating climbing fibers.

The suppression mechanism of transmitter release from parallel fibers, climbing fibers or inhibitory interneurons triggered in a postsynaptic Purkinje cell has also been reported. When a Purkinje cell is depolarized and/or the postsynaptic mGluR1 is activated, an endocannabinoid called 2-arachidonoyl glycerol (2-AG) is released from the Purkinje cell [83-87]. 2-AG suppresses the transmitter release through activation of presynaptic type 1 cannabinoid receptor (CB1R) for several tens of seconds. CB1R couples to heterotrimeric G protein, which downregulates the voltage-gated Ca^{2+} channel and increases the K^+ conductance through GIRK channel in the presynaptic terminal [88,89]. The depolarization-induced suppression of glutamate release from parallel or climbing fibers is called DSE (depolarization-induced suppression of excitation), and that of GABA from inhibitory interneurons is called DSI (depolarization-induced suppression of inhibition). 2-AG is catalyzed from DAG by DAG lipase, which is expressed in dendrites of a Purkinje cell [90,91]. The release of 2-AG depends on the depolarization-induced elevation of Ca^{2+} for DSE and DSI, and on activation of the mGluR1/PLCβ signaling cascade for the suppression induced by parallel-fiber activity [83-85,92]. Intracellular Ca^{2+} elevation to a micromolar range is required for DSE [93]. However, when mGluR1 is activated during depolarization, less intracellular Ca^{2+} elevation is sufficient to induce DSE [92]. PLCβ, which is cooperatively activated by $G_{\alpha q}$ and Ca^{2+}, plays the integrative role [94].

There is also short-term (lasting for about 10 minutes) potentiation of GABA release from inhibitory interneurons induced by depolarization of a postsynaptic Purkinje cell [95]. This phenomenon is called depolarization-induced potentiation of inhibition (DPI). DPI induction depends on activation of the presynaptic NMDA receptor. Glutamate is released from a Purkinje cell in response to depolarization, and serves as a retrograde messenger. Glutamate causes the increase in intracellular Ca^{2+} concentration in presynaptic terminals through activation of NMDA receptor, facilitating the transmitter release [95,96].

LTP has also been reported at a mossy fiber – granule cell synapse. The high frequency activation of mossy fibers paired with depolarization of the postsynaptic granule cell induces LTP [97,98]. The LTP induction requires postsynaptic activation of NMDA receptor and the consequent Ca^{2+} influx. Implication of mGluR and PKC has also been reported. This form of LTP is accompanied with the increase in amplitudes of both AMPA and NMDA receptor-mediated current. The time course of NMDA receptor-mediated current is prolonged during LTP, which could lead to the increased time window for temporal summation [97,99].

Synaptic Plasticity in the DCN

A Purkinje cell directly inhibits neurons in DCN through GABAergic synapses. Both LTP and LTD are reported at this synapse [100-102]. A DCN neuron exhibits rebound depolarization and spike bursts after the offset of hyperpolarizing current [103]. This rebound depolarization is mediated by low-threshold voltage-gated Ca^{2+} channel [104]. A Purkinje cell causes hyperpolarization and the following rebound depolarization, spike bursts and consequent Ca^{2+} influx in a DCN neuron. LTP is induced depending on the strong Ca^{2+} influx, whereas LTD is induced with a moderate Ca^{2+} influx [100]. This direction control mechanism of synaptic plasticity is similar to the BCM model at excitatory synapses [105,106].

LTP and LTD have also been reported at the mossy fiber – DCN neuron excitatory synapses [107,108]. Both AMPA and NMDA receptors are expressed at the synapse. However, unlike other synapses, NMDA receptor shows low Mg^{2+} sensitivity and weak voltage dependence. Therefore, NMDA receptor can be activated at a basal condition [109]. LTP is induced by pairing the high-frequency mossy fiber stimulation with the postinhibitory rebound depolarization of a postsynaptic DCN neuron. NMDA receptor activation and the increase in postsynaptic Ca^{2+} concentration are necessary for the induction. It was also shown that mossy fiber activity has to precede the postinhibitory rebound depolarization, implying that the LTP induction is controlled by relative timing of the mossy fiber input and the Purkinje cell input [107]. On the other hand, LTD is induced by the high-frequency burst stimulation of mossy fibers, either alone or paired with the postsynaptic depolarization [108]. The LTD induction depends on the postsynaptic Ca^{2+} increase, mGluR1 activation and protein translation.

Role of Synaptic Plasticity in Motor Learning

Adaptation of VOR and OKR

Adaptation of vestibulo-ocular reflex and opto-kinetic response (VOR and OKR, respectively) are well-studied models of motor learning which depend on the cerebellum [110-113]. Both VOR and OKR are reflex eye movement that stabilizes image on the retina during head motion. Eyes move in the opposite direction to the head movement or the same direction of visual field movement. In OKR, eye balls follow the slow visual field movement using the visual signal. In VOR, the vestibular organs in inner ears sense the head movement, and the vestibular signal drives the eye ball movement. OKR dominates in the relatively slow eye movement, and VOR plays a more important role in the relatively quick movement. They work cooperatively in a daily life. The efficacy of these reflexes during the sinusoidal rotation of an animal or visual field can be quantitatively evaluated by two parameters, the gain and the phase. The gain is the amplitude of eye movement divided by the amplitude of stimulus, the head movement in VOR and the visual field movement in OKR. The phase indicates the delay or lead of eye movement relative to the stimulus.

Adaptive changes of both VOR and OKR have been regarded as models of motor learning. Sustained stimulation of an animal with sinusoidal rotation of the visual field gradually increases the OKR gain toward one and decreases the phase toward zero. Thus, OKR adaptation minimizes the retinal slip. On the other hand, sustained sinusoidal rotation of an animal coupled with the visual field rotation changes the gain and phase of VOR. When the direction of head and visual field movement are opposite, the VOR gain increases and the phase difference decreases, which is called the gain-up VOR adaptation. When the direction of the two stimuli is the same, the VOR gain decreases, which is called the gain-down VOR adaptation. For example, when we start to wear new eyeglasses, VOR adaptation minimizes the retinal slip. Adaptation of VOR or OKR is impaired by surgical lesion, pharmacological inactivation or genetic disruption of a part of the cerebellum, suggesting that the cerebellum is required for memory formation [60,114,115]. In a *lurcher* mouse, which lacks outputs from the cerebellar cortex due to the developmental loss of Purkinje cells, neither VOR nor OKR adaptation occurs [60].

The main neural pathway controlling VOR consists of vestibular organs, vestibular nuclei and oculomotor nuclei. In addition, there is a regulatory side pathway including the flocculus and the ventral paraflocculus of cerebellum. These regions receive inputs from the vestibular organ through mossy fibers and project to the vestibular nucleus through Purkinje cell axons. Where is the motor memory for VOR adaptation stored in these neural circuits? Two candidate sites have been considered. One is the synapses between parallel fibers and Purkinje cells in the cerebellar cortex, and the other is the synapses between vestibular afferents and neurons in the vestibular nuclei. Ito proposed that the cerebellar LTD at parallel fiber – Purkinje cell synapse is responsible for VOR adaptation [111]. The correlation of retinal slip (the visual image motion on a retina) and climbing fiber activity was reported [116]. On the other hand, Lisberger and colleagues considered that the synaptic plasticity in the vestibular nucleus plays an essential role in VOR adaptation [117]. Later, implication of both forms of synaptic plasticity in the VOR adaptation has been suggested [60,113,118,119].

Eyeblink Conditioning

Eyeblink conditioning is another model task for motor learning which depends on the cerebellum, and has been studied extensively [120,121] (Figure 4).

Eyeblinking is elicited by applying aversive stimulus such as an air puff to an eye or the electrical stimulation. Such stimulus is called unconditioned stimulus (US), and the reflexive eyeblink response is called unconditioned response (UR). In eyeblink conditioning, US is preceded by a neutral stimulus that by itself does not elicit UR such as tone (conditioned stimulus, CS). Repeated CS-US pairings make an animal elicit a response similar to UR upon CS (conditioned response, CR). Two training procedures have been used. One is the delayed procedure, in which CS and US overlap in time. The other is the trace procedure with a time interval between the CS offset and the US onset. In both procedures the cerebellum is implicated. Additionally, the hippocampus plays an essential role in the trace training [120]. Lesion experiments, electrophysiological recordings and electrical stimulation of the inferior olivary nuclei have shown that US information is transmitted to the cerebellar cortex and also to the interpositus nucleus of DCN through climbing fibers. Similarly, lesion and stimulation of pontine nuclei revealed that CS information is transmitted to the cerebellar cortex and the interpositus nucleus through the mossy fiber pathway. Therefore, CS and US signals are integrated at both Purkinje cells and neurons in the interpositus nucleus .

The interpositus nucleus is involved in both UR and CR [120]. Some neurons in the interpositus nucleus discharge spikes preceding the onset of CR and in a precise temporal pattern related to the onset of CS. Lesion or reversible inactivation of the interpositus nucleus abolishes acquired CR, but not UR, in well-trained animals, and also prevents acquisition of new CR. On the other hand, inactivation of the red nucleus, which is located downstream of the interpositus nucleus, prevents expression of acquired CR without preventing CR acquisition. These results suggest that the memory trace of CR is localized in the interpositus nucleus. Infusion of a NMDA receptor antagonist or a transcription inhibitor into the interpositus nucleus also impairs acquisition of CR, but does not affect acquired CR, suggesting that the synaptic plasticity plays a role in acquisition of CR. Consistent with this view, significant increase in the number of excitatory synapses in the interpositus nucleus is observed following the eyeblink conditioning [122]. Taken together, these results suggest that LTP at mossy fiber – interpositus nucleus plays a critical role in the memory formation for the eyeblink CR.

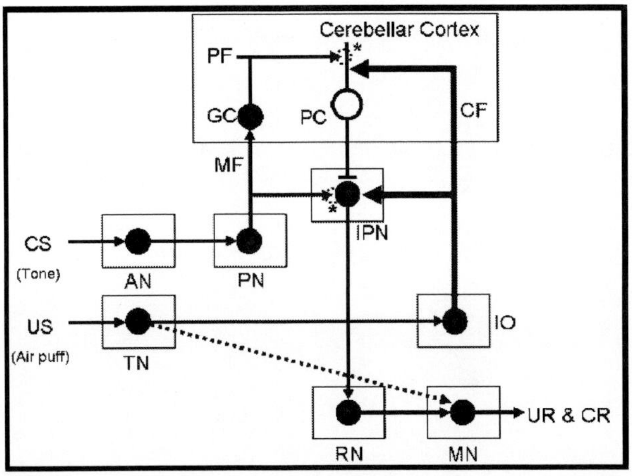

Figure 4. The neural circuits involved in the regulation of eyeblink conditioning. Filled circles and arrows show somata and axons of excitatory neurons. An open circle and a line ended with a bar indicate a soma and axon of an inhibitory neuron (Purkinje cell, PC). Broken circles marked with asterisks indicate synapses implicated in the memory formation. AN: auditory nuclei, CF: climbing fiber, GC: granule cell, IO: inferior olivary nuclei, IPN: interpositus nucleus, MF: mossy fiber, MN: motor nuclei, PC: Purkinje cell, PF: parallel fiber, PN: pontine nuclei, RN: red nucleus, TN: trigeminal nucleus. CR: conditioned response, CS: conditioned stimulus, UR: unconditioned response, US: unconditioned stimulus.

How is the cerebellar cortex involved in the eyeblink conditioning? Large lesion of the cerebellar cortex does not abolish the acquired CR, but decreases the latency and amplitude of CR in a well-trained animal. Thus, memory of CR seems not to be stored in the cerebellar cortex. In contrast, a Purkinje cell degeneration (*pcd*) mutant mouse without the cortical output shows significant deficits in the acquisition of CR, although CR is slowly acquired depending on the interpositus nucleus [123,124]. Mutant mice with impaired LTD at parallel fiber – Purkinje cell synapses such as PLCβ4 or δ2 knockout mice also show the impaired eyeblink conditioning [58,125]. In addition, a significant decrease in the AMPA binding to cerebellar cortical slices is observed after the eyeblink conditioning [126]. These results suggest that LTD at parallel fiber – Purkinje cell synapse is involved in the eyeblink conditioning. The LTD would decrease the inhibitory outputs from a Purkinje cell, which should in turn increase excitability of neurons in the interpositus nucleus and contribute to the CR expression [120,127]. After repetitive CS – US pairings, the firing rate of a Purkinje cell decreases before the US onset, implying that CR is reflected in the cortical output [128]. However, in the genetically manipulated mice in which cerebellar granule cell outputs can be blocked by administration of a drug, Purkinje cells show very low firing rates and the CR does not occur during the blockade [129]. After the removal of blockade, unexpectedly, CR occurs from the beginning of reconditioning. Taken all these information together, although cerebellar cortex is involved in some aspects of the eyeblink conditioning and that LTD at parallel fiber – Purkinje cell synapse plays a role in the conditioning, an essential memory trace seems to be formed and stored in the interpositus nucleus.

Conclusion

The cerebellar neural circuit has attracted neuroscientists over the last 40 years for its structural simplicity and homogeneity. These features might make the cerebellum the first CNS structure where the principle functioning rule and mechanism are clarified. Recent studies have shown that various forms of synaptic plasticity are induced at various synapses in the cerebellum, although their roles *in vivo* are enigmatic. Generation of mutant mice with specific deficits together with the development of new techniques to monitor and/or manipulate neuronal activity *in vivo* would contribute to the understanding of the roles of each form of synaptic plasticity.

References

[1] Fiez, J.A. (1996). Cerebellar Contributions To Cognition. *Neuron*, 16, 13-15.

[2] Cabeza, R., Nyberg, L. (2000). Imaging Cognition Ii: An Empirical Review Of 275 Pet And Fmri Studies. *J Cogn Neurosci*, 12, 1-47.

[3] Llinas, R.R., Walton, K.d., Lang, E.J. (2004). *Cerebellum*. In: Shepherd Gm (Ed). The Synaptic Organization Of The Brain: Oxford University Press; Pp. 271-309.

[4] Marr, D. (1969). A Theory Of Cerebellar Cortex. *J Physiol,* 202, 437-470.

[5] Albus J. (1971). A Theory Of Cerebellar Function. *Math Biosci*, 10, 25-61.

[6] Ito, M., Sakurai, M., Tongroach, P. (1982). Climbing Fibre Induced Depression Of Both Mossy Fibre Responsiveness And Glutamate Sensitivity Of Cerebellar Purkinje Cells. *J Physiol*, 324, 113-134.

[7] Sakurai, M. (1987). Synaptic Modification Of Parallel Fibre-Purkinje Cell Transmission In In Vitro Guinea-Pig Cerebellar Slices. *J Physiol,* 394, 463-480.

[8] Hirano, T. (1990). Depression And Potentiation Of The Synaptic Transmission Between A Granule Cell And A Purkinje Cell In Rat Cerebellar Culture. *Neurosci Lett*, 119, 141-144.

[9] Murashima, M., Hirano, T. (1999). Entire Course And Distinct Phases Of Day-Lasting Depression Of Miniature Epsc Amplitudes In Cultured Purkinje Neurons. *J Neurosci*, 19, 7326-7333.

[10] Bliss, T., Collingridge, G. (1993). A Synaptic Model Of Memory: Long-Term Potentiation In The Hippocampus. *Nature*, 361, 31-39.

[11] Llano, I., Marty, A., Armstrong, C., Konnerth, A. (1991). Synaptic- And Agonist-Induced Excitatory Currents Of Purkinje Cells In Rat Cerebellar Slices. *J Physiol*, 434, 183-213.

[12] Piochon, C., Irinopoulou, T., Brusciano, D., Bailly, Y., Mariani, J., Levenes, C. (2007). Nmda Receptor Contribution To The Climbing Fiber Response In The Adult Mouse Purkinje Cell. *J Neurosci*, 27, 10797-10809.

[13] Landsend, A., Amiry-Moghaddam, M., Matsubara, A., Bergersen, L., Usami, S., Wenthold, R. Et Al. (1997). Differential Localization Of Δ Glutamate Receptors In The Rat Cerebellum: Coexpression With Ampa Receptors In Parallel Fiber-Spine Synapses And Absence From Climbing Fiber-Spine Synapses. *J Neurosci*, 17, 834-842.

[14] Kakegawa, W., Kohda, K., Yuzaki, M. 2007). The Δ2 'Ionotropic' Glutamate Receptor Functions As A Non-Ionotropic Receptor To Control Cerebellar Synaptic Plasticity. *J Physiol*, 584, 89-96.

[15] Miyakawa, H., Lev-Ram, V., Lasser-Ross, N., Ross, W.N. (1992). Calcium Transients Evoked By Climbing Fiber And Parallel Fiber Synaptic Inputs In Guinea Pig Cerebellar Purkinje Neurons. *J Neurophysiol*, 68, 1178-1189.

[16] Oancea, E., Meyer, T. (1998). Protein Kinase C As A Molecular Machine For Decoding Calcium And Diacylglycerol Signals. *Cell,* 95, 307-318.

[17] Chung, H., Xia, J., Scannevin, R., Zhang, X., Huganir, R. (2000), Phosphorylation Of The Ampa Receptor Subunit Glur2 Differentially Regulates Its Interaction With Pdz Domain-Containing Proteins. *J Neurosci*, 20, 7258-7267.

[18] Leitges, M., Kovac, J., Plomann, M., Linden, D.J. (2004). A Unique Pdz Ligand In Pkcα Confers Induction Of Cerebellar Long-Term Synaptic Depression. *Neuron*, 44, 585-594.

[19] Osten, P., Khatri, L., Perez, J., Köhr, G., Giese, G., Daly, C. Et Al. (2000). Mutagenesis Reveals A Role For Abp/Grip Binding To Glur2 In Synaptic Surface Accumulation Of The Ampa Receptor. *Neuron*, 27, 313-325.

[20] Xia, J., Chung, H.J., Wihler, C., Huganir, R.l., Linden, D.J. (2000). Cerebellar Long-Term Depression Requires Pkc-Regulated Interactions Between Glur2/3 And Pdz Domain-Containing Proteins. *Neuron*, 28, 499-510.

[21] Steinberg, J., Takamiya, K., Shen, Y., Xia, J., Rubio, M., Yu, S. Et Al. (2006). Targeted In Vivo Mutations Of The Ampa Receptor Subunit Glur2 And Its Interacting Protein Pick1 Eliminate Cerebellar Long-Term Depression. *Neuron*, 49, 845-860.

[22] Ito, M. (2002). The Molecular Organization Of Cerebellar Long-Term Depression. *Nat Rev Neurosci,* 3, 896-902.

[23] Chen, C., Thompson, R. (1995). Temporal Specificity Of Long-Term Depression In Parallel Fiber--Purkinje Synapses In Rat Cerebellar Slice. *Learn Mem*, 2, 185-198.

[24] Wang, S.S., Denk, W., Hausser, M. (2000). Coincidence Detection In Single Dendritic Spines Mediated By Calcium Release. *Nat Neurosci*, 3, 1266-1273.

[25] Bezprozvanny, I., Watras, J., Ehrlich, B. (1991). Bell-Shaped Calcium-Response Curves Of Ins(1,4,5)P3- And Calcium-Gated Channels From Endoplasmic Reticulum Of Cerebellum. *Nature*, 351, 751-754.

[26] Doi, T., Kuroda, S., Michikawa, T., Kawato, M. (2005).Inositol 1,4,5-Trisphosphate-Dependent Ca^{2+} Threshold Dynamics Detect Spike Timing In Cerebellar Purkinje Cells. *J Neurosci*, 25, 950-961.

[27] Miyata, M., Finch, E., Khiroug, L., Hashimoto, K., Hayasaka, S., Oda, S. Et Al. (2000). Local Calcium Release In Dendritic Spines Required For Long-Term Synaptic Depression. *Neuron,* 28, 233-244.

[28] Codazzi, F., Di Cesare, A., Chiulli, N., Albanese, A., Meyer, T., Zacchetti, D. Et Al. (2006).Synergistic Control Of Protein Kinase Cγ Activity By Ionotropic And Metabotropic Glutamate Receptor Inputs In Hippocampal Neurons. *J Neurosci*, 26, 3404-3411.

[29] Tsuruno, S., Hirano, T. (2007). Persistent Activation Of Protein Kinase Cα Is Not Necessary For Expression Of Cerebellar Long-Term Depression. *Mol Cell Neurosci*, 35, 38-48.

[30] Ito, M. (2001). Cerebellar Long-Term Depression: Characterization, Signal

Transduction, And Functional Roles. *Physiol Rev*, 81, 1143-1195.
[31] Kawasaki, H., Fujii, H., Gotoh, Y., Morooka, T., Shimohama, S., Nishida, E. Et Al. (1999). Requirement For Mitogen-Activated Protein Kinase In Cerebellar Long Term Depression. *J Biol Chem*, 274, 13498-13502.
[32] Endo, S., Launey, T. (2003). Erks Regulate Pkc-Dependent Synaptic Depression And Declustering Of Glutamate Receptors In Cerebellar Purkinje Cells. *Neuropharmacology*, 45, 863-872.
[33] Linden, D. (1995). Phospholipase A2 Controls The Induction Of Short-Term Versus Long-Term Depression In The Cerebellar Purkinje Neuron In Culture. *Neuron,* 15, 1393-1401.
[34] Crepel, F., Jaillard, D. (1990). Protein Kinases, Nitric Oxide And Long-Term Depression Of Synapses In The Cerebellum. *Neuroreport*, 1, 133-136.
[35] Hartell N. (1994). Cgmp Acts Within Cerebellar Purkinje Cells To Produce Long Term Depression Via Mechanisms Involving Pkc And Pkg. *Neuroreport*, 5, 833-836.
[36] Hansel, C., De Jeu, M., Belmeguenai, A., Houtman, S., Buitendijk, G., Andreev, D. Et Al. (2006). Acamkii Is Essential For Cerebellar Ltd And Motor Learning. *Neuron*, 51, 835-843.
[37] Tanaka, K., Khiroug, L., Santamaria, F., Doi,T., Ogasawara, H., Ellis-Davies, G. Et Al. (2007). Ca^{2+} Requirements For Cerebellar Long-Term Synaptic Depression: Role For A Postsynaptic Leaky Integrator. *Neuron,* 54, 787-800.
[38] Fujii, H., Hirano, T. (2002). Calcineurin Regulates Induction Of Late Phase Of Cerebellar Long-Term Depression In Rat Cultured Purkinje Neurons. *Eur J Neurosci*, 16, 1777-1788.
[39] Fujiwara, A., Kakizawa, S., Iino, M. (2007). Induction Of Cerebellar Long-Term Depression Requires Activation Of Calcineurin In Purkinje Cells. *Neuropharmacology*, 52, 1663-1670.
[40] Kina, S., Tezuka, T., Kusakawa, S., Kishimoto, Y., Kakizawa, S., Hashimoto, K. Et Al. (2007). Involvement Of Protein-Tyrosine Phosphatase Ptpmeg In Motor Learning And Cerebellar Long-Term Depression. *Eur J Neurosci,* 26, 2269-2278.
[41] Boxall, A., Lancaster, B., Garthwaite, J. Tyrosine Kinase Is Required For Long-Term Depression In The Cerebellum. *Neuron*, (1996).16, 805-813.
[42] Hirano, T., Kasono, K., Araki, K., Shinozuka, K., Mishina, M. (1994). Involvement Of The Glutamate Receptor Δ2 Subunit In The Long-Term Depression Of Glutamate Responsiveness In Cultured Rat Purkinje Cells. *Neurosci Lett*, 182, 172-176.
[43] Casado, M., Dieudonné, S., Ascher, P. (2000). Presynaptic N-Methyl-D-Aspartate Receptors At The Parallel Fiber-Purkinje Cell Synapse. *Proc Natl Acad Sci,* USA, 97, 11593-11597.
[44] Casado, M., Isope, P., Ascher, P. Involvement Of Presynaptic N-Methyl-D-Aspartate Receptors In Cerebellar Long-Term Depression. *Neuron*, (2002). 33, 123-130.
[45] Shin, J., Linden, D. (2005). An Nmda Receptor/Nitric Oxide Cascade Is Involved In Cerebellar Ltd But Is Not Localized To The Parallel Fiber Terminal. *J Neurophysiol*, 94, 4281-4289.
[46] Boxall, A., Garthwaite, J. (1996).Long-Term Depression In Rat Cerebellum Requires Both No Synthase And No-Sensitive Guanylyl Cyclase. *Eur J Neurosci,* 8, 2209-2212.
[47] Lev-Ram, V., Nebyelul, Z., Ellisman, M., Huang, P., Tsien, R. (1997). Absence Of Cerebellar Long-Term Depression In Mice Lacking Neuronal Nitric Oxide Synthase. *Learn Mem*, 4, 169-177.
[48] Launey, T., Endo, S., Sakai, R., Harano, J., Ito, M. (2004). Protein Phosphatase 2a Inhibition Induces Cerebellar Long-Term Depression And Declustering Of Synaptic Ampa Receptor. *Proc Natl Acad Sci*, USA, 101, 676-681.

[49] Reynolds, T., Hartell, N. (2000). An Evaluation Of The Synapse Specificity Of Long-Term Depression Induced In Rat Cerebellar Slices. *J Physiol*, 527 Pt 3, 563-577.

[50] Wang, S., Khiroug, L., Augustine, G. (2000). Quantification Of Spread Of Cerebellar Long-Term Depression With Chemical Two-Photon Uncaging Of Glutamate. *Proc Natl Acad Sci*, USA, 97, 8635-8640.

[51] Hartell, N. (1996). Strong Activation Of Parallel Fibers Produces Localized Calcium Transients And A Form Of Ltd That Spreads To Distant Synapses. *Neuron*, 16, 601-610.

[52] Ogasawara, H., Doi, T., Doya, K., Kawato, M. (2007). Nitric Oxide Regulates Input Specificity Of Long-Term Depression And Context Dependence Of Cerebellar Learning. *Plos Comput Biol*, 3, E179.

[53] Araki, K., Meguro, H., Kushiya, E., Takayama, C., Inoue, Y., Mishina, M. (1993). Selective Expression Of The Glutamate Receptor Channel Δ2 Subunit In Cerebellar Purkinje Cells. *Biochem Biophys Res Commun*, 197, 1267-1276.

[54] Lomeli, H., Sprengel, R., Laurie, D., Köhr, G., Herb, A., Seeburg, P. Et Al. (1993). The Rat Δ1 And Δ2 Subunits Extend The Excitatory Amino Acid Receptor Family. *Febs Lett*, 315, 318-322.

[55] Kashiwabuchi, N., Ikeda, K., Araki, K., Hirano, T., Shibuki, K., Takayama, C. Et Al. (1995). Impairment Of Motor Coordination, Purkinje Cell Synapse Formation, And Cerebellar Long-Term Depression In Glur Δ2 Mutant Mice. *Cell*, 81, 245-252.

[56] Takayama, C., Nakagawa, S., Watanabe, M., Mishina, M., Inoue, Y. (1995). Light- And Electron-Microscopic Localization Of The Glutamate Receptor Channel Δ2 Subunit In The Mouse Purkinje Cell. *Neurosci Lett*, 188, 89-92.

[57] Hashimoto, K., Ichikawa, R., Takechi, H., Inoue, Y., Aiba, A., Sakimura, K. Et Al. (2001). Roles Of Glutamate Receptor Δ2 Subunit (Glurδ2) And Metabotropic Glutamate Receptor Subtype 1 (Mglurl) In Climbing Fiber Synapse Elimination During Postnatal Cerebellar Development. *J Neurosci*, 21, 9701-9712.

[58] Kishimoto, Y., Kawahara, S., Suzuki, M., Mori, H., Mishina, M., Kirino, Y. (2001). Classical Eyeblink Conditioning In Glutamate Receptor Subunit Δ2 Mutant Mice Is Impaired In The Delay Paradigm But Not In The Trace Paradigm. *Eur J Neurosci*, 13, 1249-1253.

[59] Yoshida, T., Katoh, A., Ohtsuki, G., Mishina, M., Hirano, T. (2004). Oscillating Purkinje Neuron Activity Causing Involuntary Eye Movement In A Mutant Mouse Deficient In The Glutamate Receptor Δ2 Subunit. *J Neurosci*, 24, 2440-2448.

[60] Katoh, A., Yoshida, T., Himeshima, Y., Mishina, M., Hirano, T. (2005). Defective Control And Adaptation Of Reflex Eye Movements In Mutant Mice Deficient In Either The Glutamate Receptor Δ2 Subunit Or Purkinje Cells. *Eur J Neurosci*, 21, 1315-1326.

[61] Yuzaki, M. (2003). New Insights Into The Structure And Function Of Glutamate Receptors: The Orphan Receptor Δ2 Reveals Its Family's Secrets. *Keio J Med*, 52, 92-99.

[62] Naur, P., Hansen, K., Kristensen, A., Dravid, S., Pickering, D., Olsen, L. Et Al. (2007). Ionotropic Glutamate-Like Receptor Δ2 Binds D-Serine And Glycine. *Proc Natl Acad Sci*, USA, 104, 14116-14121.

[63] Yawata, S., Tsuchida, H., Kengaku, M., Hirano, T. (2006). Membrane-Proximal Region Of Glutamate Receptor Δ2 Subunit Is Critical For Long-Term Depression And Interaction With Protein Interacting With C Kinase 1 In A Cerebellar Purkinje Neuron. *J Neurosci,* 26, 3626-3633.

[64] Kohda, K., Kakegawa, W., Matsuda, S., Nakagami, R., Kakiya, N., Yuzaki, M. (2007). The Extreme C-Terminus Of Glurδ2 Is Essential For Induction Of Long-Term Depression In Cerebellar Slices. *Eur J Neurosci,* 25, 1357-1362.

[65] Kakegawa, W., Miyazaki, T., Emi, K., Matsuda, K., Kohda, K., Motohashi, J. Et Al. (2008). Differential Regulation Of Synaptic Plasticity And Cerebellar Motor Learning By The C-Terminal Pdz-Binding Motif Of Glurδ2. *J Neurosci,* 28, 1460-1468.

[66] Kuroda, S., Schweighofer, N., Kawato, M. (2001). Exploration Of Signal Transduction Pathways In Cerebellar Long-Term Depression By Kinetic Simulation. *J Neurosci*, 21, 5693-5702.

[67] Crepel, F., Jaillard, D. (1991). Pairing Of Pre- And Postsynaptic Activities In Cerebellar Purkinje Cells Induces Long-Term Changes In Synaptic Efficacy In Vitro. *J Physiol*, 432, 123-141.

[68] Hirano, T. (1991). Differential Pre- And Postsynaptic Mechanisms For Synaptic Potentiation And Depression Between A Granule Cell And A Purkinje Cell In Rat Cerebellar Culture. *Synapse*, 7, 321-323.

[69] Salin, P., Malenka, R., Nicoll, R. (1996).Cyclic Amp Mediates A Presynaptic Form Of Ltp At Cerebellar Parallel Fiber Synapses. *Neuron*, 16, 797-803.

[70] Lev-Ram, V., Wong, S., Storm, D., Tsien, R. (2002). A New Form Of Cerebellar Long-Term Potentiation Is Postsynaptic And Depends On Nitric Oxide But Not Camp. *Proc Natl Acad Sci*, USA, 99, 8389-8393.

[71] Coesmans, M., Weber, J., De Zeeuw, C., Hansel, C. (2004). Bidirectional Parallel Fiber Plasticity In The Cerebellum Under Climbing Fiber Control. *Neuron*, 44, 691-700.

[72] Jörntell, H., Hansel, C. (2006). Synaptic Memories Upside Down: Bidirectional Plasticity At Cerebellar Parallel Fiber-Purkinje Cell Synapses. *Neuron*, 52, 227-238.

[73] Kano, M., Rexhausen, U., Dreessen, J., Konnerth, A. (1992). Synaptic Excitation Produces A Long-Lasting Rebound Potentiation Of Inhibitory Synaptic Signals In Cerebellar Purkinje Cells. *Nature*, 356, 601-604.

[74] Kawaguchi, S., Hirano, T. (2007). Sustained Structural Change Of $Gaba_a$ Receptor-Associated Protein Underlies Long-Term Potentiation At Inhibitory Synapses On A Cerebellar Purkinje Neuron. *J Neurosci*, 27, 6788-6799.

[75] Kano, M., Fukunaga, K., Konnerth, A. (1996). Ca^{2+}-Induced Rebound Potentiation Of Γ-Aminobutyric Acid-Mediated Currents Requires Activation Of Ca^{2+}/Calmodulin-Dependent Kinase Ii. *Proc Natl Acad Sci,* USA, 93, 13351-13356.

[76] Kawaguchi, S., Hirano, T. (2000). Suppression Of Inhibitory Synaptic Potentiation By Presynaptic Activity Through Postsynaptic $Gaba_b$ Receptors In A Purkinje Neuron. *Neuron*, 27, 339-347.

[77] Kawaguchi, S., Hirano, T. (2002). Signaling Cascade Regulating Long-Term Potentiation Of $Gaba_a$ Receptor Responsiveness In Cerebellar Purkinje Neurons. *J Neurosci,* 22, 3969-3976.

[78] Kawaguchi, S., Hirano, T. (2006). Integrin A3β1 Suppresses Long-Term Potentiation At Inhibitory Synapses On The Cerebellar Purkinje Neuron. *Mol Cell Neurosci*, 31, 416-426.

[79] Ohtsuki, G., Kawaguchi, S., Mishina, M., Hirano, T. (2004). Enhanced Inhibitory Synaptic Transmission In The Cerebellar Molecular Layer Of The Glurδ2 Knock-Out Mouse. *J Neurosci*, 24, 10900-10907.

[80] Mittmann, W., Häusser, M. (2007). Linking Synaptic Plasticity And Spike Output At Excitatory And Inhibitory Synapses Onto Cerebellar Purkinje Cells. *J Neurosci,*27, 5559-5570.

[81] Hansel, C., Linden, D.J. (2000). Long-Term Depression Of The Cerebellar Climbing Fiber-Purkinje Neuron Synapse. *Neuron,* 26, 473-482.

[82] Bosman, L.W., Takechi, H., Hartmann, J., Eilers, J., Konnerth, A. (2008). Homosynaptic Long-Term Synaptic Potentiation Of The "Winner" Climbing Fiber Synapse In Developing Purkinje Cells. *J Neurosci,* 28, 798-807.

[83] Kreitzer, A., Regehr, W. (2001). Cerebellar Depolarization-Induced Suppression Of Inhibition Is Mediated By Endogenous Cannabinoids. *J Neurosci*, 21, Rc174 (171-175).

[84] Kreitzer, A., Regehr, W. (2001). Retrograde Inhibition Of Presynaptic Calcium Influx By Endogenous Cannabinoids At Excitatory Synapses Onto Purkinje Cells. *Neuron,* 29, 717-727.

[85] Maejima, T., Hashimoto, K., Yoshida, T., Aiba, A., Kano, M. (2001). Presynaptic Inhibition Caused By Retrograde Signal From Metabotropic Glutamate To Cannabinoid Receptors. *Neuron*, 31, 463-475.

[86] Galante, M., Diana, M. (2004). Group I Metabotropic Glutamate Receptors Inhibit Gaba Release At Interneuron-Purkinje Cell Synapses Through Endocannabinoid Production. *J Neurosci*, 24, 4865-4874.

[87] Szabo, B., Urbanski, M.J., Bisogno, T., Marzo, V.D., Mendiguren, A., Baer, Wu. Et Al. (2006). Depolarization-Induced Retrograde Synaptic Inhibition In The Mouse Cerebellar Cortex Is Mediated By 2-Arachidonoylglycerol. *J Physiol*, 577, 263-280.

[88] Chevaleyre, V., Takahashi, K., Castillo, P. (2006). Endocannabinoid-Mediated Synaptic Plasticity In The Cns. *Annu Rev Neurosci,* 29, 37-76.

[89] Egertová, M., Elphick, M.R. (2000). Localisation Of Cannabinoid Receptors In The Rat Brain Using Antibodies To The Intracellular C-Terminal Tail Of Cb. *J Comp Neurol*, 422, 159-171.

[90] Bisogno, T., Howell, F., Williams, G., Minassi, A., Cascio, M.G., Ligresti, A. Et Al. (2003). Cloning Of The First Sn1-Dag Lipases Points To The Spatial And Temporal Regulation Of Endocannabinoid Signaling In The Brain. *J Cell Biol,* 163, 463-468.

[91] Yoshida, T., Fukaya, M., Uchigashima, M., Miura, E., Kamiya, H., Kano, M. Et Al. (2006). Localization Of Diacylglycerol Lipase-A Around Postsynaptic Spine Suggests Close Proximity Between Production Site Of An Endocannabinoid, 2-Arachidonoyl-Glycerol, And Presynaptic Cannabinoid Cb1 Receptor. *J Neurosci*, 26, 4740-4751.

[92] Maejima, T., Oka, S., Hashimotodani, Y., Ohno-Shosaku, T., Aiba, A., Wu, D. Et Al. (2005).Synaptically Driven Endocannabinoid Release Requires Ca^{2+}-Assisted Metabotropic Glutamate Receptor Subtype 1 To Phospholipase Cβ4 Signaling Cascade In The Cerebellum. *J Neurosci*, 25, 6826-6835.

[93] Brenowitz, S.D., Regehr, W.G. (2003). Calcium Dependence Of Retrograde Inhibition By Endocannabinoids At Synapses Onto Purkinje Cells. *J Neurosci*, 23, 6373-6384.

[94] Hashimotodani, Y., Ohno-Shosaku, T., Tsubokawa, H., Ogata, H., Emoto, K., Maejima, T. Et Al. (2005). Phospholipase Cβ Serves As A Coincidence Detector Through Its Ca^{2+} Dependency For Triggering Retrograde Endocannabinoid Signal. *Neuron,* 45, 257-268.

[95] Duguid, I., Smart, T. (2004). Retrograde Activation Of Presynaptic Nmda Receptors Enhances Gaba Release At Cerebellar Interneuron-Purkinje Cell Synapses. *Nat Neurosci*, 7, 525-533.

[96] Glitsch, M., Llano, I., Marty, A. (1996). Glutamate As A Candidate Retrograde Messenger At Interneurone-Purkinje Cell Synapses Of Rat Cerebellum. *J Physiol*, 497, 531-537.

[97] D'angelo, E., Rossi, P., Armano, S., Taglietti, V. (1999). Evidence For Nmda And Mglu Receptor-Dependent Long-Term Potentiation Of Mossy Fiber-Granule Cell Transmission In Rat Cerebellum. *J Neurophysiol*, 81, 277-287.

[98] Armano, S., Rossi, P., Taglietti, V., D'angelo, E. (2000). Long-Term Potentiation Of Intrinsic Excitability At The Mossy Fiber-Granule Cell Synapse Of Rat Cerebellum. *J Neurosci*, 20, 5208-5216.

[99] Hansel, C., Linden, D., D'angelo, E. (2001). Beyond Parallel Fiber Ltd: The Diversity Of Synaptic And Non-Synaptic Plasticity In The Cerebellum. *Nat Neurosci,* 4, 467-475.

[100]Aizenman, C., Manis, P., Linden, D. (1998). Polarity Of Long-Term Synaptic Gain Change Is Related To Postsynaptic Spike Firing At A Cerebellar Inhibitory Synapse. *Neuron*, 21, 827-835.

[101]Ouardouz, M., Sastry, B. (2000). Mechanisms Underlying Ltp Of Inhibitory Synaptic Transmission In The Deep Cerebellar Nuclei. *J Neurophysiol*, 84, 1414-1421.

[102]Morishita, W., Sastry, B. (1996). Postsynaptic Mechanisms Underlying Long-Term Depression Of Gabaergic Transmission In Neurons Of The Deep Cerebellar Nuclei. *J Neurophysiol,* 76, 59-68.

[103]Jahnsen, H. (1986). Electrophysiological Characteristics Of Neurones In The Guinea-Pig Deep Cerebellar Nuclei In Vitro. *J Physiol*, 372, 129-147.

[104]Aizenman, C., Linden, D. (1999). Regulation Of The Rebound Depolarization And Spontaneous Firing Patterns Of Deep Nuclear Neurons In Slices Of Rat Cerebellum. *J Neurophysiol,* 82, 1697-1709.

[105]Bienenstock, E., Cooper, L., Munro, P. (1982). Theory For The Development Of Neuron Selectivity: Orientation Specificity And Binocular Interaction In Visual Cortex. *J Neurosci,* 2, 32-48.

[106]Hansel, C., Artola, A., Singer, W. (1997). Relation Between Dendritic Ca^{2+} Levels And The Polarity Of Synaptic Long-Term Modifications In Rat Visual Cortex Neurons. *Eur J Neurosci*, 9, 2309-2322.

[107]Pugh, J., Raman, I. (2006). Potentiation Of Mossy Fiber Epscs In The Cerebellar Nuclei By Nmda Receptor Activation Followed By Postinhibitory Rebound Current. *Neuron,* 51, 113-123.

[108]Zhang, W., Linden, D. (2006). Long-Term Depression At The Mossy Fiber-Deep Cerebellar Nucleus Synapse. *J Neurosci,* 26, 6935-6944.

[109]Anchisi, D., Scelfo, B., Tempia, F. (2001). Postsynaptic Currents In Deep Cerebellar Nuclei. *J Neurophysiol,* 85, 323-331.

[110]Robinson, D. (1981). The Use Of Control Systems Analysis In The Neurophysiology Of Eye Movements. *Annu Rev Neurosci*, 4, 463-503.

[111]Ito, M. (1982). Cerebellar Control Of The Vestibulo-Ocular Reflex--Around The Flocculus Hypothesis. *Annu Rev Neurosci*, 5, 275-296.

[112]Nagao, S. (1988). Behavior Of Floccular Purkinje Cells Correlated With Adaptation Of Horizontal Optokinetic Eye Movement Response In Pigmented Rabbits. *Exp Brain Res*, 73, 489-497.

[113]Boyden, E., Katoh, A., Raymond, J. (2004). Cerebellum-Dependent Learning: The Role Of Multiple Plasticity Mechanisms. *Annu Rev Neurosci*, 27, 581-609.

[114]Ito, M., Jastreboff, P., Miyashita, Y. (1982). Specific Effects Of Unilateral Lesions In The Flocculus Upon Eye Movements In Albino Rabbits. *Exp Brain Res*, 45, 233-242.

[115]Luebke, A., Robinson, D. (1994). Gain Changes Of The Cat's Vestibulo-Ocular Reflex After Flocculus Deactivation. *Exp Brain Res*, 98, 379-390.

[116]Graf, W., Simpson, J.I., Leonard, C.S. (1988). Spatial Organization Of Visual Messages Of The Rabbit's Cerebellar Flocculus. Ii. Complex And Simple Spike Responses Of Purkinje Cells. *J Neurophysiol*, 60, 2091-2121.

[117]Miles, F., Lisberger, S. (1981). Plasticity In The Vestibulo-Ocular Reflex: A New Hypothesis. *Annu Rev Neurosci*, 4, 273-299.

[118]Hirata, Y., Highstein, S. (2001). Acute Adaptation Of The Vestibuloocular Reflex: Signal Processing By Floccular And Ventral Parafloccular Purkinje Cells. *J Neurophysiol,* 85, 2267-2288.

[119]Van Alphen, A.M., De Zeeuw, C.I. (2002). Cerebellar Ltd Facilitates But Is Not Essential For Long-Term Adaptation Of The Vestibulo-Ocular Reflex. *European Journal Of Neuroscience*, 16, 486-490.

[120]Christian, K., Thompson, R. (2003). Neural Substrates Of Eyeblink Conditioning: Acquisition And Retention. *Learn Mem*, 10, 427-455.

[121]Krupa, D., Thompson, J., Thompson, R. (1993). Localization Of A Memory Trace In The Mammalian Brain. *Science*, 260, 989-991.

[122]Kleim, J., Freeman, J.J., Bruneau, R., Nolan, B., Cooper, N., Zook, A. Et Al. (2002). Synapse Formation Is Associated With Memory Storage In The Cerebellum. *Proc Natl Acad Sci,* USA, 99, 13228-13231.

[123]Chen, L., Bao, S., Lockard, J., Kim, J., Thompson, R. (1996). Impaired Classical Eyeblink Conditioning In Cerebellar-Lesioned And Purkinje Cell Degeneration (Pcd) Mutant Mice. *J Neurosci*, 16, 2829-2838.

[124]Chen, L., Bao, S., Thompson, R. (1999). Bilateral Lesions Of The Interpositus Nucleus Completely Prevent Eyeblink Conditioning In Purkinje Cell-Degeneration Mutant Mice. *Behav Neurosci*, 113, 204-210.

[125]Kishimoto, Y., Hirono, M., Sugiyama, T., Kawahara, S., Nakao, K., Kishio, M. Et Al. (2001). Impaired Delay But Normal Trace Eyeblink Conditioning In Plcβ4 Mutant Mice. *Neuroreport*, 12, 2919-2922.

[126]Hauge, S., Tracy, J., Baudry, M., Thompson, R. (1998). Selective Changes In Ampa Receptors In Rabbit Cerebellum Following Classical Conditioning Of The Eyelid-Nictitating Membrane Response. *Brain Res*, 803, 9-18.

[127]Thompson, R.F. (1986). The Neurobiology Of Learning And Memory. *Science*, 233, 941-947.

[128]Jirenhed, D., Bengtsson, F., Hesslow, G. (2007). Acquisition, Extinction, And Reacquisition Of A Cerebellar Cortical Memory Trace. *J Neurosci*, 27, 2493-2502.

[129]Wada, N., Kishimoto, Y., Watanabe, D., Kano, M., Hirano, T., Funabiki, K. Et Al. (2007). Conditioned Eyeblink Learning Is Formed And Stored Without Cerebellar Granule Cell Transmission. *Proc Natl Acad Sci*, USA, 104, 16690-16695.

In: Synaptic Plasticity: New Research
Editors: Tim F. Kaiser and Felix J. Peters

ISBN: 978-1-60456-732-8

Chapter 6

SEIZURE-INDUCED SYNAPTIC PLASTICITY: UNDERSTANDING SYNAPTIC REORGANIZATION

Benedict C. Albensi *

Department of Pharmacology and Therapeutics, University of Manitoba;
St. Boniface Research Centre; Centre on Aging, University of Manitoba,
Health Sciences Centre, Manitoba Institute Child Health (MICH),
Winnipeg, Manitoba R2H 2A6 Canada

ABSTRACT

The hippocampus in epilepsy patients exhibits brain plasticity in response to seizure activity. Experimentally, brain plasticity in animals subjected to kindling or chemically-induced epilepsy, appears to be related to a long-term potentiation (LTP)-like reorganization of the neural networks. LTP is a widely accepted model of plasticity that results in activity-dependent long-term synaptic change and possibly memory encoding. Studies have further suggested that LTP induction and other activity-induced changes up-regulate various growth factors and may underlie hippocampal mossy fiber sprouting, which occurs frequently after repeated seizure activity. This article will highlight important background information, and discuss experimental models and methods that are currently being used for modeling plasticity/epilepsy and for profiling gene expression.

Keywords: plasticity, LTP, mossy fiber sprouting, epilepsy, kindling, neurotrophin, gene expression, seizure, hyperexcitability, animal model

*Correspondence: Dr. Benedict C. Albensi; St. Boniface Research Centre Division of Neurodegenerative Disorders, 351 Tache Ave./Lab 4050, Winnipeg, Manitoba R2H 2A6 Canada. balbensi@sbrc.ca204/235- 3942 office204/237- 4092 fax

INTRODUCTION

Temporal lobe epilepsy (TLE) is the most frequent type of focal epilepsy in adults [1, 2]. The seizure focus in these patients typically resides in mesial temporal regions of the brain, such as the hippocampus [3]. The surgically resected hippocampus from TLE patients very often shows neurodegenerative changes, collectively termed hippocampal sclerosis [3]. In hippocampal sclerosis, one observes gliosis and a loss of nerve cells [4]. Other changes, at a functional level, include the hypersynchronization and hyperexcitability of neurons [5, 6]. As hyperexcitability increases, an increasing number of neurons are recruited into abnormal discharge patterns, a process that has been referred to as secondary epileptogenesis or activity-induced epileptogenesis [7, 8].

Interestingly, in addition to neurodegenerative and excitability changes, the hippocampus from TLE patients shows neuronal reorganization - a form of brain plasticity in response to seizure activity or injury [7, 9, 10]. Experimentally, the long-term brain plasticity found in animals subjected to kindling, a widely-used model of epileptogenesis, or to chemically-induced epilepsy, a common method for inducing epileptic activity, appears to be related to a long-term potentiation (LTP)-like mediated reorganization of the neural networks [8]. LTP is a widely accepted model of synaptic plasticity that results in long-term activity-dependent synaptic change, a mechanism possibly involved in memory encoding [11, 12]. Data suggest that patterns of circuit reorganization can be induced depending on the location of the initial seizure activation and focus, which may depend on LTP or LTP-like mechanisms [8]. However, LTP impairments also have been reported following kindling, suggesting a complex role for LTP in epilepsy [13]. In this chapter, these ideas are discussed along with current studies that attempt to show potential links between LTP and the up-regulation of nerve growth factors (and other related molecules) in the contexts of plasticity and epilepsy. Studies of this kind may set the stage for understanding potential new drug targets for epileptic patients.

Hippocampal circuitry

There has been much interest in the hippocampal formation since it was recognized many years ago to play a major role in various forms of memory [14]. Importantly, particular regions of the hippocampus also have high seizure susceptibility, and have been shown to be especially vulnerable to the effects of ischemia and head trauma [15]. Additionally, the hippocampal formation, especially the dentate gyrus, shows some of the most profound types of structural and functional plasticity in the epileptic brain [7].

Pathways of the hippocampal formation have been characterized, showing that the overall pattern of connectivity is a trisynaptic circuit possessing primarily (but not exclusively) unidirectional serial and parallel connections [16]. Inputs to the hippocampus begin with the perforant path (lateral and medial tracts), which arise in the entorhinal cortex (layer II); the perforant path terminates in the dentate gyrus and the CA3 subfield of the hippocampus (in addition, there is an entorhinal cortex projection to CA1 arising from cells in layer III). Granule cells in the dentate gyrus give rise to mossy fibers that terminate on the dendrites of CA3 pyramidal cells. CA3 pyramidal cells project primarily to CA1 pyramidal cells along the

Schaffer collateral pathway and also to other levels of CA3. The CA1 pyramidal cells give rise to projections that terminate in the subiculum, which feeds back to the deep layers of the entorhinal cortex (layers III, IV, V), thus resulting in an entorhinal-hippocampal-entorhinal loop. The subiculum has a number of other outputs, sending projections also to the frontal cortex and the presubiculum. Presubiculum projections also connect back to the entorhinal cortex (layers III, IV, V, IV). Other minor ipsilateral pathways, as well as callosal pathways that provide communication with the contralateral hemisphere, also exist.

Long-term potentiation (LTP)

LTP is believed to contribute to synaptic plasticity in living animals, providing a basis for a highly adaptable nervous system that can be modified by activity and/or experience [12]. Because changes in synaptic strength are thought to underlie memory encoding and learning, LTP is believed to play a critical role in these processes. In fact, most theories addressing cognition regard LTP, and the reversal process long-term depression (LTD), as cellular processes responsible for memory encoding [12, 17, 18]. In experimentally induced LTP, brief high frequency bursts (e.g., ~100 Hz) of electrical stimulation initiate a long-lasting increase in the strength of synaptic transmission [19]. Under in vitro experimental conditions, applying short, high-frequency electrical stimuli to a synapse can strengthen, or potentiate, the synapse for many minutes to several hours. In living animals, LTP presumably occurs naturally or it can be induced experimentally and can last from hours to weeks. LTP has been observed in both brain slice preparations in vitro and in living animals in vivo [20]. Past studies have tried to directly link LTP with behavioral memory encoding, but most evidence to date shows indirect associations [11, 12, 21, 22]. However, more direct associations between hippocampal LTP and behaviorally defined memory have been recently shown [23, 24].

LTP and NMDA receptor activation

In most cases, LTP depends on N-methyl-D-aspartic acid (NMDA) receptor activation, and increases in intracellular calcium [11, 25, 26]. Activation of the NMDA receptor requires both glutamate and glycine binding and simultaneous depolarization of the cell membrane in order to open the associated channel that allows calcium to flow into the cell [27]. The influx of calcium through the NMDA receptor links NMDA receptor activation with calcium-dependent intracellular signaling via a variety of intracellular pathways [28]. NMDA receptor activation and NMDA-mediated downstream signaling is essential for normal synaptic function. This key rise in intracellular calcium can also be mediated through other mechanisms under different experimental conditions or in different cellular compartments (e.g., dendritic spines, mossy fiber synapses) – for example, via voltage-sensitive calcium channels [26, 29, 30] or release of calcium from intracellular stores [30]. However, most attention has been given to calcium entry through the NMDA receptor complex; since the NMDA channel opens only if there is simultaneous presynaptic glutamate release and postsynaptic membrane depolarization, the NMDA receptor has been called a synaptic "coincidence detector"[11, 12, 31]. The required depolarization in many cases appears to be mediated by the other major ionotropic glutamate receptor (the amino-3-hydroxy-5-methyl-4-isoxazole propionic acid (AMPA) receptors), which are often co-localized with NMDA receptors. NMDA receptors have slower activation kinetics, longer channel open times, and higher affinities for glutamate compared to AMPA receptors [32]. NMDA-mediated forms of LTP can be blocked with compounds such as 2-amino-5-phosphonopentanoic acid (APV), (a competitive antagonist) or MK-801, (a noncompetitive antagonist) [28]. An important exception to the above scenario is that the mossy fiber projection from the dentate to CA3 exhibits a NMDA-independent form of LTP [33, 34].

LTP induction in hippocampal brain slices

There are several aspects to LTP methodology, which cannot all be covered in this short chapter, so only some of the important LTP stimulation inducing protocols are discussed [19]. LTP can be induced by a high-frequency protocol, such as a train of 100 Hz (e.g., three bursts, with a 500 msec interval between bursts, and where each pulse of a burst is a square wave with 50 to 100 μs duration). Another experimental paradigm used in the hippocampal CA1 is primed burst (PB) potentiation. In PB, typically five pulses are used where the first pulse precedes the last 4 pulses (given at 100 Hz) by 170 ms. In addition, a very effective LTP-inducing protocol is theta-burst stimulation (TBS). In TBS, a single burst consists of 4 pulses at 100 Hz. However, this burst is typically repeated several times where some protocols consist of a train of 5 bursts each separated by 200 ms. The train can also be repeated 2 to 6 times with 10 second intervals between each train. An important characteristic of TBS protocols is the inter-burst interval of 200 msec - a time period during which inhibitory post-synaptic potentials (IPSPs) are difficult to recruit. The absence of IPSPs in this interval is due to the fact that the refractory period for IPSPs ranges from 200-500 msec - a period longer than the inter-burst interval. Without IPSP recruitment, repeated stimulation allows for more effective temporal summation of excitatory post-synaptic potentials (EPSPs). One major advantage of theta burst stimulation over standard high frequency protocols is that theta burst appears to more closely simulate the physiological activation pattern of nerve cells during theta brain wave activity as observed with EEG. Likewise in PB protocols, which are also presumably closer to normal patterns of activation, only a small number of pulses are applied (unlike high frequency protocols).

In vivo LTP

Frequencies for in vivo LTP have ranged from 100-400 Hz; however, several bursts at 400 Hz appears to be very popular [19]. In addition, it seems that early studies (ie., before 1977) reported in vivo LTP using 10-100 Hz (2-20 sec trains), but these stimuli produced strong frequency potentiation, and in unanesthetized animals generated epileptiform afterdischarges (AD). ADs can be defined as persistent trains of rhythmic ictal synchronizations, which take place after an initial spike (i.e., a fast electrographic transient). In vivo LTP can be accomplished in freely moving or anesthetized animals where the brain is left largely intact. However, patch clamping and intracellular recordings under these conditions are much more technically challenging, which promotes the continued use of methods for in vitro LTP.

Kindling model of epilepsy

Kindling is an experimental model of epilepotogenesis. The term was first proposed by Goddard et al. who performed many of the early experiments [35]. Kindling has been defined as a progressive increase in neuronal responsivity generated by spaced and repeated epileptogenic stimulation in specific brain structures [2, 13, 36-38]. Epileptogenesis has been defined as a set of progressive neurochemical, neuroanatomical, and neurophysiological changes that lead to spontaneous recurrent seizures [39, 40].

Controversy has arisen in that kindling may not be an optimal model of epilepsy or epileptogenesis since kindling does not usually result in a state of spontaneous recurrent seizures [7]. Instead a low intensity stimulus that normally produces a subtle response will give rise to seizure discharges (i.e., when a structure is "kindled."). On the other hand, kindling does allow a well-controlled experimental examination of the development of abnormal excitability, which utilizes standard stimulation protocols from animal to animal.

Kindling protocols [19] involve repeated, but intermittent, electrical stimulation or chemical exposure that eventually results in permanent nervous system change, without gross tissue damage (at the site of stimulation). The electrical stimulation protocols for kindling involve some parameters similar to those used for LTP (i.e., 50 to 100 Hz trains). However, the stimulus trains are typically longer than those used for LTP ($\sim \geq 1$ sec). Further, the stimulus intensity (often as low as 50-100 μA) is determined by the intensity level of that producing an AD. Kindling will not occur if the initial stimulus does not produce an AD.

Common sites for stimulation in kindling include the hippocampus and the amygdala, but a number of other sites have also been used with varying responsiveness [2, 36-38]. The amygdala, has been reported by many to be the most sensitive to repeated stimulation, but some studies targeting the olfactory bulb and regions of perirhinal cortex suggest otherwise and appear to be more sensitive (i.e., produce kindling with fewer trials) than the amygdala. As a whole, kindling protocols are primarily used as a model of drug-resistant epilepsy and/or for investigating developmental aspects of epilepsy.

In kindling studies with rats, electrical stimulation in the amygdala is typically repeated until the animal develops stage-5 convulsive seizures (using the 10 stage classification system developed by R. J. Racine where stage 10 is the highest [41-43]) or clonic-tonic-clonic seizures involving all four limbs. Today most common protocols utilize 60 Hz stimulation trains. Previously, Goddard tried a variety of stimulation frequencies (25, 60, and 150 Hz) and also found that the animals were maximally sensitive to 60 Hz [35]. Most kindling protocols use square wave pulse sequences, although a few have used sinusoidal waveforms.

Goddard also initially showed that varying stimulus intensity had little effect on the number of stimulations required to kindle the amygdala. However, Racine et al. later found that intensity did make a difference, since epileptiform ADs were required to produce the neural changes underlying the kindling effect [36]. Although, varying the intensity above threshold (400 vs. 1000 μA) seemed to make little difference on kindling rate. Goddard et al.

also found that the same number of stimulations were required whether they were spaced by 24 hours or 7 days.

Brain slice models of epilepsy

In addition to studies involving synaptic plasticity and LTP, the brain slice preparation has served as an important model of epilepsy providing investigators a wealth of information on seizure-like activity associated with epilepsy [15]. Past investigators, and our lab as well, have successfully used in vitro hippocampal and neocortical preparations in conjunction with a variety of recording buffer recipes or convulsant agents for inducing and modeling seizure-like events [44]. In this paradigm, the epileptiform activity observed in hippocampal slices has been compared to the interictal spike discharge seen in EEG recordings of epilepsy patients [45]. In our laboratory, we routinely use the so-called low magnesium model of epilepsy in rodent hippocampal brain slices where $MgCl_2$ is removed from our recording buffer, which results in the appearance of multiple spikes. Our current research also involves the recording of in vitro spontaneous epileptform events from human neocortical brain tissue obtained from living epileptic patients during surgery. Animal models in concert with viable human tissue create a powerful approach for recording electrical events during seizure activity.

In one application of the brain slice model, in vivo kindling stimulation was first induced and then followed by an in vitro assessment of excitability in the brain slice in an attempt to understand mechanisms responsible for kindling [46]. In this experiment, slices from the amygdala-piriform-perirhinal cortex were created after daily 60 Hz stimulation (2 secs) in the dorsal hippocampus. It was found that dorsal hippocampal kindling resulted in changes in the origin of the spontaneous discharges similar to past studies involving amygdala kindling, however, the observed changes in this case were shown in both hemispheres, thus showing a potential seizure recruitment process in this model.

The influence of in vivo kindling on in vitro LTP has also been examined in hippocampal brain slices [13]. Field potential recordings were made in brain slices obtained from kindled rats one day after the last kindling where it was found that kindling impaired primed-burst induced LTP in CA1 hippocampus. However, in some rat slices the $GABA_B$ antagonist CGP35348 was applied, suggesting that LTP is suppressed by downregulation of $GABA_B$ autoreceptors.

Collectively these studies illustrate that the analysis of epileptiform activity and events involving synaptic plasticity can be evaluated in brain slices models. This is due to the fact that the brain slice preparation retains enough intrinsic complexity to be able to manifest events such as synchronized bursts, seizure-like activity, and LTP. However, the model is simpler than in vivo models since some axons and afferents are lost upon slicing with in vitro preparations. Nevertheless, the analysis of the interictal spike in the brain slice preparation remains a powerful tool and provides great insight into epileptic mechanisms.

Kindling and plasticity

As stated above, the term "kindling" refers to the experimental procedure of inducing synchronous electrical afterdischarges and increases in susceptibility to additional electrographic and behavioral seizures by repeated small electrical or chemical stimulation to the brain [2, 35-38]. Kindling has been studied not only as a model for epilepsy, but also as a form of long-term neural plasticity since it results in a permanent change in the nervous system. It is likely that kindling protocols trigger a very large number of signaling pathways, some of which are presumably still unknown. Some of these pathways appear similar to those activated by LTP protocols, and thus investigators have hypothesized that the kindling process involves an LTP-like process.

In his pioneering work that led to the "discovery" of kindling, Goddard [35] was actually interested primarily in the effects of brain (amygdala) stimulation on learning. That kindling involves learning-related mechanisms focused much of his attention on learning. Subsequent studies on animals showed that as the

number of kindling trials increases so too do the animal's learning disabilities [2, 35-38]. The precise neurophysiological mechanisms for these learning and memory deficits seen in kindled animals - or in epileptic patients - have not yet been determined. However, one suggestion has been that alterations in the capacity of hippocampal neurons to sustain LTP could play a role in this regard [47].

Mossy fiber sprouting and plasticity

Many investigators work with the dentate gyrus subfield of the hippocampus as a model system for studies that involve plasticity and epilepsy since this region shows a great deal of functional plasticity, such as mossy fiber sprouting after repeated seizure activity [7]. In addition, mossy fiber sprouting can be examined using Timm staining [7]. The Timm method stains neuronal elements containing heavy metals such as zinc, which is predominant in the terminals of mossy fibers. Many of the types of changes that have been reported in the hippocampus have been additionally documented in the neocortex. Interestingly, past studies have reported that in vivo LTP trains (400 Hz; 1000 μA) induce mossy fiber sprouting when non-epileptogenic stimulation was applied to the perforant pathway. The results also showed that mossy fiber sprouting can be induced in the absence of neuronal degeneration, which further suggests that sprouting is dependent on neuronal activity.

Does LTP play a role in mossy fiber sprouting?

Some studies do hint at the possibility there is an association (ie., but undefined) between LTP and mossy fiber sprouting. However, there are several questions that remain to be answered about this association. For example, do LTP protocols directly induce mossy fiber sprouting? If so, is LTP-induced mossy fiber sprouting associated with neurodegeneration? Finally, what forms of LTP lead to sprouting? The first evidence that LTP stimulation protocols induce mossy fiber sprouting was produced by Adams et al. who showed that 400

Hz delivered in vivo over a series of 11 days induced sprouting in the hippocampal CA3 and intermolecular layer [48]. In addition, the study reported that mossy fiber sprouting induced by LTP trains can occur in the absence of neurodegeneration.

In another study by Hassan et al., 200 Hz in vivo stimulation was applied over a period of 10 days to the angular bundles of the dentate gyrus in rats [49]. These results confirmed the Adams study and demonstrated that both morphological and functional changes to the hippocampus, similar to what is seen after kindling stimulation, can also occur with LTP protocols used for long-lasting synaptic plasticity, but is not associated with seizure activity.

In another study by Escobar et al. [50] using male rats, it was found that 100 Hz stimulation (two 1 sec trains with intertrain interval of 20 secs) in vivo to the mossy fiber pathway (mossy fiber-CA3 synapse) resulted in bilateral synaptogenesis. In this study, animals showing any seizure activity were eliminated from the results. In agreement with past studies, the effect was NMDA-independent since the NMDA antagonist (±) CPP did not prevent LTP in this pathway.

In addition, Tim Teyler et al. have proposed a very intriguing hypothesis that may provide a partial explanation for LTP-induced mossy fiber sprouting. In a past landmark study Dr. Teyler made an important distinction between NMDA forms of LTP and voltage-dependent calcium channel (VDCC) forms of LTP where he and his student Larry Grover showed that some forms of LTP could be induced in the CA1 hippocampus without the involvement of the NMDA receptor [51]. More recently he has also suggested that activity in a primary epileptic focus is of sufficient magnitude to drive efferents from the primary focus at rates that will result in the induction of VDCC forms of LTP [8]. The hypothesis advocates that VDCC-LTP can be involved in epileptic processes even though the mechanism is also a normal component of synaptic plasticity. He further hypothesized that the synaptic enhancement mediated by VDCC-LTP leads to the activation of neurotrophins and the sprouting of aberrant connections in a secondary focus, thus hinting at the possibility that VDCC blockers might be beneficial at preventing the establishment of secondary epileptic foci.

Gene expression profiling

A review of past work identifies several important relationships between epileptic neuropathology and plasticity that are under investigation [7]. One particularly interesting area is the expression of neurotrophic factors in mossy fiber sprouting and/or during seizure activity. Studies suggest that many forms of activity-dependent changes (including LTP and ictal episodes) upregulate growth factor mRNA, transcription factors, and gene expression in the dentate and therefore function as processes that drive mossy fiber sprouting, which are dependent on the level of neural activity [7]. To this end, our laboratory is currently using DNA microarrays or "gene chips" in order to assess the potential up-regulation or downregulation of specific genes associated with various neurotrophic factors and in association with the activation of specific transcription factors, in experimental paradigms of LTP and epilepsy.

A DNA microarray is a collection of microscopic DNA sites on a grid, commonly representing single genes, arrayed on a solid surface by attachment to a chemical matrix.

DNA arrays are commonly used for monitoring expression levels of thousands of genes simultaneously. In our studies, we hypothesize that epileptic hippocampi have transcriptional changes that are different from the transcriptomes produced in non-epileptic hippocampi where we are predicting that some of the same genes that are expressed after the induction of LTP are also expressed following epileptic seizures.

In one recent study using DAN microarrays, experiments were conducted to clarify the role of various neurotrophic factors in the pilocarpine model of seizures. It was found [52] that 4 hours following pilocarpine-induced seizures, expression of nerve growth factor (NGF), brain derived neurotrophic factor (BDNF), heparin-binding epidermal growth factor-like growth factor, (HB-EGF), and fibroblast growth factor (FGF) increased in the mice manifesting tonic-clonic convulsions, but not in mice without seizures. These results suggest that brain damage in the mice having tonic-clonic seizures is accompanied by neurogenesis, which may be regulated through changes in expression of neurotrophic factors.

The regulation of gene expression by NMDA receptor activation may also be an important mechanism for plasticity in epileptogenesis. Previous studies showed that pretreatment of rodents with NMDA receptor antagonists prevented epileptogenesis in a kindling model [53, 54]. As a recent follow up, the roles of NR2A and NR2B-containing NMDA receptors in activity-dependent BDNF gene expression were examined in limbic epileptogenesis [55]. Here it was found that selectively blocking NR2A-containing NMDA receptors impaired epileptogenesis and the development of mossy fiber sprouting in the kindling and pilocarpine rat models of limbic epilepsy, whereas inhibiting NR2B-containing NMDA receptors had no effects in epileptogenesis and mossy fiber sprouting.

Another important finding is that neurotrophins themselves appear regulated by neurotrophin levels in epilepsy models. In one new study, hippocampal kindling resulted in a significant increase in levels of BDNF both in cytochrome C (control) infused and neurotrophin-3 (NT-3) infused kindled rats [56]. However, NT-3 infusion significantly reduced BDNF levels in both kindled and non-kindled hippocampi compared to their cytochrome C infused counterparts. These results demonstrate that modulation of BDNF by NT-3 occurs in naïve and kindled adult rat hippocampus.

Conclusion

One interesting aspect of these recent studies, is that the results provide a potential process and therapeutic target for blocking the progression of the epileptic state. In other words, to be able to block the recruitment of more neurons from falling into an abnormal discharge pattern, may hold clinical value for epileptic patients. Future research that involves specific treatments directed at signaling cascades that trigger gene expression or which modulate the synthesis of certain gene products, may be in order. In fact, the idea of a so-called "afterseizure" drug intervention has been entertained that would interfere with the expression of particular genes and prevent modifications that might lead to enhanced excitability.

The development of these interventions, however, will require more fundamental research using techniques such as gene arrays and other molecular methods for expanding our basic knowledge of seizure-induced gene expression. Importantly, it is essential that we identify which plastic changes are desirable and which are not before treatment strategies can be developed and attempted.

One may think that seizure activity is too variable and that each seizure model is too different to yield consistent results when evaluating seizure-induced gene expression. On the contrary, if one examines the neurotrophins, which are normally expressed in granule cells of the hippocampus and change their expression dramatically after limbic seizures, one finds that in spite of the model used (kindling, pilocarpine, kainic acid, or even brain injury models using trauma or ischemia) neurotrophins, such BDNF, are increased in every model tested. Furthermore, a number of past studies have shown that BDNF is also associated with LTP, thus potentially linking plastic processes with epileptogenesis. Given these sorts of results, the future of molecular studies involving seizure-induced gene expression and plastic responses hold great promise.

REFERENCES

[1] Duncan, J.S., and Sagar, H.J. (1987). Seizure characteristics, pathology, and outcome after temporal lobectomy. *Neurology*, 37(3), p. 405-9.

[2] Morimoto, K., Fahnestock, M., and Racine, R.J. (2004). Kindling and status epilepticus models of epilepsy: rewiring the brain. *Prog Neurobiol*, 73(1), p. 1-60.

[3] Bruton, C.J. (1988). *The neuropathology of temporal lobe epilepsy.* Oxford, UK: Oxford University Press (Maudsley Monographs).

[4] Sommer, W. (1880). *Erkrankung des Ammonshornes als aetiologisches Moment der Epilepsie. Arch Psychiatr Nervenkr*, 10, p. 631-675.

[5] Bernard, C., Marsden, D.P., and Wheal, H.V. (2001). Changes in neuronal excitability and synaptic function in a chronic model of temporal lobe epilepsy. *Neuroscience*, 103(1), p. 17-26.

[6] Wong, R.K., Miles, R., and Traub, R.D. (1984). Local circuit interactions in synchronization of cortical neurones. *J Exp Biol*, 112, p. 169-78.

[7] Scharfman, H.E. (2002). Epilepsy as an example of neural plasticity. *Neuroscientist*, 8(2), p. 154-73.

[8] Teyler, T.J. et al. (2001). Synaptic plasticity and secondary epileptogenesis. *Int Rev Neurobiol*, 45, p. 253-67.

[9] Sutula, T. et al. (1989). Mossy fiber synaptic reorganization in the epileptic human temporal lobe. *Ann Neurol*, 26(3), p. 321-30.

[10] Koyama, R., and Ikegaya, Y. (2004). Mossy fiber sprouting as a potential therapeutic target for epilepsy. *Curr Neurovasc Res*, 1(1), p. 3-10.

[11] Bliss, T.V., and Collingridge, G.L. (1993). A synaptic model of memory: long-term potentiation in the hippocampus. *Nature*, 361(6407), p. 31-9.

[12] Neves, G., Cooke, S.F., and Bliss, T.V. (2008). Synaptic plasticity, memory and the hippocampus: a neural network approach to causality. *Nat Rev Neurosci*, 9(1), p. 65-75.

[13] Leung, L.S., and Wu, C. (2003). Kindling suppresses primed-burst-induced long-term potentiation in hippocampal CA1. *Neuroreport*, 14(2), p. 211-4.

[14] Anderson, P. et al. (2007). *The Hippocampal Formation* in *The Hippocampus Book*, P. Anderson, et al. Editors. Oxford University Press: New York. p. 3-8.

[15] Anderson, P. et al. (2007). *Historical Perspective: Proposed Functions, Biological Characteristics, and Neurobiological Models of the Hippocampus*, in *The Hippocampus Book*, P. Anderson, et al., Editors. Oxford University Press: New York. p. 9-36.

[16] Amaral, D., and Lavenex, P. (2007). *Hippocampal Neuroanatomy*, in *The Hippocampus Book*, P. Anderson, et al., Editors. Oxford University Press: New York. p. 37-114.

[17] Bear, M.F., and Malenka, R.C. (1994). Synaptic plasticity: LTP and LTD. *Curr Opin Neurobiol*, 4(3), p. 389-99.

[18] Bear, M.F. (1995). Mechanism for a sliding synaptic modification threshold. *Neuron*, 15(1), p. 1-4.

[19] Albensi, B.C. et al. (2007). Electrical stimulation protocols for hippocampal synaptic plasticity and neuronal hyper-excitability: are they effective or relevant? *Exp Neurol*, 204(1), p. 1-13.

[20] Bliss, T., Collinridge, G., and Morris, R. (2007). *Synaptic plasticity in the hippocampus*, in *The Hippocampus Book*, P. Anderson, et al., Editors. Oxford University Press: New York. p. 343-474.

[21] Martin, S.J., Grimwood, P.D., and Morris, R.G. (2000). Synaptic plasticity and memory: an evaluation of the hypothesis. *Annu Rev Neurosci*, 23, p. 649-711.

[22] Otto, T. et al. (1991). Learning-related patterns of CA1 spike trains parallel stimulation parameters optimal for inducing hippocampal long-term potentiation. *Hippocampus*, 1(2), p. 181-92.

[23] Whitlock, J.R. et al. (2006). Learning induces long-term potentiation in the hippocampus. *Science*, 313(5790), p. 1093-7.

[24] Pastalkova, E. et al. (2006). Storage of spatial information by the maintenance mechanism of LTP. *Science*, 313(5790), p. 1141-4.

[25] Teyler, T.J. (1999). Use of brain slices to study long-term potentiation and depression as examples of synaptic plasticity. *Methods*, 18(2), p. 109-16.

[26] Yang, S.N., Tang, Y.G., and Zucker, R.S. (1999). Selective induction of LTP and LTD by postsynaptic [Ca2+]i elevation. *J Neurophysiol*, 81(2), p. 781-7.

[27] Kew, J.N. et al. (2000). *Functional consequences of reduction in NMDA receptor glycine affinity in mice carrying targeted point mutations in the glycine binding site.* J Neurosci, 20(11), p. 4037-49.

[28] Watkins, J.C. (1994). *The NMDA receptor concept: origins and development*. 2nd ed. The NMDA receptor, ed. Collingridge G.L., and Watkins. J.C. New York: Oxford University Press.

[29] Waxman, E.A., and Lynch, D.R. (2005). N-methyl-D-aspartate receptor subtypes: multiple roles in excitotoxicity and neurological disease. *Neuroscientist*, 11(1), p. 37-49.

[30] Emptage, N.,. Bliss, T.V., and Fine, A. (1999). Single synaptic events evoke NMDA receptor-mediated release of calcium from internal stores in hippocampal dendritic spines. *Neuron,* 22(1), p. 115-24.

[31] Wigstrom, H., and Gustafsson, B. (1986). Postsynaptic control of hippocampal long-term potentiation. *J Physiol* (Paris), 81(4), p. 228-36.

[32] Dingledine, R. et al. (1999). The glutamate receptor ion channels. *Pharmacol Rev*, 51(1), p. 7-61.

[33] Nicoll, R.A., and Schmitz, D. (2005). Synaptic plasticity at hippocampal mossy fibre synapses. *Nat Rev Neurosci*, 6(11), p. 863-76.

[34] Harris, E.W., and Cotman, C.W. (1986). Long-term potentiation of guinea pig mossy fiber responses is not blocked by N-methyl D-aspartate antagonists. *Neurosci Lett*, 70(1), p. 132-7.

[35] Goddard, G.V., McIntyre, D.C., and Leech, C.K. (1969). A permanent change in brain function resulting from daily electrical stimulation. Exp Neurol, 25(3), p. 295-330.

[36] Racine, R. (1978). Kindling: the first decade. *Neurosurgery*, 3(2), p. 234-52.

[37] Mody, I. (1993). The molecular basis of kindling. *Brain Pathol*, 3(4), p. 395-403.

[38] Weiss, S.R., and Post, R.M. (1998). Kindling: separate vs. shared mechanisms in affective disorders and epilepsy. *Neuropsychobiology*, 38(3), p. 167-80.

[39] Morrell, F. (1989). Varieties of human secondary epileptogenesis. *J Clin Neurophysiol*, 6(3), p. 227-75.

[40] Bender, R.A., and Baram, T.Z. (2007). Epileptogenesis in the developing brain: what can we learn from animal models? *Epilepsia*, 48 Suppl 5, p. 2-6.

[41] Racine, R., Okujava, V., and Chipashvili, S. (1972). Modification of seizure activity by electrical stimulation. 3. Mechanisms. *Electroencephalogr Clin Neurophysiol*, 32(3), p. 295-9.

[42] Racine, R.J. (1972). Modification of seizure activity by electrical stimulation. II. Motor seizure. *Electroencephalogr Clin Neurophysiol*, 32(3), p. 281-94.

[43] Racine, R.J. (1972). Modification of seizure activity by electrical stimulation. I. After-discharge threshold. *Electroencephalogr Clin Neurophysiol*, 32(3), p. 269-79.

[44] Kandel, E., Schwartz, J.H., and Jessell, T.M. (2000). *Seizures and Epilepsy*, in *Principles of Neural Science*, McGraw-Hill: New York. p. 918.

[45] Wong, R.K.S., Traub, R.D., and Miles, R. (1984). *Epileptogenic Mechanisms as Revealed by Studies of the Hipppcampal Slice*, in *Electrophysiology of Epilepsy*, P.A. Schwartzkroin and H.V. Wheal, Editors. Academic Press: London. p. 253-275.

[46] Schubert, M. et al. (2005). Kindling-induced changes in plasticity of the rat amygdala and hippocampus. *Learn Mem*, 12(5), p. 520-6.

[47] Palizvan, M.R., Fathollahi, Y., and Semnanian, S. (2005). Epileptogenic insult causes a shift in the form of long-term potentiation expression. *Neuroscience*, 134(2), p. 415-23.

[48] Adams, B. et al. (1997). Long-term potentiation trains induce mossy fiber sprouting. *Brain Res*, 775(1-2), p. 193-7.

[49] Hassan, H. et al. (2000). Repeated long-term potentiation induces mossy fibre sprouting and changes the sensibility of hippocampal granule cells to subconvulsive doses of pentylenetetrazol. *Eur J Neurosci*, 12(4), p. 1509-15.

[50] Escobar, M.L. et al. (1997). Opioid receptor modulation of mossy fiber synaptogenesis: independence from long-term potentiation. *Brain Res,* 751(2), p. 330-5.

[51] Grover, L.M., and Teyler, T.J. (1990). Two components of long-term potentiation induced by different patterns of afferent activation. *Nature*, 347(6292), p. 477-9.

[52] Hagihara, H. et al. (2005). Tonic-clonic seizures induce division of neuronal progenitor cells with concomitant changes in expression of neurotrophic factors in the brain of pilocarpine-treated mice. *Brain Res Mol Brain Res*, 139(2), p. 258-66.

[53] Rice, A.C., and DeLorenzo, R.J. (1998). NMDA receptor activation during status epilepticus is required for the development of epilepsy. *Brain Res*, 782(1-2), p. 240-7.

[54] Sutula, T. et al. (1996). NMDA receptor dependence of kindling and mossy fiber sprouting: evidence that the NMDA receptor regulates patterning of hippocampal circuits in the adult brain. *J Neurosci*, 16(22), p. 7398-406.

[55] Chen, Q. et al. (2007). Differential roles of NR2A- and NR2B-containing NMDA receptors in activity-dependent brain-derived neurotrophic factor gene regulation and limbic epileptogenesis. *J Neurosci*, 27(3), p. 542-52.

[56] Ullal, G.R. et al. (2007). NT-3 modulates BDNF and proBDNF levels in naive and kindled rat hippocampus. *Neurochem Int*, 50(6), p. 866-71.

In: Synaptic Plasticity: New Research
Editors: Tim F. Kaiser and Felix J. Peters

ISBN: 978-1-60456-732-8

Chapter 7

SYNAPTIC PLASTICITY IN COCAINE ADDICTION

***Margarida Corominas*[1,*]*, Carlos Roncero*[1]*, Xavier Castells*[2] *and Miquel Casas*[1]**

1 Department of Psychiaty, Vall d'Hebron Universitary Hospital,
Universitat Autonoma of Barcelona, Barcelona, Spain.
[2] Department of Pharmacology, Vall d'Hebron Universitary Hospital,
Universitat Autonoma of Barcelona, Barcelona, Spain

ABSTRACT

Addiction has been described as a pathological usurpation of the neuronal mechanisms involved in reward, motivation and reinforcement. Nevertheless, environmental stimuli closely associated with the drug can acquire the ability to elicit the emotional responses that were induced by the drug. From this perspective, addiction has something to do with long-term associative learning and memory. These effects induced by cocaine consumption account for the chronic relapse which characterizes addiction. Long-term potentiation (LTP) and long-term depression (LTD) are forms of synaptic plasticity by which chronic cocaine induces changes in the mesocorticolimbic system primarily through dopamine and glutamate transmission. Recent evidence suggests that brain-derived neurotrophic factor (BDNF) and its intracellular pathways are involved in the molecular mechanisms that modify synaptic plasticity underlying addiction.

A single dose of cocaine induces an enhancement in locomotor activity that correlates with an increase in synaptic strength (the ratio AMPAR/NMDAR) in the VTA. This effect was not increased after repeated cocaine doses, indicating that cocaine-induced synaptic plasticity in the VTA is transient and also has a ceiling effect. Adaptations in downstream circuitry, such the nucleus accumbens (NAc), are likely to be more important for the longer-lasting behavioral changes associated with drug addiction. EPSC is decreased (LTD was induced) at synapses made by prefrontal cortical afferents in spiny neurons of the NAc shell, but not in the core. This inhibitory effect appears to be induced by D1 receptor activation. These changes in synaptic plasticity disrupt goal-

* Phone: +34 (93) 489 4294 / +34 (93) 489 4295. Fax: +34 (93) 489 4587 e-mail: mcoromin@vhebron.net

directed behavior. In the dorsal striatum, LTP can be induced in physiological conditions as well as after chronic cocaine treatment. However, saline treated rats are able to reverse LTP, whereas cocaine treated rodents do not. In the dorsal striatum, LTP is induced by D1 receptor activation and enhanced by D2 receptor antagonists. In physiological conditions, the ability to reverse LTP at striatal synapses functions as a mechanism for "forgetting" maladaptive habits, thus the lack of ability to reverse LTP may have important consequences in drug addiction. Increased BDNF levels in VTA neurons during withdrawal from cocaine plays a role in synaptic remodeling. BDNF also promotes long-lasting changes in the mesolimbic dopamine system by activating mechanisms of associative learning that underlie persistent addictive behavior.

INTRODUCTION

Addiction is a chronic disorder characterized by cravings, persistent and compulsive drug-seeking behavior despite adverse consequences of use, and relapse, even after prolonged periods of abstinence (Childress et al., 1999; O'Brien et al., 1997). Addiction has been described as a pathological usurpation of the neuronal mechanisms involved in reward, motivation and reinforcement (Everitt and Robbins, 2005; Hyman and Malenka, 2001; Nestler, 1997, 2001). From this perspective, the pharmacological actions of the drug come to control the brain circuitry that regulates basic biological needs. Nevertheless, over the last decades, it has become clear that environmental contingencies closely associated to the drug, such as paraphernalia, friends and places, can acquire secondary reinforcing properties. Once conditioned, these stimuli themselves have the ability to elicit the emotional responses, such as craving, that were initially only induced by the drug during active consumption. From this perspective, an important neural substrate for the development of addiction has something to do with what is called long-term associative learning and memory.

The main substrates of addiction are the mesolimbic and mesocortical dopamine systems, which constitute the reward circuitry. These circuits arise from the ventral tegmenta area (VTA) in the midbrain and project to the nucleus accumbens (NAc) and the prefrontal cortex (PFC). The amygdala and the hippocampus are also part of this circuitry (Berke and Hyman, 2000; Everitt and Robbins, 2005; Hyman et al., 2006; Nestler, 2001). The dorsal striatum is also involved and plays an essential role in later stages of addiction (Corominas-Roso et al., 2007). Associative memories in addiction are built on the neural substrates traditionally involved in the processing of reward, incentive and motivation.

Two neurotransmitters dopamine and glutamate and their interaction are central to drug addiction (Kalivas, 2004; Kalivas and Volkow, 2005; Volkow et al., 2004). At the molecular level, the effects of addictive drugs on the different dopamine and glutamate receptors also play a role in addiction (Nogueira, 2006, Thomas and Malenka, 2003). The increased neural activity induced by cocaine consumption also modifies intracellular signaling mechanisms, which are downstream from dopamine and glutamate receptors. For example, an upregulation of the cAMP pathway and increased levels of protein kinase A (PKA) in the NAc have been described (Nestler, 1997). Cocaine also activates CREB in the same brain region (Carlezon et al., 1998; Dong et al., 2006). One common chronic action of addictive drugs is the induction of a transcription factor deltaFosB which is very stable and accumulates in the NAc and in the dorsal striatum, after repeated cocaine administration (Kelz et al., 1999; Tan et al., 2000). All these mechanisms account for part of the long-lasting, drug-induced behavioral changes.

Drugs of abuse also introduce changes in the molecular mechanisms of reward-related associative learning (Berke and Hyman, 2000) and induce long-term changes in synaptic effectiveness in critical brain areas (Thomas et al., 2001; Ungless et al., 2001; Saal et al., 2003, Thomas and Malenka, 2003). In this respect, long-term potentiation (LTP) and long-term depression (LTD) are forms of synaptic plasticity by which neuronal stimulation induces changes in synaptic connectivity, making neurons more or less responsive to future activation. LTP and LTD can lead to changes in synaptic strength that allow modification of the information flow between different structures of the reward circuitry. This includes, for example, the information flow coming from the amygdala, hippocampus or PFC to the NAc and VTA. LTP and LTD as mechanisms of synaptic plasticity may play a critical role in adaptive associative forms of learning and memory and in pathological processes such as addiction (Thomas and Malenka, 2003).

Recent evidence suggests that neurotrophins, such as brain-derived neurotrophic factor (BDNF) and its intracellular signaling pathways, including phosphatidylinositol 3-kinase (PI3-K) and the mitogen-activated protein kinase (MAPK/ERK) cascades (Heerssen and Segal, 2002; Kaplan and Miller, 2000; Patapoutian A, Reichardt, 2001), modulate the cellular mechanism of LTP and memory processes (Mizuno et al., 2003; Rattiner et al., 2005). Recent evidence suggests that BDNF and its intracellular pathways are part of the molecular mechanisms that underlie the development of addiction (Grimm et al. 2003; Lu et al., 2004; Pu et al., 2006).

The brain ability to learn by association has been recognized since the pioneering work of Ivan Pavlov (1927). Processes such as learning (Stewart and Rusakov, 1995), living in an either an isolated or complex environment (van Praag et al., 2000) or from recovery from brain damage (Biernaskie and Corbett, 2001) are forms of experience-dependent learning and give rise to behavioral changes (Kandel, 1999). These forms of learning represent critical process through which experiences shape emotion, motivation, behavior and personality (LeDoux, 2001). There is abundant experimental evidence supporting the idea that synaptic plasticity may play a role in mediating the behavioral and emotional consequences of exposure to drugs of abuse and in the development of addiction (Robinson and Berridge, 1993; Kalivas, 1995; Hyman and Malenka, 2001; Nestler, 2001).

The aim of this chapter is to review the mechanisms of synaptic plasticity, including those involving BDNF, that allow the reorganization of the neural circuits from the first contact with the drug to the development of the compulsive consumption which characterizes addiction. Additionally, the diverse neuronal processes that take place in addiction will be put into context of synaptic plasticity in order to gain a more comprehensive view of the process of addiction. Studying repeated exposure to cocaine is a useful way of investigating experience-dependent synaptic plasticity induced in different brain regions as well as its functional, emotional, and behavioral consequences. The studies of synaptic plasticity related to cocaine addiction are useful for developing possible therapeutic interventions.

Synaptic Plasticity

It is now clear that the mammalian brain is able to take advantage of the neuronal capacity to express long-lasting, activity-dependent synaptic modifications as mechanisms by which experience modifies neural circuits and behavior.

Plasticity is the ability of a structure to change its shape and/or function in response to change in environmental conditions. From the neurobiological point of view, plasticity is the capacity of neural activity to modify neural circuitry and function in response to environmental stimuli, manifesting as changes in thoughts, feelings and behavior. The term synaptic plasticity refers to the ability of the nervous system to modify the strength and the efficacy of synaptic transmission at preexisting synapses in an activity-dependent manner.

One of the first people to introduce the concept of behavior modificability was Freud in his book *Project for a Scientific Psychology* (1895), in which he explained his ideas about the neural basis of learning. Freud hypothesized a relationship between traumatic events, synaptic plasticity, memory processes and psychopathology in light of contemporary ideas about the neuronal bases of psychic symptoms and the synaptic substrate of learning and memory (Freud, 1895). Freud's interest in the neural basis of memory was based on the discoveries of Ramon y Cajal regarding the organization of the nervous system. Some years later, Ramon y Cajal in his book *Texture of the Nervous System* (1904), proposed that the ability of mammals to adapt their behavior to external conditions must be due to changes in brain anatomy, extending the notion of plasticity to the neural substrate. The concept of synaptic plasticity was articulated for the first time by Donald Hebb (1949) who proposed that associative memories can result from subtle alterations in synapses widely distributed throughout the brain. He proposed that memory is the result of the internal brain representation of an object, and is comprised of all of the cortical cells that are activated by the external stimuli. If activation of the representational group of cells persisted long enough, memory consolidation would take place. This process makes the reciprocal interconnection between involved neurons more effective in firing together. Hebb also proposed that in a synaptic cleft, the contact between the presynaptic axon and the postsynaptic neuron is strengthened when the presynaptic axon is active at the same time the postsynaptic neuron is strongly activated by other inputs. This results in a reorganization of pre-existing neural circuits, which he called synaptic plasticity (Hebb, 1949). Hebb proposed that synaptic plasticity forms a memory trace after the detection of two coincident events. This concept provides a model for the cellular and even the molecular basis underlying not only declarative memory, but also for behavioral processes such as Pavlovian and Instrumental learning. These last memory processes are associative and constitute the basis of emotions and behavior.

Later, physiological studies of the hippocampus provided experimental evidence for long-lasting changes in synaptic strength (Bliss and Lomo, 1973; Collingridge and Bliss, 1995; Cooke and Bliss 2005, 2006). Brief, high-frequency electrical stimulation of an excitatory pathway to the hippocampus was found to produce a long-lasting enhancement of the strength of the stimulated synapses (Bliss and Lomo, 1973; Bliss and Gardner-Medwin, 1973). Since the hippocampus is involved in processes such as declarative memory (Scoville and Milner, 2000; Teyler and Discenna, 1984), different authors have hypothesized that long-lasting activity-dependent synaptic changes can represent the neural basis of learning and memory (Bliss and Lomo, 1973; Morris et al., 1986). The synaptic activity that leads to changes in synaptic strength have been termed long-term potentiation (LTP) (Kuba and Kumamoto, 1990; Patterson et al., 1996; Kovalchuk et al., 2002) and long-term depression (LTD) (Bramham and Srebro, 1987; Ito, 1989; Ikegaya et al., 2002). In the hippocampus, LTD can be produced when a low-frequency train of stimulus is negatively correlated in time with a high-frequency conditioning input (Stanton and Sejnowski, 1989). The two classic forms of long-term synaptic plasticity, LTP and LTD, are widely expressed at excitatory synapses throughout the brain, possibly at every excitatory synapse in the mammalian brain, and have been widely studied in several neural systems. In the brain, most synapses that express LTP can also exhibit different forms of LTD and it is not clear that LTP and LTD are not a unitary phenomena. LTD is considered to be a normal break mechanism preventing saturation of LTP. It is now clear that there are different forms of LTP and LTD and they vary depending on the synapses and circuits in which they operate (Kauer and Malenka, 2007). Therefore, when studying synaptic plasticity, it is essential to define the types of LTP and LTD that can occur at any specific synapses (Malenka and Bear, 2004).

LTP in the hippocampus is only one of several different forms of long-term synaptic plasticity that exist in specific circuits in the mammalian brain. The prototypic form of synaptic plasticity is LTP involving glutamate and its N-tethyl-D-aspartate receptors (NMDAR) as well as its aamino-3-hydroxy-5-methyl-isoxazole propionic acid-glutamate receptors (AMPAR). Several forms of LTP, which are dependent on NMDAR, induce and increase the number of AMPAR, also expressed in the same synaptic terminal on the postsynaptic neuron (Dozmorov et al., 2006; Lu et al., 2001). As a consequence, after the induction of LTP there is also an increase in the ratio of AMPAR/NMDAR in the synaptic terminal being activated. The consequence is an increased synaptic strength between the active presynaptic and postsynaptic neurons, which become more sensitive to posterior glutamate release.

There are other structural changes as a consequence of synaptic plasticity. One of the first described was an increase in the number of synaptic spines and a decrease in spines' length, also contributing to the potentiation of synaptic contacts (Hosokawa et al., 1995; Geinisman, 2000).

BDNF is a neurotrophic factor known to promote different forms of excitatory synaptic plasticity, such as early- and late-phase long-term potentiation (LTP) in the Ca1 regions of the hippocampus (Poo et al., 2001). BDNF also blocks LTD and facilitates LTP induction (Poo et al., 2001) as well as induces neuroplastic changes in neurons promoting dendritic spine formation and sprouting (Bramham and Messaoudi, 2005), changes that underlies normal learning and memory processes. BDNF is synthesized and stored in glutamatergic neurons and can be released in an activity-dependent manner from dendrites and axon terminals (Lessmann et al., 2003). BDNF is also a key element in the survival and differentiation of the dopaminergic system (Thoenen, 1995) and its specific receptor TrkB is expressed in all mesencephalic dopaminergic neurons (Numan and Seroogy, 1999), and in brain regions such as the striatum (Yurek et al., 1996), the prefrontal cortex (Bland et al., 2005); and the amygdala (Gordon et al., 2003). All these regions are involved in drug-induced neuronal responses. Experimental evidence supports the existence of a cross-talk between the BDNF intracellular signaling mechanisms and those of the glutamate and dopamine transmission, possibly through protein kinases (PKA) and Ca2+. It has been reported that chronic cocaine treatment results in a sustained increase in ERK activity via glutamate-dependent mechanisms (Berhow et al., 1996) (see figure 1).

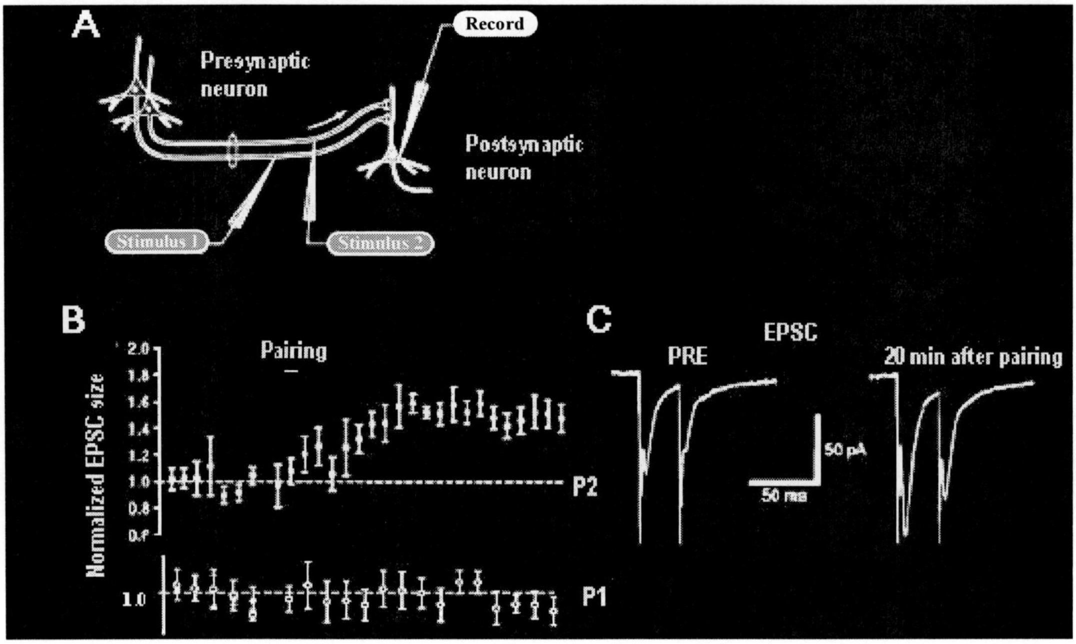

Figure 1. BDNF and the ERK intracellular signaling pathway. This figure depicts the ERK BDNF signaling cascade involved in cocaine addiction and its interaction with dopamine and glutamate intracellular messengers. There is a cross-talk between the BDNF intracellular signaling mechanism and those of the glutamate and dopamine transmission. (Source: Adapted from Corominas et al., 2007).

LTP AND LTD CAN BE INDUCED IN THE DOPAMINERGIC SYSTEM AFTER COCAINE TREATMENT

It is well accepted that dopaminergic circuitry, including midbrain dopamine cells, limbic nuclei including NAc, dorsal striatum, amygdala and hippocampus, and the PFC can undergo LTP and LTD. These cellular mechanisms involve changes in glutamate transmission and its receptors, but in the structures related with drug consumption the dopaminergic system is also involved (Calabresi et al., 1992; Centonze et al., 1999; Goto and Grace, 2005a).

To generate LTP in the lab several models have been used, some of them in vitro after the animal is sacrificed and others in vivo. The latter have the advantage of maintaining physiological conditions and patterns of neurotransmitter release, although it requires stereotaxis procedures to locate target areas to be examined. For example in a standard procedure, Sprague Dawley rats (between 14 and 42 days) were previously anesthetized and then sacrificed. Then, the brain is extracted and the block of tissue containing the midbrain VTA was sliced and prepared for cell-recording by means of electrodes (see figure 2). In a typical experiment, the effectiveness of the synapses between cells was monitored by giving a brief electrical stimulus to a bundle of presynaptic axons (afferents from the prefrontal cortex to the VTA). The electrical stimulation necessary to induce LTP is a brief burst of high-frequency electrical stimulation, typically 50-100 stimuli at a rate of 100/sec ("tetanus" or tetanic stimulation). At the same time, it is necessary to induce postsynaptic depolarization (to

0 or even positive mV) in VTA cells. As Hebb proposed, LTP requires concurrent presynaptic activity and postsynaptic depolarization. Usually, the "tetanus" induces LTP, and subsequent test stimulation evokes an EPSP that is much greater than during the initial baseline period. In other words, the "tetanus" has modified the stimulated synapses so that they are more effective. Other synaptic inputs into the same neuron that did not receive tetanic stimulation do not show LTP. Hence, LTP is input specific. LTP is a form of synaptic plasticity and it is a neurobiological mechanism for learning and memory.

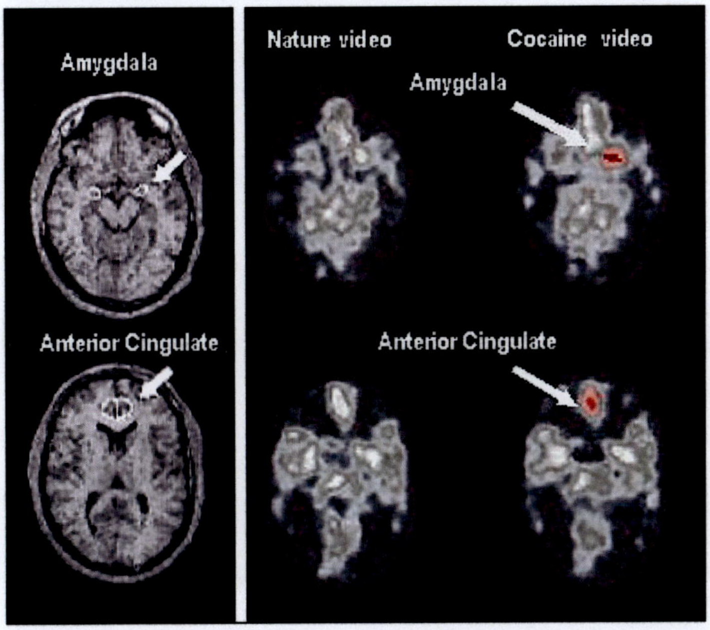

Figure 2. LTP induction requires concurrent presynaptic activity and postsynaptic depolarization. A: In the VTA dopaminergic neurons, two independent afferent pathways (P1, P2) were stimulated. P1 underwent the pairing protocol whereas P2 was not stimulated during the depolarization. B: Pairing induced potentiation of P1 (LTP), while P2 remained unchanged. C: Example traces taken immediately before and 20 minutes after pairing.

Cocaine acts as an addictive drug by increasing activity at dopamine neurons arising from the VTA, the midbrain nucleus that is the origin of the mesolimbic and mesocortical dopaminergic system. To study cocaine induced synaptic plasticity associated to LTP in the VTA neurons, Ungless et al. (2001) treated rodents by injecting them with a single dose of cocaine (experimental group) or saline (control group), and sacrificed them one day later. EPSCs from dopamine neurons present in slices of the VTA of the midbrain were evoked while holding neurons in voltage-clamp at +40 mV. The recorded EPSCs from animals treated with cocaine were greater than those of control animals, indicating that cocaine was able to induce LTP in the VTA synapses. LTP depends on NMDA receptor activation and the subsequent induced increase in AMPA receptors (Dozmorov et al., 2006; Lu et al., 2001).

Ungless et al. (2001) also explored the relative contribution of AMPA and NMDA receptors to EPSCs recorded in dopamine neurons. To do this, EPSCs were evoked both in the absence and then the presence of NMDAR antagonist AP5, and an AMPAR/NMDAR ratio was computed. If LTP were induced, a change in the relative contribution of AMPARs and NMDARs to EPSCs would reflect an increase in AMPAR function or number. Mice injected with cocaine exhibited a significantly greater AMPAR/NMDAR ratio, than mice injected with saline. These results demonstrated that cocaine can induce LTP that is related to an increase in the expression of AMPAR through NMDA mechanisms in dopamine neurons in the midbrain VTA (Ungless et al., 2001). According to these results, plasticity occurs in reward related regions of the brain, strengthening synaptic contacts on dopamine neurons and modifying its functions. There is evidence that these neuronal changes are responsible for behavioral sensitization, one of the animal models of drug addiction (Kalivas, 1995; Wolf, 1998). Consequently, a wide range of behaviors related to drug abuse such as sensitization of the incentive-motivational system, can also be affected (Robinson and Berridge, 1993; Kalivas, 1995). These results indicate that synaptic plasticity at excitatory synapses on dopamine cells may be a key neural adaptation contributing to the development of addiction.

Neuroimaging Studies Provide Evidence for Neuronal Changes in Human Addicts

To better understand synaptic plasticity and its cellular and molecular correlates, it is important to explore the evidence that neural changes are induced in addicts after cocaine abuse. Functional neuroimaging techniques have been very useful in this area and have provided evidence for the existence of neuroplastic changes involving cortical and subcortical circuitry in human addicts.

Positron emission tomography (PET) or single photon emission computed tomography (SPECT) studies have been performed in addicts during periods of abstinence. The aim of these studies was to explore the effects of repeated cocaine use in the brain. Some of these studies have assessed, at the same time, the behavioral and emotional consequences of cocaine abuse during active use and abstinence.

Volkow et al. (1992) studied 21 patients receiving treatment for cocaine addiction. Only patients that met the Diagnostic and Statistical Manual of Mental Disorders, third edition revised (DSM-III-R) criteria for cocaine dependence were included in the study. In order to isolate cocaine effects from other factors, patients with other addictions, except for tobacco, and patients with organicity or neurological abnormalities detected on PET scans were excluded from the study. Brain imaging was done 1 to 6 weeks after the last cocaine use, and a subgroup of 7 patients underwent a second scan after 3 months of abstinence. A control group with 18 normal participants paired by sex and age was selected. PET scans were obtained according to the standardized protocol at resting conditions.

Volkow et al. (1992) reported a reduced metabolism (hypofunctionality) in the prefrontal cortex (PFC) in cocaine addicts evaluated 1 to 6 weeks after last cocaine use compared with controls. It is important to note that acute cocaine use induces increased brain activity in certain areas, especially in the PFC, the same areas that were hypoactive during abstinence. Hypofunctionality during abstinence suggested neuroadaptive changes induced by the drug in those areas. Hypofunctionality in the PFC may account for the feelings of anhedonia and depression, which characterize cocaine withdrawal and often trigger cocaine craving and relapse. Changes in glucose metabolism include specifically the orbitofrontal and anterior cingulate regions, which are involved in high-order cognitive and motivational functions. Therefore, the ability to modulate the salience of a reinforcer to update reward-related information, such as learning new rewarded responses, to inhibit the response when it is no longer adaptive and to control a prepotent response are compromised in drug addicts (Volkow et al., 1992; Goldstein and Volkow 2002; Goldstein et al., 2007). In addiction, hypofrontality is a strong indicator of reduced ability to regulate drug-seeking behavior.

Reduced metabolism in the prefrontal cortex of cocaine abstinent patients was found even after 3 months of abstinence (Volkow et al., 1992). These data show that the effects of chronic cocaine use on the brain are long-lasting and suggest the possibility that these metabolic changes are induced by transient neuronal adaptation and even long-lasting neuroplastic changes. Studies using structural neuroimaging have provided evidence for a volume reduction involving cortical and subcortical limbic structures in cocaine addicts (Franklin et al., 2002). It has been suggested that this volume reduction in different brain regions (from 5% to 11%) reflects a decreased neuronal tissue as a consequence of the repeated drug consumption. These effects involving abnormalities in neuronal tissue are long-lasting and even permanent. Nevertheless, it is not known if the hypofrontality and altered cerebral tissue precedes or is a consequence of the long-term neuroadaptation induced by chronic psychostimulant use.

Other important aspects of drug addiction indicative of neuroadaptive changes as a consequence of chronic cocaine consumption are those related to the dopamine receptors. Human addicts also show reduced expression of D2 receptors in the striatum (Volkow et al., 1993, 2001) that persists some moths after the last cocaine intake (Volkow et al., 1993). This reduced density of D2 receptors can be a consequence of chronic drug consumption but can also exist previous to any contact with the drug, and hence could indicate a predisposition to addiction (Corominas-Roso et al., 2007).

Cue-stimuli induce craving and relapse in cocaine addicts

A key characteristic of addiction is that situations or stimuli (i.e., cue stimuli) previously associated with drug seeking or drug taking behavior (e.g., people, places, paraphernalia) can precipitate in abstinent abusers or addicts an intense emotional response and desire for drug, known as cravings. Craving have important clinical consequences as it frequently leads to drug seeking behavior and relapse. Cue stimuli can precipitate relapse even in individuals who have decided never to use drugs again, often without the addicted person having insight into what is happening to them (O'Brien et al., 1990, 1998). Drug conditioned cues can be environmental or can even be interoceptive body states. Cue-induced cravings are often accompanied by different signs and symptoms similar to the effects of cocaine itself, including generalized arousal, palpitations, ear ringing, and euphoria (Childress et al., 1993).

In the study of Childress et al. (1999), brain responses to cue stimuli have been conducted using PET scans or functional magnetic resonance imaging (fMRI). The protocols of obtaining such measures were similar to those used to evaluate brain responses during abstinence. But these protocols included, in addition to the scan obtained at rest conditions, one or more scans obtained with the patient engaged in watching drug-related images and non-drug related images. The non-drug images, included pictures of nature and are used as a control, whereas the drug-related images included the simulated purchase, preparation and smoking of cocaine. These protocols also include the evaluation of cocaine related states using different scales, such as the Within Session Rating Scale, a 10-item scale asking about the high, craving and withdrawal related to cocaine administered before and after each video. After the PET or fMRI sessions, each patient has a supportive "talk-down" with a trained clinician before leaving the facility, which is also useful as a form of therapy to help the patient to deal with drug-related situations in the future.

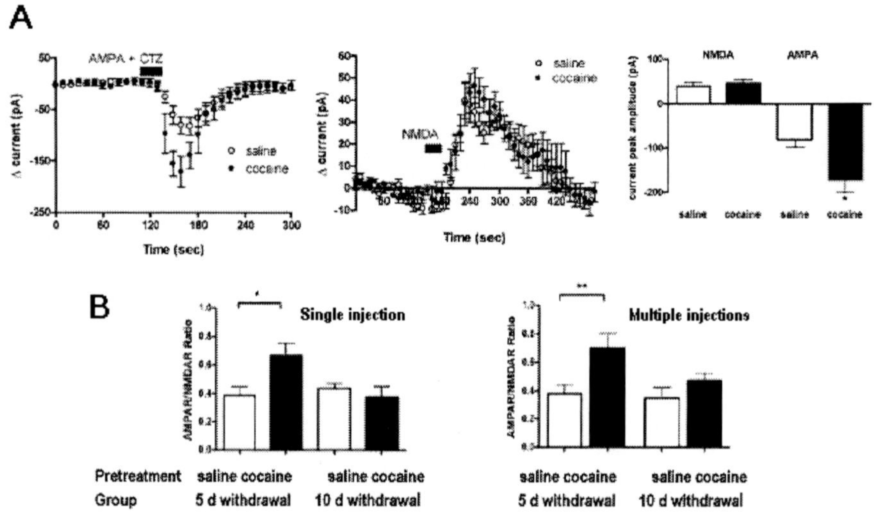

Figure 3. Functional brain activation associated with cue-induced cocaine craving in cocaine abusers. Images illustrate the differential increase in relative regional cerebral blood flow in the amygdala and anterior cingulate of a detoxified cocaine patient during a non-drug-related (nature) video and a cocaine-related video. (Source: Adapted from Childress et al., 1999).

Neuroimaging studies of response to drug conditioned cues have reported activation in different cortical and subcortical regions, including prefrontal cortical areas, especially the orbitofrontal and anterior cingulate, and the amygdala, a region involved in the stimulus-reward associations (see figure 3). Some of these studies have also found activation in the NAc and the dorsal striatum (Grant et al., 1996; Maas et al., 1998; Childress et al., 1999; Kilts et al., 2001). Interestingly, the lack of hippocampal activation suggested the subordination of explicit (factual) memory to an amygdala-driven emotional state (Squire et al., 1992). The neuronal responses obtained with neuroimaging techniques are similar to those recorded with the same techniques under the effects of psychostimulants such as cocaine. This shows that brain structures activated during cue-cocaine craving may be among those activated by cocaine itself (Goldstein and Volkow, 2002). These results support those reported during abstinence, suggesting that impaired prefrontal function characterizing addiction can be involved in relapse in drug consumption. In these studies, patient self-reports of craving correlate positively with activity in the prefrontal cortex (Childress et al., 1999; Goldstein and Volkow, 2002; Grant et al., 1996) and increased amygdala activity (Childress et al., 1999). It is important to mention that an increased response to cocaine cues persists for a long time, even throughout the life span, and can induce relapse years after the last contact with the drug. These persistent effects reflect long-term neuroplastic changes in the neural circuitry related to conditioned cocaine effects.

A crucial consequence of drug addiction, often reported by addicts in clinical settings, is the reduced interest in natural rewards, such as sex. In fact, one of the diagnostic criteria for drug addiction is the narrowing interest in different activities that previously were an important part of the person's life. When cocaine users are examined with functional neuroimaging techniques using sex images and cocaine-related images, sex (natural reward) induced less activation in cerebral circuitry than cocaine (Garavan et al., 2000). Similar results were reported in studies of cocaine self-administration in rats in which cocaine produced increases in brain stimulation reward thresholds during withdrawal (Markou and Koob, 1991). This finding has important implications and suggests that the effects of cocaine in narrowing the user's interests in life have a neurobiological background. In fact, cocaine craving is subserved by the same cerebral regions that are activated by natural rewarding and reward-evocative stimuli; this could indicate a rewriting of normal, emotionally-driven preferences. These neurobiological changes may have important consequences for decision-making because the decreased response to natural rewards may be exacerbated during craving, further increasing the desire for cocaine (Robbins and Everitt, 1999).

Together these findings suggest that the emotional and behavioral consequences in the development of addiction can result from changes in long-term synaptic plasticity, including reduced activity in the prefrontal cortex, reduced D2 expression in the striatum, increased responsiveness for cocaine related cues and decreased responsiveness for natural rewarding stimuli. These neuroplastic changes may play an important role in the feeling of craving that accompanies addiction and relapse.

Synaptic Plasticity in the Ventral Tegmental Area

Addiction is not triggered instantaneously after the exposure to cocaine. On the contrary, the development of addiction involves neural adaptations that develop with different temporal courses ranging from hours to days to months. The VTA is considered to be essential for the development of behavioral sensitization, one of the models of drug addiction. Behavioral sensitization can be defined as a progressive increase of some behavioral effects of the drug, such as locomotor activity with repeated cocaine doses. Behavioral sensitization is considered a model useful for studying the rewarding and addictive effects of cocaine (Kalivas, 1995).

The usual procedure to study behavioral sensitization is based either on passive cocaine injection of rodents (i.e. mice or rats) or intravenous self-administration of cocaine by such rodents themselves in an operant chamber. Before starting the program, spontaneous individual activity is measured in an activity chamber where the animals were placed during a stipulated time period. The program continues for approximately 6 to 15 days approximately. Each day, rodents get their programmed dose of cocaine. In the passive cocaine injection, rodents usually receive a dose of 15 mg/kg intraperitoneal (i.p.). In the self-administration program, cocaine is usually administered in doses of 0.75 mg/kg per infusion, and in each session rats get a total of 10 infusion (i.e. 7.5 mg/kg) within and hour. There is always a control group to compare with the cocaine-treated rodents. Following the sequence of repeated, intermittent drug treatment, rodents are withdrawn from the drug over several days (e.g., 3, 15 or 30 days). After the withdrawal period, rodents are placed again in the activity chamber and locomotor activity is measured over the stipulated time period after a challenge with a cocaine dose (e.g., 3 mg/kg). Locomotor activity after cocaine challenge is compared with activity measured before cocaine sensitization treatment. Behavioral sensitization of motor activity after cocaine challenge is defined as a significant increase in motor activity compared with measures of activity before cocaine treatment (Kalivas and Duffy, 1993; Phillips and Di Ciano, 1996).

Some of the cocaine sensitization studies have also assessed the levels of extracellular dopamine at the same time as measuring locomotor activity. Dopamine determinations are done through intracranial inserted cannulas, usually placed into the NAc before starting the experiment. A significant increase was found in the level of extracellular dopamine in the NAc (usually with a peak response between 20 and 40 mins after cocaine challenge). Then dopamine levels return to baseline level, approximately 80 mins after the challenge (Kalivas and Duffy, 1993). The release of dopamine in the NAc from dopaminergic projections arising in the VTA indicated that this region is required for behavioral sensitization (Kalivas, 1995).

The major cell type in the VTA is the dopaminergic neuron, which receives activating excitatory input from different cortical and subcortical regions, such as the prefrontal cortex (Omelchenko and Sesack, 2007). There is an anatomical relationship between neurons in the VTA and its projection targets, for example the NAc and the PFC. Dopamine neurons projecting to the PFC receive reciprocal input from PFC, whereas dopamine neurons projecting to the NAc do not have such reciprocal projections (Carr and Sesack, 2000). Electrophysiological experiments have demonstrated that prefrontal cortex activity plays an important role in the control of the firing pattern of dopamine neurons (White, 1996). The VTA also receives important excitatory input from the amygdala and bed nucleus of stria terminalis (Garzon et al., 1999; Georges et al., 2001). Dopaminergic neurons in the VTA are inhibited by local interneurons, which generate BAGAA receptor-mediated responses, as by GABA-ergic projections from the NAc and ventral pallidum.

In the VTA there is a close relationship between dopaminergic and glutamatergic activity. Dopamine neurons express metabotropic and ionotropic glutamate receptors, and glutamate activity on these receptors activates DA neurons in the VTA (Mercuri et al., 1992; Overton and Clark, 1997). For example, perfusion of the D1 agonist SKF-82595 in the VTA produced a dose-dependent increase in extracellular glutamate that, in turn, can be blocked by coperfusion of the D1 antagonist SCH-23390. Psychostimulants promote dopamine release into somatodendritic fields of midbrain dopamine neurons (Lacey et al., 1990; Seutin et al., 1991). For example, systemic administration of cocaine (15 mg/kg i.p.) induces a rapid increase of extracellular glutamate that lasts for 20 minutes. This increase is prevented by pre-treating the VTA with the D1 receptor antagonist SCH-23390 (Kalivas and Duffy, 1995).

Cocaine Induced Synaptic Plasticity in the VTA

Dopamine or glutamate release alone does not explain the long-lasting behavioral changes induced by repeated cocaine administration in rodents nor the development of addiction in humans. To understand the enduring and permanent effects induced by the drug, it is necessary to look at the basic mechanisms of synaptic plasticity, LTP and LTD.

Excitatory synapses on dopamine neurons in the midbrain dopamine regions, the VTA, and the substantia nigra (SN) can undergo LTP and LTD (Thomas and Malenka, 2003), the major mechanisms of synaptic plasticity. These mechanisms cause changes at the excitatory synpases in the VTA DA neurons, by potentiating some of them and depotentiating others.

The effects of cocaine within the VTA was assessed in a serial of studies done by Malenka and his colleagues (Borgland et al., 2004; Saal et al., 2003; Ungless et al., 2001). To study cocaine effects on the VTA, rodents received a single cocaine injection (15 mg/kg), the same dose used in the protocols that induce behavioral sensitization. One day later, rodents are sacrificed so that midbrain slices can be obtained and prepared to measure synaptic strength (as the magnitude of EPSCs) with whole-cell recording techniques in the manner described above. A single exposure to cocaine (15 mg/kg) enhances VTA dopamine neurons' responsiveness, measured as the magnitude of EPSCs in this brain region. Enhancement in EPSCs is due to an increase in AMPAR/NMDAR ratios, a form of LTP at excitatory synapses in the VTA DA neurons. Moreover, this enhanced AMPAR/NMDAR ratio is due to an increase in the number, function, or both, of AMPA receptors in the post-synaptic membrane of the VTA cells (Ungless et al., 2001). A similar increase in the AMPAR to NMDAR ratio was also reported in other studies after acute cocaine exposure (Borgland et al., 2004).

Cocaine-induced potentiation of excitatory synapses in the VTA can be blocked when a NMDA (Nmethyl-D-aspartate) receptor antagonist is administered with cocaine (Kalivas and Alesdatter, 1993; Ungless et al., 2001; Vezina and Queen, 2000). In a similar way, glutamatergic input to the VTA can also trigger relapse and blockade of glutamate receptors in this brain region inhibiting cocaine seeking (Vorel et al., 2001). The increased AMPAR/NMDAR ratio is specific to the VTA since it was not observed in other regions such as the hippocampus (Ungless et al., 2001). Furthermore, these neuroplastic changes appear to be specific for addictive drugs, since it was not observed after administration of non-addictive substances such as fluoxetine or carbamazepine (Saal et al., 2003).

Potentiation of synaptic activity in midbrain cells induced by cocaine is thought to be transient. To explore the length of the acute effects of cocaine on the VTA, midbrain slices were prepared 5 and 10 days after injection. The AMPAR/NMDAR was increased after 5 days of acute cocaine administration but not after 10 days (see figure 4). These results indicate that cocaine-induced potentiation of activity at VTA cells are not long-lasting. Thus, synaptic potentiation at VTA cells after cocaine administration, may only be responsible for the early stages of behavioral sensitization and the early stages of the development of human addiction (Ungless et al., 2001).

Other studies have assessed the effects of repeated and intermittent cocaine administration across 7 days on electrical VTA cell responses as well as on locomotor activity in cocaine treated rodents. The aim was to study the possible relationship between behavioral and neurobiological effects induced by repeated cocaine. In naïve animals, a single dose of cocaine induces an enhancement in locomotor activity correlated with the magnitude of synaptic enhancement (the ratio AMPAR/NMDAR on the VTA) measured 1 day after the injection (see figure 4). Nevertheless, this correlation was not found after repeated cocaine treatment (Borgland et al., 2004). When cocaine doses are administered across 7 days, the AMPAR/NMDAR ratio at the VTA synapses remained at the same level as the levels found after 24 hours of a single cocaine injection. These results suggest that cocaine-induced synaptic plasticity in the VTA is not only transient but also has a ceiling effect. (Borgland et al., 2004). Therefore, adaptations in downstream circuitry, such NAc and PFC, are likely to be more important for the longer lasting behavioral changes associated with drug addiction. As discussed below, the critical neuroplastic changes responsible for sensitization would shift from its initiation site in the VTA to its sites of expression in other brain regions, such as the NAc (Wolf, 1998; Vanderschuren and Kalivas, 2000).

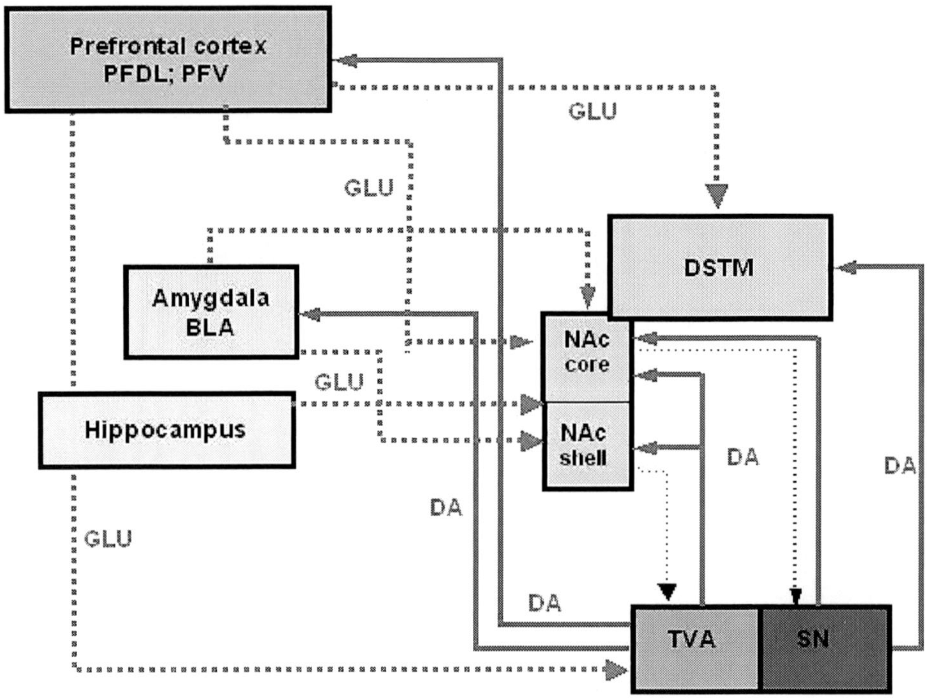

Figure 4. Involvement of NMDA and AMPA receptors in the induction of LTP. A: Potentiation of AMPAR/NMDAR after multiple injections is attributed to an increase of AMPA currents. B: Multiple injections of cocaine were found to increase the AMPAR/NMDAR ratio at 5 but not at 10 days after cocaine administration. (Source: Adapted from Borgland et al., 2004).

The above-mentioned studies have linked glutamate induced neuroplasticity in the VTA with the locomotor effects of cocaine. To study the neurochemical background of reward related learning it is possible to use a conditioned place preference to cocaine paradigm (CPP). This approach is different from the model of behavioral sensitization that uses repeated cocaine adminstration. CPP is based on operant behavior controlled by cue stimuli. CPP consists of two distinct compartments or chambers, one of them with a grid floor and black walls, and the other with a mesh floor and black and white striped walls. As a general procedure, rodents are allowed to freely explore both compartments and receive cocaine (usually intracerebral microinjections) only in one of the two compartments, so that the rodents are able to associate one of the compartments with cocaine effects. At the end of the experiment, the rodents undergo a preference test. The amount of time spend in each chamber is recorded as a measure of the rewarding effects of cocaine.

Using CPP, Harris and Aston-Jones (2003) explored the effects of glutamate release in the VTA. Rodents were first allowed to associate one of the two compartments with cocaine.

Afterwards, rats received microinjections of NMDA and AMPA glutamate receptor antagonists inside the VTA prior to each cocaine place-conditioning trial. Glutamate antagonist completely blocked the development of cocaine CPP, whereas antagonists administered outside of the VTA did not alter cocaine conditioning. These results suggest that plasticity in the VTA also plays a role in learning an association between the neutral place and the primary reward, in this case cocaine (Harris and Aston-Jones, 2003).

Although synaptic plasticity in the VTA appears to be a mechanism for up or down regulating the excitability of the entire ensemble of dopaminergic neurons (Jones et al., 2000), this brain region is not likely to be the specific site of cue-conditioning. In other words, the VTA is the site of action for transient synaptic plasticity which plays an essential role in triggering adaptations after drug exposure in regions innervated by DA neurons, including the NAc, dorsal striatum, amygdala and PFC (Nestler, 2001, 2002). These areas are involved in appetitive associative learning and all undergo activity-dependent synaptic plasticity related to cocaine consumption, which may account for long-term consequences of addiction. This proposed role for VTA is consistent with the idea that activity of dopamine neurons in the VTA are necessary for attributing motivational significance to the stimuli (Schultz, 2002). Potentiation of excitatory synapses on VTA DA neurons with repeated drug administration may contribute to the incentive salience attributed to the drugs, even for the learned association between context and drug experience (Robinson and Berridge, 1993, 2001).

Excitatory synapses on dopamine neurons of the VTA exhibit LTD as well as LTP (Thomas et al., 2000). If LTD is related to development of sensitization and to increase of strength at excitatory synapses in the VTA, psychostimulants must decrease or block LTD at VTA. In fact, Thomas et al. (2000) reported that amphetamines block LTD at VTA synapses though dopamine acting on D2 receptors in dopamine neurons. LTD also requires voltage-dependent CA2+ channels but is independent of NMDAR receptors. The inhibition of LTD makes the induction of LTP easier (Thomas et al., 2000).

Stress and Synaptic Plasticity in the VTA

Stress is a potent trigger of relapse in humans and in many animal addiction models (Marinelli and Piazza, 2002; Stewart, 2003). Individuals can be abstinent for months or even years and are still susceptible to experience cravings that can stimulate drug-seeking and relapse (O'Brien, 1997). Exposure to stress also facilitates the initial acquisition and maintenance of drug self-administration in animal models of addiction (Piazza and Le Moal, 1998; Shaham et al., 2000). From the neurobiological point of view, stress acts in a similar way to drugs of abuse, causing an increase in DA levels in the NAc and prefrontal cortex (Horger and Roth, 1996; Piazza and Le Moal, 1998). Stress also produces inhibition of LTP and enhances LTD in various brain structures, such as the hippocampus, modifying synaptic plasticity (Shors et al., 1989; Kim et al., 1996).

Acute stress, like cocaine, can also induce changes in excitatory synaptic strength on midbrain dopamine neurons. One of the studies used a forced swimming task to induce acute stress (Saal et al., 2003). Then animals were sacrificed and underwent the above-mentioned general experimental procedure to study potentiation at excitatory synapses in the VTA. The receptor mediated synaptic currents (AMPA EPSCs) to NMDA receptor mediated synaptic currents (NMDAR EPSCs) ratio on excitatory synapses in the VTA DA neurons was increased 24 hrs after animals experienced an episode of acute stress plus a saline injection when compared to animals that received only a saline injection (Saal et al., 2003). In a similar study, cocaine administration immediately after acute stress was not found to cause any additional increase in the AMPA/NMDA ratio. The interpretation of these results depends on the possibility of there being a "ceiling" effect, the maximum AMPA/NMDA ratio that can be achieved. If cocaine and stress had increased synaptic strength in the VTA by independent mechanisms, the magnitude of the increase in synaptic strength would have been greater in animals experiencing stress and cocaine combined compared to animals experiencing only stress. Thus, the results of the study suggest that drugs of abuse and stress induce LTP in the VTA through the same mechanism of action. However, these results do not allow any conclusion to be drawn about the neurobiological mechanisms underlying the increased AMPA/NMDA ratio (Dong et al., 2004).

One of the major consequences of acute stress is an enhancement in the activity of the hypothalamic-pituitary-adrenal axis (HPA) with an increased secretion of glucocorticoids and activation of their receptors (GRs). Saal et al., (2003) studied whether GR plays a role in the strengthening of synaptic plasticity induced by stress. Rodents were treated with the GR antagonist RU486 before being placed in cold water. The GR antagonist blocked LTP (i.e., increased AMPAR to NMDAR EPSC ratio) that had been induced by stress. Nevertheless, the GR antagonist did not block the LTP induced by cocaine. On the hand, Dong et al. (2004) found that administration of D1 receptor antagonists blocked those cellular mechanisms of LTP that were induced by cocaine but not those induced by stress. According to these results, although cocaine and stress are able to induce similar cellular adaptations in the VTA, potentiating activity of DA neurons in this midbrain areas, the neurobiological mechanisms of action of those effects (cocaine or stress) are different.

BDNF And Synaptic Plasticity in the VTA

The protein BDNF has been found to exert a potent effect in behavioral sensitization induced by cocaine. When BDNF is infused for two weeks into the VTA, rats showed a progressive increase in locomotor activity, compared with saline infused animals (Horger et al., 1999). However, it is during withdrawal that the expression of BDNF in the VTA is more significant, facilitating LTP induction and hence synaptic plasticity in the VTA.

The role of BDNF has been studied using animal models of cocaine craving and relapse by Grimm and his colleagues. Rats, divided in two groups, were trained to press a lever for 10 days (instrumental learning), receiving cocaine (experimental group) or sucrose (control group) as a reward. After cocaine withdrawal, behavioral measures of lever pressing during extinction were recorded over 90 days. Reward seeking, as measured by the rate of lever pressing, increased progressively over 90 days or longer. BDNF levels in the VTA were also studied during withdrawal. It was found that BDNF levels rose significantly and progressively in the VTA after ceasing cocaine, but BDNF did not increase in the same brain region and the same time period in the control group (Grimm et al., 2003). The role of BDNF in cocaine withdrawal was further studied by the same laboratory using the same animal model. This second study included, an exogenous BDNF infusion into the VTA and the SN after the training period. Intra-VTA, but not intra-SN infusions of BDNF progressively enhanced cocaine seeking after withdrawal. Cocaine-seeking responses were higher 30 days after withdrawal than 3 days after withdrawal (Lu et al., 2004). These results suggest that the increase of BDNF during psychostimulant withdrawal may mediate neuronal plasticity, leading to synaptic modifications that underlie enhanced responsiveness and compulsive drug seeking in addicts.

The role of BDNF in synaptic plasticity of the midbrain VTA dopamine neurons during cocaine withdrawal was further assessed by examining the excitatory properties of the VTA dopamine neurons. Rodents were treated with cocaine for 5-7 days and then the effectiveness of the treatment to induce sensitization was assessed through measures of locomotor activity. Brain slices were obtained sacrificing rodents 10-15 days after last cocaine injection. In VTA slices, weak presynaptic stimuli, administered on dopamine neurons, evoked persistent increases in excitatory postsynaptic potentials (EPSPs) amplitude. The enhanced VTA neuronal responses were found 10-15 days after cocaine withdrawal. However, the enhancement was not detected 1 day after withdrawal. These results suggest that during withdrawal VTA dopamine neurons become increasingly excitable and susceptible to the induction of long-term potentiation (LTP). At the same time, BDNF levels were registered in the VTA tissues and were also found to have increased after 10-15 days of withdrawal. BDNF levels in VTA were not detected 1 day after withdrawal. Moreover, when exogenous BDNF was applied to the VTA, persistent potentiation in dopamine neurons activity was observed both in naïve rats and after one day of withdrawal. These results suggested that BDNF was needed for the induction and expression of LTP in VTA synapses (Pu et al., 2006) and confirmed the role of BDNF, already described as an inductor of LTP and synaptic plasticity in the hippocampus (Poo et al., 2001).

Taken together, these data suggest that increased BDNF levels in VTA neurons during withdrawal play a role in synaptic remodeling. Moreover, the results for BDNF confirm the role of LTP in synaptic plasticity as a basic cellular mechanism underlying information storage within the neural systems (Geinisman, 2000).

Synaptic Plasticity in the Striatum

The possible use-dependent changes in synaptic efficacy in the striatum, including the ventral and dorsal striatum, have been widely studied in order to investigate the possible biochemical and cellular mechanisms that underlie memory and learning and their implications in human and non-human behavior. In cocaine addiction, it is has been proposed that strong excitatory synapses on VTA DA neurons will change the level or pattern of DA release in target structures such as the NAc and modulate DA-dependent learned associations and behaviors having remarkable consequences on human behavior and emotion (Hyman and Malenka, 2001; Kalivas and Volkow, 2005). The work in this area has revealed a remarkable plasticity in striatal cells and their cortical and subcortical projecting structures.

Structural and Functional Organization of the Striatum

The striatum is not a unitary structure, but consists of two anatomical and functional subregions, the dorsal striatum and ventral striatum, which includes the NAc. In turn, the NAc includes two different structural and functional subregions, the core and the shell (Heimer et al., 1991; Voorn et al., 1989. The core appears to be a functional extension of the dorsal striatum and there is evidence that the NAc core is involved in the control of goal-directed behavior by associative processes (Cardinal et al., 2002), in instrumental (response-reinforcement) learning (Kelley et al.,1997), and in supporting behavioral responses to motivationally significant conditioned stimuli (Bassareo and Di Chiara, 1999; Parkinson et al., 2000). The NAc shell is connected with the network of descending neuronal influences over reflexive autonomic and motor responses. The shell is a limbic structure included in the extended amygdala and seems to be involved in the processing of the primary reinforcing effect of natural rewards (Bassareo and Di Chiara, 1999) and drugs of abuse (Carlezon and Wise, 1996; Di Chiara et al., 1993), including initial stages of behavioral sensitization to cocaine (Todtenkopf et al., 2002). The NAc core and shell get excitatory input from the basolateral nucleus of the amygdala (BLA) (Wright et al.,1996; Cardinal et al., 2002). Two amygdala nuclei, the BLA and the central nucleus (Ce), are involved in emotional processes of addiction. Whereas BLA is required for Pavlovian conditioning, Ce acts as a control of brainstem arousal (see figure 5).

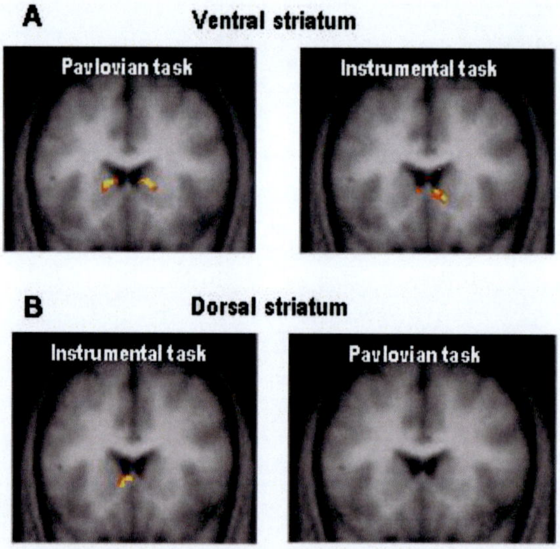

Figure 5. Basic circuitry in cocaine addiction. Includes the primary neurotransmitters, topographic organization and interconnections between the reward related pathways, learning and memory pathways, and circuits involved in cocaine seeking. The mesencephalic ventral tegmental area (VTA) projects its dopaminergic (DA) efferents to the limbic nuclei, nucleus accumbens (NAc) core and shell, amygdala and hippocampus, as well as dorsolateral prefrontal cortex (DLPF) and ventral prefrontal cortex (VPF). The hippocampus and amygdala, the latter through its basolateral subnucleus (BLA), as well as the DLPF and VPF cortex project their glutamatergic (GLU) efferents to the shell and core of the NAc. The figure also includes the dorsal striatum (DSTM) and its connexions to the substantia nigra (SN). (Source: Adapted from Corominas-Roso et al. 2007).

The dorsal striatum includes the caudate and putamen nuclei, which from the functional point of view involve the associative (caudate and central putamen) and motor striatum (dorsolateral caudate and putamen, whereas the ventral regions of the striatum constitute the limbic striatum (Haber et al., 2000).

Striatal neurons receive afferents that have their origin in the mesencephalic substantia nigra and ventral tegmental area, as well as excitatory inputs that arise from cortical and subcortical regions, and integrate glutamatergic and dopaminergic signals within the striatal cells (Kotter, 1994; Starr, 1995). The major neuronal cells in the striatum are the GABAergic medium spiny neurons which receive inputs from the PFC, amygdala and hippocampus, synapsing on the head of spiny neurons, whereas subcortical dopamine synapse on the neck or nearby dendritic shaft (Groves et al., 1994). In turn, striatal cells send projections to the VTA and substantia nigra (SN) while the midbrain dopamine cells project to the striatum. This system creates a loose topographical organization in which the VTA and the medial SN are associated with the limbic striatum whereas the lateral and ventral SN are associated with the associative and motor striatum. This structural organization provides a directional flow of information between regions that allow the ventral striatum to influence motor output, via striato-nigral-striatal pathways (Haber et al., 2000).

Sensitization and Reward-Related Learning in the Striatum

Whereas the VTA is involved in the early transient stages of cocaine sensitization, the striatum is crucial in the consolidation of drug-induced sensitization. Sensitization is an increase in locomotor activity induced by repeated cocaine intake and is essentially caused by the intrinsic properties of addictive drugs. Nevertheless, in drug addiction other processes regarding reward-related learning are also involved. This kind of learning is even more crucial than sensitization in the process that advances from initial sporadic impulsive drug intake to the compulsive consumption that characterizes addiction.

In the context of drug addiction, environmental stimuli that are closely associated in time and space with the effects of drugs of abuse can acquire secondary reinforcing properties through a process of classical conditioning. Once conditioned, these stimuli have in themselves the ability to elicit the emotional responses that were induced by the drug during active consumption. These cue-conditioned stimuli are able to maintain drug seeking behavior and relapse, even after long-term abstinence (O'Brien et al., 1992). Neuroimaging studies have revealed the neural structures activated when abstinent addicts are watching images related to drug consumption. Activation in those brain regions are involved in the feeling of craving that often leads to relapse (Childress et al., 1999; Garavan et al., 2000).

The role of conditioned stimuli in drug addiction has been widely studied through animal models of abstinence and relapse. For example, in a study by Grimm et al. (2003), rodents were trained to self-administer cocaine or sucrose as a comparative vehicle. Training was conducted with a continuous reinforcement schedule (each lever press is reinforced with cocaine) administered in six daily sessions for 10 days. Each earned reward was accompanied by a five-second tone-light cue. Afterwards, there was a withdrawal phase during which rats were housed in the animal facility. Then, rats were separated in three groups and were tested for resistance to cocaine-seeking (rate of lever-pressing) extinction and for cue-induced reinstatement (rate of lever pressing induced by the conditioned cue). These tests were conducted after 1, 30 and 90 days of withdrawal. Reinstatement of lever pressing was assessed in the absence of the discrete tone-light cue. Rats were allowed to lever-press until they had reached an extinction criterion of <15 responses per session on the active lever. Then, after the final extinction session, the test for cue-induced reinstatement was conducted. Each spontaneous lever press resulted in a presentation of the tone-light cue, that then became conditioned reinforcer. Sucrose trained rats were tested for resistance to extinction and cue-induced reinstatement after 1, 30, or 90 days of withdrawal from sucrose in the same conditions used for cocaine (Grimm et al., 2003). The results of this study will be reported later in this chapter.

Four learning processes can be identified in this experiment that also occur in human cocaine consumption and which have been found to be critical to the development of human addiction. The first is Pavlovian conditioning, represented by the discrete tone-light paired with cocaine. The tone-light begins as a neutral stimulus (NS), which after being associated with cocaine, the unconditioned stimulus (UC), becomes a conditioned stimulus (CS). The second process is a stimulus, such as the tone-light, becoming a conditioned reinforcer through the acquisition of reinforcing properties (positive or negative) by being paired with other, generally primary reinforcers, such as food, drugs, or sex. The third process taking place is instrumental reward-related learning (instrumental conditioning), by which rodents learn to perform a behavior in response a rewarding stimulus. The fourth process is Pavlovian-instrumental transfer (PIT), the modulation of instrumental performance by Pavlovian CS. For example, the tone-light cue that predicts the arrival of cocaine will enhance lever pressing for cocaine. PIT is important because it probably plays a major role in CS-precipitated reinstatement of instrumental responding, exemplified by cue-induced relapse in drug addiction (Cardinal et al., 2002).

From the neurobiological point of view, dopamine is essential in the different reward-related learning processes described above. Midbrain dopamine cells fire bursts of action potentials as a consequence of stimuli that predict the rewarding events (Mirenowicz and Schultz, 1994; Schultz, 1998). If dopamine release coincides with the solution of behavioral problems, such as obtaining food or drink, the appropriate response is to do it again and the response is learned (Ljungberg et al., 1992). Dopamine release to facilitate further learning is not necessary and does not occur after biological rewards once the most efficient behavior to obtain a reward has been learned (Schultz, 2004). However, dopamine continues to be released after a conditional stimuli once it has become a conditioned reinforcer (Schultz, 1998).

In order to be able to use the learned information the animals need a record of what has occurred at the arrival of dopamine, which acts on corticostriatal synapses and their respective striatal partners. Dopamine contributes to the creation of a new memory trace or to the change of a pre-existing one. This memory trace makes the activity of the involved set of connections more likely to be activated in similar circumstances and continues to do so for some time even in the absence of further reward. Once a behavior designed to obtain a reward or avoid a negative consequence as been learned, the role of dopamine changes. Dopamine then enables the use of the learned information to execute the adaptive behavioral response in an efficient manner (Schultz, 2004).

There is a major difference between dopamine release in response to biological reward (primary or conditioned reward) as opposed to cocaine. After a biological stimulus, tolerance develops to the release of dopamine, whereas addictive drugs release dopamine every time the drug is taken. Every administration of an addictive drug is associated with a large release of dopamine that can be expected to promote new learning (new associations between the drug and the environment). Moreover, dopamine release also cues the addict to execute an instrumental, drug-seeking behavior (i.e., relapse) (Schultz, 2004). Cocaine self-administration significantly increases extracellular levels of DA in both the NAc core and shell regions (Di Chiara et al., 1993; Carlezon and Wise, 1996). In contrast, presentation of cocaine-associated cues leads to significant increases of DA efflux in the core but not the shell of the NAc (Ito et al., 2000). Selective lesions of the core (Parkinson et al., 1999), infusions of NMDA, or dopamine receptor antagonists into the NAc core during training greatly retard the acquisition of Pavlovian approach responses to an appetitive conditioned stimulus (Di Ciano et al., 2001). These results are consistent with those that propose that DA innervation of the shell region is especially responsive to primary rewards, such as food (Tanda and Di Chiara, 1998; Bassareo and Di Chiara, 1999) and drugs of abuse (Di Chiara et al., 1993; Carlezon and Wise, 1996). In contrast, the NAc core has been involved in response-reinforcement learning (instrumental conditioning) (Kelley et al., 1997) and in behavioral responses to motivationally significant conditioned stimuli (Bassareo and Di Chiara, 1999; Parkinson et al., 1999, 2000).

These changes in DA release in different regions of the NAc during the process of cocaine intake in animal models, and also in human addicts, can have important consequences over the pattern of neuroplastic changes that are induced in the NAc. Dopamine release in different regions of the NAc has been extensively studied, however changes in this neurotransmitter by itself do not account for all the long-lasting structural and behavioral changes that occur in response to addictive drugs. A crucial point in drug addiction are the mechanisms of synaptic plasticity that underlie long-lasting functional changes in the NAc which are able to explain the progressive loss of interest for natural reward in addicts, the progressive inflexibility of the behavior which resembles a compulsive disorder, and the activity of the striatum when abstinent addicts are seeing drug-related images and experiences craving.

Cocaine Induced Synaptic Plasticity in the Nucleus Accumbens

Synaptic plasticity in the NAc, a region innervated by dopamine neurons from the midbrain VTA, plays and essential role in long-term adaptations induced by drug exposure (Nestler 2001, 2002). Both cellular mechanisms of synaptic plasticity, LTP and LTD, can be induced at excitatory synapses in the NAc. In the NAc, high-frequency tetanic stimulation of presynaptic fibers induce LTP, whereas low-frequency stimulation during depolarization of the post-synaptic neuron induce LTD (Kombian and Malenka, 1994; Bonci and Malenka, 1999; Thomas et al., 2000).

Long-term depression (LTD) in cocaine addiction

The first studies on cocaine consumption reported that repeated cocaine induced LTD in the NAc (Beurrier and Malenka, 2002; Thomas et al., 2001). In a study by Thomas et al. (2001), rodents were divided into two groups, an experimental group receiving five daily intraperitoneal cocaine injections (15 mg/kg) and a control group receiving saline injections. After two weeks of withdrawal, both groups received cocaine injections and locomotor activity was measured in an open-field chamber in order to test cocaine-induced sensitization. Rodents were then sacrificed and electrodes were placed in prepared slices of the shell and the core of the NAc to stimulate afferents from the prelimbic cortex to the NAc. The possible changes in the efficacy of AMPA (α-amino-3-hydroxy-5-methyl-4-isoxazole propionic acid) receptors to NMDA (*N*-methyl-D-aspartate) receptors after cocaine treatment were determined through measures of EPSC in different regions of the NAc. EPSC is decreased (LTD was induced) at synapses made by prefrontal cortical afferents in spiny neurons of the NAc shell, but not in the core. The decrease in EPSCs shares expression mechanisms with LTD and suggests that repeated cocaine exposure induces a decrease in synaptic strength in the shell of the NAc. In this experiment, when rodents received cocaine injections from the experimenter, there was no instrumental behavior or cue-induced cocaine seeking. This kind of experimental model would account for synaptic changes occurring in the shell but not in the core of the NAc. The shell is the primary site of cocaine action, as well as natural rewards, whereas the core is activated in response to conditioned stimuli predicting cocaine (Thomas et al., 2001). The decrease in synaptic strength in the shell of the NAc reported by Thomas et al. (2001) is consistent with previous findings that found a decrease in the responses of the NAc neurons to glutamate after a treatment of cocaine sensitization. The decrease in glutamate was reported to be present for at least 14 days following the cocaine treatment (White et al., 1995).

Since dopamine has a major role in locomotor stimulant effects induced by cocaine, the role of this neurotransmitter in the decrease of synaptic strength in the shell of the NAc after repeated cocaine treatment has been also explored (Thomas et al., 2001). Rodents underwent the same cocaine treatment described above (Thomas et al., 2001), and after repeated cocaine doses the increase in locomotor activity was recorded to assess cocaine induced sensitization. Afterwards, rodents were sacrificed and NAc slices obtained to monitor EPSCs. The ratio AMPAR/NMDAR EPSCs was measured in these slices after dopamine application to explore the involvement of this neurotransmitter in NAc cells responses. It was reported that DA caused a depression of synaptic transmission in NAc shell slices in cocaine treated rats. These results suggest that chronic in vivo cocaine treatment enhances the inhibitory actions of DA on excitatory synaptic transmission in the NAc shell. This inhibitory effects appear to be induced by D1-like receptor activation (Beurrier and Malenka, 2002).

The effects of repeated cocaine on excitatory synapses in the NAc have also been examined using cocaine self-administration (operant conditioning). In Martin et al. (2006), potentially confounding variables were controlled for using a design with four groups of rats. Rodents were trained to self-administer cocaine (cocaine rats) or food (food rats). A third group of rodents was allowed to administer non-contingent cocaine by means of a yoked design (yoked rats) with cocaine exposure matched to that of the cocaine rats. A fourth group of sham naïve rats were passively exposed to the operant chamber each day. After the corresponding treatment, all groups underwent similar surgical procedures. Synaptic plasticity was evaluated in the NAc core and shell, at day 1 and day 21 of abstinence after cocaine administration. After 1 day of abstinence, cocaine rats did not show LTD in the core or shell, suggesting that operant lever pressing for cocaine depressed LTD in both structures. Yoked rats showed similar levels of LTD as the sham-naïve rats, suggesting that the loss of LTD was not simply due the pharmacological effect of cocaine. After 21 days of abstinence, LTD could not be induced in the core of the NAc, suggesting long-lasting neuroplasticity specific to this subregion that can underlie the persistence of cocaine addiction (Martin et al., 2006). These results are consistent with the role of the core in reward-predictive stimuli (Bassareo and Di Chiara, 1999; Parkinson et al., 1999, 2000; Ito et al., 2000) and may contribute to the reduced behavioral flexibility which characterizes addicts.

Long-term potentiation (LTP) in cocaine addiction

LTP, the basic mechanism of synaptic plasticity, can be induced in the NAc core in young animals as well as in adults and has been related to NMDA glutamate receptor activation (Schramm et al., 2002). The first experiments to explore synaptic plasticity in the NAc of cocaine treated rodents reported the induction of LTD at cortical inputs (Hyman and Malenka, 2001). However, these experiments were conducted *in vitro*, where the pattern of neurotransmitter release is different from that taking place *in vivo,* because of a disconnection of the NAc from its cortical and subcortical afferents. NAc dopaminergic neurons in animals that have undertaken a treatment for cocaine sensitization exhibit an increase in dendritic branches and spines on the medium spiny neurons of the NAc (Robinson and Kolb, 1999, 2004). These changes that presumably represent a fundamental reorganization of synaptic inputs onto the intrinsic cells of the NAc, appears to be predictive of LTP rather than LTD.

Goto & Grace (2005b) investigated whether the cellular mechanisms of synaptic plasticity, LTP and LTD registered *in vivo*, were altered after a treatment of cocaine sensitization. Synaptic plasticity was studied at PFC and HPC glutamate projections on the NAc intrinsic neurons. Changes in dopamine release were also considered. Rodents underwent 6 days of cocaine sensitization (15 mg/kg per day) followed by 10-18 days of withdrawal from the drug, after which animals received a challenge with cocaine to assess locomotion. Rats were also tested with a strategy learning and a goal-directed behavior test (plus-maze task). A control group of saline treated animals was also introduced. In order to study synaptic plasticity in different brain structures, rodents were placed in a stereotaxic apparatus on 1 and 5 days following behavioral recordings. Stimulant electrodes were placed in the HPC and in the PFC to evoke LTP or LTD in anesthetized animals and the recordings were registered from the core and the shell regions of the NAc. This electrode placement was done to evaluate both the direct and indirect interactions mediated by these structures in the NAc. In saline treated animals, HPC tetanic stimulation induced LTP at HPC and LTD at the PFC inputs to the NAc shell. However, in cocaine treated animals, the same tetanic stimulation failed to induce any persistent changes in the evoked responses to the NAc. On the other hand, synaptic plasticity induced by tetanic stimulation of the PFC projections to the NAc was not different when comparing the cocaine and saline groups. These changes in synaptic plasticity disrupted goal-directed behavior as measured by a plus-maze task in such a manner that learning of a response strategy is facilitated whereas changing strategy is disrupted in cocaine sensitized rats (Goto and Grace, 2005b).

In Goto and Grace (2005b), DA modulation of synaptic plasticity was also considered. Dopamine activity in the NAc is modulated by D1 and D2 receptors. Tonic and phasic DA release was found to affect both PFC and HPC inputs into the NAc through D2 and D1 receptors, respectively. In the NAc, the dynamics of DA release were found to regulate the balance between limbic and cortical inputs through DA receptor subtypes. During HCP activation, increased tonic and phasic DA transmission activated D1 and D2 receptors, changing the balance of information flow in the NAc from the PFC to the HCP. This change facilitated the induction of LTP at HCP inputs to the NAc and LTD at PFC input to the NAc. On the other hand, when the PFC was more highly activated and the information flow went to the limbic structures, information processing in the NAc changed to a predominance of PFC activity due to the induction of LTD at limbic input and LTP at cortical input. LTP at the PFC inputs was produced only when there was a decrease in tonic D2 receptor stimulation. A decrease in D2 receptor activity would in turn decrease D2-mediated attenuation of glutamate release from PFC terminals (Goto and Grace, 2005b). Therefore, a decrease in DA release or reduced expression of DA receptors, such as in repeated cocaine consumption, would change the pattern of LTP and LTD, and hence synaptic plasticity in the NAc. The altered pattern of synaptic plasticity could account for long-term consequences of addiction.

Studies in animals and humans have revealed that D2 dopamine receptor expression has some role in determining individual vulnerability to the development of cocaine addiction. Specifically, it has been reported that reduced D2 receptors is a predisposing trait for cocaine addiction and, in turn, long-term exposure to cocaine produces a robust decrease in D2 receptor availability in primates (Nader et al., 2006) and in humans (Volkow et al.,1993, 2004). Dalley et al. (2007) reported a very interesting relationship between the levels of D2 receptor expression in rodents' NAc, behavioral impulsive traits in these animals, and their predisposition to cocaine consumption. Lister hooded rats were examined to determine their individual D2 receptor expression in the NAc. Rats were classified in two groups, Impulsive and Non-impulsive, using a five-choice serial reaction time. Impulsive rats presented a significantly reduced D2 receptor expression in the NAc but not in the dorsal striatum. After training the rats to self-administered cocaine, those in the Impulsive group showed a clear tendency for escalation of intravenous cocaine self-administration (Dalley et al., 2007). These results were consistent with those of mutant mice lacking D2-like receptors exhibiting high rates of intravenous cocaine self-administration (Caine et al., 2002). D1 and D2 dopamine receptor expression in the NAc could modulate the induction of LTP and LTD which in turn change synaptic plasticity in this structure. Whether an altered innate D1/D2 dopamine receptor balance in the NAc could have some consequences regarding synaptic plasticity in this structure is not known. However, changes in plasticity in the NAc can induce impairment in goal-directed behavior (Goto and Grace, 2005b). An innate reduced expression of D2 receptors could change the ratio D1/D2 in the NAc and would have consequences on the pattern of synaptic plasticity in this structure and on individual vulnerability to escalate from impulsive to compulsive consumption.

BDNF and Cocaine-Conditioned Stimuli

BDNF and its intracellular signaling mechanisms modulate LTP and LTD (Bramham and Messaoudi, 2005) and hence can modify synaptic plasticity (Bramham and Messaoudi, 2005) and its consequence on learning and memory (Lee et al., 2004; Yamada et al., 2002). There is also experimental evidence that BDNF can modify the reward-related properties of the conditioned stimuli in the context of cocaine addiction.

Horger et al. (1999) reported that BDNF infusions within the Nac strengthened the ability of a stimulus to act as a conditioned reinforcer and increased the cocaine-induced response to the conditioned reinforcer. The strengthening of cocaine effects in BDNF-treated rats persisted for more than a month after the BDNF infusions had finished. These results support the hypothesis that BDNF promotes long-lasting changes in the mesolimbic dopamine system by activating mechanisms of associative learning that underlie the persistent addictive behavior that endures long after withdrawal (Horger et al.,1999). The role of BDNF in drug-associated stimuli is supported by studies in heterozygous knockout mice. Using a conditioned place preference paradigm (CPP), BDNF (+/-) mice showed attenuated effects of cocaine reward and a decreased ability to learn a new association between the drug and the place where it was administered (Hall et al., 2003). Overall, these results show that BDNF modulates synaptic plasticity potentiating learning processes (Bramham and Messaoudi, 2005; Lee et al., 2004; Yamada et al., 2002) and strengthening conditioned responses to cocaine.

BDNF effects are mediated through its intracellular signal transduction systems, including the MAP kinase/ERK and PI3-kinase pathway (Kaplan and Miller, 2000; Patapoutian and Reichardt, 2001) (see figure 1). In a experimental design used by Valjent (2006) to study cocaine sensitization, mice showed an association between the effects of the drug and the context where the drug was administered. Animals displayed conditioned locomotor responses in the environment previously paired with cocaine, even in the absence of the drug. These conditioned locomotor responses have many similarities with Pavlovian conditioning, by which environmental cues become associated to the effects of the drug. The conditioned responses were completely blocked in mice pre-treated with SL327 before each injection with cocaine, suggesting a crucial role for ERK in these responses (Valjent et al., 2006). The role of ERK in the association between environmental stimuli and drugs of abuse has also been assessed with a CPP paradigm. After behavior became conditioned, ERK activity increased in the NAc core but not in the shell (Miller and Marshall, 2005). The selective increase of ERK in the NAc core is consistent with the involvement of the reward regions in conditioned emotional responses and in cue-elicited drug seeking (Cardinal et al., 2002; Ito et al., 2000). In the study of Miller and Marshall (2005), administration of U0126 intra-NAc, an inhibitor of ERK activity, prevented the activation of the ERK signaling pathway and blocked the expression of the preference for the environment previously paired with cocaine. Locomotor activity was not affected. Blockade of the place preference conditioning lasted for 14 days after the injection of different MEK inhibitors (Miller and Marshall, 2005). Taken together, these findings suggest that ERK intracellular cascade in the Nac core is part of the molecular mechanisms for drug-paired contextual cue memories, by which environmental stimuli exert a motivational influence on drug-seeking behavior.

ERK is also involved in the neurobiological and behavioral changes occurring during cocaine withdrawal and mediates the BDNF-induced potentiation of cocaine seeking in response to conditioned stimuli (Lu et al., 2004). Inhibition of ERK phosphorilation in the central amygdala (CeA) after 30 days of withdrawal decreased cocaine seeking in response to drug cues, while stimulation of ERK activity enhanced cocaine seeking induced by cues (Lu et al., 2004). These findings suggest that during withdrawal activation of the ERK pathway in response to cocaine conditioned cues is involved in synaptic plasticity. The resulting synaptic changes underlie craving and subsequent relapse during abstinence (Lu et al., 2006).

Instrumental Conditioning and Habit Forming in the Dorsal Striatum

Human drug consumption is initially a goal-directed behavior motivated by the desire to experience the rewarding effects of the drug. Nevertheless, after repetition, this goal-directed behavior quickly becomes a habit, a behavioral pattern that occurs automatically and nearly involuntarily. Automatic actions are often under the control of conditioned stimuli, such as drug-associated stimuli that have acquired the ability to motivate behavior and can trigger craving and drug seeking in addicts.

The brain structures directly involved in the control of habits are the dorsal striatum (caudate and putamen) and its reciprocal connection with the prefrontal cortex, which are necessary to conduct the sequence of actions involved in habitual drug use (Everitt and Wolf, 2002; Packard and Knowlton, 2002). Whereas the ventral striatum is implicated in reward and motivation (Cardinal et al., 2002), the dorsal striatum is implicated in cognitive control and motor function (Packard and Knowlton, 2002), specifically the learning of stimulus-response associations and the control of behavioral habits. The transition from declarative to automatic behaviors proceeds efficiently without conscious involvement while the context circumstances remain constant. If the context or the motivationally important stimulus changes, normal individuals are able to change behavior that is no longer adaptive. In this case, executive functions intrude to disrupt the habit in order to develop a new, more adaptive behavior. The ability to orient towards specific goals in the environment and maintain flexible action is a hallmark of adaptive behavior. Instrumental conditioning allows an organism to learn contingencies between its own responses and rewarding or punishing outcomes (Skinner, 1938; Mackintosh, 1983).

The involvement of the dorsal striatum in stimulus-reward-response has been studied through functional neuroimaging techniques with humans. These studies have allowed the differentiation of the role of the dorsal striatum from that of the ventral striatum, which is involved in reward prediction (motivation). O'Doherty, using an elegant design managed to identify the different neurobiological roles of this striatal regions. A reinforcement learning design called advantage learning was used and a reward prediction error signal obtained and analyzed (O'Doherty et al., 2004). Brain responses were recorded using functional resonance imaging (fMRI). To dissociate stimulus-response (S-R) learning (instrumental) from value prediction learning, which is one component of S-R learning, a Pavlovian conditioning task was used. Participants have to choose between one of two stimuli: one associated with a high probability of obtaining a reward and the other with a low probability of obtaining a reward (instrumental task). The Pavlovian task was identical to instrumental task except that the computer made the selection and the participant's task was to indicate which stimulus the computer had chosen. If the ventral striatum is involved in predicting reward, this region should show prediction error signal activity during both instrumental conditioning and Pavlovian conditioning tasks. If the dorsal striatum is involved in motor behavior, this region should manifest stronger prediction error signals during instrumental than during Pavlovian conditioning (O'Doherty et al., 2004). fMRI measures of cerebral activity were analyzed while participants were performing the tasks. Results showed that activity in the ventral striatum (NAc) is specific to processing an affective significant stimulus during a Pavlovian task. In the instrumental task, the processing of reward correlated with activity in the ventral as well as in the dorsal striatum. By subtracting reward-related responses during Pavlovian and during instrumental tasks, reward-related responses were found to be significantly enhanced in the caudate during instrumental conditioning (O'Doherty et al., 2004) (see figure 6). These results differentiate the ventral from the dorsal striatum according to their relative contribution to stimulus-reward and stimulus-response learning. At the same time, it provides experimental evidence for the involvement of the whole striatum in the process of reward-related learning. This experimental situation is equivalent to what happens in human drug consumption. Drug-associated stimuli activate the desire to take drugs, which is under the control of the ventral striatum. If craving is strong enough, drug seeking behavior executed by the dorsal striatum begins.

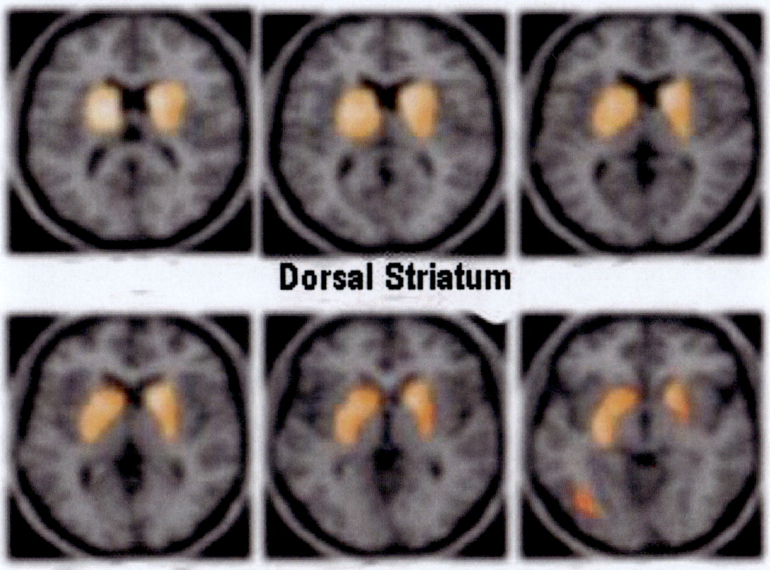

Figure 6. Dissociative roles of Ventral and Dorsal Striatum in Instrumental Conditioning. A: The Ventral Striatum is activated in Pavlovian and Instrumental Conditioning during the reward prediction task. B: The Dorsal Striatum correlates with the reward prediction signal during the Instrumental task but not during the Pavlovian task. (Source: Adapted from O'Doherty et al., 2004).

Neurochemical Evidences for the Involvement of the Dorsal Striatum in Drug Addiction

The involvement of the dorsal striatum in drug addiction may have important neurobiological implications that could be crucial in determining the clinical evolution of the disease. In fact, the dorsal striatum works together with the NAc in order to execute actions. The dorsal striatum receives dopaminergic innervation from the midbrain that can be functionally modified by chronic drug consumption. Moreover, the intrinsic neuronal cells within the dorsal striatum receive glutamatergic innervation from the PFC.

The involvement of the dorsal striatum and its dopaminergic innervation in human addiction has been detected in neuroimaging techniques. A recent study published by Volkow et al. (2006) examined the influence of stimuli paired with cocaine (conditioned stimuli) on the response of the dorsal striatum. That is, neuronal responses were registered when subjects were watching a neutral video (nature scenes) versus when they were watching a cocaine-cue video (scenes of subjects smoking cocaine). The study tested eighteen cocaine-addicted subjects that underwent PET scan using [^{11}C]raclopride as a radiolignad for dopamine D2 receptor. Patients fulfilled Diagnostic and Statistical Manual of Mental Disorders, Fourth Edition (DSM-IV) criteria for cocaine dependence and were active cocaine users for at least the previous 6 months. The feelings of craving experienced by abstinent human addicts were examined using the Brief Version of the Cocaine Craving Questionnaire (CCQ) (Tiffany et al., 1993), which evaluates current cocaine craving (desire, intention, and plan to use, anticipation of positive outcome, anticipation of relief from withdrawal or distressing symptoms, and lack of control over drug use) on a seven-point visual analog scale. The study measured dopamine release through changes in dopamine receptor availability (though PET) by comparing the specific binding of [^{11}C]raclopride when subjects were watching a neutral video (nature scenes) and when they were watching a cocaine-cue video (scenes of addicts smoking cocaine). The results showed an increase in dopamine in the dorsal striatum (caudate, putamen) in cocaine-addicted subjects when they were watching the cocaine-cue video (see figure 7). The increase in extracellular DA in the striatum was proportional to the increase in cocaine craving. Subjects with more severe addiction had larger DA increases in response to conditioned stimuli than subjects with less severe addiction. The main projection from dopaminergic cells in the midbrain to the dorsal striatum, which is involved in habit learning, arises from the substantia nigra (Haber and Fudge, 1997). This implicates the DA nigrostriatal pathway and the dorsal striatum in the subjective experience of craving that often lead to relapse (Volkow et al., 2006). The association between dorsal striatal dopaminergic activity and cue-induced cocaine craving could reflect the habit-based (automatized) nature of craving in addiction.

Consistent with the findings of Volkow (2006), various studies using animal models also reported the involvement of the dorsal striatum and its dopamine and glutamate afferences in drug addiction. Early experiences with cocaine mainly involve the limbic striatum (motivational and affective functions). In contrast, as exposure to cocaine continues, the impact of cocaine progressively affects the dorsal striatum (cognitive and sensoriomotor functions) (Porrino et al., 2004). Whereas the acquisition of the drug-seeking behavior depends on the NAc core (Di Ciano and Everitt, 2004), the control over the performance of the behavior depends on the dorsal striatum (Vanderschuren et al., 2005). Both dopamine increases in the dorsal striatum in response to cocaine cues (Ito et al., 2002) and chronic exposure to cocaine induce changes in dopamine transporters in the dorsal striatum (Letchworth et al., 2001). It has been suggested that as a behavior is repeatedly executed and becomes habitual, as is the case in drug addiction, the role of corticofugal glutamatergic circuitry from the PFC and from the amygdala to the NAc becomes less important in favor of glutamatergic projections emerging from the sensory motor cortical areas projecting into the dorsal striatum (Everitt and Robbins, 2005).

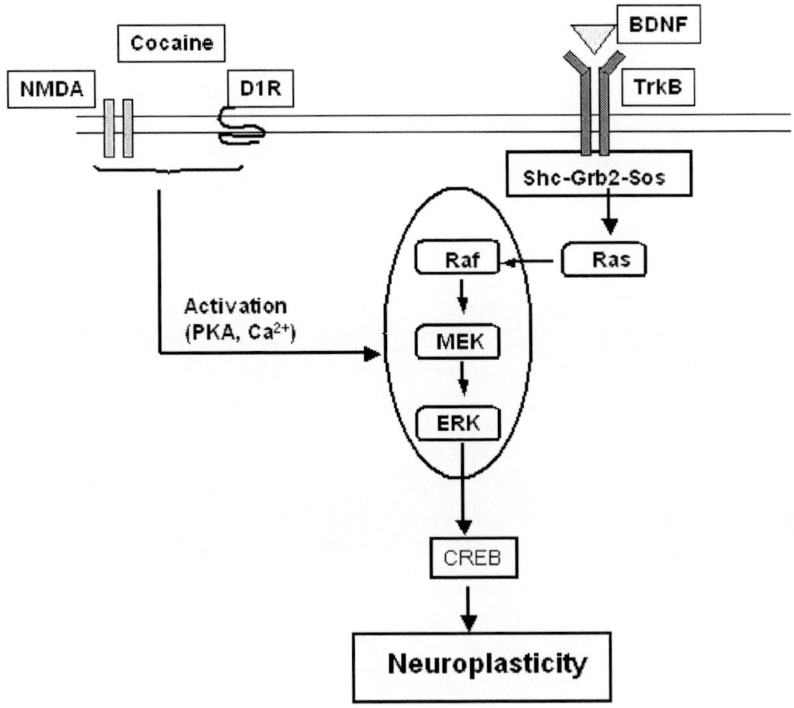

Figure 7. Functional activation in the Dorsal Striatum associated with cue-induced cocaine craving in cocaine abusers. Difference distribution of DA D2 receptor radioligand in the dorsal striatum between the neutral and the cocaine-cue conditions. The binding of the D2 radioligand is reduced in the dorsal but not in the ventral striatum during the cocaine-cue conditions. (Source: Adapted from Volkow et al., 2006).

Considering these findings, it can be proposed that as drug consumption progresses, behavior evolves from being a declarative process involving prefrontal executive functions into a habitual behavior utilizing working memory circuits (Barnes et al., 2005) and motor circuitry. In the case of drug addiction, the transition from prefrontal circuitry to habit motor circuitry is assumed to be abnormal and leads to loss of control and compulsive relapse. Thus, it is hypothesized that the dorsal striatum mediates the habitual nature of compulsive drug seeking in cocaine addiction (Tiffany, 1990; Robbins and Everitt, 1999).

Synaptic Plasticity (LTP/LTD) in the Dorsal Striatum

An important theme in research on drug addiction is to understand how the neurochemical changes involving dopamine and glutamate can modify the pattern of synaptic plasticity in the dorsal striatum. In other words, it is important to understand which mechanisms of synaptic plasticity underlie long-lasting functional changes in the dorsal striatum; moreover to study if abnormal synaptic plasticity can account for the progressive loss of interest in natural rewards and the progressive inflexibility of the behavior that resembles a compulsive disorder.

The cellular mechanisms of LTP and LTD can be evoked in the dorsal striatum. If the afferent glutamatergic projections from the cortical regions to the dorsal striatum are activated with a repetitive train of stimuli (tetanic stimulation, 100 Hz), the result is the reduction of the size of the excitatory synaptic potentials (EPSP) in the striatal cells. That is, cortical activation usually leads to long-term synaptic depression (LTD) and to a reduction in the efficacy of the synaptic input to the striatal cells (Calabresi et al., 1992; Lovinger et al., 1993; Wickens et al., 1996). The effects of applying dopamine in the dorsal striatum in brief pulses in a manner similar to the release of dopamine from midbrain cells was also investigated. This kind of dopaminergic activity is that which follows the presentation of a reward-related stimulus in vivo. When dopamine application coincides with experimentally induced presynaptic (cortical) and postsynaptic (striatal) activity, then the corticostrial synapses can show a consistent increase in EPSP amplitude LTP. These results suggest that dopamine has an enduring activity-dependent action on the efficacy of corticostriatal transmission to the dorsal striatum. This activity may be a cellular basis for long-term changes in the nigrostriatal system (Wickens et al., 1996). The involvement of dopamine in the cellular mechanisms of long-term synaptic plasticity, LTD and LTP, in the dorsal striatum, has also been reported in studies with denervated animals. Unilateral denervation of dopaminergic fibers projecting from the midbrain SN to the striatum induced by homolateral injection of 6-hydroxydopamine (6-OHDA) blocked LTP related to high-frequency stimulation (HFS) of corticostriatal fibers. In the dorsal striatum, the induction of the LTP and LTD seems to require certain levels of dopaminergic activity and the simultaneous activation of both glutamate or dopamine receptors (Centonze et al., 1999). On the other hand, endogenous adenosine acting on adenosime A1 receptors mediates the presynaptic inhibition at corticostriatal synapses, an effect that is induced by a reduction of glutamate release. Presynaptic inhibition induced by adenosine was antagonized by caffeine, a nonselective adenosine receptor antagonist (Calabresi et al., 1997a)

Centonze et al. (2006) explored the effects of acute and chronic cocaine use in the mechanisms of LTP and LTD at corticostriatal synapses. Cocaine treatment induced a significant rewarding effect measured as conditioned place preference. High-frequency stimulation of the corticostriatal projections induced LTP after 1 day of cocaine treatment and after 7 days of cocaine administration. The same results were obtained in animals treated with saline. However, saline treated rats were able to reverse LTP after 10 mins of low-frequency stimulation of corticostriatal afferents, whereas cocaine treated rodents did not. In physiological conditions, the ability to reverse LTP at striatal synapses functions as a mechanism to "forget" maladaptive habits (Picconi et al., 2003), and the lack of ability to reverse LTP may have important consequences in the drug addiction. To reverse LTP in the striatum dopamine action is required because administration D1 and D2 receptor antagonist prevented depotentiation in corticostriatal synapses (Centonze et al., 2006).

LTP is enhanced using the D2 receptor antagonist L-sulpiride whereas the D2-selective receptor agonist quinpirole not only blocks LTP but also reveals LTD (Calabresi et al., 1997b). Blockade of D1 or D5 receptors using specific antagonists stop corticostriatal LTP (Centonze et al., 2003). This suggest that stimulation of D1-like receptors is necessary for the induction of LTP in the dorsal striatum. Both D1 and D2 dopamine receptor stimulation is required for the induction of the striatal LTD (Calabresi et al., 1992, 1996), while both kind of receptors appear to act in opposition to one another during the induction of LTP (Centonzee et al., 1999). It has been proposed that the induction of LTD could require a weaker DA release in the striatum because DA has a higher affinity for the D2 receptors than the D1 receptors (for a review see Calabresi et al., 2007). Those changes in excitability and synaptic plasticity in the striatum may lead to the behavior and emotional consequences which characterize addiction. In the striatum, there is a differential distribution of the two families of DA receptors, D1-like and D2-like, which makes characterization of the role of dopamine in the long-lasting striatal synaptic plasticity difficult. In the striatum, D1 and D2 receptors seem to be segregated in to subpopulations of projecting GABA spiny neurons, which form two large efferent streams, the direct and indirect pathways. D1 receptors are found predominantly in the striatonigral neurons of the direct pathway, whereas D2 receptors are mainly expressed by the striatopallidal neurons of the indirect pathway (Gerfen et al., 1990).

A decrease of the D2 expression in the striatum of cocaine addiction, as well as in other addictive disorders such as alcohol dependence, has been repeatedly described (Volkow et al., 1993; Volkow et al., 1996). It has been proposed that a deficit of D2 could exist prior to drug abuse, a possible vulnerability trait in addicts predisposing them to substance consumption (Morgan et al., 2002). This condition is sometimes described as a reward deficit syndrome (Comings and Blum, 2000; Khantzian, 1985). In a design with mice lacking dopamaine D2 receptors, D2 has been observed playing a key role in mechanisms underlying the direction of long-term changes in synaptic efficacy and plasticity in the striatum. In fact, in rats lacking D2 in the striatum, high-frequency stimulation of corticostriatal fibers induces NMDA-dependent LTP instead of LTD. It has been suggested that reduced D2 expression might lead to loss of high-frequency activation of glutamatergic inputs. This could cause a profound shift in the direction of long-term excitability at corticostriatal synapses (Calabresi et al., 1997b) that could lead to changes in the direction of the neuroplastic organization of corticostriatocortical circuits.

Dendritic spines of striatal neurons have been proposed as being the target anatomical locus of the interaction between glutamate and dopamine, and also the site of expression of striatal synaptic plasticity (Calabresi et al., 1997c). Dopamine appears to be necessary for the maintenance of the health and functional integrity of corticostriatal synapses and it has been suggested that in the absence of dopamine some of these corticostriatal synapses disconnect and may even disappear. The loss of spines in the striatum cells takes place over the first three weeks after lesions with 6-hydroxydopamine, and these cells remain less spiny even after one year after the lesion (Ingham et al., 1993; Arbuthnott et al., 2000).

CONCLUSION

Cocaine facilitates the induction of LTP and hence synaptic plasticity in VTA dopamine neurons. Cocaine's effect on the VTA excitatory synapses is transient, has a ceiling effect, and is not likely to be the specific site of cue-induced conditioning. Therefore, synaptic plasticity at the VTA appears to be responsible only for the early stages of behavioral sensitization and human drug addiction.

Neuroplasticity in the NAc and the dorsal striatum are more important for the long-lasting behavioral and emotional changes associated with drug addiction. In the NAc, high-frequency activation from limbic and prefrontal afferents can produce either LTP or LTD in the intrinsic cells of the NAc. Repeated cocaine administration induces LTD of the glutamate synaptic transmission in the NAc. Cocaine-induced LTD involves AMPA and NMDA glutamate receptors in particular and appears to be modulated by dopamine. DA release regulates the balance between limbic and cortical input through DA receptor subtypes, and repeated cocaine changes the dynamics of DA release into mesocorticolimbic nuclei. Changes in the information flow (glutamate release) from both prefrontal cortex and limbic structures to the NAc appear to determine abnormal patterns of synaptic plasticity. The core and shell of the NAc undergo different patterns in synaptic plasticity after cocaine sensitization, and the differences between both subregions persist even after long-term abstinence. These changes in synaptic plasticity in different subregions of the NAC after cocaine sensitization appear to be responsible for disruption of goal-directed behavior.

The dorsal striatum is progressively recruited as drug consumption becomes habitual. The induction of synaptic plasticity in the striatum requires interaction between dopamine and glutamate. Both glutamate, acting specifically through AMPA and NMDA receptors, and dopamine, which acts through D1-like and D2-like receptors, influence LTP and LTD. In the striatum, both D1 and D2 receptor stimulation is required for the induction of the striatal LTD, whereas both kinds of receptor appear to have opposing effects during the induction of LTP. Repeated cocaine administration blocks the reversal of LTP at the dorsal striatal synapses and this blockade may have important consequences in drug addiction.

BDNF plays a role in modifying the mechanisms of synaptic plasticity in the VTA as well as in the NAc, even in cocaine addiction. BDNF and its intracellular signaling ERK play a role in drug-paired contextual cue memories by which environmental stimuli exert a motivational influence on drug-seeking behavior. BDNF is also part of the molecular mechanisms modulating synaptic plasticity during abstinence.

Long-lasting plasticity in the subregions of the NAc can induce functional changes in this structure that lead to the compulsive drug seeking behavior that characterizes addiction. Studying the mechanisms by which repeated cocaine change the mechanisms of synaptic plasticity in the NAc and dorsal striatum will provide new insights into the neurochemical basis of drug addiction. Moreover, exploring the mechanisms of synaptic plasticity using models of cue-controlled cocaine consumption and relapse will be important in developing an understanding of synaptic plasticity in cocaine addiction involving the limbic and cortical circuitry that is responsible for stimulus-reward-response learning.

REFERENCES

Arbuthnott, G.W., Ingham, C.A., Wickens, J.R. (2000). Dopamine and synaptic plasticity in the neostriatum. *J Anat*, 196, 587-96.

Barnes, L.L., Nelson, J.K., Reuter-Lorenz, P.A. (2001).Object-based attention and object working memory: overlapping processes revealed by selective interference effects in humans. *Prog Brain Res*, 134, 471-81.

Bassareo, V., Di Chiara, G. (1999). Differential responsiveness of dopamine transmission to food-stimuli in nucleus accumbens shell/core compartments. *Neuroscience*, 89(3), 637-41.

Berhow, M.T., Hiroi, N., Nestler, E.J. (1996).Regulation of ERK (extracellular signal regulated kinase), part of the neurotrophin signal transduction cascade, in the rat mesolimbic dopamine system by chronic exposure to morphine or cocaine. *J Neurosci*, 16(15), 4707-15.

Berke, J.D., Hyman, S.E. (2000). Addiction, dopamine, and the molecular mechanisms of memory. *Neuron*, 25(3), 515-32.

Beurrier, C., Malenka, R.C. (2002). Enhanced inhibition of synaptic transmission by dopamine in the nucleus accumbens during behavioral sensitization to cocaine. *J Neurosci*, 22(14), 817-22.

Biernaskie, J., Corbett, D. (2001). Enriched rehabilitative training promotes improved forelimb motor function and enhanced dendritic growth after focal ischemic injury. *J Neurosci*, 21(14), 5272-80.

Bland, S.T., Schmid, M.J., Der-Avakian, A., Watkins, L.R., Spencer, R.L., Maier, S.F. (2005).Expression of c-fos and BDNF mRNA in subregions of the prefrontal cortex of male and female rats after acute uncontrollable stress. *Brain Res*, 1051(1-2), 90-9.

Bliss, T.V., Lomo, T. (1973).Long-lasting potentiation of synaptic transmission in the dentate area of the anaesthetized rabbit following stimulation of the perforant path. *J Physiol*, 232(2), 331-56.

Bliss, T.V., Gardner-Medwin, A.R. (1973). Long-lasting potentiation of synaptic transmission in the dentate area of the unanaestetized rabbit following stimulation of the perforant path. *J Physiol*, 232(2), 357-74

Bonci, A., Malenka, R.C. (1999). Properties and plasticity of excitatory synapses on dopaminergic and GABAergic cells in the ventral tegmental area. *J Neurosci*, May 15, 19(10), 3723-30.

Borgland, S.L., Malenka, R.C., Bonci, A. (2004). Acute and chronic cocaine-induced potentiation of synaptic strength in the ventral tegmental area: electrophysiological and behavioral correlates in individual rats. *J Neurosci*, Aug 25, 24(34), 7482-90.

Bramham, C.R., Srebro, B. (1987). Induction of long-term depression and potentiation by low- and high-frequency stimulation in the dentate area of the anesthetized rat: magnitude, time course and EEG. *Brain Res*, 405(1), 100-7.

Bramham, C.R., Messaoudi, E. (2005).BDNF function in adult synaptic plasticity: the synaptic consolidation hypothesis. *Prog Neurobiol*, 76(2), 99-125.

Caine, S.B., Negus, S.S., Mello, N.K., Patel, S., Bristow, L., Kulagowski, J., Vallone, D., Saiardi, A., Borrelli, E. (2002). Role of dopamine D2-like receptors in cocaine self-administration: studies with D2 receptor mutant mice and novel D2 receptor antagonists. *J Neurosci*, 22(7), 2977-88.

Cajal, S.R.Y. 1999*Texture of the Nervous System of man and the vertebrates*. Original published in spanish as the Texture of of the Nervous System of man and the vertebrates (1904). Springer. pp 631.

Calabresi, P., Maj, R., Pisani, A., Mercuri, N.B., Bernardi, G. (1992). Long-term synaptic depression in the striatum: physiological and pharmacological characterization. *J Neurosci*, 12(11), 4224-33.

Calabresi, P., Maj, R., Mercuri, N.B., Bernardi, G. (1992). Coactivation of D1 and D2 dopamine receptors is required for long-term synaptic depression in the striatum. *Neurosci Lett*, 142(1), 95-9.

Calabresi, P., Centonze, D., Pisani, A., Bernardi, G. (1997a). Endogenous adenosine mediates the presynaptic inhibition induced by aglycemia at corticostriatal synapses. *J Neurosci*, 17(12),4509-16.

Calabresi, P., Saiardi, A., Pisani, A., Baik, J.H., Centonze, D., Mercuri, N.B., Bernardi, G., Borrelli, E. (1997b). Abnormal synaptic plasticity in the striatum of mice lacking dopamine D2 receptors. *J Neurosci*, 17(12), 4536-44.

Calabresi, P., Pisani, A., Centonze, D., Bernardi, G. (1997). Synaptic plasticity and physiological interactions between dopamine and glutamate in the striatum. *Neurosci Biobehav Rev*, 21(4), 519-23.

Calabresi, P., Picconi, B., Tozzi, A., Di Filippo, M. (2007). Dopamine-mediated regulation of corticostriatal synaptic plasticity. *Trends Neurosci*, 30(5), 211-9.

Cardinal, R.N., Parkinson, J.A., Hall, J., Everitt, B.J. (2002). Emotion and motivation: the role of the amygdala, ventral striatum, and prefrontal cortex. *Neurosci Biobehav Rev*, 26(3), 321-52.

Carlezon, W.A. Jr., Wise, R.A. (1996). Rewarding actions of phencyclidine and related drugs in nucleus accumbens shell and frontal cortex. *J Neurosci*, 16(9), 3112-22.

Carlezon, W.A. Jr., Thome, J., Olson ,V.G., Lane-Ladd, S.B., Brodkin, E.S., Hiroi, N., Duman, R.S., Neve, R.L., Nestler, E.J. (1998). Regulation of cocaine reward by CREB. *Science*, 282(5397), 2272-5.

Carr, D.B., Sesack, S.R. (2000). Projections from the rat prefrontal cortex to the ventral tegmental area: target specificity in the synaptic associations with mesoaccumbens and mesocortical neurons. *J Neurosci*, 15;20(10),3864-73.

Centonze, D., Gubellini, P., Picconi, B., Calabresi, P., Giacomini, P., Bernardi, G. (1999). Unilateral dopamine denervation blocks corticostriatal LTP. *J Neurophysiol*, 82(6), 3575-9.

Centonze, D., Grande, C., Saulle, E., Martin, A.B., Gubellini, P., Pavón, N., Pisani, A., Bernardi, G., Moratalla, R., Calabresi, P. (2003). Distinct roles of D1 and D5 dopamine receptors in motor activity and striatal synaptic plasticity. *J Neurosci*, 23(24), 8506-12.

Centonze, D., Costa, C., Rossi, S., Prosperetti, C., Pisani, A., Usiello, A., Bernardi, G., Mercuri, N.B., Calabresi, P. (2006). Chronic cocaine prevents depotentiation at corticostriatal synapses. *Biol Psychiatry*, 60(5), 436-43.

Childress, A.R., Hole, A.V., Ehrman, R.N., Robbins, S.J., McLellan, A.T., O'Brien, C.P. (1993). Cue reactivity and cue reactivity interventions in drug dependence. *NIDA Res Monogr*, 137, 73-95.

Childress, A.R., Mozley, P.D., McElgin, W., Fitzgerald, J., Reivich, M., O'Brien, C.P. (1999). Limbic activation during cue-induced cocaine craving. *Am J Psychiatry*, 156, 11-8.

Collingridge, G.L., Bliss, T.V. (1995). Memories of NMDA receptors and LTP. *Trends Neurosci*, 18(2), 54-6.

Comings, D.E., Blum, K. (2000). Reward deficiency syndrome: genetic aspects of behavioral disorders. *Prog Brain Res*, 126, 325-41.

Cooke, S.F., Bliss, T.V. (2005). Long-term potentiation and cognitive drug discovery. *Curr Opin Investig Drugs*, 6(1), 25-34.

Cooke, S.F., Bliss, T.V. (2006). Plasticity in the human central nervous system. *Brain*,129(Pt 7), 1659-73. Epub 2006 May 3.

Corominas, M., Roncero, C., Ribases, M., Castells, X., Casas, M. (2007). Brain-derived neurotrophic factor and its intracellular signaling pathways in cocaine addiction. *Neuropsychobiology*, 55(1), 2-13.

Corominas-Roso, M., Roncero, C., Bruguera, E., Casas, M. (2007). The dopaminergic system and addictions. *Rev Neurol*, 44(1), 23-31.

Crow, T.J., Arbuthnott, G.W. (1972). Function of catecholamine-containing neurones in mammalian central nervous system. *Nat New Biol,* 238(86), 245-6.

Nucleus accumbens D2/3 receptors predict trait impulsivity and cocaine reinforcement. (2007).Nucleus accumbens D2/3 receptors predict trait impulsivity and cocaine reinforcement. *Science*, 315(5816), 1267-70.

Di Chiara, G., Tanda, G., Frau, R., Carboni, E. (1993). On the preferential release of dopamine in the nucleus accumbens by amphetamine: further evidence obtained by vertically implanted concentric dialysis probes. *Psychopharmacology* (Berl), 112(2-3), 398-402.

Di Ciano, P., Cardinal, R.N., Cowell, R.A., Little, S.J., Everitt, B.J. (2001). Differential involvement of NMDA, AMPA/kainate, and dopamine receptors in the nucleus accumbens core in the acquisition and performance of pavlovian approach behavior. *J Neurosci*, 21(23), 9471-7.

Di Ciano, P., Everitt, B.J. (2004). Direct interactions between the basolateral amygdala and nucleus accumbens core underlie cocaine-seeking behavior by rats. *J Neurosci*, 24(32), 7167-73.

Dong, Y., Saal, D., Thomas, M., Faust, R., Bonci, A., Robinson, T., Malenka, R.C. (2004). Cocaine-induced potentiation of synaptic strength in dopamine neurons: behavioral correlates in GluRA(-/-) mice. *Proc Natl Acad Sci*, U.S.A, 101(39), 14282-7.

Dong, Y., Green, T., Saal, D., Marie, H., Neve, R., Nestler, E.J., Malenka, R.C. (2006). CREB modulates excitability of nucleus accumbens neurons. *Nat Neurosci*, 9(4), 475-7. Epub 2006 Mar 5.

Dozmorov, M., Li, R., Abbas, A.K., Hellberg, F., Farre, C., Huang, F.S., Jilderos, B., Wigström, H. (2006). Contribution of AMPA and NMDA receptors to early and late phases of LTP in hippocampal slices. *Neurosci Res*, 55(2), 182-8. Epub 2006 May 5.

Everitt, B.J., Wolf, M.E. (2002). Psychomotor stimulant addiction: a neural systems perspective. *J Neurosci,* 22(9), 3312-20.

Everitt, B.J., Robbins, T.W. (2005). Neural systems of reinforcement for drug addiction: from actions to habits to compulsion. *Nat Neurosci*, 8(11), 1481-9.

Franklin, T.R., Acton, P.D., Maldjian, J.A., Gray, J.D., Croft, J.R., Dackis, C.A., O'Brien, C.P., Childress, A.R. (2002). Decreased gray matter concentration in the insular, orbitofrontal, cingulate, and temporal cortices of cocaine patients. *Biol Psychiatry*, 51(2), 134-42.

Freud, S. (1953). *Project for a scientific Psychology*. In: The standard edition of the complete psyschological works of Sigmund Freud, Vol 3 (Strachey J, ed), pp 43-61. London, UK: Hogarth Press.

Garavan, H., Pankiewicz, J., Bloom, A., Cho, J.K., Sperry, L., Ross, T.J., Salmeron, B.J., Risinger, R., Kelley, D., Stein, E.A. (2000). Cue-induced cocaine craving: neuroanatomical specificity for drug users and drug stimuli. *Am J Psychiatry*, 157(11), 1789-98.

Garzón, M., Vaughan, R.A., Uhl, G.R., Kuhar, M.J., Pickel,V.M. (1999). Cholinergic axon terminals in the ventral tegmental area target a subpopulation of neurons expressing low levels of the dopamine transporter. *J Comp Neurol*, 410(2), 197-210.

Geinisman, Y. (2000). Structural synaptic modifications associated with hippocampal LTP and behavioral learning. *Cereb Cortex*, 10(10), 952-62.

Georges, F., Aston-Jones, G. (2001). Potent regulation of midbrain dopamine neurons by the bed nucleus of the stria terminalis. *J Neurosci*, 21(16), RC160.

Gerfen, C.R., Engber, T.M., Mahan, L.C., Susel, Z., Chase, T.N., Monsma, F.J. Jr., Sibley, D.R. (1990). D1 and D2 dopamine receptor-regulated gene expression of striatonigral and striatopallidal neurons. *Science*, 250(4986), 1429-32.

Goldstein, R.Z., Volkow, N.D. (2002). Drug addiction and its underlying neurobiological basis: neuroimaging evidence for the involvement of the frontal cortex. *Am J Psychiatry*, 159(10), 1642-52.

Goldstein, R.Z., Alia-Klein, N., Tomasi, D., Zhang, L., Cottone, L.A., Maloney, T., Telang, F., Caparelli, E.C., Chang, L., Ernst, T., Samaras, D., Squires, N.K., Volkow, N.D. (2007). Is decreased prefrontal cortical sensitivity to monetary reward associated with impaired motivation and self-control in cocaine addiction? *Am J Psychiatry*, 164(1), 43-51.

Gordon, N.S., Burke, S., Akil, H., Watson, S.J., Panksepp, J. (2003). Socially-induced brain 'fertilization': play promotes brain derived neurotrophic factor transcription in the amygdala and dorsolateral frontal cortex in juvenile rats. *Neurosci Lett*, 341(1), 17-20.

Goto, Y., Grace, A.A. (2005a). Dopaminergic modulation of limbic and cortical drive of nucleus accumbens in goal-directed behavior. *Nat Neurosci*, 8(6), 805-12.

Goto, Y., Grace, A.A. (2005b). Dopamine-dependent interactions between limbic and prefrontal cortical plasticity in the nucleus accumbens: disruption by cocaine sensitization. *Neuron*, 47(2), 255-66.

Grant, S., London, E.D., Newlin, D.B., Villemagne, V.L., Liu, X., Contoreggi, C., Phillips, R.L., Kimes, A.S., Margolin, A. (1996). Activation of memory circuits during cue-elicited cocaine craving. *Proc Natl Acad Sci*, U.S.A, 93(21), 12040-5.

Grimm, J.W., Lu, L., Hayashi, T., Hope, B.T., Su, T.P., Shaham, Y. (2003). Time-dependent increases in brain-derived neurotrophic factor protein levels within the mesolimbic dopamine system after withdrawal from cocaine: implications for incubation of cocaine craving. *J Neurosci*, 23(3), 742-7.

Groves, P.M., Linder, J.C., Young, S.J. (1994). 5-hydroxydopamine-labeled dopaminergic axons: three-dimensional reconstructions of axons, synapses and postsynaptic targets in rat neostriatum. *Neuroscience*, 58(3), 593-604.

Haber, S.N., Fudge, J.L. (1997). The primate substantia nigra and VTA: integrative circuitry and function. *Crit Rev Neurobiol*, 11(4), 323-42.

Haber, S.N., Fudge, J.L., McFarland, N.R. (2000). Striatonigrostriatal pathways in primates form an ascending spiral from the shell to the dorsolateral striatum. *J Neurosci*, 20(6), 2369-82.

Hall, F.S., Drgonova, J., Goeb, M., Uhl, G.R. (2003). Reduced behavioral effects of cocaine in heterozygous brain-derived neurotrophic factor (BDNF) knockout mice. *Neuropsychopharmacology*, 28(8), 1485-90.

Harris, G.C., Aston-Jones, G. (2003). Critical role for ventral tegmental glutamate in preference for a cocaine-conditioned environment. *Neuropsychopharmacology*, 28(1), 73-6.

Hebb, D.O.(1949). *The Organization of Behavrio*. John Wiley. New York, USA.

Heimer, L., Zahm, D.S., Churchill, L., Kalivas, P.W., Wohltmann, C.(1991). Specificity in the projection patterns of accumbal core and shell in the rat. *Neuroscience*, 41(1), 89-125.

Herrick, C.J. (1948). *The brain of the Tiger Slamander*. Chicago: University of Chicago Press.

Horger, B.A., Roth, R.H. (1996). The role of mesoprefrontal dopamine neurons in stress. *Crit Rev Neurobiol*, 10(3-4):395-418.

Horger, B.A., Iyasere, C.A., Berhow, M.T., Messer, C.J., Nestler, E.J., Taylor, J.R. (1999). Enhancement of locomotor activity and conditioned reward to cocaine by brain-derived neurotrophic factor. *J Neurosci*, 19(10), 4110-22.

Hosokawa, T., Rusakov, D.A., Bliss, T.V., Fine, A. (1995). Repeated confocal imaging of individual dendritic spines in the living hippocampal slice: evidence for changes in length and orientation associated with chemically induced LTP. *J Neurosci*, 15(8), 5560-73.

Hyman, S.E. (2005). Addiction: a disease of learning and memory. *Am J Psychiatry*, Aug, 162(8), 1414-22.

Hyman, S.E., Malenka, R.C. (2001). Addiction and the brain: the neurobiology of compulsion and its persistence. *Nat Rev Neurosci*, 2(10), 695-703.

Ingham, C.A., Hood, S.H., Arbuthnott, G.W. (1989). Spine density on neostriatal neurones changes with 6-hydroxydopamine lesions and with age. *Brain Res*, 503(2), 334-8.

Ingham, C.A., Hood, S.H., van Maldegem, B., Weenink, A., Arbuthnott, G.W. (1993). Morphological changes in the rat neostriatum after unilateral 6-hydroxydopamine injections into the nigrostriatal pathway. *Exp Brain Res,* 93(1), 17-27.

Ikegaya, Y., Ishizaka, Y., Matsuki, N. (2002). BDNF attenuates hippocampal LTD via activation of phospholipase C: implications for a vertical shift in the frequency-response curve of synaptic plasticity. *Eur J Neurosci*, 16(1), 145-8.

Ingham, C.A., Hood, S.H., van Maldegem, B., Weenink, A., Arbuthnott, G.W. (1993). Morphological changes in the rat neostriatum after unilateral 6-hydroxydopamine injections into the nigrostriatal pathway. *Exp Brain Res*, 93(1), 17-27.

Ito, M. (1989). Long-term depression. *Annu Rev Neurosci*, 12, 85-102.

Ito, R., Dalley, J.W., Howes, S.R., Robbins, T.W., Everitt, B.J. (2000). Dissociation in conditioned dopamine release in the nucleus accumbens core and shell in response to cocaine cues and during cocaine-seeking behavior in rats. *J Neurosci*, 20(19),7489-95.

Ito, R., Dalley, J.W., Robbins, T.W., Everitt, B.J. (2002). Dopamine release in the dorsal striatum during cocaine-seeking behavior under the control of a drug-associated cue. *J Neurosci*, 22(14), 6247-53.

Jones, S., Kornblum, J.L., Kauer, J.A. (2000). Amphetamine blocks long-term synaptic depression in the ventral tegmental area. *J Neurosci*, 20(15), 5575-80.

Kalivas, P.W. (1995). Interactions between dopamine and excitatory amino acids in behavioral sensitization to psychostimulants. *Drug Alcohol Depend*, Feb, 37(2), 95-100.

Kalivas, P.W. (2004). Glutamate systems in cocaine addiction. *Curr Opin Pharmacol*, 4(1), 23-9.

Kalivas, P.W., Stewart, J. (1991). Dopamine transmission in the initiation and expression of drug- and stress-induced sensitization of motor activity. *Brain Res Brain Res Rev*, 16(3), 223-44.

Kalivas, P.W., Alesdatter, J.E. (1993). Involvement of N-methyl-D-aspartate receptor stimulation in the ventral tegmental area and amygdala in behavioral sensitization to cocaine. *J Pharmacol Exp Ther*, 267(1), 486-95.

Kalivas, P.W., Duffy, P. (1993). Time course of extracellular dopamine and behavioral sensitization to cocaine. I. Dopamine axon terminals. *J Neurosci*, 13(1), 266-75.

Kalivas, P.W., Duffy, P. (1995). D1 receptors modulate glutamate transmission in the ventral tegmental area. *J Neurosci*, 15(7 Pt 2), 5379-88.

Kalivas, P.W., Volkow, N.D. (2005). The neural basis of addiction: a pathology of motivation and choice. *Am J Psychiatry*, 162(8), 1403-13.

Kalivas, P.W., Volkow, N., Seamans, J. (2005). Unmanageable motivation in addiction: a pathology in prefrontal-accumbens glutamate transmission. *Neuron*, Mar 3, 45(5), 647-50.

Kandel, E.R. (1999). Biology and the future of psychoanalysis: a new intellectual framework for psychiatry revisited. *Am J Psychiatry*, 156, 505-524.

Kaplan, D.R., Miller, F.D. (2000). Neurotrophin signal transduction in the nervous system. *Curr Opin Neurobiol*, 10(3), 381-91.

Kelley, A.E., Smith-Roe, S.L., Holahan, M.R. (1997). Response-reinforcement learning is dependent on N-methyl-D-aspartate receptor activation in the nucleus accumbens core. *Proc Natl Acad Sci*, U.S.A, 94(22), 12174-9.

Kelz, M.B., Chen, J., Carlezon, W.A. Jr., Whisler, K., Gilden, L., Beckmann, A.M., Steffen, C., Zhang, Y.J., Marotti, L., Self, D.W., Tkatch, T., Baranauskas, G., Surmeier, D.J., Neve, R.L., Duman, R.S., Picciotto, M.R., Nestler, E.J. (1999). Expression of the transcription factor deltaFosB in the brain controls sensitivity to cocaine. *Nature*, 401(6750), 272-6.

Khantzian, E.J. (1985). The self-medication hypothesis of addictive disorders: focus on heroin and cocaine dependence. *Am J Psychiatry*, 142(11), 1259-64.

Kim, J.J., Foy, M.R., Thompson, R.F. (1996). Behavioral stress modifies hippocampal plasticity through N-methyl-D-aspartate receptor activation. *Proc Natl Acad Sci*, U.S.A, 93(10), 4750-3.

Heerssen, H.M., Segal, R.A. (2002). Location, location, location: a spatial view of neurotrophin signal transduction. *Trends Neurosci,* 25, 160-5.

Kalivas, P.W. (1995). Interactions between dopamine and excitatory amino acids in behavioral sensitization to psychostimulants. *Drug Alcohol Depend*, 37(2), 95-100.

Kaplan, D.R., Miller, F.D. (2000). Neurotrophin signal transduction in the nervous system. *Curr Opin Neurobiol*, 10, 381-91.

Kauer, J.A., Malenka, R.C. (2007). Synaptic plasticity and addiction. *Nat Rev Neurosci*, 8(11), 844-58.

Kilts, C.D., Schweitzer, J.B., Quinn, C.K., Gross, R.E., Faber, T.L., Muhammad, F., Ely, T.D., Hoffman, J.M., Drexler, K.P. (2001). Neural activity related to drug craving in cocaine addiction. *Arch Gen Psychiatry*, 58(4), 334-41.

Kolb, B., Pellis, S., Robinson, T.E. (2004). Plasticity and functions of the orbital frontal cortex. *Brain Cogn*, 55(1), 104-15.

Kombian, S.B., Malenka, R.C.(1994). Simultaneous LTP of non-NMDA- and LTD of NMDA-receptor-mediated responses in the nucleus accumbens. *Nature*, 368(6468), 242-6.

Kötter, R. (1994). Postsynaptic integration of glutamatergic and dopaminergic signals in the striatum. *Prog Neurobiol*, 44(2), 163-96.

Kovalchuk, Y., Hanse, E., Kafitz, K.W., Konnerth, A. (2002). Postsynaptic Induction of BDNF-Mediated Long-Term Potentiation. *Science*, 295(5560), 1729-34.

Kuba, K., Kumamoto, E. (1990). Long-term potentiations in vertebrate synapses: a variety of cascades with common subprocesses. *Prog Neurobiol*, 34(3), 197-269.

Lacey, M.G., Mercuri, N.B., North, R.A.(1990). Actions of cocaine on rat dopaminergic neurones in vitro. *Br J Pharmacol*, 99(4), 731-5.

LeDoux, J. (2001). *Synaptic self: how our brains become sho we are*. New York, USA: Vikng Press. pp 395.

Lee, J.L., Everitt, B.J., Thomas, K.L. (2004). Independent cellular processes for hippocampal memory consolidation and reconsolidation. *Science*, 304(5672), 839-43.

Lessmann, V., Gottmann, K., Malcangio, M. (2003). Neurotrophin secretion: current facts and future prospects. *Prog Neurobiol*, 69(5), 341-74.

Letchworth, S.R., Nader, M.A., Smith, H.R., Friedman, D.P., Porrino, L.J. (2001). Progression of changes in dopamine transporter binding site density as a result of cocaine self-administration in rhesus monkeys. *J Neurosci*, 21(8), 2799-807.

Ljungberg, T., Apicella, P., Schultz, W. (1992). Responses of monkey dopamine neurons during learning of behavioral reactions. *J Neurophysiol*, 67(1), 145-63.

Lovinger, D.M., Tyler, E.C., Merritt, A.(1993). Short- and long-term synaptic depression in rat neostriatum. *J Neurophysiol*, 70(5), 1937-49.

Lu, W., Man, H., Ju, W., Trimble, W.S., MacDonald, J.F., Wang, Y.T. (2001). Activation of synaptic NMDA receptors induces membrane insertion of new AMPA receptors and LTP in cultured hippocampal neurons. *Neuron*, 29(1), 243-54.

Lu, L., Grimm, J.W., Hope, B.T., Shaham, Y. (2004). Incubation of cocaine craving after withdrawal: a review of preclinical data. *Neuropharmacology*, 47 Suppl 1, 214-26.

Lu, L., Koya, E., Zhai, H., Hope, B.T., Shaham, Y. (2006). Role of ERK in cocaine addiction. *Trends Neurosci*, 29(12), 695-703.

Maas, L.C., Lukas, S.E., Kaufman, M.J., Weiss, R.D., Daniels, S.L., Rogers, V.W., Kukes, T.J., Renshaw, P.F. (1998). Functional magnetic resonance imaging of human brain activation during cue-induced cocaine craving. *Am J Psychiatry*, 155(1), 124-6.

Mackintosh, N.J. (1983).*Conditioning and Associative Learning*. Clarendon Press. Oxford.

Malenka, R.C., Bear, M.F. (2004). LTP and LTD: an embarrassment of riches. *Neuron*, 44(1), 5-21.

Marinelli, M., Piazza, P.V. (2002). Interaction between glucocorticoid hormones, stress and psychostimulant drugs. *Eur J Neurosci*, 16(3), 387-94.

Markou, A., Koob, G.F. (1991). Postcocaine anhedonia. An animal model of cocaine withdrawal. *Neuropsychopharmacology,* 4(1), 17-26.

Martin, M., Chen, B.T., Hopf, F.W., Bowers, M.S., Bonci, A. (2006). Cocaine self-administration selectively abolishes LTD in the core of the nucleus accumbens. *Nat Neurosci*, 9(7), 868-9.

Mercuri, N.B., Stratta, F., Calabresi, P., Bernardi,G. (1992). A voltage-clamp analysis of NMDA-induced responses on dopaminergic neurons of the rat substantia nigra zona compacta and ventral tegmental area. *Brain Res*, 593(1), 51-6.

Miller, C.A., Marshall, J.F. (2005). Molecular substrates for retrieval and reconsolidation of cocaine-associated contextual memory. *Neuron*, 47(6), 873-84.

Mirenowicz, J., Schultz, W. (1994). Importance of unpredictability for reward responses in primate dopamine neurons. *J Neurophysiol*, 72(2), 1024-7.

Mizuno, M., Yamada, K., He, J., Nakajima, A., Nabeshima, T. (2003). Involvement of BDNF receptor TrkB in spatial memory formation. *Learn Mem*, 10(2), 108-15.

Morgan, D., Grant, K.A., Gage, H.D., Mach, R.H., Kaplan, J.R., Prioleau, O. et al. (2002). Social dominance in monkeys: dopamine D2 receptors and cocaine self-administration. *Nat Neurosci*, 5, 169-74.

Morris, R.G., Anderson, E., Lynch, G.S., Baudry, M. (1986). Selective impairment of learning and blockade of long-term potentiation by an N-methyl-D-aspartate receptor antagonist, AP5. *Nature*, 319(6056),774-6.

Nader, M.A., Morgan, D., Gage, H.D., Nader, S.H., Calhoun,T.L., Buchheimer, N., Ehrenkaufer, R., Mach, R.H. (2006). PET imaging of dopamine D2 receptors during chronic cocaine self-administration in monkeys. *Nat Neurosci*, 9(8), 1050-6.

Nestler, E.J. (1997). Molecular mechanisms of opiate and cocaine addiction. *Curr Opin Neurobiol*, 7(5), 713-9.

Nestler, E.J. (2001). Molecular basis of long-term plasticity underlying addiction. *Nat Rev Neurosci*, 2(2), 119-28.

Nestler, E.J. (2002). Common molecular and cellular substrates of addiction and memory. *Neurobiol Learn Mem*, 78(3), 637-47.

Nogueira, L., Kalivas, P.W., Lavin, A. (2006). Long-term neuroadaptations produced by withdrawal from repeated cocaine treatment: role of dopaminergic receptors in modulating cortical excitability. *J Neurosci*, 26(47), 12308-13.

Numan, S., Seroogy, K.B. (1999). Expression of trkB and trkC mRNAs by adult midbrain dopamine neurons: a double-label in situ hybridization study. *J Comp Neurol*, 403(3), 295-308.

O'Brien, C.P.(1997). A range of research-based pharmacotherapies for addiction. *Science*, 278, 66-70

O'Brien, C.P. (1997). A range of research-based pharmacotherapies for addiction. *Science*, 278(5335), 66-70.

O'Brien, C.P., Childress, A.R., McLellan, T., Ehrman, R. (1990). Integrating systemic cue exposure with standard treatment in recovering drug dependent patients. *Addict Behav*, 15(4), 355-65.

O'Brien, C.P., Childress, A.R., McLellan, A.T., Ehrman, R. (1992). Classical conditioning in drug-dependent humans. *Ann N Y Acad Sci*, 654, 400-15.

O'Brien, C.P., Childress, A.R., Ehrman, R., Robbins, S.J. (1998). Conditioning factors in drug abuse: can they explain compulsion? *J Psychopharmacol*, 12(1), 15-22.

O'Doherty, J., Dayan, P., Schultz, J., Deichmann, R., Friston, K., Dolan, R.J. (2004). Dissociable roles of ventral and dorsal striatum in instrumental conditioning. *Science*, 304(5669), 452-4.

Omelchenko, N., Sesack, S.R. (2007). Glutamate synaptic inputs to ventral tegmental area neurons in the rat derive primarily from subcortical sources. *Neuroscience*, 146(3),1259-74.

Overton, P.G., Clark, D. (1997). Burst firing in midbrain dopaminergic neurons. *Brain Res Brain Res Rev*, 25(3), 312-34.

Packard, M.G., Knowlton, B.J. (2002). Learning and memory functions of the Basal Ganglia. *Annu Rev Neurosci*, 25, 563-93.

Parkinson, J.A., Olmstead, M.C., Burns, L.H., Robbins, T.W., Everitt, B.J. (1999). Dissociation in effects of lesions of the nucleus accumbens core and shell on appetitive pavlovian approach behavior and the potentiation of conditioned reinforcement and locomotor activity by D-amphetamine. *J Neurosci*, 19(6), 2401-11.

Parkinson, J.A., Cardinal, R.N., Everitt, B.J. (2000). Limbic cortical-ventral striatal systems underlying appetitive conditioning. *Prog Brain Res*, 126, 263-8

Patapoutian, A., Reichardt, L.F. (2001). Trk receptors: mediators of neurotrophin action. *Curr Opin Neurobiol*, 11, 272-80.

Patterson, S.L., Abel, T., Deuel,T.A., Martin, K.C., Rose, J.C., Kandel, E.R. (1996). Recombinant BDNF rescues deficits in basal synaptic transmission and hippocampal LTP in BDNF knockout mice. *Neuron,* 16(6), 1137-45.

Pavlov, I. (1927). *Conditioned reflexes: an investigation of the physiological activity of the cerebral cortex.* London, UK: Oxford University Press.

Phillips, A.G., Di Ciano, P. (1996). Behavioral sensitization is induced by intravenous self-administration of cocaine by rats. *Psychopharmacology* (Berl), 124(3), 279-81.

Piazza, P.V., Le Moal, M. (1998). The role of stress in drug self-administration. *Trends Pharmacol Sci*, 19(2), 67-74.

Picconi, B., Centonze, D., Håkansson, K., Bernardi, G., Greengard, P., Fisone, G., Cenci, M.A., Calabresi, P. (2003). Loss of bidirectional striatal synaptic plasticity in L-DOPA-induced dyskinesia. *Nat Neurosci*, 6(5), 501-6.

Poo, M.M. (2001). Neurotrophins as synaptic modulators. *Nat Rev Neurosci*, 2(1), 24-32.

Porrino, L.J., Lyons, D., Smith, H.R., Daunais, J.B., Nader, M.A. (2004). Cocaine self-administration produces a progressive involvement of limbic, association, and sensorimotor striatal domains. *J Neurosci*, 24(14), 3554-62.

Pu, L., Liu, Q.S., Poo, M.M. (2006). BDNF-dependent synaptic sensitization in midbrain dopamine neurons after cocaine withdrawal. *Nat Neurosci*, 9(5), 605-7. Epub 2006 Apr 23.

Rattiner, L.M., Davis, M., Ressler, K.J. (2005). Brain-derived neurotrophic factor in amygdala-dependent learning. *Neuroscientist,* 11, 323-33.

Seutin, V., Verbanck, P., Massotte, L., Dresse, A. (1991). Acute amphetamine-induced subsensitivity of A10 dopamine autoreceptors in vitro. *Brain Res*, 558(1), 141-4.

Robbins, T.W., Everitt, B.J.(1999). Drug addiction: bad habits add up. *Nature*, 398(6728), 567-70.

Robinson, T.E., Berridge, K.C. (1993). The neural basis of drug craving: an incentive-sensitization theory of addiction. *Brain Res Brain Res Rev*, 18(3), 247-91.

Robinson,T.E., Berridge, K.C. (2001). Incentive-sensitization and addiction. *Addiction*, 96(1), 103-14.

Robinson, T.E., Kolb, B. (1999). Alterations in the morphology of dendrites and dendritic spines in the nucleus accumbens and prefrontal cortex following repeated treatment with amphetamine or cocaine. *Eur J Neurosci*, 11(5), 1598-604.

Robinson, T.E., Kolb, B. (2004). Structural plasticity associated with exposure to drugs of abuse. *Neuropharmacology*, 47 Suppl 1, 33-46.

Saal, D., Dong, Y., Bonci, A., Malenka, R.C. (2003). Drugs of abuse and stress trigger a common synaptic adaptation in dopamine neurons. *Neuron*, 37(4), 577-82.

Schramm, N.L., Egli, R.E., Winder, D.G. (2002). LTP in the mouse nucleus accumbens is developmentally regulated. *Synapse*, 45(4), 213-9.

Schultz, W. (1998). Predictive reward signal of dopamine neurons. *J Neurophysiol*, 80(1), 1-27.

Schultz, W. (2002). Getting formal with dopamine and reward. *Neuron*, 36(2), 241-63.

Schultz, W. (2004). Neural coding of basic reward terms of animal learning theory, game theory, microeconomics and behavioural ecology. *Curr Opin Neurobiol*, 14(2), 139-47.

Scoville, W.B., Milner, B. (2000). Loss of recent memory after bilateral hippocampal lesions. 1957. *J Neuropsychiatry Clin Neurosci,* 12(1), 103-13.

Shaham,Y., Erb, S., Stewart, J. (2000). Stress-induced relapse to heroin and cocaine seeking in rats: a review. *Brain Res Brain Res Rev*, 33(1), 13-33.

Shi, S.H., Hayashi, Y., Petralia, R.S., Zaman, S.H., Wenthold, R.J., Svoboda, K., Malinow, R. (1999). Rapid spine delivery and redistribution of AMPA receptors after synaptic NMDA receptor activation. *Science,* 284(5421), 1811-6.

Shors, T.J., Seib, T.B., Levine, S., Thompson, R.F. (1989). Inescapable versus escapable shock modulates long-term potentiation in the rat hippocampus. *Science,* 244(4901), 224-6.

Skinner, B.F. (1938).*The Behavior of Organisms*. Appleton-Century-Crofts. New York,USA.

Smith, Y., Bennett, B.D., Bolam, J.P., Parent, A., Sadikot, A.F. (1994). Synaptic relationships between dopaminergic afferents and cortical or thalamic input in the sensorimotor territory of the striatum in monkey. *J Comp Neurol*, 344(1), 1-19.

Squire, L.R., Ojemann, J.G., Miezin, F.M., Petersen, S.E., Videen, T.O., Raichle, M.E. (1992). Activation of the hippocampus in normal humans: a functional anatomical study of memory. *Proc Natl Acad Sci*, U.S.A, 89(5), 1837-41.

Stanton, P.K., Sejnowski, T. J. (1989). Associative long-term depression in the hippocampus induced by hebbian covariance. *Nature*, 339(6221), 215-8.

Starr, M.S. (1995). Glutamate/dopamine D1/D2 balance in the basal ganglia and its relevance to Parkinson's disease. *Synapse*, Apr, 19(4), 264-93.

Stewart, M.G., Rusakov, D.A. (1995). Morphological changes associated with stages of memory formation in the chick following passive avoidance training. *Behav Brain Res*, 66(1-2), 21-8.

Stewart, J. (2003). Stress and relapse to drug seeking: studies in laboratory animals shed light on mechanisms and sources of long-term vulnerability. *Am J Addict*, 12(1), 1-17.

Tan, A., Moratalla, R., Lyford, G.L., Worley, P., Graybiel, A.M. (2000). The activity-regulated cytoskeletal-associated protein arc is expressed in different striosome-matrix patterns following exposure to amphetamine and cocaine. *J Neurochem*, 74(5), 2074-8.

Tanda, G., Di Chiara, G. (1998). A dopamine-mu1 opioid link in the rat ventral tegmentum shared by palatable food (Fonzies) and non-psychostimulant drugs of abuse. *Eur J Neurosci*, 10(3), 1179-87.

Teyler, T.J., Discenna, P. (1984). Long-term potentiation as a candidate mnemonic device. *Brain Res*, 319(1), 15-28.

Thoenen, H. (1995). Neurotrophins and neuronal plasticity. *Science*, 270(5236), 593-8.

Thomas, M.J., Malenka, R.C., Bonci, A. (2000). Modulation of long-term depression by dopamine in the mesolimbic system. *J Neurosci*, Aug 1, 20(15), 5581-6.

Thomas, M.J., Beurrier, C., Bonci, A., Malenka, R.C. (2001). Long-term depression in the nucleus accumbens: a neural correlate of behavioral sensitization to cocaine. *Nat Neurosci*, 4(12),1217-23.

Thomas, M.J., Malenka, R.C. (2003). Synaptic plasticity in the mesolimbic dopamine system. *Philos Trans R Soc Lond B Biol Sci*, 358(1432), 815-9.

Tiffany, S.T. (1990). A cognitive model of drug urges and drug-use behavior: role of automatic and nonautomatic processes. *Psychol Rev,* 97(2), 147-68.

Tiffany, S.T., Singleton, E., Haertzen, C.A., Henningfield, J.E. (1993). The development of a cocaine craving questionnaire. *Drug Alcohol Depend*, 34(1), 19-28.

Todtenkopf, M.S., Carreiras, T., Melloni, R.H., Stellar, J.R. (2002). The dorsomedial shell of the nucleus accumbens facilitates cocaine-induced locomotor activity during the induction of behavioral sensitization. *Behav Brain Res*, 131(1-2), 9-16.

Ungless, M.A., Whistler, J.L., Malenka, R.C., Bonci, A. (2001). Single cocaine exposure in vivo induces long-term potentiation in dopamine neurons. *Nature*, 411(6837), 583-7.

Valjent, E., Corvol, J.C., Trzaskos, J.M., Girault, J.A., Hervé, D. (2006). Role of the ERK pathway in psychostimulant-induced locomotor sensitization. *BMC Neurosci*, 7, 20.

Van Praag, H., Kempermann, G., Gage, F.H. (2000). Neural consequences of environmental enrichment. *Nat Rev Neurosci*, 1(3),191-8.

Vanderschuren, L.J., Kalivas, P.W. (2000). Alterations in dopaminergic and glutamatergic transmission in the induction and expression of behavioral sensitization: a critical review of preclinical studies. *Psychopharmacology* (Berl), 151(2-3), 99-120

Vanderschuren, L.J., Di Ciano, P., Everitt, B.J. (2005). Involvement of the dorsal striatum in cue-controlled cocaine seeking. *J Neurosci*, 25(38), 8665-70.

Vezina, P., Queen, A.L. (2000). Induction of locomotor sensitization by amphetamine requires the activation of NMDA receptors in the rat ventral tegmental area. *Psychopharmacology* (Berl), 151(2-3), 184-91.

Volkow, N.D., Hitzemann, R., Wang, G.J., Fowler, J.S., Wolf, A.P., Dewey, S.L., Handlesman, L. (1992). Long-term frontal brain metabolic changes in cocaine abusers. *Synapse*, 11(3), 184-90.

Volkow, N.D., Fowler, J.S., Wang, G.J., Hitzemann, R., Logan, J., Schlyer, D.J. et al. (1993). Decreased dopamine D2 receptor availability is associated with reduced frontal metabolism in cocaine abusers. *Synapse*, 14, 169-77.

Volkow, N.D.,Wang, G.J., Fowler, J.S., Logan, J., Hitzemann, R., Ding, Y.S., Pappas, N., Shea, C., Piscani, K. (1996). Decreases in dopamine receptors but not in dopamine transporters in alcoholics. *Alcohol Clin Exp Res*, 20(9), 1594-8.

Volkow, N.D., Fowler, J.S. (2000). Addiction, a disease of compulsion and drive: involvement of the orbitofrontal cortex. *Cereb Cortex*, 10(3), 318-25.

Volkow, N.D., Chang, L., Wang, G.J., Fowler, J.S., Ding, Y.S., Sedler, M., Logan, J., Franceschi, D., Gatley, J., Hitzemann, R., Gifford, A., Wong, C., Pappas, N. (2001). Low level of brain dopamine D2 receptors in methamphetamine abusers: association with metabolism in the orbitofrontal cortex. *Am J Psychiatry*, 158(12), 2015-21.

Volkow, N.D., Fowler, J.S., Wang, G.J., Swanson, J.M. (2004). Dopamine in drug abuse and addiction: results from imaging studies and treatment implications. *Mol Psychiatry*, 9(6), 557-69.

Volkow, N.D., Wang, G.J., Ma,Y., Fowler, J.S., Wong, C., Ding, Y.S., Hitzemann, R., Swanson, J.M., Kalivas, P. (2005). Activation of orbital and medial prefrontal cortex by methylphenidate in cocaine-addicted subjects but not in controls: relevance to addiction. *J Neurosci*, Apr 13, 25(15), 3932-9.

Volkow, N.D., Wang, G.J., Telang, F., Fowler, J.S., Logan, J., Childress, A.R., Jayne, M., Ma, Y., Wong, C. (2006). Cocaine cues and dopamine in dorsal striatum: mechanism of craving in cocaine addiction. *J Neurosci*, Jun 14, 26(24), 6583-8.

Voorn, P., Gerfen, C.R., Groenewegen, H.J. (1989). Compartmental organization of the ventral striatum of the rat: immunohistochemical distribution of enkephalin, substance P, dopamine, and calcium-binding protein. *J Comp Neurol*, Nov 8, 289(2), 189-201.

Vorel, S.R., Liu, X., Hayes, R.J., Spector, J.A., Gardner, E.L. (2001). Relapse to cocaine-seeking after hippocampal theta burst stimulation. *Science*, 292(5519):1175-8.

Yurek, D.M., Lu, W., Hipkens, S., Wiegand, S.J. (1996). BDNF enhances the functional reinnervation of the striatum by grafted fetal dopamine neurons. *Exp Neurol*, 137(1), 105-18.

White, F.J. (1996). Synaptic regulation of mesocorticolimbic dopamine neurons. *Annu Rev Neurosci*, 19, 405-36.

White, F.J., Hu, X.T., Zhang, X.F., Wolf, M.E.(1995). Repeated administration of cocaine or amphetamine alters neuronal responses to glutamate in the mesoaccumbens dopamine system. *J Pharmacol Exp Ther*, 273(1), 445-54.

Wickens, J.R., Begg, A.J., Arbuthnott, G.W. (1996). Dopamine reverses the depression of rat corticostriatal synapses which normally follows high-frequency stimulation of cortex in vitro. *Neuroscience*, 70(1), 1-5.

Wolf, M.E. (1998).The role of excitatory amino acids in behavioral sensitization to psicomotor stimulants. *Prog Neurobiol*, 54(6), 679-720.

Wright, C.I., Beijer, A.V., Groenewegen, H.J. (1996). Basal amygdaloid complex afferents to the rat nucleus accumbens are compartmentally organized. *J Neurosci*, 16(5), 1877-93.

Yamada, K., Mizuno, M., Nabeshima, T. (2002). Role for brain-derived neurotrophic factor in learning and memory. *Life Sci*, 70(7), 735-44.

Zhang, X.F., Hu, X.T., White, F.J., Wolf, M.E. (1997). Increased responsiveness of ventral tegmental area dopamine neurons to glutamate after repeated administration of cocaine or amphetamine is transient and selectively involves AMPA receptors. *J Pharmacol Exp Ther*, May, 281(2), 699-706.

In: Synaptic Plasticity: New Research
Editors: Tim F. Kaiser and Felix J. Peters
ISBN: 978-1-60456-732-8

Chapter 8

SYNAPTIC PLASTICITY IN THE MEDIAL PREFRONTAL CORTEX

E.S. Louise Faber
Queensland Brain Institute, The University of Queensland, Brisbane, Australia

ABSTRACT

Synaptic plasticity in the medial prefrontal cortex is essential for shaping the responsiveness of neuronal networks involved in executive and cognitive functions. This chapter will review the current literature on synaptic plasticity in this brain region. It will begin with an overview of the basic circuitry in the medial prefrontal cortex. It will then describe the multiple forms of short-term plasticity exhibited by pyramidal neurons in the medial prefrontal cortex. The cellular and molecular mechanisms underlying long-term synaptic changes will next be described, including long-term potentiation, long-term depression and spike timing-dependent plasticity, in addition to how these forms of long-term synaptic changes are modulated by neuromodulators such as dopamine. Synaptic plasticity at connections between the hippocampus and the medial prefrontal cortex will be examined, together with a discussion on the role of interactions between the medial prefrontal cortex and the amygdala. Finally I will explore the physiological function of synaptic plasticity in the medial prefrontal cortex, including the role it plays in working memory, in determining rules to shape behavioural patterns, in consolidation of memories, in neurological disorders, and in drug addiction.

ABBREVIATIONS

2-AG – 2-acylglycerol
AM-251 – N-(Piperidin-1-yl)-5-(4-iodophenyl)-1-(2,4-dichlorophenyl)-4-methyl-1H-pyrazole-3-carboxamide
AMPA – α-amino-3-hydroxy-5-methyl-4-issoxazoleproprionic acid

AP5 – 2-amino-5-phosphonobutyric acid
BDA – biotinylated dextran amine
BDNF – brain derived neurotrophic factor
CB1 – cannabinoid receptor 1
CREB – cyclic AMP response element binding protein
D1 – dopamine 1 class receptors
D2 – dopamine 2 class receptors
DA – dopamine
DARP-32 – dopamine and cAMP regulated phosphoprotein (Mr 32)
DHPG – dihydroxyphenylglycine
ERK1/2 – extracellular signal-regulated kinase 1/2
EPSP – excitatory postsynaptic potential
fMRI – functional magnetic resonance imaging
IL – infralimbic cortex
IP_3 – inositol triphosphate
IPSP – inhibitory postsynaptic potential
LTD – long-term depression
LTP – long-term potentiation
MAP kinase – mitogen activated protein kinase
MCPG - methyl-4-carboxyphenylglycine
MD – mediodorsal thalamic nucleus
mGluR – metabotropic glutamate receptor
MPEP - 2-methyl-6-phenylethynyl pyridine hydrochloride
mPFC – medial prefrontal cortex
NMDA – N-methyl-D-aspartate
PFC – prefrontal cortex
PKC – protein kinase C
PL – prelimbic cortex
PLC – phospholipase C
PLD – phospholipase D
PSA-NCAM - polysialylated form of nerve cell adhesion molecule
PTP – post-tetanic potentiation
STDP – spike timing-dependent plasticity
STP – short-term potentiation
Δ^9THC - Δ^9tetrahydrocannabinol
VTA – ventral tegmental area

1. Introduction

The prefrontal cortex (PFC) occupies 30% of the human brain, and is the most recently evolved brain region. It is a neocortical structure involved in higher cognitive, mnemonic and executive functions, such as planning and sequencing of actions, and attention (Goldman-Rakic 1999). Fuster (Fuster 2001) has described the function of the PFC is as a "perception-action interface", as it receives detailed information pertaining to the environment and internal milieu, and uses this information, together with a set of learnt "rules" (Wise et al. 1996), to guide appropriate behaviour. The afferent and efferent connections of the PFC, together with intrinsic connectivity, endow it with this range of functions. For example, the PFC is involved in integrating highly processed sensory information received from afferents arising from association cortical regions in the temporal and parietal lobes, and in mnemonic and emotional processing, due to its connectivity with limbic structures (Groenewegen and Uylings 2000). Reciprocal connections with the hypothalamus and brainstem afford the PFC with visceral functions.

One aspect of executive function is working memory, the ability to maintain information "in mind" for a short period of time in the presence of distracting stimuli (Goldman-Rakic 1995). The cellular basis for working memory is a persistent firing of networks of PFC neurons with shared stimulus properties (Goldman-Rakic 1995). While neurons in other brain regions also show repetitive firing during working memory, PFC neurons are unique in their ability to maintain firing in the presence of distractions (Miller and Cohen 2001). At present the persistent firing underlying working memory is thought to be mediated by a combination of reverberant synaptic activity in networks of neurons, and activation of intrinsic conductances in pyramidal neurons, such as plateau potentials (Wang 2001; Milojkovic et al. 2005; Durstewitz and Seamans 2006; Wang et al. 2006). Computational models suggest the requirement for both reverberating activity within the PFC and intrinsic bistability ("up and down" states; Marder et al. 1996; Wang 2001). In primates, executive functions are performed by the dorsolateral region of the PFC. In rodents, this function is performed by the medial prefrontal cortex (mPFC), which includes the prelimbic and infralimbic regions (Heidbreder and Groenewegen 2003). The prelimbic region is primarily associated with working memory tasks (Zahrt et al. 1997; Birrell and Brown 2000), while the infralimbic region is primarily involved in regulation of emotions (see below; Quirk and Mueller 2008). Despite some controversy in the past, it is now widely accepted that the rodent provides a viable model for studying PFC function. The early criterion for classification of the mPFC was based solely on connections with the mediodorsal thalamic nucleus, which led some to doubt the presence of a functional mPFC in the rodent (Preuss and Kaas 1999). However more recent analyses of the structure, based on neurochemical, functional and developmental studies, have yielded convincing data showing that the mPFC in the rodent is the anatomical correlate of the dorsolateral PFC in the primate (Uylings et al. 2003; Povysheva et al. 2006).

While early studies on the mPFC focused on its role in short-term forms of memory such as working memory, more recent work has established a role for the mPFC in long-term memory, such as the laying down of "rules" to shape behavioural responses and consolidation of memories. The underlying mechanisms for these forms of long-term memory are thought to be synaptic plasticity. This chapter will provide an overview of the current literature on synaptic plasticity in the mPFC, primarily at excitatory synapses in the rodent mPFC.

2. Synaptic Circuitry in the PFC

As with other neocortical regions, the mPFC is a laminated structure consisting of layers 1-6, with the majority of excitatory pyramidal neurons located in layer 2/3 and layer 5. In rats the mPFC lacks a layer 4. Three main types of pyramidal neuron have been identified in the rat mPFC in vivo according to their firing properties in response to current injection; regular firing, inactivating bursting and non-inactivating bursting (Degenetais et al. 2002). Similar firing properties were recorded in vitro (Yang et al. 1996). In addition, several types of interneuron have been identified (Kawaguchi and Kubota 1997).

Horizontal cortico-cortical connections are made between layer 2/3 pyramidal neurons in the prelimbic and infralimbic cortices (Lewis and Gonzalez-Burgos 2000; Gabbott et al. 2003). In primates, layer 3 neurons in the PFC form "stripes" when axons are labelled with biotinylated dextran amine (BDA), revealing reciprocal connections (Melchitzky et al. 2001). Fifty percent of the local connections made within these stripes are to interneurons, while 90% are to excitatory neurons in other stripes, suggesting that layer 3 neurons in the PFC function in modules. Indeed in primates, synaptic reverberation contributing to working memory is thought occur at cortico-cortical synapses in layer 3 (Levitt et al. 1993; Kritzer and Goldman-Rakic 1995; Gonzalez-Burgos et al. 2000; Lewis and Gonzalez-Burgos 2000). As with other cortical regions, layer 5 pyramidal neurons are the output cells of the PFC and project to many other cortical and subcortical regions. In addition to local inputs, afferents terminating in layer 2/3 also arise from other cortical regions, such as the contralateral mPFC, the entorhinal cortex and association cortices, the mediodorsal nucleus of the thalamus (Kuroda et al. 1998), the hippocampus and the amygdala. Afferents terminating in layer 5 arise intrinsically, together with afferents from other cortical regions, the hippocampus, the amygdala and the thalamus (Jay and Witter 1991; Gonzalez Burgos et al. 2007).

Dual recordings from pairs of pyramidal neurons in other regions of the neocortex have shown that connections between layer 2/3 pyramidal neurons and layer 5 pyramidal neurons are mostly made on the apical dendrites of layer 5 neurons, whereas connections between layer 5 pyramidal neurons are made on the basal dendrites of layer 5 neurons (Letzkus et al. 2006; Sjostrom and Hausser 2006). To date, connectivity between layer 5 pyramidal neurons has only been examined in the ferret mPFC. These connections were also made on the basal dendrites, and occurred in approximately 12% of pairs of neurons, similar to the connection rate observed in the visual cortex (Wang et al. 2006). However the incidence of reciprocal connections in these pairs was double that seen in the visual cortex, and was most frequently observed between pyramidal neurons with similar firing properties and synaptic properties (Wang et al. 2006). This may be attributable to the substantially higher number of dendritic spines on mPFC pyramidal neurons compared to visual cortical pyramidal neurons, providing the mPFC with advanced computational abilities (Elston 2003). Paired recordings have yet to be made between layer 2/3 and layer 5 pyramidal neurons in the mPFC, thus the properties of these connections are currently unknown. However, synapses on pyramidal neurons in the mPFC at both inputs express both α-amino-3-hydroxy-5-methyl-4-issoxazoleproprionic acid (AMPA) and N-methyl-D-aspartate (NMDA) receptors (Hirsch and Crepel 1991; Kang 1995).

3. Short-Term Plasticity in the PFC

Short-term plasticity is the change in strength of synaptic responses over a short time period that occurs with repetitive stimulation. There are several types of short-term plasticity. Over a period of milliseconds, during a train of excitatory postsynaptic potentials (EPSPs), facilitation or depression can occur. Depression of synaptic responses is typical of a high presynaptic release probability, while the converse is true for facilitation (Atzori et al. 2001; Rozov et al. 2001). On a longer time scale, synaptic augmentation, which lasts up to tens of milliseconds, and post-tetanic potentiation (PTP), which lasts up to several minutes, can occur. Both of these are measured by evoking an EPSP after a delay period following a train of stimuli, and both are thought to result from a build up of presynaptic calcium in the afferent terminal (Zucker and Regehr 2002). Finally, short-term potentiation (STP) can occur. This is an enhancement of synaptic responses that lasts up to ten minutes, and is due to postsynaptic effects such as receptor saturation or desensitisation (Xu-Friedman and Regehr 2004).

Both synaptic depression and facilitation have been reported at layer 5 pyramidal neuron synapses during trains of EPSPs in the rat (Hempel et al. 2000; Huang et al. 2004) and ferret (Wang et al. 2006). At layer 3 inputs to layer 5 pyramidal neurons in the rat, synaptic depression was observed in the majority of synapses (at frequencies of 1-50 Hz), with a minority of synapses showing facilitation followed by depression (Hempel et al. 2000). At layer 5-layer 5 synapses in the ferret mPFC, facilitation was observed in the majority of neurons at low frequencies (approximately 10 Hz), while at higher frequencies (20-50 Hz) these synapses displayed an initial facilitation followed by depression (Wang et al. 2006). Depressing synapses and synapses that showed equal facilitation and depression were also observed, but in lesser proportions (Wang et al. 2006). Pyramidal neurons with facilitating synapses and with synapses where facilitation balanced depression tended to have a bifurcated apical dendrite, while depressing synapses had a single apical dendrite, similar to pyramidal neurons in other brain regions (Wang et al. 2006). It is unclear whether the differences in proportions of depressing versus facilitating synapses are a feature of the different inputs (layer 2/3 versus layer 5 inputs) or due to species differences. However since pyramidal neurons with bifurcating dendrites have not been described in the rat, this may be a specific feature of pyramidal neurons in the ferret mPFC.

Following a brief tetanus, inputs to layer 5 pyramidal neurons from layer 2/3 and layer 5 both show frequency-dependent synaptic augmentation, lasting up to several hundred milliseconds (Hempel et al. 2000; Wang et al. 2006). Augmentation is unaffected by the NMDA receptor antagonist, 2-amino-5-phosphonobutyric acid (AP5; Hempel et al. 2000), consistent with the notion that synaptic augmentation is likely to be due to a build up of residual calcium in the presynaptic terminal during the tetanic stimulation (Zucker and Regehr 2002). Both short-term depression and synaptic augmentation have also been observed during paired recordings from layer 5 pyramidal neurons, discounting the possibility that activation of afferents containing neuromodulators or polysynaptic activity underlies these processes.

PTP and STP have also been observed at synapses on layer 5 pyramidal neurons in the rat prelimbic mPFC. Short-term plasticity at layer 3 and layer 5 inputs to layer 5 pyramidal neurons is frequency- and layer-dependent, and determined by the activity of the neuron prior to tetanic stimulation (15 stimuli at 50 Hz delivered twice; Young and Yang 2005). Following baseline stimulation at 0.5 Hz, PTP was evoked that lasted for approximately 1 minute at layer 3 but not layer 5 inputs. The same tetanus delivered following a baseline recording frequency of 0.067 Hz evoked STP at both layer 3 and layer 5 inputs, although this was longer lasting at layer 5 inputs (6 minutes versus 4 minutes). In contrast, in the ferret, PTP lasting up to a few minutes was observed only at layer 5-layer 5 synapses following tetanic stimulation (15 action potentials at 50 Hz, repeated 4 times), following baseline stimulation at 0.5 Hz (Wang et al. 2006). This could be attributable to the greater number of tetanic repetitions given, or alternatively could be suggestive of a distinct synaptic subtype in the ferret, since it only occurred at facilitating synapses. PTP evoked in the rat was enhanced by a dopamine type-1 (D1) receptor antagonist (Young and Yang 2005), suggesting that endogenous release of dopamine during the induction protocol suppresses PTP, presumably via a presynaptic suppression of glutamate release (Gao et al. 2001; Seamans et al. 2001). In contrast STP was suppressed by a D1 antagonist at layer 5 inputs, instead revealing long-term depression (LTD), and thereby suggesting a requirement for endogenous dopamine to evoke both STP and long-term potentiation (LTP; see below). In vivo, STP is reduced by both D1 and dopamine type-2 (D2) receptor antagonists, following stimulation of the superficial layers of the PFC with trains of stimuli at 40 Hz (Goto and Grace 2007).

Facilitating or depressing synapses behave as high- and low-band filters, respectively, endowing a postsynaptic neuron with an optimum frequency range for presynaptic inputs (Fuhrmann et al. 2002). Furthermore, synaptic augmentation allows neurons in the mPFC to reach action potential threshold repetitively during activation of recurrent synapses. Computer simulations have shown that a balance between augmentation and synaptic depression is important for sustaining persistent activity at a level observed in vivo in behaving animals during working memory tasks (approximately 50 Hz) (Funahashi et al. 1989). Consistent with this, during synaptic depression evoked with a "natural" spike train i.e. with a variable temporal pattern of firing mimicking in vivo recordings, postsynaptic depolarisation is maintained (Gonzalez-Burgos et al. 2004). Such diversity in short-term plasticity exhibited by pyramidal neuron synapses in the mPFC is likely to be advantageous for its role in executive function and mnemonic processing, since it allows greater flexibility than, for example, LTP, and has a lesser metabolic load. Short-term plasticity also enables rapid switching of attention, essential for the functioning of the PFC in cognitive processing.

4. Long-Term Plasticity

As well as being important in working memory, the PFC is also important in long-term memories, such as declarative memory in humans and associative learning in rodents (see below) (Otani 2002). As in other brain regions, the process underlying the formation of these memories is thought to be synaptic plasticity. The next section will describe what is known about the mechanisms underlying long-term synaptic plasticity in the prelimbic mPFC.

(i) LTP and LTD in the PFC

Early studies examining plasticity at layer 2/3 and layer 5 inputs to layer 5 pyramidal neurons found that at synapses where plasticity could be evoked, which constituted approximately two thirds of synapses, either LTP or LTD was elicited in relatively equal proportions (Hirsch and Crepel 1990; 1991; Law-Tho et al. 1995; Auclair et al. 2000; Guzman et al. 2005). This was induced by tetanic stimulation (4 trains of stimuli at 50-100 Hz for 1-2 seconds) in the presence of GABAergic blockers. LTP and LTD evoked in this way require a rise in postsynaptic calcium (Hirsch and Crepel 1992). However there is controversy as to the role of NMDA receptors in synaptic plasticity in the mPFC. While early studies showed that LTP is converted to LTD in the presence of AP5 (Hirsch and Crepel 1991; Law-Tho et al. 1995), later studies found that AP5 blocked both LTP and LTD at layer 2/3 inputs (Vickery et al. 1997; Otani et al. 2002; see below).

(a) LTD induction

LTD can be induced in several ways at layer 5 synapses following stimulation of the superficial layers. Firstly, LTD can be induced by tetanic stimulation (4 trains of 100 stimuli at 50 Hz) in the presence of a high concentration of dopamine (100 μM; Otani et al. 1998). Secondly, LTD can be evoked by tetanic stimulation in the presence of a group 1 metabotropic glutamate receptors (mGluR) agonist (Otani et al. 1999). Thirdly, two types of chemical LTD that do not require tetanic stimulation can be evoked. One can be induced by application of a group 2 mGluR agonist alone (Otani et al. 2002; Barbara et al. 2003), while the other can be evoked by dopamine in the presence of an mGluR1 agonist (Otani et al. 2002; Barbara et al. 2003). Finally, LTD can be evoked by low frequency stimulation (3 Hz stimulation for 15 minutes), in the presence of a very high concentration of dopamine (200 μM; Huang et al. 2004).

LTD evoked by tetanic stimulation in the presence of dopamine is blocked by antagonists at both D1 and dopamine type-2 (D2) receptors, antagonists of either group 1 and group 2 mGluRs, and by chelating postsynaptic calcium (Otani et al. 1998; Otani et al. 1999). However this type of LTD is not NMDA receptor-mediated. In contrast, mGluR2-evoked LTD (in the absence of tetanic stimulation) can be blocked by AP5 (Otani et al. 2002). This form of LTD is induced postsynaptically through activation of phospholipase C, which releases calcium from inositol triphosphate (IP_3)-sensitive intracellular stores, and activates phospholipase D, protein kinase C (PKC) and protein kinase A (PKA; Otani et al. 2002). However it is expressed presynaptically, as shown by a sustained increase in the paired pulse ratio, and can be occluded by a cannabinoid CB1 receptor agonist, suggesting that cannabinoids mediate the presynaptic expression (see below; Barbara et al. 2003). The link between NMDA receptor activation and group 2 mGluRs has not been ascertained, but is likely to be due to a critical concentration of calcium being reached at the synapse.

The common mechanism for tetanic stimulation-evoked and group 1 mGluR-induced LTD is via convergent activation of mitogen-activated protein kinases (MAP kinases). These forms of LTD are blocked by a MAP kinase inhibitor, and phosphorylation of MAP kinases is observed in the presence of dopamine and group 1 mGluR agonists (Otani et al. 1999). The function of MAP kinases in the PFC is currently unknown, but in the hippocampus MAP kinases are necessary for phosphorylation of cyclic AMP response element-binding protein (CREB) by PKA and PKC (Roberson et al. 1999), for triggering transcription, and for modifying spine shape (Wu et al. 2001).

Finally, LTD evoked by low frequency stimulation is blocked by both D1 and D2 receptor antagonists, a PKA inhibitor and by the mGluR antagonist methyl-4-carboxyphenylglycine (MCPG), but not by AP5 (Huang et al. 2004), similar to LTD evoked by dopamine coupled with tetanic stimulation at 50 Hz (Otani et al. 1998). The generation of LTD in the presence of dopamine with this stimulation protocol is blocked in the D1 receptor heterozygote knockout mice, which express 50% of the wildtype levels of D1 receptors, showing the action of dopamine is mediated by D1 receptors.

(b) LTP induction

In spite of early reports that tetanic stimulation evokes LTP (Hirsch and Crepel 1990; 1991; Law-Tho et al. 1995), subsequent studies have been unable to replicate this finding (Vickery et al. 1997; Otani et al. 1998). However, more recent studies have evoked LTP in the mPFC by using very high frequency tetanic stimulation, by using a burst stimulation protocol instead of tetanic stimulation, or by "priming" the mPFC with a prior application of dopamine. These are discussed below.

Theta burst stimulation (4 stimuli at 100 Hz, repeated 10 times at 5 Hz) has been found to be effective in evoking LTP following stimulation of superficial layers (Vickery et al. 1997; Morris et al. 1999; Otani and Kolomiets 2003) and deep layers of the mPFC (Vickery et al. 1997; Morris et al. 1999; Young and Yang 2005) but not following stimulation of layer 3 (Young and Yang 2005). This form of LTP is mediated by mGluRs since it is blocked by the MCPG (Vickery et al. 1997) and facilitated by the group 1 mGluR agonist dihydroxyphenylglycine (DHPG; Morris et al. 1999). During burst stimulation more action potentials and a larger depolarisation are evoked than during tetanic stimulation (Otani and Kolomiets 2003), likely leading to a greater increase in calcium, and thereby facilitating the induction of LTP (Dudek and Bear 1992; Artola and Singer 1993; Hansel et al. 1996; Cormier et al. 2001). Alternatively, LTP may be evoked more readily under these conditions because short bursts of stimulation "prime" the dendrites to optimise NMDA receptor activation (Larson and Lynch 1988). However in the presence of dopamine, burst firing evoked LTD (Otani and Kolomiets 2003).

LTP is also evoked in rodent layer 5 field EPSPs by very high tetanic stimulation of layer 2 (300 Hz for 0.5 second). Delivering the tetanic stimulation once evokes LTP that persists for approximately 60 minutes (early phase LTP), while delivering the tetanus five times evokes LTP that is sustained for 3 hours (late phase LTP; Huang et al. 2004). Late phase LTP is blocked by AP5 and anisomycin, and attenuated by a D1 receptor antagonist, while early phase LTP is converted to late phase LTP in the presence of a D1 receptor agonist. This suggests that D1 receptor activation is required for long lasting LTP. Consistent with this, in D1 heterozygote knockout mice application of a D1 agonist failed to convert early phase LTP to late phase LTP (Huang et al. 2004).

In agreement with the above finding that dopamine facilitates LTP, dopamine release following stimulation of the ventral tegmental area (VTA) combined with tetanic stimulation leads to LTP in vivo (Gurden et al, 1999; 2000). However this contrasts with experiments coupling low frequency tetanic stimulation (50 Hz) with dopamine exposure in vitro (Otani et al. 1998), which evokes LTD. This discrepancy may be due to the very low ambient dopamine concentrations in vitro compared to a substantial background dopamine tone in vivo (Takahata and Moghaddam 2000). Consistent with this, transient exposure to dopamine in vitro, prior to tetanic stimulation, leads to LTP, when the 50 Hz tetanic stimulation is subsequently delivered in the presence of dopamine (Blond et al. 2002; Matsuda et al. 2006). This was not due to enhanced postsynaptic depolarisation during the LTP protocol following "priming", since this was actually less than that observed when LTD was evoked. Instead this "priming" effect of dopamine application requires activation of both D1 and D2 receptors (Matsuda et al. 2006), and may be due to metaplastic changes (Abraham and Bear 1996). Applying AP5 during "priming" or during the tetanus blocks LTP, as does buffering intracellular calcium or hyperpolarising the cell during the LTP induction protocol (Matsuda et al. 2006), suggesting that calcium influx through NMDA receptors is required for this form of LTP.

(c) Spike timing-dependent plasticity

Spike timing-dependent plasticity (STDP) is a paradigm that pairs presynaptically evoked EPSPs with postsynaptic action potentials (Dan and Poo 2004; Letzkus et al. 2007). This is highly likely to occur physiologically since both the pre- and postsynaptic neurons are invariably simultaneously active in vivo (Letzkus et al. 2007). During this Hebbian form of plasticity, pairing needs to occur within a specific temporal window, and the direction of plasticity depends on the timing of the presynaptic activity in relation to the postsynaptic activity, generating a "tuning" curve. In general, pairing trains of action potentials before trains of EPSPs leads to LTD, whereas pairing action potentials after EPSPs leads to LTP (Dan and Poo 2004; Letzkus et al. 2007).

A few studies have examined STDP in the mPFC. Pairing action potentials 5 ms after the start of a train of EPSPs (50 times repeated at 0.1 Hz) evokes LTP at layer 2/3 inputs to layer 5 pyramidal neurons in mice (Couey et al. 2007; Meredith et al. 2007). However a delay of 10 ms between the EPSP onset and the action potentials fails to evoke LTP, both in mice (Meredith et al. 2007) and rats (evoked by EPSP-spike pairings of 10 bursts of 5 stimuli at 20 Hz; Huang et al. 2007a). In mice, when the action potential precedes the EPSP by 0-10 ms or 40-70 ms, LTD is evoked, with no plasticity evoked at intermediate delays (Meredith et al. 2007). It remains to be seen if a similar temporal profile of STDP is seen in layer 5 pyramidal neurons in the rat. LTP evoked by STDP requires a rise in intracellular calcium, and can be blocked by application of nicotine (10 μM), via activation of GABAergic interneurons. This subsequently decreases the dendritic calcium rise (Couey et al. 2007), which is essential for eliciting STDP (Magee and Johnston 1997; Koester and Sakmann 1998).

In summary, while the majority of synapses in the mPFC are plastic, there appears to be a delicate balance between LTP and LTD, with one often masking the other (Hirsch and Crepel 1991; Law-Tho et al. 1995; Otani et al. 1998; Auclair et al. 2000; Matsuda et al. 2006). Thus the same induction protocol can evoke either LTP or LTD. This contrasts with other brain regions where high frequency stimulation (50-100 Hz) typically evokes LTP, while low frequency stimulation (1 Hz) typically evokes LTD. The reason for this is not clear, but calcium imaging studies would help to elucidate what underlies these mechanistic discrepancies.

Synaptic plasticity is differentially regulated by dopamine, depending on the induction mechanism and prior exposure. These findings may be confounded by the release of endogenous dopamine in the slice during the stimulation protocol (Calabresi et al. 1995; Young and Yang 2005), with the amount of residual dopamine in the brain slice depending on the timing of recording following the brain dissection (Otani et al. 2003; Young and Yang 2005), and with bursts more likely to evoke higher concentrations of transmitter release from dopaminergic afferent fibres (Goto et al. 2007). Therefore in future studies it would be useful to investigate the action of selective dopamine receptor antagonists alone on these forms of synaptic plasticity, to investigate plasticity at a range of times following dissection, and to investigate the effects of a range of concentrations of dopamine (i.e. 3 μM versus 100 μM; Seamans and Yang 2004). Indeed, Matsuda and colleagues found that 3 μM dopamine did not trigger LTD when combined with tetanic stimulation (Matsuda et al. 2006).

In addition, synaptic plasticity in the PFC may also depend on the membrane potential of layer 5 pyramidal neurons. Under anaesthesia, neurons in the PFC exhibit a bistability in vivo, oscillating between up and down states at a frequency of approximately 1 Hz (Branchereau et al. 1996; Lewis and O'Donnell 2000). Furthermore, stimulation of the VTA, which releases dopamine into the mPFC, triggers up states (Lewis and O'Donnell 2000). Since during in vitro slice recordings the resting membrane potential mimics a down state, this may be an explanation for the greater ease of evoking LTD than LTP with tetanic stimulation (Law-Tho et al. 1995; Otani et al. 1998; Takita et al. 1999). In contrast, LTP may be more likely to be evoked from depolarised potentials that mimic the up state in vivo (Gurden et al. 1999; Gurden et al. 2000), due to greater activation of NMDA receptors at these membrane potentials.

(ii) PFC-hippocampal connections

The CA1 region of the hippocampus, apart from the most dorsal region, together with the subiculum, send direct inputs via the fornix and fimbria to the prelimbic, infralimbic, lateral, and medial orbital areas of the mPFC (Jay and Witter 1991). Hippocampal fibres innervate all cell layers of the mPFC, but most densely innervate layer 5 of the prelimbic mPFC in an ipsilateral and unidirectional manner (Sesack et al. 1989). Hippocampal fibres form asymmetrical synapses on dendritic spines of pyramidal neurons and on dendrites of GABAergic interneurons (Carr and Sesack 1996; Gabbott et al. 2002; Tierney et al. 2004), where they release glutamate to activate AMPA and NMDA receptors to evoke an EPSP with a latency of approximately 16 ms (Jay et al. 1992; Gigg et al. 1994; Thierry et al. 2000; Degenetais et al. 2003). Intracellular recordings in vivo have shown that stimulation of CA1 can evoke complex EPSP/ inhibitory postsynaptic potential (IPSP) waveforms in pyramidal neurons in the prelimbic mPFC (Degenetais et al. 2003), presumably via disynaptic activation of pyramidal neurons and interneurons. Inputs from the hippocampus have been shown to provide information about context during extinction of fear memories (see below; Kim and Fanselow 1992; Phillips and LeDoux 1992), and spatial working memory (see below; Floresco et al. 1997; Seamans et al. 1998), and LTP at inputs to the prelimbic mPFC in the awake rat can last for days (Doyere et al. 1993; Jay et al. 1996). As well as being crucial for the retrieval of stored information during working memory tasks, hippocampal inputs are also important for the generation of up and down states in the mPFC, since lesioning of the ventral hippocampus prevents up transitions in the mPFC (O'Donnell et al. 2002).

Plasticity at inputs from the hippocampus, including those travelling via the subiculum, has been well studied, with the function of plasticity at these synapses thought to be involved in stabilising the storage of learned events in the cortex, and with providing retrospective information for future planning (Goto and Grace 2007). High frequency stimulation of the ventral hippocampus (250 Hz in bursts of 200 ms) evokes LTP of field EPSP recorded in the deep layers of the prelimbic mPFC in vivo (Jay et al. 1995; Laroche et al. 2000; Hotte et al. 2007), and LTP of both EPSPs and IPSPs recorded intracellularly (Degenetais et al. 2003), which persists for several hours in both anaesthetised animals and awake freely moving animals (Jay et al. 1996). Similarly, tetanic stimulation of the fornix also evokes LTP in the prelimbic mPFC (Mulder et al. 1997). This form of LTP requires activation of NMDA receptors for induction but not maintenance since induction can be blocked by infusion of AP5 into the prelimbic PFC (Laroche et al. 1990; Jay et al. 1995; 1996).

Dopaminergic input from the VTA is also required for LTP at hippocampal-mPFC synapses. Jay and colleagues showed that lesioning the VTA reduced LTP, while stimulating the VTA enhanced LTP evoked with a moderate induction protocol (Gurden et al. 1999). Consistent with this, infusion of a D1 agonist enhanced LTP, while infusion of a D1 antagonist blocked LTP at these inputs (Gurden et al. 2000; Matsumoto et al. 2008). The actions of DA acting on D1 receptors is presumably via activation of PKA, since LTP at these inputs was blocked by the PKA inhibitor Rp-cAMPs (Gurden et al. 2000). A recent study showed that D1 receptors are also required for short-term plasticity at hippocampal-PFC synapses in vivo (Goto and Grace 2007).

LTD has also been evoked at hippocampal-PFC synapses, by low frequency tetanic stimulation (trains of 5 stimuli at 250 Hz, repeated 900 times at 1 Hz; Takita et al. 1999; Izaki et al. 2001). This was reversible upon high frequency stimulation (50 pulses at 250 Hz, repeated 12 times; Takita et al. 1999). In contrast to the traditional induction protocol that induces LTD in other brain regions (single stimuli at 1 Hz repeated 900 times for 15 minutes; Dudek and Bear 1992; Kirkwood et al. 1993; Dudek and Friedlander 1996; Manabe 1997)), this protocol failed to induce LTD in the mPFC but instead led to depotentiation of evoked LTP in vivo (Burette et al. 1997).

Neurons in the hippocampus oscillate in the theta (4-10 Hz) range during exploratory behaviour and REM sleep (Green and Arduini 1954; Vanderwolf 1969; Buzsaki 2002), both of which are thought to be involved in memory formation. Furthermore the mPFC is entrained to theta rhythms in the hippocampus in freely behaving rats (Siapas et al. 2005) and during spatial working memory tasks (Jones and Wilson 2005). Despite this, however, only one study has examined plasticity at hippocampal-PFC synapses using theta burst stimulation. In this study only STP was evoked with moderate strength theta burst stimulation (Goto and Grace 2007). Neuronal firing rates have also been measured at 1 Hz in CA1 pyramidal neurons in the awake rat, and ripple activity has been observed at approximately 250 Hz, suggesting that these frequencies, which have been used for inducing longer-term plasticity, are also behaviourally relevant (Suzuki and Smith 1988; Ylinen et al. 1995). The implications for plasticity at hippocampal-mPFC synapses are discussed below.

(iii) PFC-amygdala interactions

The amygdala is involved in generating emotions and emotional memories, in particular fear-related memories, in response to sensory inputs (Sah et al. 2003). The mPFC and the amygdala have reciprocal connections (Cassell and Wright 1986; Cassell et al. 1989; McDonald 1991; 1996; McDonald et al. 1996) and this circuit has been shown to be crucial for integrating emotionally salient stimuli and regulating emotional memories (Milad and Quirk 2002; Ochsner and Gross 2005; Laviolette and Grace 2006). Medial PFC neurons can inhibit (Rosenkranz and Grace 1999; 2001; 2002) or excite (Likhtik et al. 2005) amygdala neurons, and project directly to inhibitory intercalated cells in the amygdala (McDonald et al. 1996). Conversely, amygdala neurons excite parvalbumin-containing interneurons in the mPFC (Gabbott et al. 2006), but stimulation of the basolateral amygdala evokes both inhibitory and excitatory responses in the mPFC (Perez-Jaranay and Vives 1991). NMDA receptor-dependent LTP can be evoked in the prelimbic mPFC following theta burst stimulation (10 trains of ten stimuli at 100 Hz, repeated 3 times) of the rat basolateral amygdala in vivo (Maroun and Richter-Levin 2003).

Emotional memory formation has been widely studied using a form of Pavlovian associative learning, fear conditioning. This involves pairing an unconditioned stimulus, which evokes fear, with a neutral conditioned stimulus, such that subsequent exposure to the conditioned stimulus elicits a fear response (Pavlov 1927). Plasticity underlying this effect is known to occur within the amygdala (LeDoux 2000), since lesions or inactivation of the amygdala before conditioning prevent the animal from learning fear associations (Iwata et al. 1986; Goosens and Maren 2003), while lesions of the amygdala following conditioning prevent the expression of the fear response (Anglada-Figueroa and Quirk 2005). While initial experiments showed that lesioning the mPFC had no effect on the acquisition or expression of conditioned fear (Rosen et al. 1992; Quirk et al. 2000), recent evidence suggests that the mPFC is involved in the expression of fear conditioning. Inactivation of the prelimbic mPFC suppresses fear responses following conditioning (Blum et al. 2006; Corcoran and Quirk 2007), and the prelimbic mPFC shows increased firing following conditioning (Baeg et al. 2001; Gilmartin and McEchron 2005; Laviolette et al. 2005). Furthermore microstimulation of the prelimbic mPFC enhances conditioned fear responses (Vidal-Gonzalez et al. 2006). Thus the results of the initial lesioning experiments may have been confounded by compensatory measures occurring following lesioning, and do not discount the possibility that the intact mPFC contributes to expression of fear conditioning (Quirk and Mueller 2008). In view of the excitatory projections from the mPFC to the basolateral amygdala (McDonald et al. 1996), and the finding that firing in the prelimbic mPFC precedes that in the amygdala, this suggests that the prelimbic mPFC may drive the basolateral amygdala during expression of fear responses (Vertes 2004; Likhtik et al. 2005).

The mPFC also plays an important role in extinction of fear conditioning. Extinction to a conditioned stimulus occurs when exposure to the conditioned stimulus is repeated in the absence of the unconditioned stimulus, thereby eliminating the fear memory (Pavlov 1927; Myers and Davis 2002). Extinction involves new learning as opposed to "unlearning" of the fear memory (Pavlov 1927; Bouton et al. 2006; Myers and Davis 2007). There are three phases of extinction: acquisition, consolidation, and retrieval. Acquisition is the initial learning, consolidation follows for several hours afterwards and involves cellular and molecular mechanisms of memory storage, and retrieval occurs during a subsequent testing (Quirk and Mueller 2008).

The mPFC is not required for acquisition of extinction, since mPFC lesions have no effect on the acquisition of extinction in rodents (Gewirtz et al. 1997; Quirk et al. 2000; Vouimba et al. 2000), and no association has been found between extinction acquisition and plasticity in the mPFC (Herry and Garcia 2002). However one study did show an acceleration of extinction acquisition when tetanic stimulation of the infralimbic cortex was combined with presentations of the conditioned stimulus alone (Milad and Quirk 2002). The amygdala is the primary area that has been attributed with the acquisition of extinction, demonstrated through lesioning studies and infusion of compounds that inhibit synaptic plasticity into the basolateral region of the amygdala (for review see Quirk and Mueller 2008).

A number of studies have implicated the infralimbic mPFC in the consolidation of extinction (Quirk et al. 2000; Weible et al. 2000; Fernandez Espejo 2003; Morgan et al. 2003; Lebron et al. 2004). For example, lesioning the infralimbic mPFC prevents retrieval of the memory the following day (Quirk et al. 2000). However, other investigators have failed to observe this effect (Gewirtz et al. 1997; Farinelli et al. 2006; Garcia et al. 2006). Again, compensatory mechanisms following lesioning may be a confounding issue, as a number of investigators have since found that a more transient inactivation of the infralimbic mPFC, by infusing compounds into the infralimbic mPFC before extinction training, blocks retrieval of extinction. For example, infusion of the sodium channel blocker tetrodotoxin (TTX)(Sierra-Mercado et al. 2006), the NMDA receptor antagonist CPP (Burgos-Robles et al. 2007), a PKA inhibitor, a beta adrenoceptor antagonist (Mueller et al. 2008), the protein synthesis inhibitor anisomycin (Santini et al. 2004; Mueller et al. 2008), or the transcription inhibitor actinomycin (Mueller et al. 2008) into the infralimbic mPFC block retrieval of extinction. Furthermore infusion of a MAP kinase inhibitor (Hugues et al. 2004; Hugues et al. 2006) or CPP (Burgos-Robles et al. 2007) immediately following acquisition of training also blocked extinction retrieval the following day. Enhancing metabolism in the infralimbic mPFC (Gonzalez-Lima and Bruchey 2004), enhancing brain-derived neurotrophic factor (BDNF) activity (Bredy et al. 2007) or the activity of AMPA receptors (Zushida et al. 2007) augments consolidation of extinction. Finally, an increase in the expression of c-fos, an immediate early gene implicated in synaptic plasticity, is observed in the mPFC following extinction (Santini et al. 2004), All of these molecular markers point to a role of synaptic plasticity in the mPFC in the consolidation of extinction memories.

When animals are re-exposed to a conditioned stimulus on days subsequent to the acquisition of extinction, they can either exhibit the fear memory or the extinction memory, which are mediated by distinct neural substrates (Bouton 1993; Rescorla 2001; Garcia 2002). A large body of evidence indicates a role for the mPFC in the retrieval of the extinction memory. Firstly, an increase in evoked potentials in the mPFC (Herry and Garcia 2002; Farinelli et al. 2006; Hugues and Garcia 2007), and the degree of synaptic potentiation displayed by neurons in the mPFC following extinction training, has been shown to correlate with the degree of extinction memory exhibited (Herry and Garcia 2002; Barrett et al. 2003). Similarly, high frequency firing of mPFC neurons correlates with the degree of extinction (Milad and Quirk 2002), and predicts retrieval of the fear memory after extinction training the following day (Burgos-Robles et al. 2007). In contrast synaptic depression in the mPFC is associated with expression of the fear memory (Herry and Garcia 2002; 2003). Secondly, lesioning the infralimbic mPFC results in only the fear memory being exhibited on re-exposure to the conditioned stimulus (Quirk et al. 2000). Thirdly, enhancing activity in the mPFC, by triggering LTP in the prelimbic mPFC with high frequency stimulation of the mediodorsal thalamic nucleus (Herry and Garcia 2002) or the hippocampus (Farinelli et al. 2006), or by stimulating the infralimbic mPFC directly (Milad and Quirk 2002; Milad et al. 2004; Vidal-Gonzalez et al. 2006) facilitates extinction expression. Moreover stimulating the mediodorsal thalamic nucleus with low frequency stimulation to evoke LTD in the prelimbic mPFC facilitates expression of the fear memory (Herry and Garcia 2002). In contrast with these findings, it has recently shown that rats show normal expression of extinction of fear memories with mPFC lesions (Garcia et al. 2006). Again, however, the discrepancy in the literature lies with studies examining the effects of lesioning, suggesting methodological issues.

Thus while some groups have found the association between activity and the extinction memory to occur in the prelimbic mPFC (Herry and Garcia 2002; Farinelli et al. 2006; Hugues and Garcia 2007), others have attributed this function only to the infralimbic mPFC

(Milad and Quirk 2002; Barrett et al. 2003; Burgos-Robles et al. 2007). Since increases in activity in the prelimbic mPFC have been observed during expression of conditioned fear responses (Baeg et al. 2001; Gilmartin and McEchron 2005; Laviolette et al. 2005; Vidal-Gonzalez et al. 2006), this suggests that the correlations between synaptic plasticity and retrieval of the extinction versus fear memory may be confounded by other factors. For example the field recordings used in these experiments are average responses of many neurons. It is possible that there are distinct populations of pyramidal neurons within the prelimbic mPFC that encode fear versus extinction memories.

Since most inputs from the mPFC to the amygdala are excitatory (Smith et al. 2000; Likhtik et al. 2005) and neurons in the basolateral amygdala still fire during extinction, despite the animal showing less fear (Repa et al. 2001), this suggests that enhanced activity of the mPFC has effects on the amygdala that are downstream of the basolateral amygdala. This may be via direct activation of intercalated neurons in the amygdala (McDonald et al. 1996), which could act to inhibit fear memory expression in the amygdala (Maren and Quirk 2004; Pare et al. 2004). Intercalated neurons are GABAergic neurons that act as an inhibitory gate between the basolateral amygdala, which receives inputs containing information regarding the conditioned stimulus, and the central amygdala, the output station of the amygdala that projects to the brainstem to initiate the fear response (Royer et al. 1999; Sah et al. 2003). Stimulation of the infralimbic mPFC evokes c-fos expression in intercalated neurons (Berretta et al. 2005), and inhibits the responsiveness of central amygdala neurons to stimulation of the basolateral amygdala (Quirk et al. 2003). Furthermore, intercalated neurons show both LTP and LTD (Royer and Pare 2002), suggesting that plasticity at mPFC inputs to intercalated neurons may underlie extinction.

Connections between the mPFC and hippocampus have also been implicated in fear conditioning and extinction. For example, fear memories overcome extinction memories when presented in a new context. Furthermore hippocampal inputs and outputs both show prolonged synaptic plasticity associated with traumatic memories, which outlasts extinction of the memory, and hippocampal synaptic efficacy is altered during re-exposure to the conditioned stimulus (Garcia and Jaffard 1996; Garcia et al. 1998). When development of LTP at hippocampal-mPFC synapses following extinction training is prevented by low frequency stimulation of the ventral hippocampus, recall of the extinction memory is impaired (Farinelli et al. 2006). Furthermore long-term changes are seen in the hippocampus during consolidation of extinction in the inhibitory avoidance paradigm. These are dependent on NMDA receptors, MAP kinase, PKA, gene expression and protein synthesis (for review see Quirk and Mueller 2008), suggesting that synaptic plasticity in the hippocampus, or at hippocampal inputs to the mPFC, also contributes to the consolidation of extinction.

In summary, the mPFC is involved in both the expression of fear memories, and the expression and retrieval of extinction (Vidal-Gonzalez et al. 2006). Changes that occur in the mPFC during extinction expression and retrieval involve regulation by many molecular markers and receptors that are involved in synaptic plasticity, implicating synaptic plasticity in the mPFC and at connections between the mPFC, the amygdala and the hippocampus as the cellular basis of extinction memories. While synaptic plasticity can be induced in the prelimbic mPFC following stimulation of the basolateral amygdala (Maroun and Richter-Levin 2003), few studies to date have investigated the mechanisms underlying synaptic plasticity in the infralimbic mPFC and at connections between the infralimbic mPFC and the amygdala (Maroun 2006), which may be more relevant to extinction. Understanding these cellular mechanisms is important for developing treatments for post-traumatic stress disorder and anxiety disorders, since they are thought to result from the inability to extinguish fear memories (see below).

5. Neuromodulation of Synaptic Plasticity in the PFC

Removing catecholamines from the PFC is as detrimental to the functioning of the PFC as removal of the PFC itself (Brozoski et al. 1979), pointing to the vital role that neuromodulators serve in the functioning of this brain region. In addition, a large body of evidence has shown that neuromodulators play an important role in regulating synaptic plasticity. These are discussed below.

While all cortical regions receive inputs from monoaminergic and cholinergic systems, leading to the release of dopamine, noradrenaline, 5-hydroxytryptamine (5-HT) and acetylcholine, it is only the mPFC that sends projections back to these brainstem structures, endowing the mPFC with control over the functioning of these neuromodulator systems (Arnsten 1997; Everitt and Robbins 1997). Serotonergic neurons arise in the raphe nuclei project to the mPFC (Azmitia and Segal 1978). Lesioning these inputs with 5,7-dihydroxytryptamine (5,7-DHT) augments LTP of field EPSPs in the prelimbic mPFC, evoked by high frequency stimulation of CA1 (50 trains at 250 Hz; Ohashi et al. 2003). This suggests that 5-HT attenuates LTP at hippocampal-mPFC synapses, potentially via a depression of NMDA receptor-mediated currents (Staubli and Otaky 1994; Edagawa et al. 1999).

Afferents from the locus coeruleus densely innervate the mPFC, where they release noradrenaline (Levitt and Moore 1978; Lindvall et al. 1978; Morrison et al. 1978; Aoki et al. 1998). Noradrenaline is important for extinction of fear memories, as it has been shown that noradrenaline is released into the mPFC during fear extinction (Hugues et al. 2007), and depletion of forebrain noradrenaline impairs extinction retrieval (Mason and Iversen 1977). Furthermore activation of beta adrenoceptors in the mPFC is required for consolidation of extinction (Mueller et al. 2008) and odour reward memories (see below; (Tronel et al. 2004)), suggesting that activation of beta adrenoceptors may facilitate LTP. In contrast, recent evidence suggests that activation of alpha adrenoceptors promotes LTD. Activation of both □1 and □2 adrenoceptors by noradrenaline evokes LTD, and this is mediated by activation of NMDA receptors, PKC and extracellular signal-regulated kinase 1/2 (ERK1/2; Marzo et al. 2007).

(i) Dopamine

Dopamine levels in the mPFC are essential for normal functioning, for example in working memory. Dopamine exhibits an inverted U-shaped dose response curve, whereby levels of dopamine that are either too low or too high impair proper functioning (Vijayraghavan et al. 2007). As well as being essential for working memory (Sawaguchi and Goldman-Rakic 1991; 1994; Seamans et al. 1998; Floresco and Phillips 2001; Seamans and Yang 2004), dopaminergic systems are also involved in predicting the reward value of a stimulus (Brozoski et al. 1979; Simon et al. 1980; Robbins and Everitt 1996; Schultz 2002). The dopamine signal in the mPFC is highly tuned to signal the reward value of an event and its precise coincident release into the mPFC may signal such an event by evoking plasticity of the ongoing glutamatergic activity (Schultz 2002).

There are two broad classes of dopamine receptor, classified according to their genetic sequence and pharmacology: D1-type, comprising D1 and D5 receptors, and D2-type, comprising D2, D3 and D4 receptors (Civelli et al. 1993). The predominant type of dopamine receptor in the mPFC is D1-type receptors, which outnumber D2-type receptors several fold (Smiley et al. 1994). D1 receptors are expressed mainly on pyramidal neurons in layer 5 (Gaspar et al. 1995) where they are located on the spines and dendrites of neurons (Smiley et al. 1994; Bergson et al. 1995), and presynaptically on afferent terminals where they depress transmitter release (Gao et al. 2001; Seamans et al. 2001; Paspalas and Goldman-Rakic 2005). Dopaminergic afferents to the mPFC arise in the VTA (Thierry et al. 1973), where they synapse onto dendritic spines and shafts of layer 5 and 6 neurons (Van Eden et al. 1987; Sesack et al. 1995). Some dopaminergic terminals form synaptic "triads", where a dopaminergic terminal targets both a postsynaptic dendritic spine and an excitatory terminal of another afferent (Van Eden et al. 1987; Goldman-Rakic et al. 1989; Verney et al. 1990; Sesack et al. 1995), although the main form of transmission is thought to be via volume transmission (Garris and Wightman 1994). In addition to the phasic release of dopamine from VTA afferents, for example during expectation of reward (Schultz 2002), slow tonic activity maintains ambient levels of dopamine in the PFC (Bassareo and Di Chiara 1997; Takahata and Moghaddam 2000). This may regulate the sensitivity of PFC neurons to forthcoming inputs (Williams and Goldman-Rakic 1995).

The effects of dopamine on basal synaptic transmission in the PFC have been extensively studied in vitro, yielding somewhat conflicting data (see Seamans and Yang 2004). However the general consensus is that dopamine depresses single EPSPs evoked by local stimulation in vitro (Gao et al. 2001; Seamans et al. 2001) or hippocampal stimulation in vivo (Gurden et al. 1999), but enhances NMDA receptor-mediated responses evoked with repetitive stimulation (Seamans et al. 2001; Seamans and Yang 2004). Stimulation of the VTA in vivo evokes a transition of layer 5 pyramidal neurons into an up state, while at the same time decreasing the number of evoked action potentials (Lewis and O'Donnell 2000).

The effects of dopamine on synaptic plasticity in the mPFC are discussed above. In summary, however, dopamine can facilitate either LTD or LTP. LTD is facilitated by dopamine at layer 2/3 inputs to layer 5 pyramidal neurons, through a mechanism involving mGluRs and activation of MAP kinase (Otani et al. 1998; Otani et al. 1999). Alternatively, prior exposure to dopamine can "prime" synapses to evoke LTP (Blond et al. 2002; Matsuda et al. 2006). At hippocampal inputs, the effect of dopamine is a facilitation of LTP. For example, infusion of dopamine into the mPFC enhances LTP following tetanic stimulation of the hippocampus (Jay et al. 1996). Furthermore, tetanic stimulation of the VTA at 50 Hz for 2 seconds, which releases dopamine into the mPFC (Garris et al. 1993) prior to stimulation of the hippocampus, leads to a persistently enhanced LTP at hippocampal-mPFC synapses (Gurden et al. 1999). Moreover disruption of the mesocortical dopaminergic projection from the VTA to the PFC impairs LTP induction at hippocampal-mPFC synapses (Gurden et al. 1999; Gurden et al. 2000). This effect is mediated by D1 receptors, demonstrated by the fact that infusion of a D1 agonist into the PFC prior to tetanic stimulation of the hippocampus enhances LTP, while infusion of a D1 antagonist into the PFC blocks LTP (Gurden et al.

2000). Furthermore, LTP at hippocampal inputs is associated with a sustained enhancement in the release of dopamine in the PFC, measured by microdialysis (Gurden et al. 2000).

The mechanism of D1 receptor-mediated enhancement of LTP is likely to be via PKA (Jay et al. 1998), which phosphorylates the AMPA receptor GluR1 subunit (Lee et al. 2000b) and stimulates trafficking of GluR1 receptors into the postsynaptic density (Hu et al. 2007; Man et al. 2007). Activation of PKA leads to activation of DARP-32 (Snyder et al. 1998) and CREB, both of which have been found to be upregulated during late LTP at hippocampal-mPFC synapses (Hotte et al. 2007), leading to gene transcription. Moreover, activation of PKA by D1 receptors has also been shown to phosphorylate NMDA receptors, a process which is involved in the D1-mediated activation of CREB (Dudman et al. 2003). Finally, activation of D1 receptors can trigger insertion of AMPA receptors into the synaptic membrane, when activated in conjunction with NMDA receptors (Sun et al. 2005). Thus, activation of D1 receptors may increase the availability of extrasynaptic membrane-bound AMPA receptors for synaptic insertion during LTP. This action in particular may contribute to the "priming" effect of dopamine (Matsuda et al. 2006). In contrast, activation of D2 receptors reduces the surface expression of GluR1 AMPA receptors, suggesting a possible mechanism for dopamine facilitation of LTD (Sun et al. 2005).

(ii) Cannabinoids

Activation of cannabinoid receptors, for example by inhalation of marijuana, is known to produce cognitive and mnemonic deficits, together with alterations in sensory perception and emotional processing (Ameri 1999; Sullivan 2000). Some of these effects may be mediated by an action in the mPFC. For example, infusion of agonist Δ^9THC (Δ^9tetrahydrocannabinol) into the PFC has been shown to impair working memory tasks (Jentsch et al. 1997; Jentsch et al. 1998), and cannabinoids have also been implicated in emotional learning (Marsicano et al. 2002; Chhatwal et al. 2005; Varvel et al. 2005; Laviolette and Grace 2006). Furthermore, elevations in the endocannabioid system have been implicated in schizophrenia (Leweke et al. 1999; Ujike and Morita 2004). CB1 receptors, the cannabinoid receptor found in the brain, are abundantly expressed in the mPFC (Herkenham et al. 1990; Marsicano and Lutz 1999; Moldrich and Wenger 2000). As with other brain regions, CB1 receptors are localised on excitatory terminals where they act presynaptically to reduce glutamate release (Auclair et al. 2000; Ferraro et al. 2001; Lafourcade et al. 2007). However their effectiveness at suppressing inhibitory transmission is yet to be demonstrated in the mPFC.

CB1 receptors both mediate and facilitate LTD at inputs to layer 5 pyramidal neurons in the mPFC. Following tetanic stimulation (4 trains of 100 stimuli at 100 Hz), activation of CB1 receptors facilitates LTD induction over LTP induction at layer 5 to layer 5 synapses in the rat prelimbic mPFC, while application of a CB1 receptor antagonist alone favours LTP (Auclair et al. 2000). Moreover, a CB1 receptor-mediated LTD can be evoked at layer 2/3 and layer 5/6 inputs to layer 5/6 neurons in the prelimbic mPFC of the mouse by tetanic stimulation at moderate frequencies (10 Hz for 10 minutes; Lafourcade et al. 2007). LTD evoked in this way is mediated by activation of postsynaptic mGluR5 receptors, leading to a rise in intracellular calcium and activation of phospholipase C, and is expressed presynaptically as a long-term reduction in transmitter release, mediated by the release of the endogenous cannabinoid 2-acylglycerol (2-AG; Lafourcade et al. 2007). It is independent of

NMDA receptors and D1 and D2 receptors, but instead can be blocked by the cannabinoid antagonist AM251 or by the mGluR5 antagonist MPEP (Lafourcade et al. 2007).

Actions of endocannabinoids in the mPFC also play a role in the expression of olfactory fear conditioning. Infusion of a CB1 receptor agonist into the mPFC potentiates the fear response in this paradigm, while infusion of a CB1 antagonist blocks the fear response (Laviolette and Grace 2006). This correlates with single unit recordings in vivo, which showed an increase in burst firing in mPFC neurons that receive inputs from the basolateral amygdala during presentations of a conditioned stimulus. Burst firing was potentiated by microinfusions of a CB1 receptor agonist into the mPFC but blocked by a CB1 receptor antagonist (Laviolette and Grace 2006), showing that cannabinoid receptor activation in the mPFC is necessary for this form of emotional learning. Since cannabinoids mediate LTD of excitatory inputs in the mPFC in vitro (Lafourcade et al. 2007), these data present an apparent disparity between in vitro and in vivo studies. Thus the cellular basis of the actions of cannabinoids in olfactory fear conditioning remains to be elucidated, however this effect may be specific to afferents from the basolateral amygdala to the mPFC.

6. Roles Of Plasticity in the PFC

There are a number of lines of evidence pointing to a role of the mPFC in long-term memory. In humans, neuropsychological and neuroimaging studies have provided this evidence (Janowsky et al. 1989; Shimamura 1995; Buckner and Koutstaal 1998), while imaging and electrophysiological studies have shown a role for the mPFC in humans and primates in long-term recognition memory (Parkin et al. 1996; Schacter et al. 1996; Tulving et al. 1996; Kopelman and Stanhope 1998; Cabeza and Nyberg 2000; Lee et al. 2000a; Cadoret et al. 2001; Dobbins et al. 2002; Kikyo et al. 2002; Konishi et al. 2002; Petrides et al. 2002; Rugg et al. 2002; Xiang and Brown 2004). Disruption of PFC function with transcranial magnetic stimulation impairs formation of a visual recognition memory during episodic memory learning tasks, providing direct evidence a role for the PFC in the storage of long-term memories (Rossi et al. 2001; Rossi et al. 2006). Furthermore patients with damage to the PFC show similar impairments in remembering contextual details to patients with temporal lobe damage (Shimamura et al. 1990; Simons et al. 2002).

Initial evidence for the role of the PFC in long-term memory formation in animals derives from the observation that only trained animals show persistent firing during the delay period of a spatial working memory task (see below; Fuster 1973). This suggests that learning the working memory task involves plastic changes. Furthermore during operant conditioning rats exhibit either long-term decreases or increases in neuronal activity in the mPFC (Mulder et al. 2000). This requires simultaneous activation of D1 receptors, NMDA receptors and PKA in the mPFC (Baldwin et al. 2002), consistent with in vitro and in vivo studies of LTP in the mPFC (Hirsch and Crepel 1991; Gurden et al. 2000). In addition, long-term changes in the activity of mPFC neurons are involved in extinction of conditioned fear responses (see above). Specific roles of long-term memory in the mPFC are discussed below.

(i) Stimulus-action coupling

In 1949 Hebb proposed that development of the PFC is particularly important for developing schemas to solve problems that will be encountered later in life (Hebb 1949). These are learnt during the relatively late period of development of the PFC, with respect to other brain structures, and contribute to appropriate behavioural responses that, in humans, are learnt during early adulthood. Through its anatomical connections with other regions, including inputs from other cortical regions pertaining to visual, tactile and olfactory cues, as well as information about the internal milieu of the organism carried from subcortical structures, the PFC is able integrate an array of information to develop such schemas. This information can be used to plan the sequence of forthcoming actions according to the current sensory context and internal state (Shallice 1982; Kolb 1984; Robbins 1996; Shallice and Burgess 1996; Floresco et al. 1997).

Neurons in the primate dorsolateral PFC increase their firing during the delay period in a delayed response task, a model for working memory (Fuster and Alexander 1971; Kubota and Niki 1971; Kojima and Goldman-Rakic 1982). While some neurons fire at the beginning of the delay period, others fire as the delay progresses (Fuster 1995). The neurons that fire during and immediately after the cue have been attributed with encoding recent perceptual stimuli. These neurons are thought to then project to a neighbouring group of neurons that fire during the delay, encoding projections towards a future action. The latter group only display enhanced firing following learning of a particular delay-related task (Fuster 1973). These findings led Fuster to suggest that these neurons form a cortical network that encodes a stimulus-action memory (Fuster et al. 2000). In keeping with this, during learning of a spatial navigation task in rats, increased correlated firing was observed in the prelimbic mPFC, and this firing persisted after learning (Baeg et al. 2007).

As a continuation of the seminal studies by Fuster, Miller and Cohen suggested that the PFC provides a "bias" signal to the perception-action cycle (Miller and Cohen 2001). Subsequently, Otani proposed that the mPFC behaves as a "cognitive switch", coupling a particular set of stimuli with a particular set of actions, and proposed that synaptic plasticity in the mPFC is the neural trace underlying the permanent storage of these rules (Otani 2002). Consistent with this, during repeated training of working memory tasks, an improvement in performance is observed (McNamara and Scott 2001). This is thought to be mediated by synaptic plasticity in the mPFC. For example blockade of protein synthesis by infusion of anisomycin in the mPFC impairs the improvement in learning (Touzani et al. 2007). In this way declarative memories (involving the hippocampus) are linked with procedural memories (involving the striatum), thereby contributing to systematic behavioural patterns. Thus plasticity in the PFC is involved in the laying down of a repertoire of actions that have been learnt as appropriate ways to respond to a particular set of cues, in a particular behavioural context. In humans, improvements in working memory with repeated tasks may be of relevance for learning strategies to deal with complex behaviours.

(ii) Short-term memory

While the cellular basis of working memory is the persistent firing of neurons in the mPFC over delays up to 20 seconds, delays of minutes in these tasks require short-term memory storage (Runyan and Dash 2005), suggesting that short-term synaptic plasticity may underlie these effects. This has been studied in rats in the radial maze, using the delayed non-matching to place paradigm, a delayed spatial task. Connections between the hippocampus and the PFC are known to be important for this task (Floresco et al. 1997; Seamans et al. 1998). Hippocampal inputs provide spatial information for executive function in this short-term memory task over a 30 minute delay period, and are regulated by dopamine since infusion of a D1 receptor antagonist into the prelimbic mPFC before the test phase impairs performance in this task (Seamans et al. 1998). However infusion of lidocaine into the mPFC in this task does not impair behavioural performance in a short-term spatial memory paradigm, showing that the information for this task is not actively maintained in the mPFC but instead stored in the hippocampus (Seamans et al. 1995; 1998).

In addition to playing a role in learning and utilising "rules", in which the mPFC accesses long-term memories stored in other brain regions for use with working memory to guide actions, the mPFC is also important for conflict resolution in order to suppress habitual responses. This is termed behavioural flexibility, and one example of this is extinction of fear conditioning. Another is the delayed match to place task, which can be studied using an adjusted Morris water maze test where the platform is moved following training and testing (Runyan and Dash 2005). (The mPFC plays no role in spatial learning using a standard Morris water maze (de Bruin et al. 1994; Compton et al. 1997).) In this delayed match to place task, the mPFC has been shown to be important not just for working memory (lasting up to 20 seconds) but for short-term memory that requires conflict resolution (lasting minutes). This was shown to require activation of PKA because the short-term memory was blocked by infusing a PKA inhibitor into the mPFC (Runyan and Dash 2005). In contrast working memory is blocked by activation of PKA in the mPFC, showing distinct molecular mechanisms underlying working memory and short-term memory in the mPFC (Taylor et al. 1999; Runyan and Dash 2005).

(iii) Consolidation of memories

In addition to the involvement of the mPFC in the consolidation of extinction of fear memories (see above), the mPFC is also involved in the consolidation of other forms of memory. Early evidence for the role of the mPFC in consolidation of memories was provided by studies examining synaptic transmission at hippocampal-mPFC inputs, which showed a delayed but sustained potentiation of this pathway following an associative learning task (Doyere et al. 1993). Furthermore, expression of syntaxin-1B, a presynaptic protein that is a marker for LTP, is also elevated in the mPFC following a spatial memory task (Davis et al. 1996).

The infralimbic and prelimbic mPFC are important in consolidation and reconsolidation i.e. the stabilisation of long term memories once formed, of recognition memories (Akirav and Maroun 2006). This function has been assessed using an object discrimination task, which involves examining the spontaneous exploratory behaviour of a rat by measuring the time spent exploring novel versus familiar objects. Rats usually spend more time exploring novel objects, thus an impairment in memory formation is shown by rats exploring familiar objects to the same extent as novel objects. Infusion of AP5 or a protein synthesis inhibitor into the mPFC immediately following training impairs object recognition, as does infusion immediately following reactivation, showing blockade of consolidation and reconsolidation, respectively (Akirav and Maroun 2006). In contrast the mPFC has not been found to be required for short-term recognition memory, since drug infusions 3 hours after training (Akirav and Maroun 2006), which is the time scale for short-term memories in behavioural tasks (McGaugh 1966; Dudai 2004), fails to impair memory retention.

In addition to recognition memory, the prelimbic mPFC also plays a role in reward learning. Activation of c-fos is observed in the prelimbic mPFC following odour reward learning (Tronel and Sara 2002), and activation of NMDA receptors in the prelimbic mPFC is required for consolidation since infusion of AP5 into the prelimbic mPFC impairs retention of the reward memory (Tronel and Sara 2003). Consolidation of odour reward memory also requires activation of beta adrenoceptors, since infusion of a beta adrenoceptor antagonist into the prelimbic mPFC two hours after training impairs retrieval of the memory, while microdialysis showed that noradrenaline is released into the prelimbic mPFC during the consolidation period (Tronel et al. 2004).

A growing body of evidence also implicates the mPFC in the consolidation of hippocampal memories, which is thought to involve the transferral of the memory from the hippocampus to the neocortex (Wiltgen et al. 2004; Paz et al. 2007). For example, lesions of the mPFC or microinfusion of an NMDA receptor antagonist produce deficits in performance in long-term recall of trace eyeblink conditioning a month after training, while hippocampal lesions only cause a deficit within the first month (Takehara et al. 2003; Takehara-Nishiuchi et al. 2006). Furthermore remote (i.e. more than a month after training) contextual fear conditioning tasks evoke an increase in the immediate early gene zif268 in the mPFC (Frankland et al. 2004).

(iv) Neurological disorders

The prefrontal cortex has been implicated in many neurological disorders, including schizophrenia, psychosis and drug addiction, and emotional disorders, such as anxiety, depression, bipolar disorder, obsessive-compulsive disorder, sleep disorders and eating disorders. Cognitive impairments, such as a deficit in working memory, is a feature of many of these disorders (Mattes 1980; Weinberger et al. 1986; Deutch 1993; Fibiger 1995), and many of these are associated with malfunctions in dopamine signalling (Lange et al. 1992; Dolan et al. 1994; Tanda et al. 1994). There is now a growing body of evidence suggesting that disruption of synaptic plasticity in the mPFC may contribute to the pathology of these neurological disorders.

For example, in transgenic mice overexpressing amyloid precursor protein (APP) and presenilin-1, the animal model for Alzheimer's disease, LTP (evoked by tetanic stimulation at 300 Hz) is impaired at layer 5 inputs to layer 5 pyramidal neurons, due to attenuation in NMDA receptor function (Battaglia et al. 2007). Patients with Fragile X syndrome, the most commonly inherited form of mental retardation, show deficits in cognitive function (Kooy 2003). Consistent with the role of the PFC in cognitive function, spine morphology in layer 2/3 pyramidal neurons in the mPFC is altered, and the threshold for plasticity in the mPFC is raised due to malfunctions in calcium signalling and impaired L-type calcium channel function (Chen et al. 2003; Meredith et al. 2007). This impairment can be overcome by exposure to an enriched environment (Meredith et al. 2007), which has been shown to enhance dendritic growth and spine numbers in the mPFC.

(a) Schizophrenia

Disruption of cognitive function, including working memory, is a key feature of schizophrenia (Carter et al. 1998; Manoach 2003; Elvevag and Goldberg 2000). Bilateral hypofunction of the PFC has been shown to occur in schizophrenia patients, leading to profound deficits in working memory and attention (Weinberger et al. 1986; Arnsten 2007). In patients with schizophrenia, synaptic connectivity in the PFC is altered, particularly in layer 3 (Lewis and Anderson 1995; Lewis and Gonzalez-Burgos 2008), and layer 3 pyramidal neurons show reduced soma size and have reduced inhibitory inputs (Lewis and Gonzalez-Burgos 2000). Aberrations in the dopamine system in the mPFC are considered a major feature in the pathology of schizophrenia (Grace 1991; Carlsson et al. 2001). Moreover functional connectivity between the hippocampus and the mPFC is likely to be impaired given that a common symptom of schizophrenia is the inability to integrate contextual information (Bazin et al. 2000; Harrow et al. 2000; Stratta et al. 2000). Consistent with this, neonatal lesions of the ventral hippocampus, which sends a heavy projection to the mPFC, serve as an animal model for schizophrenia (Lipska and Weinberger 2002). Finally, clozapine, the atypical antipsychotic drug which at present is the most effect treatment for schizophrenia, has been shown to facilitate synaptic plasticity at hippocampal inputs to the mPFC (Dupin et al. 2006; Matsumoto et al. 2008). Together, these findings suggest that aberrations in synaptic plasticity in the mPFC may contribute to the pathology of schizophrenia. Future studies examining synaptic plasticity in the mPFC in animal models of schizophrenia will help to elucidate the cellular basis of such aberrations.

(b) Anxiety disorders, stress and post-traumatic stress disorder

Stress has a deleterious effect on cognitive function, and impairs working memory (McEwen and Sapolsky 1995). These deficits can be overcome by modulating DA levels in the mPFC (Murphy et al. 1996a; Murphy et al. 1996b). Stress can either precipitate or exacerbate other neurological disorders, such as depression, schizophrenia and Parkinson's disease (Schwab and Zieper 1965). The mPFC plays a key role in the neurocircuitry underlying responses to stress. For example it has been shown to modulate neuroendocrine responses during stress (Meaney and Aitken 1985; McEwen et al. 1986), it is selectively activated by both psychological and social stressors (Thierry et al. 1976), and acute stress induces higher glutamate release into the mPFC. Glucocorticoids released during chronic stress can cause atrophy of pyramidal cell apical dendrites and dendritic spines in layer 2/3 of the mPFC (Wellman 2001; Radley et al. 2004; Brown et al. 2005; Cerqueira et al. 2007b) and stress can impair spatial memory tasks and behavioural flexibility (Mizoguchi et al. 2000; Cerqueira et al. 2007b). Thus submitting rats to acute stress by placing them on an elevated platform for 30 minutes impairs LTP at hippocampal-PFC synapses, when evoked in vivo within 180 minutes of the acute stress treatment. This effect can be reversed by antidepressant treatment (Rocher et al. 2004). Chronic stress also impairs LTP at hippocampal-prelimbic mPFC inputs (evoked by 10 trains of stimuli at 250 Hz; Goto and Grace 2006; Cerqueira et al. 2007a). Conversely, stress evoked for only 10 minutes (by exposure to cold), facilitates LTP at these inputs (evoked by 10 trains of stimuli at 250 Hz; Goto and Grace 2006).

Pathways between the amygdala and the mPFC are also involved in the response to stress. Acute stress blocks LTP at inputs from the basolateral amygdala to the prelimbic mPFC (Maroun and Richter-Levin 2003). Conversely, stress reduces LTD (evoked by low frequency stimulation) and facilitates LTP at inputs from the prelimbic and infralimbic mPFC to the basolateral amygdala (Maroun 2006). Thus it appears that higher order processing in the mPFC is impaired during stress to allow more autonomic-type responses, mediated by plasticity in the amygdala. Functionally, it is now widely viewed that phobias and post-traumatic stress disorder result from an inability to extinguish fear memories. For example, patients with post-traumatic stress disorder have reduced activity in the mPFC during recall of the traumatic event (Bremner et al. 1999), but increases in mPFC activity following successful therapeutic treatment (Fernandez et al. 2001). Consistent with this, stress can impair extinction (Miracle et al. 2006), and has been shown to increase dendritic branching and spine numbers in the basolateral amygdala (Vyas et al. 2002; Mitra et al. 2005; Vyas et al. 2006), but to decrease dendritic branching in the infralimbic PFC (Izquierdo et al. 2006).

(c) Depression

Evidence from post-mortem studies and fMRI has suggested that antidepressants such as fluoxetine ("Prozac") act by enhancing neurogenesis and structural plasticity, leading to the "neurotoxic hypothesis" (Manji and Duman 2001; Santarelli et al. 2003; Fossati et al. 2004). This hypothesis states that depression results from an impairment in establishing new neuronal adaptations, synaptic connections and synaptic plasticity, in addition to changes in neurotransmitter concentrations and receptor levels. Some of this "neurotoxicity" is likely to reside in the mPFC and in connections between the hippocampus and mPFC. For example, prolonged depression is associated with atrophy of the prefrontal cortex, particularly dendritic atrophy in layer 2/3 (Ongur et al. 1998; Cook and Wellman 2004; Fossati et al. 2004; Radley et al. 2004), in addition to atrophy of the hippocampus (Bremner et al. 2000). A reduction in metabolic activity in the mPFC (Dolan et al. 1994; Drevets et al. 1997), in association with cognitive dysfunction (Dolan et al. 1992), is also seen during depression, and can be reversed by treatment by selective serotonin reuptake inhibitors (SSRI; Kennedy et al. 2001). Furthermore, chronic antidepressant treatment evokes increases in the expression of molecules associated with synaptic plasticity in the mPFC, namely CREB, synaptophysin and the polysialylated form of nerve cell adhesion molecule (PSA-NCAM; Tiraboschi et al. 2004; Laifenfeld et al. 2005; Sairanen et al. 2007; Varea et al. 2007a; Varea et al. 2007b). Finally, and consistent with the notion that connections between the hippocampus and the mPFC may be impaired in depression, treatment with an SSRI also enhances synaptic transmission and LTP at hippocampal-mPFC synapses in vivo (Ohashi et al. 2002).

(v) Drugs of abuse

Many drugs of abuse have been shown to exert actions in the mPFC. For example, many drugs cause cognitive impairments (Moghaddam et al. 1997; Bisagno et al. 2002; Nordahl et al. 2003). The psychotomimetic drugs ketamine and phencyclidine have been shown to increase glutamate and dopamine levels in the rat mPFC, which is associated with an impairment of working memory (Nishijima et al. 1994; Moghaddam et al. 1997; Adams and

Moghaddam 1998), and which can be reversed by blocking glutamate release (Moghaddam and Adams 1998).

Over the longer term, behavioural sensitisation, the process by which the behavioural effect of a drug is enhanced with repeated applications, and which may contribute to drug addiction and craving (Robinson and Berridge 1993; Hyman 1996), has been postulated to be mediated by synaptic or structural plasticity in the mPFC. Treatment of animals with amphetamine leads to a marked enhancement of dendritic length and spine density (Uranova et al. 1989; Robinson and Kolb 1999). 3,4-methylenedioxymetamphetamine (MDMA)-induced behavioural sensitisation is prevented by blocking $5HT_{2C}$ receptors in the mPFC (Ramos et al. 2005a) or by lesioning the mPFC (Ramos et al. 2005b). Repetitive treatment with methamphetamine impairs LTP evoked by tetanic stimulation (10 trains of stimuli at 250 Hz for 200 ms) of hippocampal inputs to the mPFC in vivo, an effect that can be blocked by a D1 receptor antagonist (Ishikawa et al. 2005).

Lesioning the PFC also prevents the development of cocaine-induced behavioural sensitisation (Tzschentke 2001). However, in contrast to methamphetamine, repeated cocaine administration, at a level sufficient to induce behavioural sensitisation, facilitates the induction of LTP (evoked by bursts of EPSP-spike pairs) at layer 2/3 inputs to layer 5 pyramidal neurons in the prelimbic mPFC in vitro. This action is mediated by a reduction in inhibitory drive through activation of D1 receptors, PKA and a subsequent reduction in the surface expression of the $GABA_A$ □1 subunit (Huang et al. 2007a). Repeated treatment with cocaine also impairs LTD mediated by group 2 mGluRs at layer 5 inputs to layer 5 pyramidal neurons (Huang et al. 2007b). This latter effect of cocaine is mediated by activation of D1 receptors, leading to elevations in cAMP. Cyclic AMP is subsequently broken down to adenosine, which then acts at adenosine A_3 receptors to activate PKC, inhibiting group 2 mGluR function, possibly by uncoupling the receptors from their G proteins. The functional significance of the opposite effects of amphetamine and cocaine on plasticity in the mPFC is not known at present.

Finally, acute treatment of lysergic acid diethylamine (LSD) or nicotine induces expression of a number of genes in the PFC that encode proteins that have been shown to play a role in synaptic plasticity. These include c-fos and activity related cytoskeletal protein (arc; Nichols et al. 2003; Schochet et al. 2005).

7. CONCLUSION

In summary, synapses in the mPFC are highly plastic, displaying several types of short-term as well as long-term plasticity. Short-term plasticity is observed during trains of EPSPs as well as during repetitive suprathreshold stimulation, and is therefore likely to be induced during basal transmission and during the repetitive firing observed during working memory tasks. Such heterogeneity of short-term plasticity in the mPFC is likely to be important for its role in the rapid switching of attention during cognitive processing, reducing distractions and endowing the mPFC with highly flexible computational abilities. Long-term synaptic plasticity is important for learning sequences of behavioural responses, or "rules" to different sensory contexts, and for consolidation of memories that are acquired elsewhere in the brain, such as in the hippocampus or amygdala. Thus it is now well established that in addition to short-term memory tasks such as working memory, the mPFC also plays an important role in long-term memories.

The cellular mechanisms underlying synaptic plasticity at mPFC synapses are similar to those in other brain regions where synaptic plasticity has been well studied, such as the hippocampus. Both LTD and LTP require a both rise in postsynaptic calcium, and they both generally require activation of NMDA receptors. Furthermore, activation of PKA, MAP kinase, CREB phosphorylation, and protein synthesis point to similar molecular mechanisms underlying plasticity. While neuromodulation by dopamine has been well studied, the effects of other neuromodulators such as 5-HT, acetylcholine and noradrenaline remain largely elusive. Given that 5-HT in the mPFC is known to be essential for mood regulation, and acetylcholine for cognitive abilities, elucidating the effects of these neuromodulators on synaptic plasticity may provide insights into the cellular basis of these cognitive functions.

The most striking difference between synaptic plasticity in the mPFC and in other brain regions is the similarity in induction protocols that induce LTP and LTD in the mPFC. All but two studies (Milad and Quirk 2002; Huang et al. 2004) have evoked LTD with the same high frequency stimulation both in vitro (Hirsch and Crepel 1990; Auclair et al. 2000) and in vivo (Takita et al. 1999) that can induce LTP. The relationship between LTP and LTD in other brain areas, such as the hippocampus and other cortical regions, is determined by the amount of calcium influx during the induction protocol, with greater calcium rises associated with LTP and lesser calcium rises associated with LTD (Dudek and Bear 1992; Kirkwood et al. 1993; Dudek and Friedlander 1996; Manabe 1997). The reason for the disparity in LTD induction in the mPFC is not clear, but may be due to a higher NMDA receptor-mediated contribution to basal synaptic transmission at synapses in the mPFC (Faber, unpublished observations; Wang 2001), shifting the rules for synaptic plasticity induction. An investigation into the properties of spike timing-dependent plasticity, in addition to calcium imaging of spines and dendrites undergoing synaptic plasticity, would help to elucidate these discrepancies.

Disorders of synaptic plasticity in the mPFC may contribute to the pathology of a range of psychiatric disorders, including Alzheimer's disease, mental retardation, depression, anxiety disorders, and drug addiction. Therefore it is crucial to understand the cellular mechanisms underlying synaptic plasticity in the mPFC, to understand not only the mechanisms underlying normal cognitive processes, the functioning of the mind and "conscious" thought processes, but also to pave the way to the development of improved therapies of neurological disorders, for which the current treatments are very poor.

ACKNOWLEDGEMENTS

I would like to thank Jeremy Seamans and Satoru Otani for their useful comments on this chapter.

REFERENCES

Abraham, W.C., Bear, M.F. (1996). Metaplasticity: the plasticity of synaptic plasticity. *Trends Neurosci*, 19 (4), 126-130.

Adams, B., Moghaddam, B. (1998). Corticolimbic dopamine neurotransmission is temporally dissociated from the cognitive and locomotor effects of phencyclidine. *J Neurosci*, 18 (14), 5545-5554.

Akirav, I., Maroun, M. (2006). Ventromedial prefrontal cortex is obligatory for consolidation and reconsolidation of object recognition memory. *Cereb Cortex*, 16 (12), 1759-1765.

Ameri, A. (1999). The effects of cannabinoids on the brain. *Prog Neurobiol*, 58 (4), 315-348.

Anglada-Figueroa, D., Quirk, G.J. (2005). Lesions of the basal amygdala block expression of conditioned fear but not extinction. *J Neurosci*, 25 (42), 9680-9685.

Aoki, C., Venkatesan, C., Kurose, H. (1998). Noradrenergic modulation of the prefrontal cortex as revealed by electron microscopic immunocytochemistry. *Adv Pharmacol*, 42, 777-780.

Arnsten, A.F. (1997). Catecholamine regulation of the prefrontal cortex. *J Psychopharmacol*, 11 (2), 151-162.

Arnsten, A.F. (2007). Catecholamine and second messenger influences on prefrontal cortical networks of "representational knowledge": a rational bridge between genetics and the symptoms of mental illness. *Cereb Cortex*, 17 Suppl 1, i6-15.

Artola, A., Singer, W. (1993). Long-term depression of excitatory synaptic transmission and its relationship to long-term potentiation. *Trends Neurosci*, 16 (11), 480-487.

Atzori, M., Lei, S., Evans, D.I., Kanold, P.O., Phillips-Tansey. E., McIntyre, O., McBain, C.J. (2001). Differential synaptic processing separates stationary from transient inputs to the auditory cortex. *Nat Neurosci*, 4 (12), 1230-1237.

Auclair, N., Otani, S., Soubrie, P., Crepel, F.(2000). Cannabinoids modulate synaptic strength and plasticity at glutamatergic synapses of rat prefrontal cortex pyramidal neurons. *J Neurophysiol*, 83 (6), 3287-3293.

Azmitia, E.C., Segal, M. (1978). An autoradiographic analysis of the differential ascending projections of the dorsal and median raphe nuclei in the rat. *J Comp Neurol*, 179 (3), 641-667.

Baeg, E.H., Kim, Y.B., Jang, J., Kim, H.T., Mook-Jung, I., Jung, M.W. (2001). Fast spiking and regular spiking neural correlates of fear conditioning in the medial prefrontal cortex of the rat. *Cereb Cortex*, 11 (5), 441-451.

Baeg, E.H., Kim, Y.B., Kim, J., Ghim, J.W., Kim, J.J., Jung, M.W. (2007). Learning-induced enduring changes in functional connectivity among prefrontal cortical neurons. *J Neurosci*, 27 (4), 909-918.

Baldwin, A.E., Sadeghian, K., Kelley, A.E. (2002). Appetitive instrumental learning requires coincident activation of NMDA and dopamine D1 receptors within the medial prefrontal cortex. *J Neurosci*, 22 (3), 1063-1071.

Barbara, J.G., Auclair, N., Roisin, M.P., Otani, S., Valjent, E., Caboche, J., Soubrie, P., Crepel, F. (2003). Direct and indirect interactions between cannabinoid CB1 receptor and group II metabotropic glutamate receptor signalling in layer V pyramidal neurons from the rat prefrontal cortex. *Eur J Neurosci*, 17 (5), 981-990.

Barrett, D., Shumake, J., Jones, D., Gonzalez-Lima, F. (2003). Metabolic mapping of mouse brain activity after extinction of a conditioned emotional response. *J Neurosci*, 23 (13), 5740-5749.

Bassareo, V., Di Chiara, G. (1997). Differential influence of associative and nonassociative learning mechanisms on the responsiveness of prefrontal and accumbal dopamine transmission to food stimuli in rats fed ad libitum. *J Neurosci*, 17 (2), 851-861.

Battaglia, F., Wang, H.Y., Ghilardi, M.F., Gashi, E., Quartarone, A., Friedman, E., Nixon, R.A. (2007). Cortical plasticity in Alzheimer's disease in humans and rodents. *Biol Psychiatry*, 62 (12), 1405-1412.

Bazin, N., Perruchet, P., Hardy-Bayle, M.C., Feline, A. (2000). Context-dependent information processing in patients with schizophrenia. *Schizophr Res*, 45 (1-2), 93-101.

Bergson, C., Mrzljak, L., Lidow, M.S., Goldman-Rakic, P.S., Levenson, R. (1995). Characterization of subtype-specific antibodies to the human D5 dopamine receptor: studies in primate brain and transfected mammalian cells. *Proc Natl Acad Sci USA*, 92 (8), 3468-3472.

Berretta, S., Pantazopoulos, H., Caldera, M., Pantazopoulos, P., Pare, D. (2005). Infralimbic cortex activation increases c-Fos expression in intercalated neurons of the amygdala. *Neuroscience*, 132 (4), 943-953.

Birrell, J.M., Brown, V.J. (2000). Medial frontal cortex mediates perceptual attentional set shifting in the rat. *J Neurosci*, 20 (11), 4320-4324.

Bisagno, V., Ferguson, D., Luine, V.N. (2002). Short toxic methamphetamine schedule impairs object recognition task in male rats. *Brain Res*, 940 (1-2), 95-101.

Blond, O., Crepel, F., Otani, S. (2002). Long-term potentiation in rat prefrontal slices facilitated by phased application of dopamine. *Eur J Pharmacol*, 438 (1-2), 115-116.

Blum, S., Hebert, A.E., Dash, P.K. (2006). A role for the prefrontal cortex in recall of recent and remote memories. *Neuroreport*, 17 (3), 341-344.

Bouton, M.E. (1993). Context, time, and memory retrieval in the interference paradigms of Pavlovian learning. *Psychol Bull*, 114 (1), 80-99.

Bouton, M.E., Westbrook, R.F., Corcoran, K.A., Maren, S. (2006). Contextual and temporal modulation of extinction: behavioral and biological mechanisms. *Biol Psychiatry*, 60 (4), 352-360.

Branchereau, P., Van Bockstaele, E.J., Chan, J., Pickel, V.M. (1996). Pyramidal neurons in rat prefrontal cortex show a complex synaptic response to single electrical stimulation of the locus coeruleus region: evidence for antidromic activation and GABAergic inhibition using in vivo intracellular recording and electron microscopy. *Synapse*, 22 (4), 313-331.

Bredy, T.W., Wu, H., Crego, C., Zellhoefer, J., Sun, Y.E., Barad, M. (2007). Histone modifications around individual BDNF gene promoters in prefrontal cortex are associated with extinction of conditioned fear. *Learn Mem*, 14 (4), 268-276.

Bremner, J.D., Narayan, M., Anderson, E.R., Staib, L.H., Miller, H.L., Charney, D.S. (2000). Hippocampal volume reduction in major depression. *Am J Psychiatry*, 157 (1), 115-118.

Bremner, J.D., Staib, L.H., Kaloupek, D., Southwick, S.M., Soufer, R., Charney, D.S. (1999). Neural correlates of exposure to traumatic pictures and sound in Vietnam combat veterans with and without posttraumatic stress disorder: a positron emission tomography study. *Biol Psychiatry*, 45 (7), 806-816.

Brown, S.M., Henning, S., Wellman, C.L. (2005). Mild, short-term stress alters dendritic morphology in rat medial prefrontal cortex. *Cereb Cortex*, 15 (11), 1714-1722.

Brozoski, T.J., Brown, R.M., Rosvold, H.E., Goldman, P.S. (1979). Cognitive deficit caused by regional depletion of dopamine in prefrontal cortex of rhesus monkey. *Science*, 205 (4409), 929-932.

Buckner, R.L., Koutstaal, W. (1998). Functional neuroimaging studies of encoding, priming, and explicit memory retrieval. *Proc Natl Acad Sci USA*, 95 (3), 891-898.

Burette, F., Jay, T.M., Laroche, S. (1997). Reversal of LTP in the hippocampal afferent fiber system to the prefrontal cortex in vivo with low-frequency patterns of stimulation that do not produce LTD. *J Neurophysiol*, 78 (2), 1155-1160.

Burgos-Robles, A., Vidal-Gonzalez, I., Santini, E., Quirk, G.J. (2007). Consolidation of fear extinction requires NMDA receptor-dependent bursting in the ventromedial prefrontal cortex. *Neuron*, 53 (6), 871-880.

Buzsaki, G. (2002). Theta oscillations in the hippocampus. *Neuron*, 33 (3), 325-340.

Cabeza, R., Nyberg, L. (2000). Imaging cognition II: An empirical review of 275 PET and fMRI studies. *J Cogn Neurosci*, 12 (1), 1-47.

Cadoret, G., Pike, G.B., Petrides, M. (2001). Selective activation of the ventrolateral prefrontal cortex in the human brain during active retrieval processing. *Eur J Neurosci*, 14 (7), 1164-1170.

Calabresi, P., Fedele, E., Pisani, A., Fontana, G., Mercuri, N.B., Bernardi, G., Raiteri, M. (1995). Transmitter release associated with long-term synaptic depression in rat corticostriatal slices. *Eur J Neurosci*, 7 (9), 1889-1894.

Carlsson, A., Waters, N., Holm-Waters, S., Tedroff, J., Nilsson, M., Carlsson, M.L. (2001). Interactions between monoamines, glutamate, and GABA in schizophrenia: new evidence. *Annu Rev Pharmacol Toxicol*, 41, 237-260.

Carr, D.B., Sesack, S.R. (1996). Hippocampal afferents to the rat prefrontal cortex: synaptic targets and relation to dopamine terminals. *J Comp Neurol*, 369 (1), 1-15.

Carter, C.S., Perlstein, W., Ganguli, R., Brar, J., Mintun, M., Cohen, J.D. (1998). Functional hypofrontality and working memory dysfunction in schizophrenia. *Am J Psychiatry*, 155 (9), 1285-1287.

Cassell, M.D., Chittick, C.A., Siegel, M.A., Wright, D.J. (1989). Collateralization of the amygdaloid projections of the rat prelimbic and infralimbic cortices. *J Comp Neurol*, 279 (2), 235-248.

Cassell, M.D., Wright, D.J. (1986). Topography of projections from the medial prefrontal cortex to the amygdala in the rat. *Brain Res Bull*, 17 (3), 321-333.

Cerqueira, J.J., Mailliet, F., Almeida, O.F., Jay, T.M., Sousa, N. (2007a). The prefrontal cortex as a key target of the maladaptive response to stress. *J Neurosci*, 27 (11), 2781-2787.

Cerqueira, J.J., Taipa, R., Uylings, H.B., Almeida, O.F., Sousa, N. (2007b). Specific configuration of dendritic degeneration in pyramidal neurons of the medial prefrontal cortex induced by differing corticosteroid regimens. *Cereb Cortex*, 17 (9), 1998-2006.

Chen, L., Yun, S.W., Seto, J., Liu, W., Toth, M. (2003). The fragile X mental retardation protein binds and regulates a novel class of mRNAs containing U rich target sequences. *Neuroscience*, 120 (4), 1005-1017.

Chhatwal, J.P., Davis, M., Maguschak, K.A., Ressler, K.J. (2005). Enhancing cannabinoid neurotransmission augments the extinction of conditioned fear. *Neuropsychopharmacology*, 30 (3), 516-524.

Civelli, O., Bunzow, J.R., Grandy, D.K. (1993). Molecular diversity of the dopamine receptors. *Annu Rev Pharmacol Toxicol*, 33, 281-307.

Compton, D.M., Griffith, H.R., McDaniel, W.F., Foster, R.A., Davis, B.K. (1997). The flexible use of multiple cue relationships in spatial navigation: a comparison of water maze performance following hippocampal, medial septal, prefrontal cortex, or posterior parietal cortex lesions. *Neurobiol Learn Mem*, 68 (2), 117-132.

Cook, S.C., Wellman, C.L. (2004). Chronic stress alters dendritic morphology in rat medial prefrontal cortex. *J Neurobiol*, 60 (2), 236-248.

Corcoran, K.A., Quirk, G.J. (2007). Activity in prelimbic cortex is necessary for the expression of learned, but not innate, fears. *J Neurosci*, 27 (4), 840-844.

Cormier, R.J., Greenwood, A.C., Connor, J.A. (2001). Bidirectional synaptic plasticity correlated with the magnitude of dendritic calcium transients above a threshold. *J Neurophysiol*, 85 (1), 399-406.

Couey, J.J., Meredith, R.M., Spijker, S., Poorthuis, R.B., Smit, A.B., Brussaard, A.B., Mansvelder, H.D. (2007). Distributed network actions by nicotine increase the threshold for spike-timing-dependent plasticity in prefrontal cortex. *Neuron*, 54 (1), 73-87.

Dan, Y., Poo, M.M. (2004). Spike timing-dependent plasticity of neural circuits. *Neuron*, 44 (1), 23-30.

Davis, S., Rodger, J., Hicks, A., Mallet, J., Laroche, S. (1996). Brain structure and task-specific increase in expression of the gene encoding syntaxin 1B during learning in the rat: a potential molecular marker for learning-induced synaptic plasticity in neural networks. *Eur J Neurosci*, 8 (10), 2068-2074.

de Bruin, J.P., Sanchez-Santed, F., Heinsbroek, R.P., Donker, A., Postmes, P. (1994). A behavioural analysis of rats with damage to the medial prefrontal cortex using the Morris water maze: evidence for behavioural flexibility, but not for impaired spatial navigation. *Brain Res*, 652 (2), 323-333.

Degenetais, E., Thierry, A.M., Glowinski, J., Gioanni, Y. (2002). Electrophysiological properties of pyramidal neurons in the rat prefrontal cortex: an in vivo intracellular recording study. *Cereb Cortex*, 12 (1), 1-16.

Degenetais, E., Thierry, A.M., Glowinski, J., Gioanni, Y. (2003). Synaptic influence of hippocampus on pyramidal cells of the rat prefrontal cortex: an in vivo intracellular recording study. *Cereb Cortex*, 13 (7), 782-792.

Deutch, A.Y. (1993). Prefrontal cortical dopamine systems and the elaboration of functional corticostriatal circuits: implications for schizophrenia and Parkinson's disease. *J Neural Transm Gen Sect*, 91 (2-3), 197-221.

Dobbins, I.G., Foley, H., Schacter, D.L., Wagner, A.D. (2002). Executive control during episodic retrieval: multiple prefrontal processes subserve source memory. *Neuron*, 35 (5), 989-996.

Dolan, R.J., Bench, C.J., Brown, R.G., Scott, L.C., Frackowiak, R.S. (1994). Neuropsychological dysfunction in depression: the relationship to regional cerebral blood flow. *Psychol Med*, 24 (4), 849-857.

Dolan, R.J., Bench, C.J., Brown, R.G., Scott, L.C., Friston, K.J., Frackowiak, R.S. (1992). Regional cerebral blood flow abnormalities in depressed patients with cognitive impairment. *J Neurol Neurosurg Psychiatry*, 55 (9), 768-773.

Doyere, V., Burette, F., Negro, C.R., Laroche, S. (1993). Long-term potentiation of hippocampal afferents and efferents to prefrontal cortex: implications for associative learning. *Neuropsychologia*, 31 (10), 1031-1053.

Drevets, W.C., Price, J.L., Simpson, J.R. Jr., Todd, R.D., Reich, T., Vannier, M., Raichle, M.E. (1997). Subgenual prefrontal cortex abnormalities in mood disorders. *Nature*, 386 (6627), 824-827.

Dudai, Y. (2004). The neurobiology of consolidations, or, how stable is the engram? *Annu Rev Psychol*, 55, 51-86.

Dudek, S.M., Bear, M.F. (1992). Homosynaptic long-term depression in area CA1 of hippocampus and effects of N-methyl-D-aspartate receptor blockade. *Proc Natl Acad Sci USA*, 89 (10), 4363-4367.

Dudek, S.M., Friedlander, M.J. (1996). Developmental down-regulation of LTD in cortical layer IV and its independence of modulation by inhibition. *Neuron*, 16 (6), 1097-1106.

Dudman, J.T., Eaton, M.E., Rajadhyaksha, A., Macias, W., Taher, M., Barczak, A., Kameyama, K., Huganir, R., Konradi, C. (2003). Dopamine D1 receptors mediate CREB phosphorylation via phosphorylation of the NMDA receptor at Ser897-NR1. *J Neurochem*, 87 (4), 922-934.

Dupin, N., Mailliet, F., Rocher, C., Kessal, K., Spedding, M., Jay, T.M. (2006). Common efficacy of psychotropic drugs in restoring stress-induced impairment of prefrontal plasticity. *Neurotox Res*, 10 (3-4), 193-198.

Durstewitz, D., Seamans, J.K. (2006). Beyond bistability: biophysics and temporal dynamics of working memory. *Neuroscience*, 139 (1), 119-133.

Edagawa, Y., Saito, H., Abe, K. (1999). Stimulation of the 5-HT1A receptor selectively suppresses NMDA receptor-mediated synaptic excitation in the rat visual cortex. *Brain Res*, 827 (1-2), 225-228.

Elston, G.N. (2003). Cortex, cognition and the cell: new insights into the pyramidal neuron and prefrontal function. *Cereb Cortex*, 13 (11), 1124-1138.

Elvevag, B., Goldberg, T.E. (2000). Cognitive impairment in schizophrenia is the core of the disorder. *Crit Rev Neurobiol*, 14 (1), 1-21.

Everitt, B.J., Robbins, T.W. (1997). Central cholinergic systems and cognition. *Annu Rev Psychol*, 48, 649-684.

Farinelli, M., Deschaux, O., Hugues, S., Thevenet, A., Garcia, R. (2006). Hippocampal train stimulation modulates recall of fear extinction independently of prefrontal cortex synaptic plasticity and lesions. *Learn Mem*, 13 (3), 329-334.

Fernandez Espejo, E. (2003). Prefrontocortical dopamine loss in rats delays long-term extinction of contextual conditioned fear, and reduces social interaction without affecting short-term social interaction memory. *Neuropsychopharmacology*, 28 (3), 490-498.

Fernandez, M., Pissiota, A., Frans, O., von Knorring, L., Fischer, H., Fredrikson, M. (2001). Brain function in a patient with torture related post-traumatic stress disorder before and after fluoxetine treatment: a positron emission tomography provocation study. *Neurosci Lett*, 297 (2), 101-104.

Ferraro, L., Tomasini, M.C., Gessa, G.L., Bebe, B.W., Tanganelli, S., Antonelli, T. (2001). The cannabinoid receptor agonist WIN 55,212-2 regulates glutamate transmission in rat cerebral cortex: an in vivo and in vitro study. *Cereb Cortex*, 11 (8), 728-733.

Fibiger, H.C. (1995). Neurobiology of depression: focus on dopamine. *Adv Biochem Psychopharmacol*, 49, 1-17.

Floresco, S.B., Phillips, A.G. (2001). Delay-dependent modulation of memory retrieval by infusion of a dopamine D1 agonist into the rat medial prefrontal cortex. *Behav Neurosci*, 115 (4), 934-939.

Floresco, S.B., Seamans, J.K., Phillips, A.G. (1997). Selective roles for hippocampal, prefrontal cortical, and ventral striatal circuits in radial-arm maze tasks with or without a delay. *J Neurosci*, 17 (5), 1880-1890.

Fossati, P., Radtchenko, A., Boyer, P. (2004). Neuroplasticity: from MRI to depressive symptoms. *Eur Neuropsychopharmacol*, 14 Suppl 5, S503-510.

Frankland, P.W., Bontempi, B., Talton, L.E., Kaczmarek, L., Silva, A.J. (2004). The involvement of the anterior cingulate cortex in remote contextual fear memory. *Science*, 304 (5672), 881-883.

Fuhrmann, G., Segev, I., Markram, H., Tsodyks, M. (2002). Coding of temporal information by activity-dependent synapses. *J Neurophysiol*, 87 (1), 140-148.

Funahashi, S., Bruce, C.J., Goldman-Rakic, P.S. (1989). Mnemonic coding of visual space in the monkey's dorsolateral prefrontal cortex. *J Neurophysiol*, 61 (2), 331-349.

Fuster, J.M. (1973). Unit activity in prefrontal cortex during delayed-response performance: neuronal correlates of transient memory. *J Neurophysiol*, 36 (1), 61-78.

Fuster, J.M. (1995). Memory in the Cerebral Cortex. Cambridge, Massachusetts: MIT Press.

Fuster, J.M. (2001). The prefrontal cortex--an update: time is of the essence. *Neuron*, 30 (2), 319-333.

Fuster, J.M., Alexander, G.E. (1971). Neuron activity related to short-term memory. *Science*, 173 (997), 652-654.

Fuster, J.M., Bodner, M., Kroger, J.K. (2000). Cross-modal and cross-temporal association in neurons of frontal cortex. *Nature*, 405 (6784), 347-351.

Gabbott, P., Headlam, A., Busby, S. (2002). Morphological evidence that CA1 hippocampal afferents monosynaptically innervate PV-containing neurons and NADPH-diaphorase reactive cells in the medial prefrontal cortex (Areas 25/32) of the rat. *Brain Res*, 946 (2), 314-322.

Gabbott, P.L., Warner, T.A., Busby, S.J. (2006). Amygdala input monosynaptically innervates parvalbumin immunoreactive local circuit neurons in rat medial prefrontal cortex. *Neuroscience*, 139 (3), 1039-1048.

Gabbott, P.L., Warner, T.A., Jays, P.R., Bacon, S.J. (2003). Areal and synaptic interconnectivity of prelimbic (area 32), infralimbic (area 25) and insular cortices in the rat. *Brain Res*, 993 (1-2), 59-71.

Gao, W.J., Krimer, L.S., Goldman-Rakic, P.S. (2001). Presynaptic regulation of recurrent excitation by D1 receptors in prefrontal circuits. *Proc Natl Acad Sci USA*, 98 (1), 295-300.

Garcia, R. (2002). Postextinction of conditioned fear: between two CS-related memories. *Learn Mem*, 9 (6), 361-363.

Garcia, R., Chang, C.H., Maren, S. (2006). Electrolytic lesions of the medial prefrontal cortex do not interfere with long-term memory of extinction of conditioned fear. *Learn Mem*, 13 (1), 14-17.

Garcia, R., Jaffard, R. (1996). Changes in synaptic excitability in the lateral septum associated with contextual and auditory fear conditioning in mice. *Eur J Neurosci*, 8 (4), 809-815.

Garcia, R., Tocco, G., Baudry, M., Thompson, R.F. (1998). Exposure to a conditioned aversive environment interferes with long-term potentiation induction in the fimbria-CA3 pathway. *Neuroscience*, 82 (1), 139-145.

Garris, P.A., Collins, L.B., Jones, S.R., Wightman, R.M. (1993). Evoked extracellular dopamine in vivo in the medial prefrontal cortex. *J Neurochem*, 61 (2), 637-647.

Garris, P.A., Wightman, R.M. (1994). Different kinetics govern dopaminergic transmission in the amygdala, prefrontal cortex, and striatum: an in vivo voltammetric study. *J Neurosci*, 14 (1), 442-450.

Gaspar, P., Bloch, B., Le Moine, C. (1995). D1 and D2 receptor gene expression in the rat frontal cortex: cellular localization in different classes of efferent neurons. *Eur J Neurosci*, 7 (5), 1050-1063.

Gewirtz, J.C., Falls, W.A., Davis, M. (1997). Normal conditioned inhibition and extinction of freezing and fear-potentiated startle following electrolytic lesions of medical prefrontal cortex in rats. *Behav Neurosci*, 111 (4), 712-726.

Gigg, J., Tan, A.M., Finch, D.M. (1994). Glutamatergic hippocampal formation projections to prefrontal cortex in the rat are regulated by GABAergic inhibition and show convergence with glutamatergic projections from the limbic thalamus. *Hippocampus*, 4 (2), 189-198.

Gilmartin, M.R., McEchron, M.D. (2005). Single neurons in the medial prefrontal cortex of the rat exhibit tonic and phasic coding during trace fear conditioning. *Behav Neurosci*, 119 (6), 1496-1510.

Goldman-Rakic, P.S. (1995). Cellular basis of working memory. *Neuron*, 14 (3), 477-485.

Goldman-Rakic, P.S. (1999). The "psychic" neuron of the cerebral cortex. *Ann N Y Acad Sci*, 868, 13-26.

Goldman-Rakic, P.S., Leranth, C., Williams, S.M., Mons, N., Geffard, M. (1989). Dopamine synaptic complex with pyramidal neurons in primate cerebral cortex. *Proc Natl Acad Sci U S A*, 86(22), 9015-9019.

Gonzalez Burgos, G., Kroener, S., Seamans, J.K. Cellular Mechanisms of Working Memory and its Modulation by Dopamine in the Prefrontal Cortex of Primates and Rats. In: KY Tseng, M Atzori, (Eds.) Monoaminergic modulation of cortical excitability (1st edition, pp125-152)

Gonzalez-Burgos, G., Barrionuevo, G., Lewis, D.A. (2000). Horizontal synaptic connections in monkey prefrontal cortex: an in vitro electrophysiological study. *Cereb Cortex,* 10 (1), 82-92.

Gonzalez-Burgos, G., Krimer, L.S., Urban, N.N., Barrionuevo, G., Lewis, D.A. (2004). Synaptic efficacy during repetitive activation of excitatory inputs in primate dorsolateral prefrontal cortex. *Cereb Cortex*,14 (5), 530-542.

Gonzalez-Lima, F., Bruchey, A.K. (2004). Extinction memory improvement by the metabolic enhancer methylene blue. *Learn Mem*, 11 (5), 633-640.

Goosens, K.A., Maren, S. (2003). Pretraining NMDA receptor blockade in the basolateral complex, but not the central nucleus, of the amygdala prevents savings of conditional fear. *Behav Neurosci*, 117 (4), 738-750.

Goto, Y., Grace, A.A. (2006). Alterations in medial prefrontal cortical activity and plasticity in rats with disruption of cortical development. *Biol Psychiatry*, 60 (11), 1259-1267.

Goto, Y., Grace, A.A. (2007). Dopamine Modulation of Hippocampal Prefrontal Cortical Interaction Drives Memory-Guided *Behavior. Cereb Cortex*.

Goto, Y., Otani, S., Grace, A.A. (2007). The Yin and Yang of dopamine release: a new perspective. *Neuropharmacology*, 53 (5), 583-587.

Grace, A.A. (1991). Phasic versus tonic dopamine release and the modulation of dopamine system responsivity: a hypothesis for the etiology of schizophrenia. *Neuroscience*, 41 (1), 1-24.

Green, J.D., Arduini, A.A. (1954). Hippocampal electrical activity in arousal. *J Neurophysiol*, 17 (6), 533-557.

Groenewegen, H.J., Uylings, H.B. (2000). The prefrontal cortex and the integration of sensory, limbic and autonomic information. *Prog Brain Res*, 126, 3-28.

Gurden, H., Takita, M., Jay, T.M. (2000). Essential role of D1 but not D2 receptors in the NMDA receptor-dependent long-term potentiation at hippocampal-prefrontal cortex synapses in vivo. *J Neurosci*, 20 (22), RC106.

Gurden, H., Tassin, J.P., Jay, T.M. (1999). Integrity of the mesocortical dopaminergic system is necessary for complete expression of in vivo hippocampal-prefrontal cortex long-term potentiation. *Neuroscience*, 94 (4), 1019-1027.

Guzman, S.J., Gerevich, Z., Hengstler, J.G., Illes, P., Kleemann, W. (2005). P2Y1 receptors inhibit both strength and plasticity of glutamatergic synaptic neurotransmission in the rat prefrontal cortex. *Synapse*, 57 (4), 235-238.

Hansel, C., Artola, A., Singer, W. (1996). Different threshold levels of postsynaptic [Ca2+]i have to be reached to induce LTP and LTD in neocortical pyramidal cells. *J Physiol Paris*, 90 (5-6), 317-319.

Harrow, M., Green, K.E., Sands, J.R., Jobe, T.H., Goldberg, J.F., Kaplan, K.J., Martin, E.M. (2000). Thought disorder in schizophrenia and mania: impaired context. *Schizophr Bull*, 26 (4), 879-891.

Hebb, D.O. (1949). The Organisation of Behaviour. New York: John Wiley and Sons.

Heidbreder, C.A., Groenewegen, H.J. (2003). The medial prefrontal cortex in the rat: evidence for a dorso-ventral distinction based upon functional and anatomical characteristics. *Neurosci Biobehav Rev*, 27 (6), 555-579.

Hempel, C.M., Hartman, K.H., Wang, X.J., Turrigiano, G.G., Nelson, S.B. (2000). Multiple forms of short-term plasticity at excitatory synapses in rat medial prefrontal cortex. *J Neurophysiol*, 83 (5), 3031-3041.

Herkenham, M., Lynn, A.B., Little, M.D., Johnson, M.R., Melvin, L.S., de Costa, B.R., Rice, K.C. (1990). Cannabinoid receptor localization in brain. *Proc Natl Acad Sci USA*, 87 (5), 1932-1936.

Herry, C., Garcia, R. (2002). Prefrontal cortex long-term potentiation, but not long-term depression, is associated with the maintenance of extinction of learned fear in mice. *J Neurosci*, 22 (2), 577-583.

Herry, C., Garcia, R. (2003). Behavioral and paired-pulse facilitation analyses of long-lasting depression at excitatory synapses in the medial prefrontal cortex in mice. *Behav Brain Res*, 146 (1-2), 89-96.

Hirsch, J.C., Crepel, F. (1990). Use-dependent changes in synaptic efficacy in rat prefrontal neurons in vitro. *J Physiol*, 427, 31-49.

Hirsch, J.C., Crepel, F. (1991). Blockade of NMDA receptors unmasks a long-term depression in synaptic efficacy in rat prefrontal neurons in vitro. *Exp Brain Res*, 85 (3), 621-624.

Hirsch, J.C., Crepel, F. (1992). Postsynaptic calcium is necessary for the induction of LTP and LTD of monosynaptic EPSPs in prefrontal neurons: an in vitro study in the rat. *Synapse*, 10 (2), 173-175.

Hotte, M., Thuault, S., Dineley, K.T., Hemmings, H.C.Jr., Nairn, A.C., Jay, T.M. (2007). Phosphorylation of CREB and DARPP-32 during late LTP at hippocampal to prefrontal cortex synapses in vivo. *Synapse*, 61 (1), 24-28.

Hu, H., Real, E., Takamiya, K., Kang, M.G., Ledoux, J., Huganir, R.L., Malinow, R. (2007). Emotion enhances learning via norepinephrine regulation of AMPA-receptor trafficking. *Cell* 2007, 131 (1), 160-173.

Huang, C.C., Lin, H.J., Hsu, K.S. (2007a). Repeated cocaine administration promotes long-term potentiation induction in rat medial prefrontal cortex. *Cereb Cortex*, 17 (8), 1877-1888.

Huang, C.C., Yang, P.C., Lin, H.J., Hsu, K.S. (2007b). Repeated cocaine administration impairs group II metabotropic glutamate receptor-mediated long-term depression in rat medial prefrontal cortex. *J Neurosci*, 27 (11), 2958-2968.

Huang, Y.Y., Simpson, E., Kellendonk, C., Kandel, E.R. (2004). Genetic evidence for the bidirectional modulation of synaptic plasticity in the prefrontal cortex by D1 receptors. *Proc Natl Acad Sci USA*, 101 (9), 3236-3241.

Hugues, S., Chessel, A., Lena, I., Marsault, R., Garcia, R. (2006). Prefrontal infusion of PD098059 immediately after fear extinction training blocks extinction-associated prefrontal synaptic plasticity and decreases prefrontal ERK2 phosphorylation. *Synapse*, 60 (4), 280-287.

Hugues, S., Deschaux, O., Garcia, R. (2004). Postextinction infusion of a mitogen-activated protein kinase inhibitor into the medial prefrontal cortex impairs memory of the extinction of conditioned fear. *Learn Mem*, 11 (5), 540-543.

Hugues, S., Garcia, R. (2007). Reorganization of learning-associated prefrontal synaptic plasticity between the recall of recent and remote fear extinction memory. *Learn Mem*, 14 (8), 520-524.

Hugues, S., Garcia, R., Lena, I. (2007). Time course of extracellular catecholamine and glutamate levels in the rat medial prefrontal cortex during and after extinction of conditioned fear. *Synapse*, 61 (11), 933-937.

Hyman, S.E. (1996). Addiction to cocaine and amphetamine. *Neuron*, 16 (5), 901-904.

Ishikawa, A., Kadota, T., Kadota, K., Matsumura, H., Nakamura, S. (2005). Essential role of D1 but not D2 receptors in methamphetamine-induced impairment of long-term potentiation in hippocampal-prefrontal cortex pathway. *Eur J Neurosci*, 22 (7), 1713-1719.

Iwata, J., LeDoux, J.E., Meeley, M.P., Arneric, S., Reis, D.J. (1986). Intrinsic neurons in the amygdaloid field projected to by the medial geniculate body mediate emotional responses conditioned to acoustic stimuli. *Brain Res*, 383 (1-2), 195-214.

Izaki, Y., Takita, M., Jay, T.M., Kaneko, H., Suzuki, S.S., Nomura, M. (2001). Effect of long-term potentiation induction on gamma-band electroencephalograms in prefrontal cortex following stimulation of rat hippocampus in vivo. *Neurosci Lett*, 305 (1), 57-60.

Izquierdo, A., Wellman, C.L., Holmes, A. (2006). Brief uncontrollable stress causes dendritic retraction in infralimbic cortex and resistance to fear extinction in mice. *J Neurosci*, 26 (21), 5733-5738.

Janowsky, J.S., Shimamura, A.P., Kritchevsky, M., Squire, L.R. (1989). Cognitive impairment following frontal lobe damage and its relevance to human amnesia. *Behav Neurosci*, 103 (3), 548-560.

Jay, T.M., Burette, F., Laroche, S. (1995). NMDA receptor-dependent long-term potentiation in the hippocampal afferent fibre system to the prefrontal cortex in the rat. *Eur J Neurosci*, 7 (2), 247-250.

Jay, T.M., Burette, F., Laroche, S. (1996). Plasticity of the hippocampal-prefrontal cortex synapses. *J Physiol Paris*, 90 (5-6), 361-366.

Jay, T.M., Gurden, H., Yamaguchi, T. (1998). Rapid increase in PKA activity during long-term potentiation in the hippocampal afferent fibre system to the prefrontal cortex in vivo. *Eur J Neurosci*, 10 (10), 3302-3306.

Jay, T.M., Thierry, A.M., Wiklund, L., Glowinski, J. (1992). Excitatory Amino Acid Pathway from the Hippocampus to the Prefrontal Cortex. Contribution of AMPA Receptors in Hippocampo-prefrontal Cortex Transmission. *Eur J Neurosci*, 4 (12), 1285-1295.

Jay, T.M., Witter, M.P. (1991). Distribution of hippocampal CA1 and subicular efferents in the prefrontal cortex of the rat studied by means of anterograde transport of Phaseolus vulgaris-leucoagglutinin. *J Comp Neurol*, 313 (4), 574-586.

Jentsch, J.D., Andrusiak, E., Tran, A., Bowers, M.B. Jr., Roth, R.H. (1997). Delta 9-tetrahydrocannabinol increases prefrontal cortical catecholaminergic utilization and impairs spatial working memory in the rat: blockade of dopaminergic effects with HA966. *Neuropsychopharmacology*, 16 (6), 426-432.

Jentsch, J.D., Wise, A., Katz, Z., Roth, R.H. (1998). Alpha-noradrenergic receptor modulation of the phencyclidine- and delta9-tetrahydrocannabinol-induced increases in dopamine utilization in rat prefrontal cortex. *Synapse*, 28 (1), 21-26.

Jones, M.W., Wilson, M.A. (2005). Theta rhythms coordinate hippocampal-prefrontal interactions in a spatial memory task. *PLoS Biol*, 3 (12), e402.

Kang, Y. (1995). Differential paired pulse depression of non-NMDA and NMDA currents in pyramidal cells of the rat frontal cortex. *J Neurosci*, 15 (12), 8268-8280.

Kawaguchi, Y., Kubota, Y. (1997). GABAergic cell subtypes and their synaptic connections in rat frontal cortex. *Cereb Cortex*, 7 (6), 476-486.

Kennedy, S.H., Evans, K.R., Kruger, S., Mayberg, H.S., Meyer, J.H., McCann, S., Arifuzzman, A.I., Houle, S., Vaccarino, F.J. (2001). Changes in regional brain glucose metabolism measured with positron emission tomography after paroxetine treatment of major depression. *Am J Psychiatry*, 158 (6), 899-905.

Kikyo, H., Ohki, K., Miyashita, Y. (2002). Neural correlates for feeling-of-knowing: an fMRI parametric analysis. *Neuron*, 36 (1), 177-186.

Kim, J.J., Fanselow, M.S. (1992). Modality-specific retrograde amnesia of fear. *Science*, 256 (5057), 675-677.

Kirkwood, A., Dudek, S.M., Gold, J.T., Aizenman, C.D., Bear, M.F. (1993). Common forms of synaptic plasticity in the hippocampus and neocortex in vitro. *Science*, 260 (5113), 1518-1521.

Koester, H.J., Sakmann, B. (1998). Calcium dynamics in single spines during coincident pre- and postsynaptic activity depend on relative timing of back-propagating action potentials and subthreshold excitatory postsynaptic potentials. *Proc Natl Acad Sci USA*, 95 (16), 9596-9601.

Kojima, S., Goldman-Rakic, P.S. (1982). Delay-related activity of prefrontal neurons in rhesus monkeys performing delayed response. *Brain Res*, 248 (1), 43-49.

Kolb, B. (1984). Functions of the frontal cortex of the rat: a comparative review. *Brain Res*, 320 (1), 65-98.

Konishi, S., Uchida, I., Okuaki, T., Machida, T., Shirouzu, I., Miyashita, Y. (2002). Neural correlates of recency judgment. *J Neurosci*, 22 (21), 9549-9555.

Kooy, R.F. (2003). Of mice and the fragile X syndrome. *Trends Genet*, 19 (3), 148-154.

Kopelman, M.D., Stanhope, N. (1998). Recall and recognition memory in patients with focal frontal, temporal lobe and diencephalic lesions. *Neuropsychologia*, 36 (8), 785-795.

Kritzer, M.F., Goldman-Rakic, P.S. (1995). Intrinsic circuit organization of the major layers and sublayers of the dorsolateral prefrontal cortex in the rhesus monkey. *J Comp Neurol*, 359 (1), 131-143.

Kubota, K., Niki, H. (1971). Prefrontal cortical unit activity and delayed alternation performance in monkeys. *J Neurophysiol*, 34 (3), 337-347.

Kuroda, M., Yokofujita, J., Murakami, K. (1998). An ultrastructural study of the neural circuit between the prefrontal cortex and the mediodorsal nucleus of the thalamus. *Prog Neurobiol*, 54 (4), 417-458.

Lafourcade, M., Elezgarai, I., Mato, S., Bakiri, Y., Grandes, P., Manzoni, O.J. (2007). Molecular components and functions of the endocannabinoid system in mouse prefrontal cortex. *PLoS ONE*, 2(1), e709.

Laifenfeld, D., Karry, R., Grauer, E., Klein, E., Ben-Shachar, D. (2005). Antidepressants and prolonged stress in rats modulate CAM-L1, laminin, and pCREB, implicated in neuronal plasticity. *Neurobiol Dis*, 20 (2), 432-441.

Lange, K.W., Robbins, T.W., Marsden, C.D., James, M., Owen, A.M., Paul, G.M. (1992). L-dopa withdrawal in Parkinson's disease selectively impairs cognitive performance in tests sensitive to frontal lobe dysfunction. *Psychopharmacology* (Berl), 107 (2-3), 394-404.

Laroche, S., Davis, S., Jay, T.M. (2000). Plasticity at hippocampal to prefrontal cortex synapses: dual roles in working memory and consolidation. *Hippocampus*, 10 (4), 438-446.

Laroche, S., Jay, T.M., Thierry, A.M. (1990). Long-term potentiation in the prefrontal cortex following stimulation of the hippocampal CA1/subicular region. *Neurosci Lett*, 114 (2), 184-190.

Larson, J., Lynch, G. (1988). Role of N-methyl-D-aspartate receptors in the induction of synaptic potentiation by burst stimulation patterned after the hippocampal theta-rhythm. *Brain Res*, 441 (1-2), 111-118.

Laviolette, S.R., Grace, A.A. (2006). Cannabinoids Potentiate Emotional Learning Plasticity in Neurons of the Medial Prefrontal Cortex through Basolateral Amygdala Inputs. *J Neurosci*, 26 (24), 6458-6468.

Laviolette, S.R., Lipski, W.J., Grace, A.A. (2005). A subpopulation of neurons in the medial prefrontal cortex encodes emotional learning with burst and frequency codes through a dopamine D4 receptor-dependent basolateral amygdala input. *J Neurosci*, 25 (26), 6066-6075.

Law-Tho, D., Desce, J.M., Crepel, F. (1995). Dopamine favours the emergence of long-term depression versus long-term potentiation in slices of rat prefrontal cortex. *Neurosci Lett*, 188 (2), 125-128.

Lebron, K., Milad, M.R., Quirk, G.J. (2004). Delayed recall of fear extinction in rats with lesions of ventral medial prefrontal cortex. *Learn Mem*, 11 (5), 544-548.

LeDoux, J.E. (2000). Emotion circuits in the brain. *Annu Rev Neurosci*, 23, 155-184.

Lee, A.C., Robbins, T.W., Owen, A.M. (2000a). Episodic memory meets working memory in the frontal lobe: functional neuroimaging studies of encoding and retrieval. *Crit Rev Neurobiol*, 14 (3-4), 165-197.

Lee, H.K., Barbarosie, M., Kameyama, K., Bear, M.F., Huganir, R.L. (2000b). Regulation of distinct AMPA receptor phosphorylation sites during bidirectional synaptic plasticity. *Nature*, 405 (6789), 955-959.

Letzkus, J.J., Kampa, B.M., Stuart, G.J. (2006). Learning rules for spike timing-dependent plasticity depend on dendritic synapse location. *J Neurosci*, 26 (41), 10420-10429.

Letzkus, J.J., Kampa, B.M., Stuart, G.J. (2007). Does spike timing-dependent synaptic plasticity underlie memory formation? *Clin Exp Pharmacol Physiol*, 34 (10), 1070-1076.

Levitt, J.B., Lewis, D.A., Yoshioka, T., Lund, J.S. (1993). Topography of pyramidal neuron intrinsic connections in macaque monkey prefrontal cortex (areas 9 and 46). *J Comp Neurol*, 338 (3), 360-376.

Levitt, P., Moore, R.Y. (1978). Noradrenaline neuron innervation of the neocortex in the rat. *Brain Res*, 139 (2), 219-231.

Leweke, F.M., Giuffrida, A., Wurster, U., Emrich, H.M., Piomelli, D. (1999). Elevated endogenous cannabinoids in schizophrenia. *Neuroreport*, 10 (8), 1665-1669.

Lewis, B.L., O'Donnell, P. (2000). Ventral tegmental area afferents to the prefrontal cortex maintain membrane potential 'up' states in pyramidal neurons via D(1) dopamine receptors. *Cereb Cortex*, 10 (12), 1168-1175.

Lewis, D.A., Anderson, S.A. (1995). The functional architecture of the prefrontal cortex and schizophrenia. *Psychol Med*, 25 (5), 887-894.

Lewis, D.A., Gonzalez-Burgos, G. (2000. Intrinsic excitatory connections in the prefrontal cortex and the pathophysiology of schizophrenia. *Brain Res Bull*, 52 (5), 309-317.

Lewis, D.A., Gonzalez-Burgos, G. (2008). Neuroplasticity of neocortical circuits in schizophrenia. *Neuropsychopharmacology*, 33 (1), 141-165.

Likhtik, E., Pelletier, J.G., Paz, R., Pare, D. (2005). Prefrontal control of the amygdala. *J Neurosci*, 25 (32), 7429-7437.

Lindvall, O., Bjorklund, A., Divac, I. (1978). Organization of catecholamine neurons projecting to the frontal cortex in the rat. *Brain Res*, 142 (1), 1-24.

Lipska, B.K., Weinberger, D.R. (2002). A neurodevelopmental model of schizophrenia: neonatal disconnection of the hippocampus. *Neurotox Res*, 4 (5-6), 469-475.

Magee, J.C., Johnston, D. (1997). A synaptically controlled, associative signal for Hebbian plasticity in hippocampal neurons. *Science*, 275 (5297), 209-213.

Man, H.Y., Sekine-Aizawa, Y., Huganir, R.L. (2007). Regulation of {alpha}-amino-3-hydroxy-5-methyl-4-isoxazolepropionic acid receptor trafficking through PKA phosphorylation of the Glu receptor 1 subunit. P*roc Natl Acad Sci USA*, 104 (9), 3579-3584.

Manabe, T. (1997). Two forms of hippocampal long-term depression, the counterpart of long-term potentiation. *Rev Neurosci*, 8 (3-4), 179-193.

Manji, H.K., Duman, R.S. (2001). Impairments of neuroplasticity and cellular resilience in severe mood disorders: implications for the development of novel therapeutics. *Psychopharmacol Bull*, 35 (2), 5-49.

Manoach, D.S. (2003). Prefrontal cortex dysfunction during working memory performance in schizophrenia: reconciling discrepant findings. *Schizophr Res*, 60 (2-3), 285-298.

Marder, E., Abbott, L.F., Turrigiano. G.G., Liu, Z., Golowasch, J. (1996). Memory from the dynamics of intrinsic membrane currents. *Proc Natl Acad Sci USA*, 93 (24), 13481-13486.

Maren, S., Quirk, G.J. (2004). Neuronal signalling of fear memory. *Nat Rev Neurosci*, 5 (11), 844-852.

Maroun, M. (2006). Stress reverses plasticity in the pathway projecting from the ventromedial prefrontal cortex to the basolateral amygdala. *Eur J Neurosci*, 24 (10), 2917-2922.

Maroun, M., Richter-Levin, G. (2003). Exposure to acute stress blocks the induction of long-term potentiation of the amygdala-prefrontal cortex pathway in vivo. *J Neurosci*, 23 (11), 4406-4409.

Marsicano, G., Lutz, B. (1999). Expression of the cannabinoid receptor CB1 in distinct neuronal subpopulations in the adult mouse forebrain. *Eur J Neurosci*, 11 (12), 4213-4225.

Marsicano, G., Wotjak, C.T., Azad, S.C., Bisogno, T., Rammes, G., Cascio, M.G., Hermann, H., Tang, J., Hofmann, C., Zieglgansberger, W., Di Marzo, V., Lutz, B. (2002). The endogenous cannabinoid system controls extinction of aversive memories. *Nature*, 418 (6897), 530-534.

Marzo, A., Vanhoutte, P., Otani, S. (2007). Noradrenaline induces long-term synaptic depression in rat prefrontal cortex: involvement of alpha1- and alpha2-adrenoceptors, NMDA receptors and MAP kinases, *39th Annual European Brain and Behaviour Society*.

Mason, S.T., Iversen, S.D. (1977). Effects of selective forebrain noradrenaline loss on behavioral inhibition in the rat. *J Comp Physiol Psychol*, 91 (1), 165-173.

Matsuda, Y., Marzo, A., Otani, S. (2006). The presence of background dopamine signal converts long-term synaptic depression to potentiation in rat prefrontal cortex. *J Neurosci*, 26 (18), 4803-4810.

Matsumoto, M., Shikanai, H., Togashi, H., Izumi, T., Kitta, T., Hirata, R., Yamaguchi, T., Yoshioka, M. (2008). Characterization of clozapine-induced changes in synaptic plasticity in the hippocampal-mPFC pathway of anesthetized rats. *Brain Res*, doi: 10.1016/*j.brainres,* 2007.12.010.

Mattes, J.A. (1980). The role of frontal lobe dysfunction in childhood hyperkinesis. *Compr Psychiatry*, 21 (5), 358-369.

McDonald, A.J. (1991). Organization of amygdaloid projections to the prefrontal cortex and associated striatum in the rat. *Neuroscience*, 44 (1), 1-14.

McDonald, A.J. (1996). Glutamate and aspartate immunoreactive neurons of the rat basolateral amygdala: colocalization of excitatory amino acids and projections to the limbic circuit. *J Comp Neurol*, 365 (3), 367-379.

McDonald, A.J., Mascagni, F., Guo, L. (1996). Projections of the medial and lateral prefrontal cortices to the amygdala: a Phaseolus vulgaris leucoagglutinin study in the rat. *Neuroscience*, 71 (1), 55-75.

McEwen, B.S., De Kloet, E.R., Rostene, W. (1986). Adrenal steroid receptors and actions in the nervous system. *Physiol Rev*, 66 (4), 1121-1188.

McEwen, B.S., Sapolsky, R.M. (1995). Stress and cognitive function. *Curr Opin Neurobiol*, 5 (2), 205-216.

McGaugh, J.L. (1966). Time-dependent processes in memory storage. *Science*, 153 (742), 1351-1358.

McNamara, D.S., Scott, J.L. (2001). Working memory capacity and strategy use. *Mem Cognit*, 29 (1), 10-17.

Meaney, M.J., Aitken, D.H. (1985). [3H]Dexamethasone binding in rat frontal cortex. *Brain Res*, 328 (1), 176-180.

Melchitzky, D.S., Gonzalez-Burgos, G., Barrionuevo, G., Lewis, D.A. (2001). Synaptic targets of the intrinsic axon collaterals of supragranular pyramidal neurons in monkey prefrontal cortex. *J Comp Neurol*, 430 (2), 209-221.

Meredith, R.M., Holmgren, C.D., Weidum, M., Burnashev, N., Mansvelder, H.D. (2007). Increased threshold for spike-timing-dependent plasticity is caused by unreliable calcium signaling in mice lacking fragile X gene FMR1. *Neuron*, 54 (4), 627-638.

Milad, M.R., Quirk, G.J. (2002). Neurons in medial prefrontal cortex signal memory for fear extinction. *Nature*, 420 (6911), 70-74.

Milad, M.R., Vidal-Gonzalez, I., Quirk, G.J. (2004). Electrical stimulation of medial prefrontal cortex reduces conditioned fear in a temporally specific manner. *Behav Neurosci*, 118 (2), 389-394.

Miller, E.K., Cohen, J.D. (2001). An integrative theory of prefrontal cortex function. *Annu Rev Neurosci*, 24, 167-202.

Milojkovic, B.A., Radojicic, M.S., Antic, S.D. (2005). A strict correlation between dendritic and somatic plateau depolarizations in the rat prefrontal cortex pyramidal neurons. *J Neurosci*, 25 (15), 3940-3951.

Miracle, A.D., Brace, M.F., Huyck, K.D., Singler, S.A., Wellman, C.L. (2006). Chronic stress impairs recall of extinction of conditioned fear. *Neurobiol Learn Mem*, 85 (3), 213-218.

Mitra, R., Jadhav, S., McEwen, B.S., Vyas, A., Chattarji, S. (2005). Stress duration modulates the spatiotemporal patterns of spine formation in the basolateral amygdala. *Proc Natl Acad Sci USA*, 102 (26), 9371-9376.

Mizoguchi, K., Yuzurihara, M., Ishige, A., Sasaki, H., Chui, D.H., Tabira, T. (2000). Chronic stress induces impairment of spatial working memory because of prefrontal dopaminergic dysfunction. *J Neurosci*, 20 (4), 1568-1574.

Moghaddam, B., Adams, B., Verma, A., Daly, D. (1997). Activation of glutamatergic neurotransmission by ketamine: a novel step in the pathway from NMDA receptor blockade to dopaminergic and cognitive disruptions associated with the prefrontal cortex. *J Neurosci*, 17 (8), 2921-2927.

Moghaddam, B., Adams, B.W. (1998). Reversal of phencyclidine effects by a group II metabotropic glutamate receptor agonist in rats. *Science*, 281 (5381), 1349-1352.

Moldrich, G., Wenger, T. (2000). Localization of the CB1 cannabinoid receptor in the rat brain. An immunohistochemical study. *Peptides*, 21 (11), 1735-1742.

Morgan, M.A., Schulkin, J., LeDoux, J.E. (2003). Ventral medial prefrontal cortex and emotional perseveration: the memory for prior extinction training. *Behav Brain Res*, 146 (1-2), 121-130.

Morris, S.H., Knevett, S., Lerner, E.G., Bindman, L.J. (1999). Group I mGluR agonist DHPG facilitates the induction of LTP in rat prelimbic cortex in vitro. *J Neurophysiol*, 82 (4), 1927-1933.

Morrison, J.H., Grzanna, R., Molliver, M.E., Coyle. J.T. (1978). The distribution and orientation of noradrenergic fibers in neocortex of the rat: an immunofluorescence study. *J Comp Neurol*, 181 (1), 17-39.

Mueller, D., Porter, J.T., Quirk, G.J. (2008). Noradrenergic signaling in infralimbic cortex increases cell excitability and strengthens memory for fear extinction. *J Neurosci*, 28 (2), 369-375.

Mulder, A.B., Arts, M.P., Lopes da Silva, F.H. (1997). Short- and long-term plasticity of the hippocampus to nucleus accumbens and prefrontal cortex pathways in the rat, in vivo. *Eur J Neurosci*, 9 (8), 1603-1611.

Mulder, A.B., Nordquist, R., Orgut, O., Pennartz, C.M. (2000). Plasticity of neuronal firing in deep layers of the medial prefrontal cortex in rats engaged in operant conditioning. *Prog Brain Res*, 126, 287-301.

Murphy, B.L., Arnsten, A.F., Goldman-Rakic, P.S., Roth, R.H. (1996a). Increased dopamine turnover in the prefrontal cortex impairs spatial working memory performance in rats and monkeys. *Proc Natl Acad Sci USA*, 93 (3), 1325-1329.

Murphy, B.L., Arnsten, A.F., Jentsch, J.D., Roth, R.H. (1996b). Dopamine and spatial working memory in rats and monkeys: pharmacological reversal of stress-induced impairment. *J Neurosci*, 16 (23), 7768-7775.

Myers, K.M., Davis, M. (2002). Behavioral and neural analysis of extinction. *Neuron*, 36 (4), 567-584.

Myers, K.M., Davis, M. (2007). Mechanisms of fear extinction. *Mol Psychiatry*, 12 (2), 120-150.

Nichols, C.D., Garcia, E.E., Sanders-Bush, E. (2003). Dynamic changes in prefrontal cortex gene expression following lysergic acid diethylamide administration. *Brain Res Mol Brain Res*, 111 (1-2), 182-188.

Nishijima, K., Kashiwa, A., Nishikawa, T. (1994). Preferential stimulation of extracellular release of dopamine in rat frontal cortex to striatum following competitive inhibition of the N-methyl-D-aspartate receptor. *J Neurochem*, 63 (1), 375-378.

Nordahl, T.E., Salo, R., Leamon, M. (2003). Neuropsychological effects of chronic methamphetamine use on neurotransmitters and cognition: a review. *J Neuropsychiatry Clin Neurosci*, 15 (3), 317-325.

O'Donnell, P., Lewis, B.L., Weinberger, D.R., Lipska, B.K. (2002). Neonatal hippocampal damage alters electrophysiological properties of prefrontal cortical neurons in adult rats. *Cereb Cortex*, 12 (9), 975-982.

Ochsner, K.N., Gross, J.J. (2005). The cognitive control of emotion. *Trends Cogn Sci*, 9 (5), 242-249.

Ohashi, S., Matsumoto, M., Otani, H., Mori, K., Togashi, H., Ueno, K., Kaku, A., Yoshioka, M. (2002). Changes in synaptic plasticity in the rat hippocampo-medial prefrontal cortex pathway induced by repeated treatments with fluvoxamine. *Brain Res*, 949 (1-2), 131-138.

Ohashi, S., Matsumoto, M., Togashi, H., Ueno, K., Yoshioka, M. (2003). The serotonergic modulation of synaptic plasticity in the rat hippocampo-medial prefrontal cortex pathway. *Neurosci Lett*, 342 (3), 179-182.

Ongur, D., Drevets, W.C., Price, J.L. (1998). Glial reduction in the subgenual prefrontal cortex in mood disorders. *Proc Natl Acad Sci USA*, 95 (22), 13290-13295.

Otani, S. (2002). Memory trace in prefrontal cortex: theory for the cognitive switch. *Biol Rev Camb Philos Soc*, 77 (4), 563-577.

Otani, S., Auclair, N., Desce, J.M., Roisin, M.P., Crepel, F. (1999). Dopamine receptors and groups I and II mGluRs cooperate for long-term depression induction in rat prefrontal cortex through converging postsynaptic activation of MAP kinases. *J Neurosci*, 19 (22), 9788-9802.

Otani, S., Blond, O., Desce, J.M., Crepel, F. (1998). Dopamine facilitates long-term depression of glutamatergic transmission in rat prefrontal cortex. *Neuroscience*, 85 (3), 669-676.

Otani, S., Daniel, H., Roisin, M.P., Crepel, F. (2003). Dopaminergic modulation of long-term synaptic plasticity in rat prefrontal neurons. *Cereb Cortex*, 13 (11), 1251-1256.

Otani, S., Daniel, H., Takita, M., Crepel, F. (2002). Long-term depression induced by postsynaptic group II metabotropic glutamate receptors linked to phospholipase C and intracellular calcium rises in rat prefrontal cortex. *J Neurosci*, 22 (9), 3434-3444.

Otani, S., Kolomiets, B. (2003). Induction properties of synaptic plasticity in rat prefrontal neurons. In: Otani, S. (Ed.) *Prefrontal cortex. From synaptic plasticity to cognition.* Kluwer Academic Publishers, pp. 85-106

Pare, D., Quirk, G.J., Ledoux, J.E. (2004). New vistas on amygdala networks in conditioned fear. *J Neurophysiol*, 92 (1), 1-9.

Parkin, A.J., Bindschaedler, C., Harsent, L., Metzler, C. (1996). Pathological false alarm rates following damage to the left frontal cortex. *Brain Cogn*, 32 (1), 14-27.

Paspalas, C.D., Goldman-Rakic, P.S. (2005). Presynaptic D1 dopamine receptors in primate prefrontal cortex: target-specific expression in the glutamatergic synapse. *J Neurosci*, 25 (5), 1260-1267.

Pavlov, I.P. (1927). Conditioned Reflexes. Oxford, UK: Oxford University Press.

Paz, R., Bauer, E.P., Pare, D. (2007). Learning-related facilitation of rhinal interactions by medial prefrontal inputs. *J Neurosci*, 27 (24), 6542-6551.

Perez-Jaranay, J.M., Vives, F. (1991). Electrophysiological study of the response of medial prefrontal cortex neurons to stimulation of the basolateral nucleus of the amygdala in the rat. *Brain Res*, 564 (1), 97-101.

Petrides, M., Alivisatos, B., Frey, S. (2002). Differential activation of the human orbital, mid-ventrolateral, and mid-dorsolateral prefrontal cortex during the processing of visual stimuli. *Proc Natl Acad Sci USA*, 99 (8), 5649-5654.

Phillips, R.G., LeDoux, J.E. (1992). Differential contribution of amygdala and hippocampus to cued and contextual fear conditioning. *Behav Neurosci*, 106 (2), 274-285.

Povysheva, N.V., Gonzalez-Burgos, G., Zaitsev, A.V., Kroner, S., Barrionuevo, G., Lewis, D.A., Krimer, L.S. (2006). Properties of excitatory synaptic responses in fast-spiking interneurons and pyramidal cells from monkey and rat prefrontal cortex. *Cereb Cortex*, 16 (4), 541-552.

Preuss, T.M., Kaas, J.M. Human Brain Evolution. In: Zigmond, M.J., Bloom, F.E., Landis, S.C., Roberts, J.L., Squire, L.R. (Eds.) *Fundamentals in Neuroscience*, San Diego, Academic Press. pp 1283-1311.

Quirk, G.J., Likhtik, E., Pelletier, J.G., Pare, D. (2003). Stimulation of medial prefrontal cortex decreases the responsiveness of central amygdala output neurons. *J Neurosci*, 23 (25), 8800-8807.

Quirk, G.J., Mueller, D. (2008). Neural mechanisms of extinction learning and retrieval. *Neuropsychopharmacology*, 33 (1), 56-72.

Quirk, G.J., Russo, G.K., Barron, J.L., Lebron, K. (2000). The role of ventromedial prefrontal cortex in the recovery of extinguished fear. *J Neurosci*, 20 (16), 6225-6231.

Radley, J.J., Sisti, H.M., Hao, J., Rocher, A.B., McCall, T., Hof. P.R., McEwen, B.S., Morrison, J.H. (2004). Chronic behavioral stress induces apical dendritic reorganization in pyramidal neurons of the medial prefrontal cortex. *Neuroscience*, 125 (1), 1-6.

Ramos, M., Goni-Allo, B., Aguirre, N. (2005a). Administration of SCH 23390 into the medial prefrontal cortex blocks the expression of MDMA-induced behavioral sensitization in rats: an effect mediated by 5-HT2C receptor stimulation and not by D1 receptor blockade. *Neuropsychopharmacology*, 30 (12), 2180-2191.

Ramos, M., Goni-Allo, B., Aguirre, N. (2005b). Ibotenic acid lesions of the medial prefrontal cortex block the development and expression of 3,4-methylenedioxymethamphetamine-induced behavioral sensitization in rats. *Behav Brain Res*, 160 (2), 304-311.

Repa, J.C., Muller, J., Apergis, J., Desrochers, T.M., Zhou, Y., LeDoux, J.E. (2001). Two different lateral amygdala cell populations contribute to the initiation and storage of memory. *Nat Neurosci*, 4 (7), 724-731.

Rescorla, R.A. (2001). Retraining of extinguished Pavlovian stimuli. *J Exp Psychol Anim Behav Process*, 27 (2), 115-124.

Robbins, T.W. (1996). Dissociating executive functions of the prefrontal cortex. *Philos Trans R Soc Lond B Biol Sci*, 351 (1346), 1463-1470, discussion 1470-1461.

Robbins, T.W., Everitt, B.J. (1996). Neurobehavioural mechanisms of reward and motivation. *Curr Opin Neurobiol*, 6 (2), 228-236.

Roberson, E.D., English, J.D., Adams, J.P., Selcher, J.C., Kondratick, C., Sweatt, J.D. (1999). The mitogen-activated protein kinase cascade couples PKA and PKC to cAMP response element binding protein phosphorylation in area CA1 of hippocampus. *J Neurosci*, 19 (11), 4337-4348.

Robinson, T.E., Berridge, K.C. (1993). The neural basis of drug craving: an incentive-sensitization theory of addiction. *Brain Res Brain Res Rev*, 18 (3), 247-291.

Robinson, T.E., Kolb, B. (1999). Alterations in the morphology of dendrites and dendritic spines in the nucleus accumbens and prefrontal cortex following repeated treatment with amphetamine or cocaine. *Eur J Neurosci*, 11 (5), 1598-1604.

Rocher, C., Spedding, M., Munoz, C., Jay, T.M. (2004). Acute stress-induced changes in hippocampal/prefrontal circuits in rats: effects of antidepressants. *Cereb Cortex*, 14 (2), 224-229.

Rosen, J.B., Hitchcock, J.M., Miserendino, M.J., Falls, W.A., Campeau, S., Davis, M. (1992). Lesions of the perirhinal cortex but not of the frontal, medial prefrontal, visual, or insular cortex block fear-potentiated startle using a visual conditioned stimulus. *J Neurosci*, 12 (12), 4624-4633.

Rosenkranz, J.A., Grace, A.A. (1999). Modulation of basolateral amygdala neuronal firing and afferent drive by dopamine receptor activation in vivo. *J Neurosci*, 19 (24), 11027-11039.

Rosenkranz, J.A., Grace, A.A. (2001). Dopamine attenuates prefrontal cortical suppression of sensory inputs to the basolateral amygdala of rats. *J Neurosci*, 21 (11), 4090-4103.

Rosenkranz, J.A., Grace, A.A. (2002). Cellular mechanisms of infralimbic and prelimbic prefrontal cortical inhibition and dopaminergic modulation of basolateral amygdala neurons in vivo. *J Neurosci*, 22 (1), 324-337.

Rossi, S., Cappa, S.F., Babiloni, C., Pasqualetti, P., Miniussi, C., Carducci, F., Babiloni, F., Rossini, P.M. (2001). Prefrontal cortex in long-term memory: an "interference" approach using magnetic stimulation. *Nat Neurosci*, 4 (9), 948-952.

Rossi, S., Pasqualetti, P., Zito, G., Vecchio, F., Cappa, S.F., Miniussi, C., Babiloni, C., Rossini, P.M. (2006). Prefrontal and parietal cortex in human episodic memory: an interference study by repetitive transcranial magnetic stimulation. *Eur J Neurosci*, 23 (3), 793-800.

Royer, S., Martina, M., Pare, D. (1999). An inhibitory interface gates impulse traffic between the input and output stations of the amygdala. *J Neurosci*, 19 (23), 10575-10583.

Royer, S., Pare, D. (2002). Bidirectional synaptic plasticity in intercalated amygdala neurons and the extinction of conditioned fear responses. *Neuroscience*, 115 (2), 455-462.

Rozov, A., Burnashev, N., Sakmann, B., Neher, E. (2001). Transmitter release modulation by intracellular Ca2+ buffers in facilitating and depressing nerve terminals of pyramidal cells in layer 2/3 of the rat neocortex indicates a target cell-specific difference in presynaptic calcium dynamics. *J Physiol*, 531 (Pt 3), 807-826.

Rugg, M.D., Otten, L.J., Henson, R.N. (2002). The neural basis of episodic memory: evidence from functional neuroimaging. *Philos Trans R Soc Lond B Biol Sci*, 357 (1424), 1097-1110.

Runyan, J.D., Dash, P.K. (2005). Distinct prefrontal molecular mechanisms for information storage lasting seconds versus minutes. *Learn Mem*, 12 (3), 232-238.

Sah, P., Faber, E.S., Lopez De Armentia, M., Power, J. (2003). The amygdaloid complex: anatomy and physiology. *Physiol Rev*, 83 (3), 803-834.

Sairanen, M., O'Leary, O.F., Knuuttila, J.E., Castren, E. (2007). Chronic antidepressant treatment selectively increases expression of plasticity-related proteins in the hippocampus and medial prefrontal cortex of the rat. *Neuroscience*, 144 (1), 368-374.

Santarelli, L., Saxe, M., Gross, C., Surget, A., Battaglia, F., Dulawa, S., Weisstaub, N., Lee, J., Duman, R., Arancio, O., Belzung, C., Hen, R. (2003). Requirement of hippocampal neurogenesis for the behavioral effects of antidepressants. *Science*, 301 (5634), 805-809.

Santini, E., Ge, H., Ren, K., Pena de Ortiz, S., Quirk, G.J. (2004). Consolidation of fear extinction requires protein synthesis in the medial prefrontal cortex. *J Neurosci*, 24 (25), 5704-5710.

Sawaguchi, T., Goldman-Rakic, P.S. (1991). D1 dopamine receptors in prefrontal cortex: involvement in working memory. *Science*, 251 (4996), 947-950.

Sawaguchi, T., Goldman-Rakic, P.S. (1994). The role of D1-dopamine receptor in working memory: local injections of dopamine antagonists into the prefrontal cortex of rhesus monkeys performing an oculomotor delayed-response task. *J Neurophysiol*, 71 (2), 515-528.

Schacter, D.L., Curran, T., Galluccio, L., Milberg, W.P., Bates, J.F. (1996). False recognition and the right frontal lobe: a case study. *Neuropsychologia*, 34 (8), 793-808.

Schochet, T.L., Kelley, A.E., Landry, C.F. (2005). Differential expression of arc mRNA and other plasticity-related genes induced by nicotine in adolescent rat forebrain. *Neuroscience*, 135 (1), 285-297.

Schultz, W. (2002). Getting formal with dopamine and reward. *Neuron*, 36 (2), 241-263.

Schwab, R.S., Zieper, I. (1965). Effects of mood, motivation, stress and alertness on the performance in Parkinson's disease. *Psychiatr Neurol* (Basel), 150 (6), 345-357.

Seamans, J.K., Durstewitz, D., Christie, B.R., Stevens, C.F., Sejnowski, T.J. (2001). Dopamine D1/D5 receptor modulation of excitatory synaptic inputs to layer V prefrontal cortex neurons. *Proc Natl Acad Sci USA*, 98, (1), 301-306.

Seamans, J.K., Floresco, S.B., Phillips, A.G. (1995). Functional differences between the prelimbic and anterior cingulate regions of the rat prefrontal cortex. *Behav Neurosci*, 109 (6), 1063-1073.

Seamans, J.K., Floresco, S.B., Phillips, A.G. (1998). D1 receptor modulation of hippocampal-prefrontal cortical circuits integrating spatial memory with executive functions in the rat. *J Neurosci*, 18 (4), 1613-1621.

Seamans, J.K., Yang, C.R. (2004). The principal features and mechanisms of dopamine modulation in the prefrontal cortex. *Prog Neurobiol*, 74 (1), 1-58.

Sesack, S.R., Deutch, A.Y., Roth, R.H., Bunney, B.S. (1989). Topographical organization of the efferent projections of the medial prefrontal cortex in the rat: an anterograde tract-tracing study with Phaseolus vulgaris leucoagglutinin. *J Comp Neurol*, 290 (2), 213-242.

Sesack, S.R., Snyder, C.L., Lewis, D.A. (1995). Axon terminals immunolabeled for dopamine or tyrosine hydroxylase synapse on GABA-immunoreactive dendrites in rat and monkey cortex. *J Comp Neurol*, 363 (2), 264-280.

Shallice, T. (1982). Specific impairments of planning. *Philos Trans R Soc Lond B Biol Sci*, 298 (1089), 199-209.

Shallice, T., Burgess, P. (1996). The domain of supervisory processes and temporal organization of behaviour. *Philos Trans R Soc Lond B Biol Sci*, 351 (1346), 1405-1411.

Shimamura, A.P. In: MS Gazzaniga (Ed.) *The Cognitive Neuroscience*, Cambridge Massachusetts, MIT Press, pp 803-813.

Shimamura, A.P., Janowsky, J.S., Squire, L.R. (1990). Memory for the temporal order of events in patients with frontal lobe lesions and amnesic patients. *Neuropsychologia*, 28 (8), 803-813.

Siapas, A.G., Lubenov, E.V., Wilson, M.A. (2005). Prefrontal phase locking to hippocampal theta oscillations. *Neuron*, 46 (1), 141-151.

Sierra-Mercado, D.Jr., Corcoran, K.A., Lebron-Milad, K., Quirk, G.J. (2006). Inactivation of the ventromedial prefrontal cortex reduces expression of conditioned fear and impairs subsequent recall of extinction. *Eur J Neurosci*, 24 (6), 1751-1758.

Simon, H., Scatton, B., Moal, M.L. (1980). Dopaminergic A10 neurones are involved in cognitive functions. *Nature*, 286 (5769), 150-151.

Simons, J.S., Verfaellie, M., Galton, C.J., Miller, B.L., Hodges, J.R., Graham, K.S. (2002). Recollection-based memory in frontotemporal dementia: implications for theories of long-term memory. *Brain*, 125 (Pt 11), 2523-2536.

Sjostrom, P.J., Hausser, M. (2006). A cooperative switch determines the sign of synaptic plasticity in distal dendrites of neocortical pyramidal neurons. *Neuron*, 51 (2), 227-238.

Smiley, J.F., Levey, A.I., Ciliax, B.J., Goldman-Rakic, P.S. (1994). D1 dopamine receptor immunoreactivity in human and monkey cerebral cortex: predominant and extrasynaptic localization in dendritic spines. *Proc Natl Acad Sci USA*, 91 (12), 5720-5724.

Smith, Y., Pare, J.F., Pare, D. (2000). Differential innervation of parvalbumin-immunoreactive interneurons of the basolateral amygdaloid complex by cortical and intrinsic inputs. *J Comp Neurol*, 416 (4), 496-508.

Snyder, G.L., Fienberg, A.A., Huganir, R.L., Greengard, P. (1998). A dopamine/D1 receptor/protein kinase A/dopamine- and cAMP-regulated phosphoprotein (Mr 32 kDa)/protein phosphatase-1 pathway regulates dephosphorylation of the NMDA receptor. *J Neurosci*, 18 (24), 10297-10303.

Staubli, U., Otaky, N. (1994). Serotonin controls the magnitude of LTP induced by theta bursts via an action on NMDA-receptor-mediated responses. *Brain Res*, 643 (1-2), 10-16.

Stratta, P., Daneluzzo, E., Bustini, M., Prosperini, P., Rossi, A. (2000). Processing of context information in schizophrenia: relation to clinical symptoms and WCST performance. *Schizophr Res*, 44 (1), 57-67.

Sullivan, J.M. (2000). Cellular and molecular mechanisms underlying learning and memory impairments produced by cannabinoids. *Learn Mem*, 7 (3), 132-139.

Sun, X., Zhao, Y., Wolf, M.E. (2005). Dopamine receptor stimulation modulates AMPA receptor synaptic insertion in prefrontal cortex neurons. *J Neurosci*, 25 (32), 7342-7351.

Suzuki, S.S., Smith, G.K. (1988). Spontaneous EEG spikes in the normal hippocampus. II. Relations to synchronous burst discharges. *Electroencephalogr Clin Neurophysiol*, 69 (6), 532-540.

Takahata, R., Moghaddam, B. (2000). Target-specific glutamatergic regulation of dopamine neurons in the ventral tegmental area. *J Neurochem*, 75 (4), 1775-1778.

Takehara, K., Kawahara, S., Kirino, Y. (2003). Time-dependent reorganization of the brain components underlying memory retention in trace eyeblink conditioning. *J Neurosci*, 23 (30), 9897-9905.

Takehara-Nishiuchi, K., Nakao, K., Kawahara, S., Matsuki, N., Kirino, Y. (2006). Systems consolidation requires postlearning activation of NMDA receptors in the medial prefrontal cortex in trace eyeblink conditioning. *J Neurosci*, 26 (19), 5049-5058.

Takita, M., Izaki, Y., Jay, T.M., Kaneko, H., (1999). Suzuki SS. Induction of stable long-term depression in vivo in the hippocampal-prefrontal cortex pathway. *Eur J Neurosci*, 11 (11), 4145-4148.

Tanda, G., Carboni, E., Frau, R., Di Chiara, G. (1994). Increase of extracellular dopamine in the prefrontal cortex: a trait of drugs with antidepressant potential? *Psychopharmacology* (Berl), 115 (1-2), 285-288.

Taylor, J.R., Birnbaum, S., Ubriani, R., Arnsten, A.F. (1999). Activation of cAMP-dependent protein kinase A in prefrontal cortex impairs working memory performance. *J Neurosci*, 19 (18), RC23.

Thierry, A.M., Blanc, G., Sobel, A., Stinus, L., Golwinski, J. (1973). Dopaminergic terminals in the rat cortex. *Science*, 182 (4111), 499-501.

Thierry, A.M., Gioanni, Y., Degenetais, E., Glowinski, J. (2000). Hippocampo-prefrontal cortex pathway: anatomical and electrophysiological characteristics. *Hippocampus*, 10 (4), 411-419.

Thierry, A.M., Tassin, J.P., Blanc, G., Glowinski, J. (1976). Selective activation of mesocortical DA system by stress. *Nature*, 263 (5574), 242-244.

Tierney, P.L., Degenetais, E., Thierry, A.M., Glowinski, J., Gioanni, Y.(2004). Influence of the hippocampus on interneurons of the rat prefrontal cortex. *Eur J Neurosci*, 20 (2), 514-524.

Tiraboschi, E., Tardito, D., Kasahara, J., Moraschi, S., Pruneri, P., Gennarelli, M., Racagni, G., Popoli, M. (2004). Selective phosphorylation of nuclear CREB by fluoxetine is linked to activation of CaM kinase IV and MAP kinase cascades. *Neuropsychopharmacology*, 29 (10), 1831-1840.

Touzani, K., Puthanveettil, S.V., Kandel, E.R. (2007). Consolidation of learning strategies during spatial working memory task requires protein synthesis in the prefrontal cortex. *Proc Natl Acad Sci USA*, 104 (13), 5632-5637.

Tronel, S., Feenstra, M.G., Sara, S.J. (2004). Noradrenergic action in prefrontal cortex in the late stage of memory consolidation. *Learn Mem*, 11 (4), 453-458.

Tronel, S., Sara, S.J. (2002). Mapping of olfactory memory circuits: region-specific c-fos activation after odor-reward associative learning or after its retrieval. *Learn Mem*, 9 (3), 105-111.

Tronel, S., Sara, S.J. (2003). Blockade of NMDA receptors in prelimbic cortex induces an enduring amnesia for odor-reward associative learning. *J Neurosci*, 23 (13), 5472-5476.

Tulving, E., Markowitsch, H.J., Craik, F.E., Habib, R., Houle, S. (1996). Novelty and familiarity activations in PET studies of memory encoding and retrieval. *Cereb Cortex*, 6 (1), 71-79.

Tzschentke, T.M. (2001). Pharmacology and behavioral pharmacology of the mesocortical dopamine system. *Prog Neurobiol*, 63 (3), 241-320.

Ujike, H., Morita, Y. (2004). New perspectives in the studies on endocannabinoid and cannabis: cannabinoid receptors and schizophrenia. *J Pharmacol Sci*, 96 (4), 376-381.

Uranova, N.A., Klintzova, A.J., Istomin, V.V., Haselhorst, U., Schenk, H. (1989). The effects of amphetamine on synaptic plasticity in rat's medial prefrontal cortex. *J Hirnforsch*, 30 (1), 45-50.

Uylings, H.B., Groenewegen, H.J., Kolb, B. (2003). Do rats have a prefrontal cortex? *Behav Brain Res*, 146 (1-2), 3-17.

Van Eden, C.G., Hoorneman, E.M., Buijs, R.M., Matthijssen, M.A., Geffard, M., Uylings, H.B. (1987). Immunocytochemical localization of dopamine in the prefrontal cortex of the rat at the light and electron microscopical level. *Neuroscience*, 22 (3), 849-862.

Vanderwolf, C.H. (1969). Hippocampal electrical activity and voluntary movement in the rat. *Electroencephalogr Clin Neurophysiol*, 26 (4), 407-418.

Varea, E., Blasco-Ibanez, J.M., Gomez-Climent, M.A., Castillo-Gomez, E., Crespo, C., Martinez-Guijarro, F.J., Nacher, J. (2007a). Chronic fluoxetine treatment increases the expression of PSA-NCAM in the medial prefrontal cortex. *Neuropsychopharmacology*, 32 (4), 803-812.

Varea, E., Castillo-Gomez, E., Gomez-Climent, M.A., Blasco-Ibanez, J.M., Crespo, C., Martinez-Guijarro, F.J., Nacher, J. (2007b). Chronic antidepressant treatment induces contrasting patterns of synaptophysin and PSA-NCAM expression in different regions of the adult rat telencephalon. *Eur Neuropsychopharmacol*, 17 (8), 546-557.

Varvel, S.A., Anum, E.A., Lichtman, A.H. (2005). Disruption of CB(1) receptor signaling impairs extinction of spatial memory in mice. *Psychopharmacology* (Berl), 179 (4), 863-872.

Verney, C., Alvarez, C., Geffard, M., Berger, B. (1990). Ultrastructural Double-Labelling Study of Dopamine Terminals and GABA-Containing Neurons in Rat Anteromedial Cerebral Cortex. *Eur J Neurosci*, 2 (11), 960-972.

Vertes, R.P. (2004). Differential projections of the infralimbic and prelimbic cortex in the rat. *Synapse*, 51 (1), 32-58.

Vickery, R.M., Morris, S.H., Bindman, L.J. (1997). Metabotropic glutamate receptors are involved in long-term potentiation in isolated slices of rat medial frontal cortex. *J Neurophysiol*, 78 (6), 3039-3046.

Vidal-Gonzalez, I., Vidal-Gonzalez, B., Rauch, S.L., Quirk, G.J. (2006). Microstimulation reveals opposing influences of prelimbic and infralimbic cortex on the expression of conditioned fear. *Learn Mem*, 13 (6), 728-733.

Vijayraghavan, S., Wang, M., Birnbaum, S.G., Williams, G.V., Arnsten, A.F. (2007). Inverted-U dopamine D1 receptor actions on prefrontal neurons engaged in working memory. *Nat Neurosci*, 10 (3), 376-384.

Vouimba, R.M., Garcia, R., Baudry, M., Thompson, R.F. (2000). Potentiation of conditioned freezing following dorsomedial prefrontal cortex lesions does not interfere with fear reduction in mice. *Behav Neurosci*, 114 (4), 720-724.

Vyas, A., Jadhav, S., Chattarji, S. (2006). Prolonged behavioral stress enhances synaptic connectivity in the basolateral amygdala. *Neuroscience*, 143 (2), 387-393.

Vyas, A., Mitra, R., Shankaranarayana Rao, B.S., Chattarji, S. (2002). Chronic stress induces contrasting patterns of dendritic remodeling in hippocampal and amygdaloid neurons. *J Neurosci*, 22 (15), 6810-6818.

Wang, X.J. (2001). Synaptic reverberation underlying mnemonic persistent activity. *Trends Neurosci*, 24 (8), 455-463.

Wang, Y., Markram, H., Goodman, P.H., Berger, T.K., Ma, J., Goldman-Rakic, P.S. (2006). Heterogeneity in the pyramidal network of the medial prefrontal cortex. *Nat Neurosci*, 9 (4), 534-542.

Weible, A.P., McEchron, M.D., Disterhoft, J.F. (2000). Cortical involvement in acquisition and extinction of trace eyeblink conditioning. *Behav Neurosci*, 114 (6), 1058-1067.

Weinberger, D.R., Berman, K.F., Zec, R.F. (1986). Physiologic dysfunction of dorsolateral prefrontal cortex in schizophrenia. I. Regional cerebral blood flow evidence. *Arch Gen Psychiatry*, 43 (2), 114-124.

Wellman, C.L. (2001). Dendritic reorganization in pyramidal neurons in medial prefrontal cortex after chronic corticosterone administration. *J Neurobiol*, 49 (3), 245-253.

Williams, G.V., Goldman-Rakic, P.S. (1995). Modulation of memory fields by dopamine D1 receptors in prefrontal cortex. *Nature*, 376 (6541), 572-575.

Wiltgen, B.J., Brown, R.A., Talton, L.E., Silva, A.J. (2004). New circuits for old memories: the role of the neocortex in consolidation. *Neuron*, 44 (1), 101-108.

Wise, S.P., Murray, E.A., Gerfen, C.R. (1996). The frontal cortex-basal ganglia system in primates. *Crit Rev Neurobiol*, 10 (3-4), 317-356.

Wu, G.Y., Deisseroth, K., Tsien, R.W. (2001). Spaced stimuli stabilize MAPK pathway activation and its effects on dendritic morphology. *Nat Neurosci*, 4 (2), 151-158.

Xiang, J.Z., Brown, M.W. (). Neuronal responses related to long-term recognition memory processes in prefrontal cortex. *Neuron* 2004, 42 (5), 817-829.

Xu-Friedman, M.A., Regehr, W.G. (2004). Structural contributions to short-term synaptic plasticity. *Physiol Rev*, 84 (1), 69-85.

Yang, C.R., Seamans, J.K., Gorelova, N. (1996). Electrophysiological and morphological properties of layers V-VI principal pyramidal cells in rat prefrontal cortex in vitro. *J Neurosci*, 16 (5), 1904-1921.

Ylinen, A., Bragin, A., Nadasdy, Z., Jando, G., Szabo, I., Sik, A., Buzsaki, G. (1995). Sharp wave-associated high-frequency oscillation (200 Hz) in the intact hippocampus: network and intracellular mechanisms. *J Neurosci*, 15 (1 Pt 1), 30-46.

Young, C.E., Yang, C.R. (2005). Dopamine D1-like receptor modulates layer- and frequency-specific short-term synaptic plasticity in rat prefrontal cortical neurons. *Eur J Neurosci*, 21 (12), 3310-3320.

Zahrt, J., Taylor, J.R., Mathew, R.G., Arnsten, A.F. (1997). Supranormal stimulation of D1 dopamine receptors in the rodent prefrontal cortex impairs spatial working memory performance. *J Neurosci*, 17 (21), 8528-8535.

Zucker, R.S., Regehr, W.G. (2002). Short-term synaptic plasticity. *Annu Rev Physiol*, 64, 355-405.

Zushida, K., Sakurai, M., Wada, K., Sekiguchi, M. (2007). Facilitation of extinction learning for contextual fear memory by PEPA: a potentiator of AMPA receptors. *J Neurosci*, 27 (1), 158-166.

In: Synaptic Plasticity: New Research
Editors: Tim F. Kaiser and Felix J. Peters

ISBN: 978-1-60456-732-8

Chapter 9

CELLULAR COGNITION: A FOCUS ON LTP AND LTD IN THE LATERAL NUCLEUS OF THE AMYGDALA

Doris Albrecht and Oliver von Bohlen und Halbach

ABSTRACT

Synaptic plasticity is a fundamental process underlying learning and memory formation. Long-term potentiation (LTP) and long-term depression (LTD) are the predominant experimental models used for studying the mechanisms of synaptic plasticity. This chapter focuses on signal molecules and signaling cascades involved in pre- and postsynaptic mechanisms that contribute to the induction of LTP and LTD in a key structure of the limbic system, the lateral nucleus of the amygdala (LA). The amygdala is a component of the limbic system that plays a central role in emotional behavior predominantly in fear conditioning. Moreover, the amygdala is involved in certain psychopathologies, like epilepsy or major depression. The amygdala is a complex structure, composed of different brain nuclei, whereby the LA seems to play an essential role for the amygdala, since the LA represents the main input station of the amygdala. Since a large body of literature highlights the role of the amygdala in fear learning, we will therefore focus primarily on differences and similarities in long-term transmission changes recorded in coronal and horizontal brain slices of mice and rats. Topics include the four cardinal features of synaptic plasticity in the LA (cooperativity, associativity, persistence, and input-specificity). Further topics include the modulatory actions of various transmitter systems on amygdaloid plasticity, evidences for upregulated postsynaptic mechanisms in LTP, and the role of gene expression regulation in the maintenance of LTP. Moreover, we will shed light onto the paradigms used to induce synaptic plasticity, since, depending on the used stimulation protocols, multiple, different forms of LTP and LTD can be induced in the LA. Furthermore, it is known that the efficiency of transmission across synapses can be potentiated or depressed in response to a prior history of stimulation. We will present data that support the finding that this phenomenon, called metaplasticity, is not restricted to the cortex and hippocampus, but can also be observed at the level of the amygdala. Last, but not least, we will also briefly discuss the impact of age and gender on LTP and LTD within the LA.

I. Introduction

In recent years, functional neuroimaging and neuropsychological studies have begun to refine our understanding of the functions of the human amygdala. Studies in animals have implicated the amygdala in emotional and social behaviors (LeDoux 2000), especially those related to fear and aggression, whereby emotionally valenced stimuli need not reach conscious awareness to engage amygdala processing. Lesion and functional imaging studies in humans have demonstrated the participation of the amygdala in recognizing emotional facial expressions. After anterior temporal lobectomy or selective amygdalo-hippocampectomy in drug-resistant temporal lobe epilepsy patients, it has been also shown that subjects with considerable amygdala damage were significantly impaired in learning emotional facial expressions when compared with control subjects (Orman and Stewart 2007)

In addition, the amygdala appears to be an important component of the neural systems that help retrieve socially relevant knowledge on the basis of facial appearance (Adolphs et al. 1998). Recently, it has been shown that complete amygdala lesions result in a severe reduction in direct eye contact during conversations with real people, together with an abnormal increase in gaze to the mouth (Spezio et al. 2007). These novel findings from real social interactions are consistent with the hypothesized role for the amygdala in autism (Baron-Cohen et al. 2000; Sweeten et al. 2002). Imaging studies have also revealed that the amygdala response during facial recognition is altered in patients with schizophrenia (Kosaka et al. 2002). In humans, as well as animals, activation of the amygdala has been shown to be closely correlated with memory for both aversive and pleasant stimuli (Hamann et al. 1999; LeDoux and Muller 1997). Data suggest that the amygdala is not a critical long-term information storage site but that its role is to regulate memory consolidation in other brain regions (McGaugh 2002).

Emotion is central to the quality and range of everyday human experience. It is known that emotional items when presented in a neutral context interfere with episodic encoding of temporally contiguous non-emotional items, resulting in dissociable valence-dependent retrograde and arousal-dependent anterograde modulatory effects. By studying two rare patients with congenital lipoid proteinosis (Urbach-Wiethe) and a focal disease emphasis on the basolateral nucleus of the amygdala (BLA), it has been demonstrated that this bidirectional modification of episodic encoding by emotion depends on the integrity of the amygdala, as both retrograde and anterograde modulatory effects are absent (Hurlemann et al. 2007). These findings implicate the amygdala in a neural circuitry that orchestrates rapid retrograde and anterograde regulation of episodic memory access upon criteria of behavioral significance.

Long-term potentiation (LTP) is a mnemonic model in which particular patterns of activation of incoming excitatory fibers (representing the learning experience) may induce long-lasting enhancement of the communication between the involved pre- and post-synapses (representing the memory) (Richter-Levin and Yaniv 2001). Hippocampal LTP, the most prominent cellular model of memory formation, can be modulated by stimulation of the BLA in its induction and early maintenance. It has been shown that specific areas of the rat amygdala project to the entorhinal cortex, hippocampus, subiculum, and parasubiculum (Pikkarainen et al. 1999) and that the amygdala differently controls hippocampal subregions as well as memory processes involving the hippocampal CA1 region of the hippocampus and the dentate gyrus (Vouimba et al. 2007). Recent data obtained by stimulation of the BLA in freely moving rats (Frey et al. 2001) support the view that hippocampal sensory information can be stabilized by amygdaloidal influences. Activation of BLA inputs also facilitates LTP induction at corticostriatal synapses (Popescu et al. 2007).

Beside the ability of LA and BLA neurons to develop long-term plasticity changes, which will be discussed below, LTP can be also induced in the medial (Shindou et al. 1993; Watanabe et al. 1995b) and the central nucleus of the amygdala (Ce) (Fu et al. 2007; Lopez de and Sah 2007; Pollandt et al. 2006; Samson and Pare 2005). In addition, low- and high-frequency stimulation of basolateral afferents, respectively, induce LTD and LTP of responses in GABAergic intercalated cells of the amygdala (Royer and Pare 2002).

II. LTP in the Lateral Nucleus of the Amygdala and Fear Conditioning

Pavlovian fear conditioning has emerged as a leading behavioral paradigm for studying the neurobiological basis of learning and memory (Schafe et al. 2001).

Fear conditioning is a form of classical conditioning that depends on the amygdala (LeDoux 2000; Maren 2001). The conditioned fear response is considered to be acquired by rodents when a neutral conditioned stimulus (tone information) is combined with that of an unconditioned stimulus (typically an electrical foot shock). The lateral nucleus of the amygdala (LA) receives direct sensory inputs from the thalamus and cortex, and serves as the sensory input station of the amygdala (Pitkanen et al. 1997). The LA sends direct and indirect projections to the Ce, which in turn project to brainstem and to hypothalamic regions that govern defensive behaviors and accompanying autonomic and endocrine responses (Pitkanen et al. 1997). It is proposed that the LA activation as a sensory interface is limited to relatively simple, unimodal conditioned stimulus features, whereas the BLA may serve as an amygdaloid sensory interface for complex, configural conditioned stimulus information (Yaniv et al. 2004).

The LA is a crucial site of neural changes that occur during fear conditioning. LTP within the LA as an experience-dependent form of neural plasticity is believed to involve mechanisms that underlie fear memory formation. A number of studies indicate that both fear conditioning-induced neuronal plasticity and LTP at amygdaloid synapses share common mechanisms of induction and expression (McKernan and Shinnick-Gallagher 1997; Rogan et al. 1997). For example, McKernan and Shinnick-Gallagher (1997) have shown that fear-potentiated startle training enhances the amplitude of synaptic currents in LA neurons in-vitro. Fear conditioning also reduced paired pulse facilitation, in which the evoked response to the second stimulus of a pair is larger than that to the first stimulus. This indicates that fear-potentiated startle training had increased transmitter release in the thalamo-LA pathway. In addition, Rogan et al. (1997) have demonstrated that auditory evoked potentials in the thalamo-amygdaloid pathway are also augmented during the acquisition of auditory fear conditioning. Furthermore, it was also observed that fear conditioning produces an LTP-like enhancement of neurotransmitter release in the cortico-amygdaloid pathways, while reducing LTP-induced enhancement of synaptic plasticity (Tsvetkov et al. 2002).

III. Properties and Mechanisms of LTP and LTD Induction in LA Projection Neurons

In recent years, important progress has been made in delineating the cellular and molecular mechanisms of LA-LTP. These data show that there are great similarities in the induction, maintenance, and expression mechanisms of LTP in the LA to LTP recorded in the hippocampal area CA1, which has become the prototypical site of mammalian LTP studies.

LTP in the amygdala has been characterized in-vivo using tetanic stimulation of a number of afferents, including the piriform cortex (Racine et al. 1983), the medial geniculate body (Clugnet and LeDoux 1990), and the hippocampus (Maren and Fanselow 1995). In anesthetized rats LA-LTP can be induced by theta burst stimulation (TBS) of thalamic afferents (Yaniv et al. 2001). LA-LTP can be also induced in freely moving animals (Doyere et al. 2003), where it has been shown that LA-LTP at cortical inputs exhibited the largest change at early time points (24 h) but faded within 3 days. In contrast, LTP at thalamic inputs, though smaller initially than cortical LTP, remained stable until at least six days. Similarly, in freely behaving Wistar rats the BLA is able to sustain entorhinal cortex-induced LTP for seven days (Vouimba et al. 2004).

A. Afferent pathways that support LTP and LTD in the lateral amygdala

Although cellular mechanisms of LA-LTP have been nearly exclusively investigated in coronal brain slices (Figure 1B), LA-LTP was first characterized in-vitro in horizontal brain slices (Chapman et al. 1990) by stimulating fibers running through the external capsule (EC) (Figure 1A). In horizontal brain slices, EC stimulation activates excitatory afferents from cortical structures, including the lateral entorhinal and perirhinal cortices, that course through the EC and synapse in the LA and the BLA (von Bohlen und Halbach and Albrecht 2002). In contrast to EC stimulation, stimulation within the LA (intranuclear stimulation site) not only causes stable LA-LTP but also reliable LA-LTD (Drephal et al. 2006; Kaschel et al. 2004). It can be suggested that, in addition to activation of cortical fibers, the intranuclear stimulation also activates local connections within the LA and afferents from other amygdaloid nuclei. These connections are preserved in horizontal brain slices (von Bohlen und Halbach and Albrecht 1998c).

In coronal brain slices synaptic responses are either elicited by stimulation of thalamic fibers (Fendt and Schmid 2002; Lee et al. 2002; Schafe et al. 2000; Weisskopf et al. 1999) or by stimulation of EC fibers (Abe et al. 1996; Lin et al. 2003a; Schroeder and Shinnick-Gallagher 2004; Tsvetkov et al. 2002), which in coronal slices contains amygdala afferents from higher-order sensory cortices (deOlmos et al. 1985). Much of the work in coronal slices has involved the auditory modality (Medina et al. 2002), whereas findings concerning the somatosensory and visual afferents are rare.

We have learned that LA-LTP exhibits the main properties, initially described for hippocampal neurons: rapid induction, input specificity, cooperativity and associativity. The characteristics of LTP, cooperativity, associativity, input specificity as well as the durability or persistence of LTP have been identified as solid arguments that support the hypothesis that LTP may be a biological substrate for at least some forms of memory (Lynch 2004). Once induced, LTP at one synapse is usually not arbitrarily propagated to adjacent synapses; rather LTP is input specific. In most cases LA-LTP is only propagated to those synapses according to the rules of associativity and cooperativity.

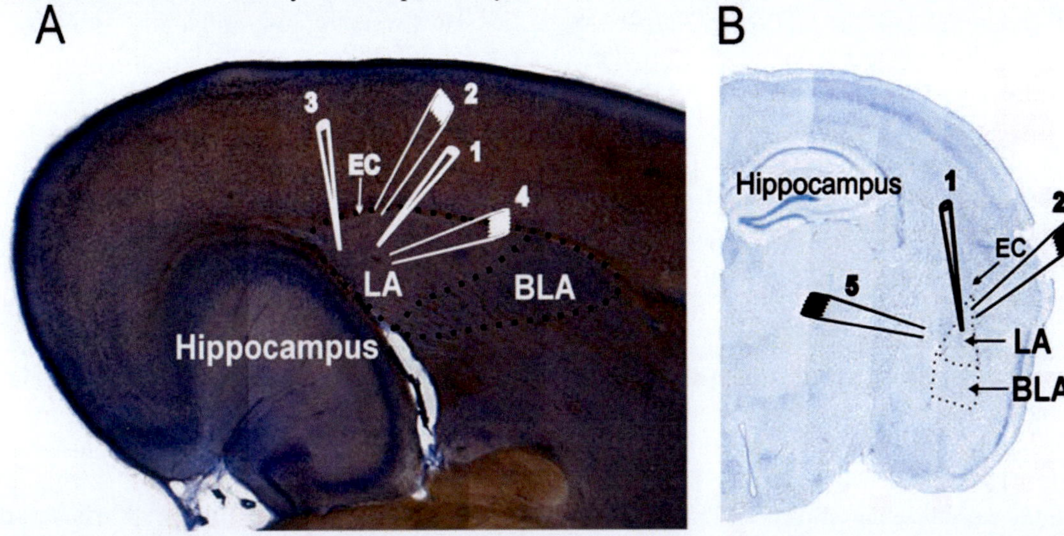

Figure 1. Horizontal and coronal sections of the rodent brain. Recording (1;3) and stimulation electrodes (2;4;5) are schematically shown. A. Bielshowsky-impregnated horizontal section of a rat brain. B. Coronal section of a mouse brain (DAPI-staining).
LA – lateral nucleus of the amygdala; BLA – basolateral nucleus of the amygdala; EC – external capsule.

In brain slices LA-LTP can be rapidly induced by applying brief tetanic stimuli (high frequency stimulation – HFS) to a presynaptic input in both, horizontal (Chapman and Bellavance 1992b; Schubert et al. 2005) and coronal brain slices (Gean et al. 1993). It can be supposed that inhibitory mechanisms in horizontal slices are weaker than those in coronal slices (Samson et al. 2003). Therefore, we could establish stable HFS-induced LA-LTP without bath application of GABA receptor antagonists by stimulating either EC or intranuclear afferences. Tetanic stimulation applied within the LA could represent a stronger stimulus than tetanic EC stimulation because of the involvement of intraamydaloid glutamatergic afferences from the basolateral and medial amygdala to the LA. This leads to a greater depolarization of the postsynaptic neurons, greater postsynaptic calcium entry and thus enhanced LTP.

Studies done in coronal brain slices showed that the use of high frequency stimulation needed an additional depolarization of cells (Weisskopf et al. 1999) or was only effective by perfusing the slices with GABA receptor antagonists (Rammes et al. 2000; Watanabe et al. 1995a). Although the intrinsic connectivities within the amygdala are poorly understood, it has been shown that stimulation of the LA effectively induces LTP in the basolateral amygdala in coronal slices (Azad et al. 2004; DeBock et al. 2003).

TBS can be considered as a weak tetanic stimulus and considering the different architecture of LA in comparison to the layered architecture of the hippocampus this stimulation paradigm is not always strong enough to activate pre- and postsynaptic sites. TBS is sufficient to induce LA-LTP at least in horizontal slices in young rats and mice when intranuclear afferents were stimulated (Albrecht et al. 2003; Drephal et al. 2006; Pollandt et al. 2003). In older rats (> 16 weeks) we could not induce TBS-induced LA-LTP. In addition, whereas both TBS and HFS of afferents running through the LA induced stable LA-LTP, TBS failed to induce LTP of EC-inputs to the LA. However, the low probability to induce TBS-induced in an non-laminated structure as the LA confirm data obtained in coronal slices, where TBS-induced LTP was dependent on additional stimulation of serotonin HT2 receptors (Chen et al. 2003).

Many studies have shown that LTP can be induced in the amygdala (Chapman and Chattarji 2000), however, only few studies indicate that LTD did occur in neurons of the LA. LTD, as a use-dependent decrease in synaptic strength, may increase the flexibility of neuronal circuits within the amygdala. The first study which has documented LA-LTD in coronal slices (Heinbockel and Pape 2000) used theta pulse stimulation (TPS; 8 Hz for 150 sec) of thalamic input fibers. This stimulation resulted in LA-LTD in 21% of the tested neurons. The same stimulation delivered to cortical afferents (stimulation of EC fibers) did not provoke long-term depression of LA activity. We found that TPS of afferents within the LA caused a weaker LTD in horizontal slices than low frequency stimulation (900 pulses, 1 Hz – LFS) (Schubert et al. 2005). Although we have shown that the stimulation of EC fibers did not produce significant LTD in rats (Kaschel et al. 2004), we tested LFS of EC fibers in mice. In accordance with our previous results (Kaschel et al. 2004) as well as with results obtained in coronal slices (Heinbockel and Pape 2000) we did not observe LTD of field potential amplitudes when single pulse EC stimulation was used. However, using low frequency paired pulse stimulation of EC fibers with an interstimulus interval of 40 ms, LA-LTD can be provoked at least in the majority of recordings (unpublished observations). These data suggest that excitatory afferents from the entorhinal cortex also activate GABAergic interneurons within the LA. Paired pulse stimulation seems to cause a higher increase in intracellular calcium and thereby facilitates the induction of LA-LTD. LTD within the LA could enhance the relative effect of LTP at neighbouring synapses, by increasing the signal-to-noise ratio as shown recently for the amygdala (Royer and Pare 2003).

B. NMDARs, voltage-gated calcium channels (VGCCs) and mGluRs

Glutamatergic transmission is mediated by ionotropic and metabotropic glutamate receptors. Ionotropic glutamate receptors are subdivided into three groups: α-amino-3-hydroxy-5-methyl-4-isoxazole propionic acid (AMPA), N-methyl-D-aspartate (NMDA) and kainate receptors. Metabotropic glutamate receptors (mGluRs) are divided into eight known subtypes and three groups based on sequence homology, second messenger coupling and pharmacology (Dingledine et al. 1999). In previous experiments we could show that field potentials in horizontal slices of the LA were largely blocked by the AMPA and kainate receptor antagonist 6-cyano-7-nitroquinoxaline-2,3-dione (CNQX) (Pollandt et al. 2003). Similar results were obtained in coronal slices (Lin et al. 2001). These results support the conclusion that glutamate is the main transmitter at excitatory LA-synapses (Huang et al. 2000; Weisskopf et al. 1999).

It is known that the NMDA receptor (NMDAR) subtype of glutamate-gated ion channels is co-agonized by glycine and possesses high calcium permeability as well as a voltage-dependent block by extracellular magnesium. NMDA receptors show unique properties depending on their subunit composition (NR1, NR2A, NR2B, and NR2C and NR2D) (Cull-Candy et al. 2001; Dingledine et al. 1999). These subunits are structurally related, with less than 20% sequence identity, to other excitatory amino acid receptor subunits (Monyer et al. 1992). Pyramidal cells of the LA receive convergent inputs from the cortex, thalamus and basal nuclei. At all inputs, AMPA, kainate and NMDA receptors are active and co-localized in the postsynaptic density (Mahanty and Sah 1999). In both, cortical (Farb and LeDoux 1999) and thalamic (Farb and LeDoux 1997) afferent synapses anatomical evidence for NMDARs has been found. The role of NMDARs is discussed controversially in basal synaptic transmission and in LTP in the amygdala (for review, see Chapman and Chattarji 2000). The disparities may be explained by differences in inputs stimulated and experimental paradigms. Since in very young animals excitatory postsynaptic potentials (EPSPs) or field potentials included some NMDA receptor mediated activity (Aroniadou-Anderjaska et al. 2001; Mahanty and Sah 1999; Weisskopf and LeDoux 1999), an age-dependent shift can be suggested. In adult rats we did not observe an involvement of NMDA receptors in basal transmission (Drephal et al. 2006). The lack of effects of the NMDA receptor antagonist APV on normal synaptic transmission in the LA of adult rodents was also observed in coronal slices during EC stimulation (Huang and Kandel 1998; Schroeder and Shinnick-Gallagher 2004).

Although it was suggested that HFS-induced LTP is not NMDA dependent (Chapman and Bellavance 1992a; Watanabe et al. 1995a), our results suggest that both TBS- and HFS-induced LA-LTP are dependent on NMDARs (Drephal et al. 2006). APV reduced HFS-induced LTP in all our studies in accordance with studies in coronal slices (Huang and Kandel 1998; Schroeder and Shinnick-Gallagher 2004; Tsvetkov et al. 2002). Since we obtained similar results for both, intracellular and extracellular recordings, it can be suggested that field potentials in the LA authentically reflect synaptic events.

In coronal slices, postsynaptically induced forms of homosynaptic LA-LTP were described at cortical (Huang and Kandel 1998) as well as thalamic inputs (Bauer et al. 2002). At thalamic input synapses LTP can be induced by using a pairing protocol in which weak presynaptic stimulation of thalamo-amygdala afferents is presented concurrently with brief depolarization of the postsynaptic cell by current injection (Bauer et al. 2001; Bauer et al. 2002; Schafe et al. 2000; Weisskopf et al. 1999).

Two pharmacologically distinct forms of LTP can be distinguished at thalamic input synapses to the LA: LTP dependent on L-type VGCCs or on NMDARs. It has been suggested that back-propagating action potentials invade the dendrites during pairing and interact with EPSPs, leading to calcium entry through VGCCs. When trains of 10 stimuli at 30 Hz were paired with 1 nA, 5 ms depolarizations given 5-10 ms after the onset of each EPSP in the train, then this pattern yields an action potential at the peak of each EPSP of the train (Bauer et al. 2002). NMDA dependent LTP can be induced by a 30 Hz tetanus (100 stimuli, given twice with a 20s interval) (Bauer et al. 2002). This protocol did not trigger action potentials but rather produced a long depolarization of the postsynaptic cell. Recently, it has been shown that large dendritic spines contacted by thalamic afferents exhibited larger Ca^{2+} transients during action potential backpropagation than did small dendritic spines contacted by cortical afferents (Humeau et al. 2005).

It is known that NMDA receptor blockade leads to a deficit in long- and short-term memory of fear conditioning (Walker and Davis 2000). Whereas intra-amygdala blockade of the NR2B subunit of the NMDA receptor disrupts the acquisition but not the expression of fear conditioning (Rodrigues et al. 2001), mutant mice lacking NR2A exhibit normal responses to tone-dependent, hippocampal-independent fear response (Kiyama et al. 1998).

Synapses in the LA contain receptors composed of both NR2A and NR2B subunits (Sah and Lopez 2003). It has been shown that LA-LTP is dependent on NR2B subunits, since the selective antagonist ifenprodil impaired tetanus-induced LTP at thalamic input synapses (Bauer et al. 2002). Using different NMDA subunit antagonists (NVP-AAM 077, Co 101244, Ro 04-5595), we have demonstrated in horizontal slices derived from adult mice that NR2B and NR2A subunits are involved in LA-LTP at cortical input synapses and that LA-LTD is dependent on NR2B and to a lesser extent on NR2A subunits (unpublished observations).

In horizontal slices, EC-induced LA-LTP was also dependent on L-type voltage-gated calcium channels (Drephal et al. 2006), whereas LA-LTP induced by stimulation of fibers within the LA was not altered by the L-type calcium antagonist nifedipine. These results support data obtained in coronal slices indicating that plasticity changes in the amygdala show input-specific properties.

By application of the glutamate antagonist APV we showed for the first time that NMDA receptors are required for the LFS-induced LTD in the LA (Kaschel et al. 2004). In addition, our group (Kaschel et al. 2004) and others (Heinbockel and Pape 2000) could show that LA-LTD is dependent on group II mGluRs in both, horizontal and coronal brain slices.

In coronal slices an involvement of VGCCs in spike-timing dependent LA-LTD has been suggested (Humeau et al. 2005). Using in horizontal slices we were able to demonstrate that L-type calcium channels are involved in the mechanisms of LFS-induced LTD-induction, since nifedipine nearly completely blocks the intranuclear-induced LA-LTD (Tchekalarova and Albrecht 2007).

Comparable results were obtained in the CA1 region of the hippocampus. Induction of homosynaptic LTD depends on postsynaptic increases in calcium (Bear and Abraham 1996; Bear and Malenka 1994; Kerr and Abraham 1996) brought about by different mechanisms that include activation of NMDA receptors (Abraham and Wickens 1991; Mulkey and Malenka 1992) or mGlu receptors (Oliet et al. 1997) Similarly, LFS of the LA induces two distinct forms of LTD in the BLA, which depend either on the Ca^{2+} influx through NMDARs (Wang and Gean 1999) or on the activation of mGluRs (Lin et al. 2000). Concerning the BLA, it has been also shown that a preconditioning HFS operating via activation of group II mGluR altered the response to LFS from the induction of NMDAR-dependent LTP to LTD (Li et al. 1998). These data represent an example of metaplasticity in the amygdala, since the induction of synaptic plasticity could be modulated by previous/preconditioning synaptic activity.

It has been evidenced that metabotrop glutamate 5 receptors (mGLUR5) are localized to dendritic shafts and spines in the LA and are postsynaptic to auditory thalamic inputs (Rodrigues et al. 2002). In the thalamo-amygdala pathway mGluR5 are involved in LA-LTP induction (Rodrigues et al. 2002) besides NMDA receptors and L-type calcium channels, whereas the mGluR1 antagonist CPCCOEt failed to show any effects on LA-LTP induction (Lee et al. 2002). In a similar approach induction of LA-TP but not synaptic transmission was disrupted by the mGLUR5 receptor antagonist MPEP (Fendt and Schmid 2002).

C. Presynaptic involvement

LTP can be induced either by strong tetanic stimulation of a single pathway to a synapse, or cooperatively via a weaker stimulation of many. This is due to the presence of a stimulus threshold that must be reached in order to induce LTP. Associativity refers to the observation that when weak stimulation of a single pathway is insufficient for the induction of LTP, simultaneous strong stimulation of another pathway will induce LTP at both pathways. Simultaneous activation of converging cortical and thalamic afferents specifically induced associative, NMDA-receptor-dependent LTP at cortical, but not at thalamic, inputs (Humeau et al. 2003). The induction of associative LTP at cortical inputs was found to be completely independent of postsynaptic activity, including depolarization, postsynaptic NMDA receptor activation or increases in postsynaptic Ca^{2+} concentration, and did not require network activity. LTP expression was mediated by a persistent increase in presynaptic release probability at cortical afferents. Thus, the authors demonstrated the presynaptic induction and expression of heterosynaptic and associative synaptic plasticity on simultaneous activity of converging afferents. These data suggest that input specificity of associative LTP can be determined exclusively by presynaptic properties, although it has been also demonstrated for the amygdala that near coincidental pre- and postsynaptic action potentials induce associative LTP or LTD, depending on the order of their timing. A presynaptic involvement in LA-LTP induction was also described (Tsvetkov et al. 2002), when the EC-LA pathway was stimulated in coronal slices. In this context, it is noteworthy to add that by immuno-electron microscopy the existence of presynaptic NMDARs in the LA has been evidenced (Farb et al. 1995).

Interestingly, inhibition of glutamate transporters leads to a loss of input specificity of LTP in the amygdala slices, as assessed by monitoring synaptic responses at two independent inputs converging on a single postsynaptic neuron. Diffusion of glutamate ("spillover") from stimulated synapses, paired with postsynaptic depolarization, is sufficient to induce LTP in the heterosynaptic pathway, whereas an enzymatic glutamate scavenger abolishes this effect. These results establish active glutamate uptake as a crucial mechanism maintaining the pathway specificity of LTP in the neural circuitry of fear conditioning (Tsvetkov et al. 2004).

Furthermore, using a combined genetic and electrophysiological approach, it recently has been shown that the lack of a specific $GABA_B$ receptor subtype, $GABA_B$(1a,2), unmasks a nonassociative, NMDA receptor-independent form of presynaptic LTP at cortico-amygdala afferents (Shaban et al. 2006). Moreover, these authors show that the level of presynaptic $GABA_B$(1a,2) receptor activation, and hence the balance between associative and nonassociative forms of LTP, could be dynamically modulated by local inhibitory activity. At the behavioral level, genetic loss of $GABA_B$(1a) resulted in a generalization of conditioned fear to nonconditioned stimuli.

In addition to the recently demonstrated presynaptic location of NMDA receptors, it is well known that the group II mGluRs, mGluR 2 and 3, are found in a high concentration presynaptically and also at a lower concentration postsynaptically. In the BLA presynaptic (Neugebauer et al. 1997) as well postsynaptic effects (Rainnie et al. 1994) of group II mGluR agonists have been shown. It has been demonstrated that LTD can be also induced by activation of group II mGLURs in the BLA. This chemically-induced LTD was NMDA-independent and required synaptic activation and presynaptic, but not postsynaptic, Ca^{2+} increase and was associated with an increase in paired pulse facilitation (Lin et al. 2000). In accordance with data from Lin et al. (2000), but in contrast to data from Wang and Gean (1999), we found that LA-LTD induced by intranuclear stimulation was accompanied by an enhancement in the paired pulse ratio, indicating that LA-LTD results from an decrease in transmitter release probability (unpublished observation). This implicates an involvement of a presynaptic expression mechanism of LA-LTD. These results and other findings described for BLA neurons support the hypothesis that two forms of LTD coexist at the same LA synapses. Both, induction and expression mechanisms appear to be different; one is dependent on group II mGluRs and seems to be predominantly expressed presynaptically, whereas the other is NMDA receptor-dependent and seems to be expressed postsynaptically.

D. Depotentiation of LA-LTP and reversal of LA-LTD

The question arose whether LTP or LTD in the LA passes through a consolidation period during which it is susceptible to disruption. When delivered to the intranuclear pathway 10 min after LTP induction, a 15 min episode of LFS (1 Hz) permanently erased LTP. However, when administered at a delay of 20 min, the same treatment did not have a strong impact on established LTP. These results provide the first evidence of the limited vulnerability of LA-LTP to be reversed by LFS and may support the assumption that LTP stabilization mechanisms in the LA take less than 20 min at least when intranuclear fibers were stimulated. When EC fibers were stimulated to induce LTP in the BLA, a LFS-induced depotentiation was even possible 35 min after HFS (Aroniadou-Anderjaska et al. 2001). Therefore, we repeated the depotentiation experiments using EC-stimulation. In contrast to intranuclear stimulation, LFS was not able to erase LTP, when delivered to the EC pathway 10 min after LTP induction. However, LFS given 20 min after LTP induction permanently erased LTP (Drephal et al. 2006). Therefore, LTP in the LA exhibits vulnerability at different time windows in dependence of the kind of used afferents. In contrast to the BLA (Aroniadou-Anderjaska et al. 2001) LFS did not cause a complete depotentiation when applied 35 min after LTP induction in the LA.

In some instances, low-frequency stimuli that are normally subthreshold for inducing homosynaptic LTD can induce LTD, if the pathway has been previously potentiated. This effect has been reported for LFS in coronal slices from the BLA (Aroniadou-Anderjaska et al. 2000; Li et al. 1998). It can be supposed that the induction of LTP, like priming stimulation, lowers the threshold for the subsequent induction of homosynaptic LTD. Our data indicate that the reversal of LTD can be induced by TBS as well as by HFS when the stimulus was delivered $\leq$ 20 min after LFS at these synapses. The delivery of weak TBS enhanced depressed fEPSPs to approximately pre-LFS control levels. The delivery of HFS resulted not only in a reversal, but it potentiated fEPSPs at a higher degree than HFS-induced LTP delivered in naive ("non-primed") slices (Kaschel et al. 2004). Our results also support previous data that induction of synaptic plasticity can be influenced by prior neuronal activity

It is known that several neurotransmitter systems are implicated in the mediation of depotentiation. When LFS is delivered 10 min after HFS to the EC-LA pathway, depotentiation is dependent on the serine/threonine protein phosphatase calcineurin (Lin et al. 2003b) along with the involvement of NMDARs. It is to note that GABA antagonists were used in the study of Lin et al. (2003b). However, since we did not find a depotentiation of LTP when LFS was delivered 10 min after HFS, it can be suggested that susceptibility to disruption of LA-LTP by LFS could also be due to different kinds of afferents running through the EC in coronal and horizontal slices.

E. LTP in interneurons of the LA

The lateral amygdala contains several subpopulations of inhibitory interneurons that represent nearly 25% of the neurons in the LA (McDonald and Augustine 1993) and can be distinguished on the basis of their content of calcium-binding proteins or peptides. Interneurons can also identified morphologically by their aspiny dendritic trees and physiologically by their ability to generate high frequency, non-adapting spike trains in response to depolarizing current pulses (Lang and Pare 1998; Rainnie et al. 1991; Sah et al. 2003). It is well known that the ability to induce LTP in LA projection neurons in vitro depends on the strength of the local inhibitory network. At least in the BLA, GABAergic local circuit neurons might possess AMPA receptors with higher calcium permeability on average than pyramidal cells, as it has been suggested for hippocampus (He et al. 1999). An involvement of GABAergic interneurons in NMDA-dependent LTP in the amygdala is controversially discussed. Whereas Mahanty and Sah (1998) reported that LTP in GABAergic interneurons in the BLA is AMPAR-dependent, Bauer and LeDoux (2004) demonstrated an involvement of NMDA receptors in LA-LTP of GABAergic interneurons.

F. Retrograde signaling

As described above LA-LTP and LA-LTD are triggered postsynaptically and, at least in part, their expressions depend on presynaptic mechanisms. From the hippocampus it is known that different retrograde messengers exist that can be released from the postsynaptic dendrite and diffuse back across the synapse to increase neurotransmitter release. Several candidates including lipid mediators such as arachidonic acid or one of its lipoxygenase metabolites, platelet-activating factor, and neuroactive gaseous substances, such as nitric oxide (NO) and carbon monoxide, have attracted much interest (Medina and Izquierdo 1995). Real progress has been made in clarifying the possible role of nitric oxide as a retrograde messenger. We and others have shown that TBS-induced CA1-LTP is NO-dependent, since CA1-LTP is blocked by the unspecific NO-synthetase inhibitor N^G-nitro-L-arginine-methyl-ester (L-NAME). We used the dye 1,2-diaminoanthraquinone (DAQ) to demonstrate NO production in rat brain slices in relation to induction of LTP. We found that DAQ induced fluorescence is elevated within a limited area of about 40000 μm^2 during LTP-induction in the hippocampal area CA1 (von Bohlen und Halbach et al. 2002). L-NAME was able to inhibit the induction of LTP, accompanied by a strong reduction of DAQ induced fluorescence.

Although the neuronal nitric oxide synthetase (n-NOS) is localized in the LA (Schafe et al. 2005), EC-induced LA-LTP recorded in coronal slices was unaffected by inhibition of endogenous NO (Watanabe et al. 1995b). We recently studied LA-LTP which was induced in horizontal brain slices of wild types mice (C57BL/6J), mice homozygous for disruption of the endothelial nitric oxide synthetase gene ($eNOS^{-/-}$) and the nNOS gene ($nNOS^{-/-}$). HFS of EC fibers caused a reduced LA-LTP in both $e\text{-}NOS^{-/-}$ and the $n\text{-}NOS^{-/-}$ mice (unpublished observation). Along this line, a decrease in the magnitude of hippocampal LTP has been shown in brain slices derived either from eNOS$^{-/-}$ or nNOS$^{-/-}$ mice (Kantor et al. 1996; O'Dell et al. 1994).

Interestingly, we could demonstrate that increasing NO concentration by the NO-donor SNAP caused LFS-induced LTD in wild-type mice, when EC fibers were stimulated (Albrecht 2007), whereas LFS of EC fibers did not produce long-term reduction of synaptic activity in drug-free slices as described above. In addition, Schafe and coworkers (2005) showed that NO signalling is required for LTP at thalamic inputs to the LA and for the long-term consolidation of auditory fear conditioning. Changes in NO production during fear conditioning were also found by Sato and colleagues (2006). NO is known to affect synaptic plasticity in various regions of the brain via the cGMP-cGMP-dependent protein kinase (PKG) pathway. It has been found that the compound 3-(5-hydroxymethyl-2-furyl)-1-benzyl-indazole (YC-1), a drug known to modulate the response of soluble guanylyl cyclase to NO, greatly potentiated LTP in the amygdala (Chien et al. 2003). Therefore, the above mentioned results suggest that LA-LTP and LA-LTD depends on NO-sensitive processes.

It is known from different studies that produced NO influences cyclooxygenase-2 (COX-2) activity. We recently could recognized that there is a molecular cross-talk between COX-2 and NO that may regulate synaptic plasticity in the LA (Albrecht 2007). COX is a key enzyme that converts arachidonic acid to prostaglandins. It has been revealed that selective COX-2 inhibitors significantly reduced postsynaptic membrane excitability, back-propagating dendritic action potential-associated Ca^{2+} influx, and LTP induction in hippocampal dentate granule neurons and CA1 neurons, while COX-1 inhibitors were ineffective (Chen et al. 2002; Murray and O'Connor 2003; Slanina et al. 2005). In addition, recent behavioral data indicate that COX-2 is a required biochemical component mediating the consolidation of hippocampus-dependent memory (Teather et al. 2002).

The functional significance of COX-2 in the amygdala is unclear, although it is expressed at high levels (Kaufmann et al. 1996). A comparably high packing density of COX-2 positive neurons has been also observed in the LA (Bidmon et al. 2000). Our recent data provide the first evidence that COX-2 contributes to plasticity changes in the amygdala. We demonstrated that the selective COX-2 inhibitor NS-398 significantly reduced the probability of LA-LTP induction. The involvement of COX-2 in mediating of LA-LTP is supported by the decrease in LA-LTP in animals lacking the inducible enzyme COX-2 (Albrecht 2007). The reduced paired pulse facilitation obtained in our experiments in heterozygous COX-2 deficient mice and in NS-398-treated mice suggests an involvement of presynaptic mechanisms. COX-2 might act as a retrograde signal that participates in presynaptic aspects of plasticity in the LA. In this way the impairment of LTP in homozygous COX-2 deficient mice could be explained by a reduced glutamate release.

In addition, recent data provide solid evidence for retrograde endocannabinoid signalling at least in the BLA and also indicate that this retrograde signalling requires only a postsynaptic neuron and attached synaptic boutons (Zhu and Lovinger 2005). Endocannabinoids are fatty acid derivatives that have a variety of biological actions, most notably via activation of the cannabinoid receptors. These receptors are also targets for drugs derived from Cannabis sativa. In the nervous system, endocannabinoids act as neuromodulators that depress neurotransmitter release at presynaptic terminals. In the amygdala, endocannabinoid signalling has been implicated in learning and memory, specifically in extinction of aversive memories (Marsicano et al. 2002). It has been also shown that amphetamine-induced LA-LTD can be blocked by the cannabinoid CB1 receptor antagonist AM251 (Huang et al. 2003).

IV. Signaling Events That Follow LA-LTP Induction

LTP is a complex mechanism consisting of distinct phases that involve different molecular mechanisms. The early phase (E-LTP) is independent on protein synthesis, while the more persistent long-lasting LTP (L-LTP), which lasts several hours in vitro and days and weeks in vivo, requires synthesis of new proteins. Some authors also distinguish an intermediate phase (Matthies et al. 1990).

Much of the work on NMDAR-dependent LTP or LTD in the LA has focused on the mechanisms responsible for the initial increase in synaptic strength lasting 30-60 min. Of greater interest and importance are, however, the mechanisms that allow LTP or LTD to persist hours, days, or even weeks. It is now well established that late LA-LTP requires gene transcription and the synthesis of new proteins. In contrast to L-LTP studies, studies of late LA-LTD in the LA are currently largely unknown.

A. Ca^{2+}/calmodulin-dependent protein kinase II

After the discovery that increased calcium concentration in the postsynaptic cell, as a consequence of NMDA receptor activation, is a critical factor in the induction of LA-LTP, the analysis of the downstream cellular consequences of this calcium influx has gained considerable interest. Ca^{2+}/calmodulin-dependent protein kinase II (CaMKII) is known to play a critical role in synaptic plasticity and memory formation in a variety of learning systems and species. Consistent with the evidence that fear conditioning results in an increase of the autophosphorylated (active) form of CaMKII-alpha in LA dendritic spines (Rodrigues et al. 2004), the bilateral post-training intracerebral infusion of KN62, a specific inhibitor of CAMKII, causes retrograde amnesia in rats (Wolfman et al. 1994). The intra-amygdala infusion of KN-62, dose-dependently impaired the acquisition, but not the expression, of auditory and contextual fear conditioning. In accordance with these behavioral data the NMDA-dependent form of LTP at thalamic input synapses to the LA was impaired by KN-62 administration (Rodrigues et al. 2004). CaMKII-alpha is postsynaptic to auditory thalamic inputs and co-localizes with the NR2B subunit of the NMDA receptor (Rodrigues et al. 2004). It is known that the NR2B subunit of the NMDA receptor is tyrosine-phosphorylated in the brain, with Tyr-1472 being the major phosphorylation site. Mice with a knock-in mutation of the Tyr-1472 site to phenylalanine (Y1472F) show impaired fear-related learning, reduced LA-LTP, and impaired NMDAR-mediated CaMKII signaling (Nakazawa et al. 2006). In addition, in NMDA receptor-deficient mice it has been shown that CaMKII-beta and CaMKII-alpha activation involves the NR2A subunit in the lateral/basolateral amygdala during memory retrieval following auditory fear conditioning. These results suggest that auditory fear conditioning also involves a linkage between NR2A of NMDAR and the CaMKII cascade (Moriya et al. 2000). Moreover, an up-regulation in the expression of the endogenous inhibitor gene CaMKIIN-alpha during consolidation of fear memory has been demonstrated by quantitative real-time PCR (Lepicard et al. 2006). These results suggest that the CaMKIIN-alpha inhibitor has a physiological role in controlling CaMKII activity from an early stage of memory consolidation.

B. AMPA receptors

Although AMPAR functions - dependent on their subunit composition, associated proteins (TARPs) and interacting proteins – could be very diverse, there is compelling evidence that trafficking of AMPA receptors to and away from the synapse alters synaptic strengths and plays an essential role in both, LTP and LTD (Malenka 2003). LTP at hippocampal synapses is thought to involve the insertion of AMPA receptors into the postsynaptic membrane. There is evidence implicating postsynaptic as well as presynaptic changes in this process. These changes include:

(i) addition of AMPA channels to the extrasynaptic membrane and diffusional equilibrium of extrasynaptic receptors with synaptic receptors,
(ii) sudden addition of AMPA channels to the synapse in large groups,
(iii) a change in the mode of glutamate release (presumably from kiss-and-run to full fusion), and
(iv) a delayed increase in the number of vesicles released (Lisman and Raghavachari 2006).

It now appears safe to state that one of the essential mechanisms for the expression of LA-LTP involves increasing the number of AMPARs in the membrane at synapses via activity-dependent changes in AMPAR trafficking. Fear conditioning, for example, drives AMPA receptors into the synapse of a large fraction of postsynaptic neurons in the LA (Rumpel et al. 2005). Furthermore, Rumpel and colleagues have demonstrated that memory was reduced if AMPA receptor synaptic incorporation was blocked in as few as 10 to 20% of LA neurons.

Concerning the composition of the AMPA receptors, immunoreactivity for different subunits of the AMPA receptor (GluR1, GluR2/3, and GluR4) has been shown for the amygdala. Immunoreactivity for GluR1 and Glu2/3 is predominantly localized to dendritic shafts and seems to be more intense than that of GluR4 due to heavy labeling of proximal portions of dendrites. The distribution of GluR4 immunoreactivity is very similar to that of NMDAR1: GluR4 was seen in presynaptic terminals, glia, and dendrites and was primarily localized to spines (Farb et al. 1995). Whereas high expression of GluR2 mRNA has been correlated with low calcium entry, recent work reveals that LTP in the amygdala and Pavlovian fear conditioning induce similar changes in postsynaptic AMPA-type glutamate receptors and that occluding these changes by viral-mediated overexpression of a dominant-negative GluR1 construct attenuates both LTP and fear memory in rats (Maren 2005). Furthermore, it recently has been shown in GluR1 and GluR3 gene deficient mice that GluR1 and GluR3 contributed to LTP in the cortico-LA pathway, whereas LTP at thalamic inputs to LA projection neurons and at glutamatergic synapses in the basal amygdala was completely absent in GluR1$^{-/-}$ mice (Humeau et al. 2007). Since both auditory and contextual fear conditioning were selectively impaired in GluR1$^{-/-}$, but not GluR3$^{-/-}$ mice, the authors conclude that GluR1-dependent synaptic plasticity is the dominant form of LTP underlying the acquisition of auditory and contextual fear conditioning, and that plasticity in distinct amygdala pathways differentially contributes to aversive conditioning.

C. PKA, MAPK and CREB

The dependence of different forms of LA plasticity on cAMP/proteinkinase A (PKA) has been widely investigated. For instance, LA-LTP can be inhibited by the PKA inhibitor Rp-8-Cl-cAMPS (Schafe et al. 2000). Activation of PKA was also shown to accompany contextual fear conditioning (Schafe et al. 1999). In coronal slices it has been demonstrated that besides PKA mitogen-activated protein kinase (MAPK) is also critical for the expression of early BLA-LTP (Merino and Maren 2006) as well as for the late phase of LTP in the LA (Huang et al. 2000). In horizontal brain slices we have shown that the p38 mitogen-activated protein (MAP) kinase inhibitor SKF 86002, provoke a reduction in LA-LTP (Schubert et al. 2007). MAPK is also required for memory reconsolidation of auditory fear conditioning (Duvarci et al. 2005).

It is known that the small GTPases of the Ras subfamily are activated by multiple extracellular stimuli and, via a complex array of downstream effectors, control a variety of cellular events that culminate in gene transcription. Mice that lack the neuronal-specific Ras regulator, Ras-GRF (guanine-releasing factor), have severely impaired LTP in the amygdala and display corresponding deficits in long-term memory for aversive events (Orban et al. 1999). Tetanus or forskolin-induced activation of MAPK can be blocked by phosphatidylinositol 3-kinase (PI-3 kinase) inhibitors, which also inhibits cAMP response element binding protein (CREB) phosphorylation (Lin et al. 2001). These results provide novel evidence of a requirement of PI-3 kinase activation in the amygdala for synaptic plasticity and memory consolidation, and this activation may occur at a point upstream of MAPK activation.

As revealed by immunocytochemical studies, aversive training induced extracellular signal-regulated kinase (ERK) phosphorylation and c-Fos expression specifically in the ventral but not dorsal tip of LA (Radwanska et al. 2002). These data show for the first time molecular differences between subdivisions of LA as well as they also strengthen the idea that neurons in the ventral tip of LA are involved in storage of long-lasting changes associated with formation of fear memories. The brain-specific striatal-enriched protein tyrosine phosphatase (STEP) plays a key role in neuroplasticity and fear memory formation by its ability to regulate ERK1/2 activation. STEP co-localizes with ERKs within LA neurons. A substrate-trapping STEP protein binds to ERKs and prevents their nuclear translocation after glutamate stimulation in primary cell cultures. Administration of TAT-STEP into the LA disrupts LA-LTP and selectively disrupts fear memory consolidation (Paul et al. 2007).

CREB-mediated transcriptional regulation involves several signaling pathways, known to mediate nuclear responses to diverse behavioral stimuli, along with coordinated interactions with multiple other transcription activators, coactivators and repressors. Although fear memory retrieval induces CREB phosphorylation and Fos expression within the amygdala (Hall et al. 2001) and CREB-mediated transcription and protein synthesis are required for instance for conditioned taste aversion memory (Josselyn et al. 2004; Lamprecht et al. 1997), transgenic mice expressing a dominant-negative form of cAMP response element-binding protein (CREBA133), show unaltered expression of LTP and depotentiation in the BLA (Rammes et al. 2000). In Figure 2 the above discussed mechanisms of LA-LTP and LA-LTD are schematically summarized.

Recent results suggest that calcium influx through NMDA receptors and VDCCs during fear conditioning activates PKA and CaMK IV resulting in CREB phosphorylation. The phosphorylated CREB binds to BDNF promoter and up-regulates the expression of BDNF in the amygdala, which helps the consolidation of fear memory (Ou and Gean 2007). BDNF acts through the high-affinity receptor trkB. This receptor is highly expressed in the amygdala (Krause et al. 2007) and activation of trkB trough BDNF has been shown to induce a specific form of LTP, at least in the hippocampus (Bramham and Messaoudi 2005) Thus, a link between synaptic plasticity and BDNF may exist also on the level of the amygdala. Along this line, it has been shown that expression of conditioned fear is positively related to BDNF levels in the amygdala, but not in the hippocampus (Yee et al. 2007).

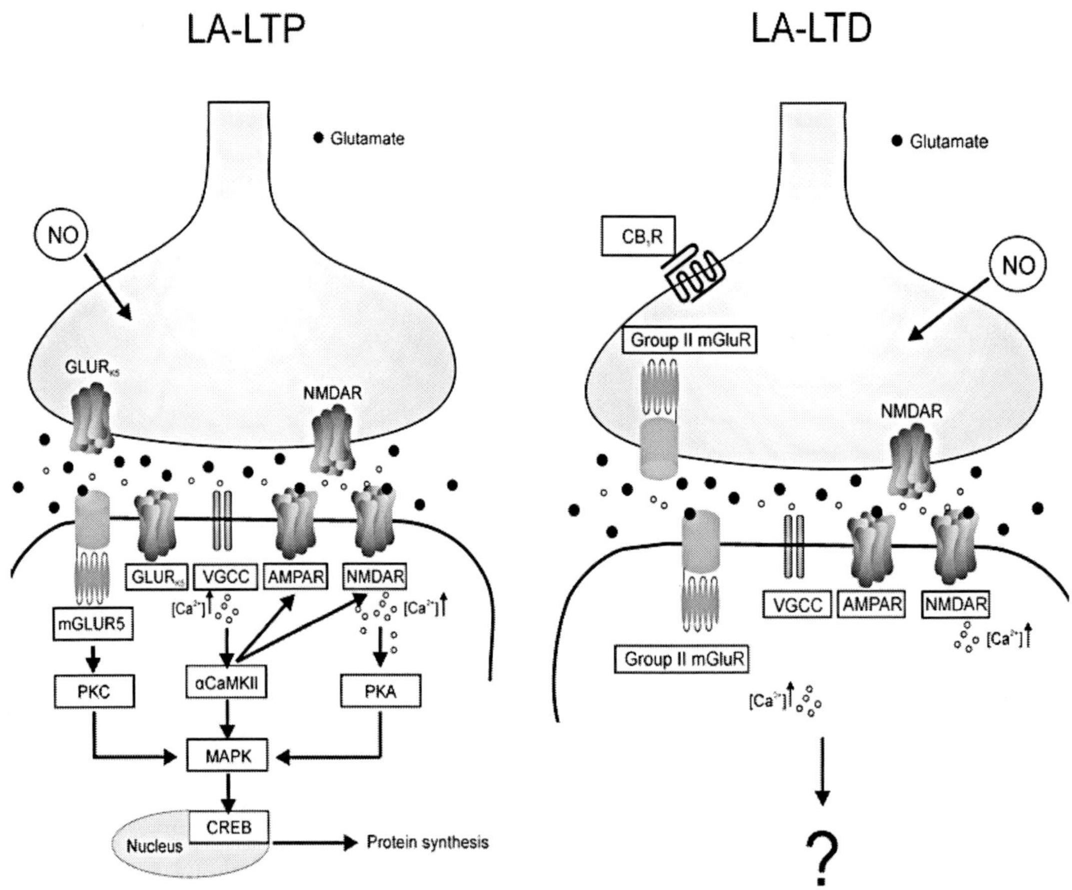

Figure 2. Models of LTP and LTD in the lateral nucleus (LA) of the amygdala (for a detailed escription, see text)

V. Gender Differences

Most of the studies in the amygdala neglected female rats. However, since hippocampal LTP and fear conditioning is known to differ in males and females (Maren et al. 1994) we were interested in getting insight in a possible gender-dependence of neuronal plasticity within the LA. We were not able to demonstrate gender specific differences in HFS-induced LA-LTP (Drephal et al. 2006) or in LFS-induced LA-LTD (Kaschel et al. 2004). However, in agreement with data obtained in the dentate gyrus of urethane anesthetized rats (Maren et al. 1994; Maren 1995) we could demonstrate gender specific differences in LA-LTP magnitude when TBS was applied (Drephal et al. 2006). The small, but significant higher magnitude of TBS-induced LA-LTP in females in comparison to males was also found in the BLA when TBS was applied to induce LTP (Krezel et al. 2001). It is known that TBS is more sensitive to pharmacological manipulations and age-dependent factors than HFS (Diamond et al. 1996; Hellner et al. 2005; Moore et al. 1993). It is further known that gonadal steroids have a profound impact on the morphology of dendrites and patterns of synaptic connectivity (Cooke and Woolley 2005; Pozzo-Miller et al. 1999; Romeo et al. 2005). Comparable to the results obtained in the hippocampus, we have shown that the magnitude of LA-LTP depends on the phase of the estrus cycle (Schubert et al. 2007). Additionally, we found gender-dependent changes in the magnitude of LA-LTP after stimulation of kainate GLU_{K5} receptors by the specific agonist ATPA.

Kainate receptors are hetero-oligomeric receptor channels composed of the subunits glutamate receptor GLU_{K5}, GLU_{K6}, GLU_{K7}, GLU_{K1} and GLU_{K2} (Huettner 2003). They appear to play a specific role in the regulation of synaptic network activity, such as mediation of excitatory synaptic transmission (Clarke and Collingridge 2002; Li and Rogawski 1998) or the modulation of neurotransmitter release (Braga et al. 2003; Frerking and Nicoll 2000). GLU_{K5} kainate receptors are, compared to the hippocampus, highly expressed in the adult amygdala (Bettler et al. 1990; Li et al. 2001). Low concentrations of ATPA reduced high-frequency-induced LA-LTP in males, while it enhanced LTP in females during certain phases of the estrus cycle. The ATPA-induced changes of LA-LTP could be blocked with the specific GLU_{K5} kainate receptor antagonist UBP296. The gender-specific effects of ATPA on LA-LTP could be due to the influences of sex hormones, which may alter GLU_{K5} receptor expression or GLU_{K5}-induced currents. Thus, our results could be interpreted as molecular and neurophysiological correlates of gender- and hormone-specific alterations in behavior and functional memory, and may represent one explanation for gender differences seen in epilepsy (Christensen et al. 2005). In addition, Mitsushima and co-authors have found sex differences in the extracellular levels of serotonin and dopamine in the BLA and their responses to restraint stress. For instance, the mean extracellular levels of serotonin or dopamine in the BLA were higher in male than in female rats (Mitsushima et al. 2006). These differences may not only contribute to the sex-specific emotional response at the behavioural level, but also to sex-specific differences in mechanisms of learning and memory.

VI. AGE-DEPENDENCE OF LA-LTP AND LA-LTD

Most patch-clamp and intracellular studies elucidating the mechanisms of plasticity changes in the LA were performed in brain slices of very young animals. Therefore, recordings of neuronal activity in brain slices of aged rodents are to our knowledge not performed yet. Although several studies on aging and hippocampal LTP failed to demonstrate any age-related deficits using HFS (Lanahan et al. 1997), TBS revealed age-related deficits in the induction of LTP (Moore et al. 1993). The type of CA1-LTP induced by HFS seems to be genuinely different from LTP induced by learning processes or theta-patterned stimulation. Moreover, TBS-induced LTP in the CA1 region of the hippocampus depends only on NMDARs (Larson and Lynch 1988) and NMDA receptor-dependent LTP appears to decline in the CA1 area of aged rats (Shankar et al. 1998).

Recently, we compared changes in the magnitude of LA-LTP with those of CA1-LTP in 24-months-old rats. Since the LA does not have a layered architecture like the hippocampus, and since TBS was not able to induce stable LA-LTP in aged mice, we used HFS of EC fiber stimulation to induce LA-LTP. In case of the hippocampal CA1 region, TBS of Schaffer collateral stimulation was used. In both structures we found an age-dependent decrease in LTP magnitude (in comparison to 9-months-old rats; unpublished observation).

Concerning LTD in aged rodents it is known that hippocampal slices from very young animals show robust LTD, whereas slices from adult animals lack, or show attenuated LTD after LFS (Battistin and Cherubini 1994; Kemp and Bashir 1999). In agreement with these data we obtained that LA-LTD can be easily induced in 8-week-old mice or 8-16 week old rats, whereas LFS of fibers within the LA failed to induce LA-LTD in 12-months-old mice as shown in Fig. 3.

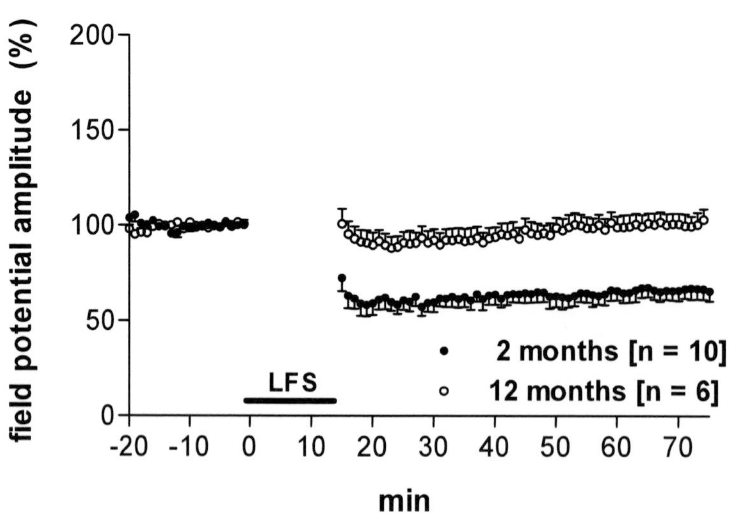

Figure 3. Age-dependency of LA-LTD. Low frequency stimulation (1 Hz, 15 min; LFS) of afferents within the LA. Data points represent averaged amplitudes (mean ± SEM) normalized in relation to baseline values

VII. Modulation of the Magnitude of LA-LTP Under Special Consideration of Stress-Related Neuromodulators

In addition to the signaling pathways described above, LTP in the basolateral complex of the amygdala can be modulated by a variety of molecules (Table 1). Behavioral experiments have shown the involvement of additional transmitters in amygdala-mediated learning mechanisms (Adamec 1997; Guterman and Richter-Levin 2006; Izquierdo et al. 1995; Rattiner et al. 2005; Roozendaal et al. 2007).

Extensive evidence indicates that stress hormones may affect memory storage and memory consolidation via noradrenergic mechanisms in the amygdala. Dopamine increases the excitability of inhibitory interneurons in the LA. Using whole-cell recordings from LA projection neurons in coronal mouse brain slices, it has been found that dopamine strongly increased the frequency of spontaneous inhibitory postsynaptic currents (sIPSCs). In addition, dopamine application induced low-frequency (2-6 Hz) oscillatory activity of inhibitory circuits in the absence of excitatory input. The increase in sIPSC frequency required activation of D1-like receptors. Unlike D1 receptor-mediated transmission in other brain areas, this effect was independent of the cAMP/PKA signal transduction cascade, but involved activation of the protein tyrosine kinase Src (Guarraci et al. 1999). Dopamine transmission within the amygdala contributes to the acquisition and expression of Pavlovian fear conditioning (Inglis and Moghaddam 1999). In addition, dopaminergic innervation of the amygdala may be more responsive to stress than other dopamine-innervated regions of the limbic system (e.g. the prefrontal cortex), implicating that amygdaloid dopamine in normal and pathophysiological processes subserves an organism's response to stress (Johnson et al. 2005).

It is known that the LA is a region specifically implicated in the formation of memories for stressful experiences. Recent findings suggest that endocannabinoid CB1 receptors in the BLA contribute to stress-induced analgesia (Connell et al. 2006). In addition, using electron microscopy, glucocorticoid receptors has been found localized to non-genomic sites in rat lateral amygdala, glia processes, presynaptic terminals, neuronal dendrites, and dendritic spines including spine organelles and postsynaptic membrane densities (Goussakov et al. 2006). By studying the effects of stress and corticosterone in vivo, it could be demonstrated that the BLA mediates the effects of stress on memory-related processes. The design of such a study can be the following: rats were exposed to an acute elevated-platform stress and administered with vehicle or 5 mg/kg, 10 mg/kg, or 25 mg/kg of corticosterone systemically. Thereafter, they were anesthetized and prepared for field potential recording in the BLA, in response to stimulation of the entorhinal cortex. Using such an approach, it could be demonstrated that the elevated platform stress enhanced baseline responses in BLA and plasma corticosterone but inhibited amygdaloid LTP (Kavushansky and Richter-Levin 2006). In contrast, predator stress enhanced LTP in BLA (Vouimba et al. 2006). Thus, many factors, including the type of stress, the phase of the stress response, the type of LTP, and the life history of the organism determine in which direction LTP will be changed. These results may have consequences for the understanding of the posttraumatic stress disorder or of depression, considering that posttraumatic stress disorder is the pathological replay of emotional memory formed in response to painful, life-threatening, or horrifying events, whereas depression is often precipitated by more social context-related stressors (Post et al. 1998).

Table 1. Effects of drug manipulations on the magnitude of LA-LTP (↑ increase; ↓ decrease)

Substance	Ltp	Nucleus	References
Kainate GLUR$_{K5}$	↑↓	LA	gender-dependent (Schubert et al. 2007)
GABA$_A$ agonists GABA$_A$ antagonists	↓ ↑		(Izquierdo and Medina 1995) (Schubert and Albrecht 2007)
cytoskeletal-regulatory proteins myosin light chain kinase	↓	LA	(Lamprecht et al. 2006)
SK channels	↓	LA	(Boucsein et al. 2001)
Serotonin 5HT1A 5HT2 5HT4	↓ ↑ ↑	LA BLA LA	(Pollandt et al. 2003) (Chen et al. 2003) (Huang and Kandel 2007b)
Dopamine	↑	LA	(Bissiere et al. 2003)
Norepinephrine α_2 ß	↑ ↑ ↓ ↑	BLA LA BLA LA	(Izquierdo and Medina 1995; Tully et al. 2007) (DeBock et al. 2003) (Huang et al. 2000)
ACh (muscarinergic)	↑	LA	(Watanabe et al. 1995a)
NO	↑	LA	(Schafe et al. 2005)
COX-2	↑	LA	(Albrecht 2007)
cannabinoid system CB1	↓	LA	(Azad et al. 2005)
gastrin-releasing peptide	↓	LA	(Shumyatsky et al. 2002)
corticosterone	↓	BLA	(Kavushansky and Richter-Levin 2006)
Renin-Angiotensin system Angiotensin II Angiotensin IV Angiotensin-(1-7)	↓ ↑ ↑	LA LA LA	(von Bohlen und Halbach and Albrecht 1998a; von Bohlen und Halbach and Albrecht 2006) (Albrecht 2007)

VIII. Pathophysiological Changes in Plasticity

A. Addiction to drugs

The amygdala plays key roles in several aspects of addiction to drugs of abuse. This brain structure has been implicated in behaviors that reflect drug reward, drug seeking, and the aversive effects of drug withdrawal.Using an animal model that involves repeated cocaine injections to approximate 'binge' intoxication, it has been shown in rats that, during cocaine withdrawal, the impact of rewarding brain stimulation is attenuated, as quantified by alterations in intracranial self-stimulation (ICSS) behavior. These behavioral signs of withdrawal were accompanied by enhancements of glutamatergic synaptic transmission within the LA that occlude electrically induced LTP in brain slices. Synaptic enhancements during periods of cocaine withdrawal were similar to LTP induced with electrical stimulation in control slices, as both forms of synaptic plasticity involve an increase in glutamate release. These results suggest that mechanisms of LTP within the amygdala are recruited during withdrawal from repeated exposure to cocaine (Goussakov et al. 2006). As such, the authors discuss the possibility that the development and maintenance of addictive behaviors may involve, at least in part, mechanisms of synaptic plasticity within specific amygdala circuits.

Similar data we found in the LA after alcohol withdrawal of rats (Little et al. 2005; Stephens et al. 2005). In rats, repeated episodes of alcohol consumption and withdrawal (RWD) not only impair the formation of conditioned associations between discrete cues and aversive unconditioned stimuli, but also reduced subsequent induction of LTP in EC - LA and Schaffer collateral–hippocampal CA1 pathways. We speculate that reduced capacity for LTP reflects RWD-induced synaptic saturation. Such synaptic strengthening might also allow unconditioned stimuli access to pathways underlying previously-conditioned responses, giving rise to broad stimulus generalization. Rats conditioned prior to RWD, but not controls, showed generalization of conditioned fear from the training stimulus to a neutral control stimulus, and a novel tone. These data indicate marked effects of binge-like drinking on conditioning mechanisms, and suggest that such drinking patterns result in inappropriate generalization of fear responses. In conclusion, repeated cycles of alcohol intoxication and withdrawal such as are experienced by detoxified alcoholic patients, and even bouts of binge drinking in social drinkers, have effects on neurotransmission that may account for increased sensitivity to seizures in alcoholics undergoing detoxification and increased withdrawal-induced anxiety.

B. Temporal lobe epilepsy

Temporal lobe epilepsy (TLE) is a common form of epilepsy and the amygdala is often involved. TLE patients frequently show emotional disturbances ranging from mild fear to pathological levels of anxiety and depression as well as memory impairment (Kalynchuk 2000). Kindling is a widely studied animal model of TLE in which daily electrical stimulation of certain brain regions results in the gradual progression and intensification of limbic motor seizures (Goddard et al. 1969). These recurrent seizures induced by repeated electrical stimulation develop much faster in the amygdala than in the hippocampus (Goddard et al. 1969; McIntyre and Racine 1986). Although kindling has been extensively investigated in the context of its clinical relevance to epilepsy, limited numbers of studies have investigated plasticity changes after the kindling procedure. We have shown that kindling of the BLA resulted in a significant impairment in the overall magnitude of LTP in the LA, the magnitude of which was dependent on the number of prior stage V seizures. (Schubert et al. 2005). In pilocarpine-treated rats we also found a reduced LA-LTP in comparison with sham-treated controls. These data are in agreement with data obtained from tissue of TLE patients, showing a strong suppression of NMDAR-dependent LTP in the dentate gyrus as compared to non-epileptic tissue (Beck et al. 2000). Along this line, we have recently obtained data indicating that saturation of LA-LTP, assessed through repeated spaced delivery of HFS, occurred at lower levels in kindled as compared to sham-implanted animals, consistent with the hypothesis of reduced capacity of further synaptic strengthening (Fig. 4). Similar data we have found after alcohol withdrawal (see above).

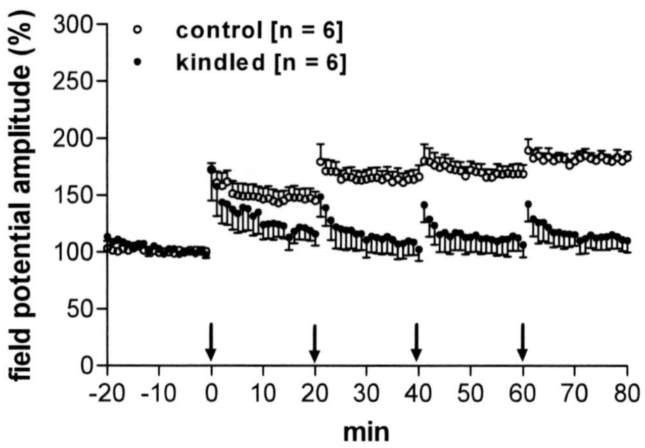

Figure 4. Saturation in kindled and control animals. Different saturation level of LA-LTP in kindled rats and in sham-implanted animals (control) in response to repeated spaced high frequency stimulation of afferents within the LA (four times 2 x 100 Hz, interval 30 s with the spaced interval of 20 min). Data points represent averaged amplitudes (mean ± SEM) of field potential amplitudes normalized with respect to baseline values

It is commonly observed that repeated delivery of HFS leads to a gradually increasing degree of induction of LTP up to saturation, and that an excessively large number of stimulus trains is deleterious to LTP (Abraham and Huggett 1997). Therefore, for the first time we have shown that the kindling procedure acts like a depotentiation process in the LA. Given the phenomenon of metaplasticity, that is the capacity for LTP itself to change (Abraham and Bear 1996), our data show that the kindling procedure as kind of metaplasticity influences the saturation level in the amygdala. It has been shown for the hippocampal CA1 region that over-stimulation transiently inhibits subsequent LTP induction through activation of VGCC and of NMDA receptors (Abraham and Huggett 1997). A potential mechanism for this LTP inhibition might be a long-lasting reduction in NMDA receptor-mediated responses by prior stimulation. Our electrophysiological data in kindled rats provide an interesting parallel to the conditioning deficits seen after kindling (Hannesson and Corcoran 2000; Ripley et al. 2003). The entire set of electrophysiological and behavioral data might be reconciled by suggesting that kindling increases efficiency of synaptic connections, leading to reduced capacity for further plasticity. Furthermore, theta pulse stimulation (TPS) elicited LA-LTD in controls, whereas the same stimulation protocol caused LTP in kindled rats (Schubert et al. 2005). Similar results we have found in the hippocampal region CA1. In controls, TPS-induced LTD can be reversed by HFS, whereas in kindled animals the strength of TPS-induced LA-LTP was further increased by the subsequent HFS.

The intracellular calcium concentration seems to be a crucial determinant of the polarity and magnitude of long-term synaptic plasticity, in that low levels of calcium via activation of calcium-dependent phosphatases facilitate LTD, whereas a shift towards higher calcium levels triggers LTP via protein kinase pathways (Kirkwood and Bear 1995). Interestingly, recently it has been shown that LFS also elicited a long-lasting potentiation in the LA in slices derived from fear-conditioned rats (Schroeder and Shinnick-Gallagher 2004). Therefore, kindling differentially affects the magnitude, saturation and polarity of LTP in LA and CA1, respectively, most likely indicating an activity-dependent mechanism in the context of synaptic metaplasticity. Kindling-evoked seizure activity may thus prime synapses via calcium-dependent mechanisms, thereby affecting threshold, magnitude and saturation of long-term plasticity at these synapses. This sort of metaplasticity may then contribute to the alteration in memory performance and emotional behaviour observed in TLE patients.

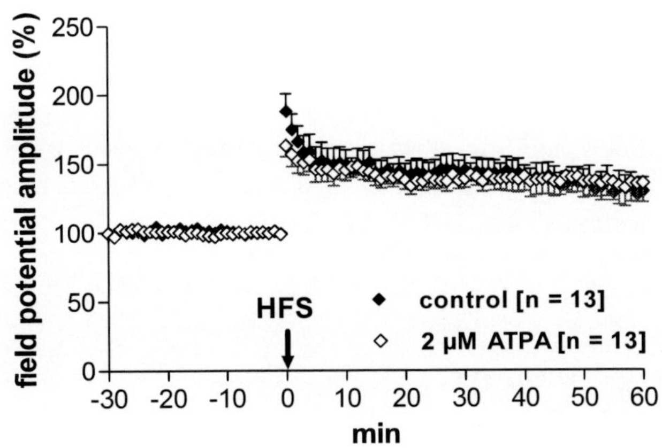

Figure 5. Stimulation of kainate GLUK5 receptors by ATPA did not change the magnitude of LA-LTP induced by high frequency stimulation of afferents within the LA of brain slices derived from pilocarpine-treated, chronic epileptic rats. Data points represent averaged amplitudes (mean ± SEM) normalized with respect to baseline values.

Although a significant reduction of cell density and the appearance of degenerated fibers was evident in the LA after 15 times stage V seizures in BLA-kindled rats (von Bohlen und Halbach et al. 2004), the observed impairment of LA-LTP in kindled animals might also be a result of functional changes such as the up- or down-regulation of transmitter receptors, involved in mediation of plasticity in the amygdala. Although different transmitter systems are modified after kindling, we focused on the role of GLU_{K5} kainate receptors in kindled animals. It is known that GLU_{K5} kainate receptor antagonists prevent hippocampal seizures induced by pilocarpine or electrical stimulation in rats, both in vitro and in vivo (Smolders et al. 2002). High concentrations of the selective GLU_{K5} kainate receptor agonist ATPA induce spontaneous epileptiform bursting in rat amygdala slices (Li et al. 2001) and limbic status epilepticus when infused intravenously or when applied directly into the rat amygdala (Kaminski et al. 2004; Rogawski et al. 2003). We used intra- and extracellular recordings of LA neurons to study the role of kainate GLU_{K5} receptors as modulators of synaptic transmission and plasticity in brain slices derived from age-matched controls and from kindled animals 48 hours after the last of 7 consecutive stage-five seizures. In our experiments the stimulation of GLU_{K5} kainate receptors by ATPA caused a decrease in LA-LTP in slices derived from male control animals. However, ATPA rescues kindling-induced impairment of LA-LTP. The partial blockade of GABAergic transmission enhanced the induction of LA-LTP in controls, but did not compensate for kindling-induced changes in the magnitude of LTP (Schubert and Albrecht 2007). The LTP-enhancing effect of ATPA in kindled animals suggests an up-regulation of GLU_{K5} kainate receptors on projection neurons similar to that described for the kainate model of epilepsy in the hippocampus (Ullal et al. 2005). As shown in Figure 5, we did not find that GLU_{K5} stimulation enhanced LA-LTP in pilocarpine-treated rats. Therefore, the LTP-enhancing effect of ATPA seems to be specific to the kindling procedure.

C. The CNS renin-angiotensin system (RAS)

Aside from the classical functions of the renin-angiotensin system (RAS) in salt and water homeostasis and in the regulation of blood pressure, the RAS in the CNS is also involved in the regulation of multiple functions in the brain, including processes of sensory information, learning and memory as well as regulation of emotional responses. Moreover, there are growing evidences that the RAS is also involved in several neurodegenerative diseases.

We could demonstrate that angiotensin II (Ang II) binds to neurons in the LA (von Bohlen und Halbach and Albrecht 1998d). Furthermore, the presence of AT1 (von Bohlen und Halbach and Albrecht 1998b), AT2 (Albrecht et al. 2000) and AT4 receptors within the LA has been described (von Bohlen und Halbach and Albrecht 2000). Neuronal AT1 receptors mediate the stimulatory actions of Ang II on blood pressure, water and salt intake, and secretion of vasopressin. In contrast, neuronal AT2 receptors have been implicated in the stimulation of apoptosis and as being antagonistic to AT1 receptors. In accordance with the role of AT2 receptors in development, we have shown that cell densities in the LA are higher in adult AT2-deficient in comparison to wildtype mice (von Bohlen und Halbach et al. 2001).

The amygdala is discussed in terms of its role in receiving afferent sensory input and in processing information related to hydromineral balance. Angiotensin acts on and through the amygdala to stimulate thirst and sodium appetite (Johnson and Thunhorst 1997). In normotensive Sprague-Dawley rats, iontophoretically ejected Ang II induced a significant increase in the discharge rate in responsive amygdaloid neurons. In contrast, in hypertensive, transgenic [TGR(mREN-2)27] rats with higher brain Ang II level, Ang II more often caused inhibitory effects on the amygdaloid firing rate in comparison to controls. Moreover, we have shown that the responsiveness of amygdaloid neurons was significantly higher in transgenic rats in comparison to controls (Albrecht et al. 2000). In addition, we have observed that Ang II causes a suppression of LA-LTP (Albrecht et al. 2003; von Bohlen und Halbach and Albrecht 1998a) as well as of LA-LTD (Tchekalarova and Albrecht 2007), whereas angiotensin-(1-7) enhances LA-LTP (Albrecht 2007) through the G-protein-coupled receptor Mas (Hellner et al. 2005). Actions of the RAS on synaptic plasticity seems not to be restricted to the amygdala, since it has been shown that Ang II and angiotensin IV also influence hippocampal LTP (Armstrong et al. 1996; Denny et al. 1991; Kramar et al. 2001; Wayner et al. 2001).

Considering the Mas receptor as one of the receptors for Ang-(1-7), it is important to note that Mas can hetero-oligomerize with the AT1 receptor and, by doing so, inhibits the actions of Ang II (Kostenis et al. 2005). This is a novel demonstration that a G-protein-coupled receptor acts as a physiological antagonist of a previously characterized receptor. These data also support our results obtained in the LA. We analyzed whether field potentials are altered by Ang II in brain slices. Opposite actions of Ang II were obtained in mice lacking the Mas-protooncogene, in comparison to wildtype mice. The use of different angiotensin receptor antagonists provided the in vitro evidence for a functional interaction between the Mas-protooncogene and the AT1 receptor (von Bohlen und Halbach et al. 2000). Consequently, the AT1-Mas complex could be of great importance as a target for pharmacological intervention in cardiovascular diseases. Our experiments also revealed that both NO and COX-2 are involved in the mediation of angiotensin 1-7-induced effect on LA-LTP (Albrecht 2007).

In summary, based on the enhanced cognitive performance mediated by ACE inhibitors (see for review von Bohlen und Halbach and Albrecht 2006), capable of crossing the blood-brain barrier, manipulation of the CNS angiotensin system might be considered as a novel therapeutic target in the treatment of cognitive dysfunctions.

IX. Conclusion

The present paper has presented a review of the current status of our knowledge of the mechanisms of plasticity changes in the lateral amygdala. Though this knowledge is still fragmentary, much more is known about the neuroscience of Pavlovian conditioning than about any other form of learning and memory. We show that most of the mechanisms responsible for plasticity changes in the LA have great similarities with that of CA1 region of the hippocampus, including the main mechanisms of induction and persistence of LA-LTP and LA-LTD. Therefore, we cannot agree with the generalized statement that, concerning the synaptic plasticity and synaptic physiology, the amygdala is not the hippocampus (Chapman 2001). This conclusion was mainly based on the experiments done by Li et al. (2001). These authors have shown that LFS of EC afferents to basolateral amygdala neurons results in enduring enhancement of excitatory synaptic responses. The induction of this form of synaptic plasticity was eliminated by one of the selective antagonists of kainate GLU_{K5} receptors and could be mimicked by the GLU_{K5} agonist ATPA. As described above, the level of GLU_{K5} receptors is higher in the amygdala than that in the hippocampus. A LFS-induced enhancement of excitatory synaptic responses in the LA can be only obtained when very high concentrations of ATPA (10 μM) are used. In drug-free control slices, LFS of EC fibers did not provoke LTP-like changes in EPSP amplitude in our experiments. However, as shown recently (Huang and Kandel 2007b; Huang and Kandel 2007a) we often observed a late (about 50 min after LFS), long-lasting facilitation lasting >5 h in slice recordings.

The forthcoming years will undoubtedly bring further clarification to diverse LTP and LTD mechanisms in the amygdala and will allow getting more insight in the mode how they contribute to adaptive brain function. Understanding the synaptic adaptations elicited and regulated by different transmitter systems will not only provide mechanistic information about how neural circuit modifications mediate experience-dependent plasticity but also will accelerate our understanding of the pathophysiology of neuropsychiatric disorders, ranging from different kinds of emotional disturbances to drug addiction and to Alzheimer's disease.

References

Abe, K., Watanabe, Y., And Saito, H. (1996).. Differential Role Of Nitric Oxide In Long-Term Potentiation In The Medial And Lateral Amygdala. *Eur. J. Pharmacol*, 297, 43-46.

Abraham, W. C., And Bear, M. F. (1996).. Metaplasticity: The Plasticity Of Synaptic Plasticity. *Trends Neurosci*, 19, 126-130.

Abraham, W. C., And Huggett, A. (1997). Induction And Reversal Of Long-Term Potentiation By Repeated High-Frequency Stimulation In Rat Hippocampal Slices. *Hippocampus*, 7, 137-145.

Abraham, W. C., And Wickens, J. R. (1991). Heterosynaptic Long-Term Depression Is Facilitated By A Blockade Of Inhibition In Area CA1 Of The Hippocampus. *Brain Res*, 546, 336-340.

Adamec, R. (1997). Transmitter Systems Involved In Neural Plasticity Underlying Increased Anxiety And Defense--Implications For Understanding Anxiety Following Traumatic Stress. *Neurosci. Biobehav. Rev*, 21, 755-765.

Adolphs, R., Tranel, D., And Damasio, A. R. (1998). The Human Amygdala In Social Judgment. *Nature*, 393, 470-474.

Albrecht, D. (2007). Angiotensin-(1-7)-Induced Plasticity Changes In The Lateral Amygdala Are Mediated By COX-2 And NO. *Learn. Mem*, 14, 177-184.

Albrecht, D., Hellner, K., Walther, T., And Von Bohlen Und Halbach, O. (2003). Angiotensin II And The Amygdala. *Ann. N. Y. Acad. Sci*, 985, 498-500.

Albrecht, D., Nitschke, T., And Von Bohlen Und Halbach, O. (2000). Various Effects Of Angiotensin II On Amygdaloid Neuronal Activity In Normotensive Control And Hypertensive Transgenic [TGR(Mren-2)27] Rats. *FASEB J*, 14, 925-931.

Armstrong, D. L., Garcia, E. A., Ma, T., Quinones, B., And Wayner, M. J. (1996). Angiotensin II Blockade Of Long-Term Potentiation At The Perforant Path--Granule Cell Synapse In Vitro. *Peptides*, 17, 689-693.

Aroniadou-Anderjaska, V., Post, R. M., Rogawski, M. A., And Li, H. (2001). Input-Specific LTP And Depotentiation In The Basolateral Amygdala. *Neuroreport*, 12, 635-640.

Aroniadou-Anderjaska, V., Post, R. M., Rogawski, M. A., And Li, H. (2000). Input-Specific LTP And Depotentiation In The Basolateral Amygdala. *Neuroreport*, 12, 635-640.

Azad, S. C., Huge, V., Schops, P., Hilf, C., Beyer, A., Dodt, H. U., Rammes, G., And Zieglgansberger, W. (2005). [Endogenous Cannabinoid System. Effect On Neuronal Plasticity And Pain Memory]. *Schmerz*, 19, 521-527.

Azad, S. C., Monory, K., Marsicano, G., Cravatt, B. F., Lutz, B., Zieglgansberger, W., And Rammes, G. (2004). Circuitry For Associative Plasticity In The Amygdala Involves Endocannabinoid Signaling. *J. Neurosci*, 24, 9953-9961.

Baron-Cohen, S., Ring, H. A., Bullmore, E. T., Wheelwright, S., Ashwin, C., And Williams, S. C. R. (2000). The Amygdala Theory Of Autism. *Neurosci. Biobehav. Rev*, 24, 355-364.

Battistin, T., And Cherubini, E. (1994). Developmental Shift From Long-Term Depression To Long-Term Potentiation At The Mossy Fibre Synapses In The Rat Hippocampus. *Eur. J. Neurosci*, 6, 1750-1755.

Bauer, E. P., And Ledoux, J. E. (2004). Heterosynaptic Long-Term Potentiation Of Inhibitory Interneurons In The Lateral Amygdala. *J. Neurosci*, 24, 9507-9512.

Bauer, E. P., Ledoux, J. E., And Nader, K. (2001). Fear Conditioning And LTP In The Lateral Amygdala Are Sensitive To The Same Stimulus Contingencies. *Nat. Neurosci*, 4, 687-688.

Bauer, E. P., Schafe, G. E., And Ledoux, J. E. (2002). NMDA Receptors And L-Type Voltage-Gated Calcium Channels Contribute To Long-Term Potentiation And Different Components Of Fear Memory Formation In The Lateral Amygdala. *J. Neurosci*, 22, 5239-5249.

Bear, M. F., And Abraham, W. C. (1996). Long-Term Depression In Hippocampus. *Annu. Rev. Neurosci*, 19, 437-462.

Bear, M. F., And Malenka, R. C. (1994). Synaptic Plasticity: LTP And LTD. *Curr. Opin. Neurobiol*, 4, 389-399.

Beck, H., Goussakov, I. V., Lie, A., Helmstaedter, C., And Elger, C. E. (2000). Synaptic Plasticity In The Human Dentate Gyrus. *J. Neurosci*, 20, 7080-7086.

Bettler, B., Boulter, J., Hermans-Borgmeyer, I., O'Shea-Greenfield, A., Deneris, E. S., Moll, C., Borgmeyer, U., Hollmann, M., And Heinemann, S. (1990). Cloning Of A Novel Glutamate Receptor Subunit, Glur5: Expression In The Nervous System During Development. *Neuron*, 5, 583-5895.

Bidmon, H. J., Oermann, E., Schiene, K., Schmitt, M., Kato, K., Asayama, K., Witte, O. W., And Zilles, K. (2000). Unilateral Upregulation Of Cyclooxygenase-2 Following Cerebral, Cortical Photothrombosis In The Rat: Suppression By MK-801 And Co-Distribution With Enzymes Involved In The Oxidative Stress Cascade. *J. Chem. Neuroanat*, 20, 163-176.

Bissiere, S., Humeau, Y., And Luthi, A. (2003). Dopamine Gates LTP Induction In Lateral Amygdala By Suppressing Feedforward Inhibition. *Nat. Neurosci*, 6, 587-592.

Boucsein, K., Weniger, G., Mursch, K., Steinhoff, B. J., And Irle, E. (2001). Amygdala Lesion In Temporal Lobe Epilepsy Subjects Impairs Associative Learning Of Emotional Facial Expressions. *Neuropsychologia*, 39, 231-236.

Braga, M. F., Aroniadou-Anderjaska, V., Xie, J., And Li, H. (2003). Bidirectional Modulation Of GABA Release By Presynaptic Glutamate Receptor 5 Kainate Receptors In The Basolateral Amygdala. *J. Neurosci*, 23, 442-452.

Bramham, C. R., And Messaoudi, E. (2005). BDNF Function In Adult Synaptic Plasticity: The Synaptic Consolidation Hypothesis. *Prog. Neurobiol*, 76, 99-125.

Chapman, P. F. (2001). The Diversity Of Synaptic Plasticity. *Nat. Neurosci*, 4, 556-558.

Chapman, P. F., And Bellavance, L. L. (1992b). Induction Of Long-Term Potentiation In The Basolateral Amygdala Does Not Depend On NMDA Receptor Activation. *Synapse*, 11, 310-318.

Chapman, P. F., And Bellavance, L. L. (1992a). NMDA Receptor-Independent LTP In The Amygdala. *Synapse*, 11, 310-318.

Chapman, P. F., And Chattarji, S. (2000). Synaptic Plasticity In The Amygdala. In 'The Amygdala: A Functional Analysis'. (Ed J. P. Aggleton) Pp. 117-153. (University Press: Oxford).

Chapman, P. F., Kairiss, E. W., Keenan, C. L., And Brown, T. H. (1990). Long-Term Synaptic Potentiation In The Amygdala. *Synapse*, 6, 271-278.

Chen, A., Hough, C. J., And Li, H. (2003). Serotonin Type II Receptor Activation Facilitates Synaptic Plasticity Via N-Methyl-D-Aspartate-Mediated Mechanism In The Rat Basolateral Amygdala. *Neuroscience*, 119, 53-63.

Chen, C., Magee, J. C., And Bazan, N. G. (2002). Cyclooxygenase-2 Regulates Prostaglandin E2 Signaling In Hippocampal Long-Term Synaptic Plasticity. *J. Neurophysiol*, 87, 2851-2857.

Chien, W. L., Liang, K. C., Teng, C. M., Kuo, S. C., Lee, F. Y., And Fu, W. M. (2003). Enhancement Of Long-Term Potentiation By A Potent Nitric Oxide-Guanylyl Cyclase Activator, 3-(5-Hydroxymethyl-2-Furyl)-1-Benzyl-Indazole. *Mol. Pharmacol*, 63, 1322-1328.

Christensen, J., Kjeldsen, M. J., Andersen, H., Friis, M. L., And Sidenius, P. (2005). Gender Differences In Epilepsy. *Epilepsia*, 46, 956-960.

Clarke, V. R., And Collingridge, G. L. (2002). Characterisation Of The Effects Of ATPA, A GLU(K5) Receptor Selective Agonist, On Excitatory Synaptic Transmission In Area CA1 Of Rat Hippocampal Slices. *Neuropharmacology*, 42, 889-902.

Clugnet, M. C., And Ledoux, J. E. (1990). Synaptic Plasticity In Fear Conditioning Circuits: Induction Of LTP In The Lateral Nucleus Of The Amygdala By Stimulation Of The Medial Geniculate Body. *J. Neurosci*, 10, 2818-2824.

Connell, K., Bolton, N., Olsen, D., Piomelli, D., And Hohmann, A. G. (2006). Role Of The Basolateral Nucleus Of The Amygdala In Endocannabinoid-Mediated Stress-Induced Analgesia. *Neurosci. Lett*, 397, 180-184.

Cooke, B. M., And Woolley, C. S. (2005). Gonadal Hormone Modulation Of Dendrites In The Mammalian CNS. *J. Neurobiol*, 64, 34-46.

Cull-Candy, S., Brickley, S., And Farrant, M. (2001). NMDA Receptor Subunits: Diversity, Development And Disease. *Curr. Opin. Neurobiol*, 11, 327-335.

Debock, F., Kurz, J., Azad, S. C., Parsons, C. G., Hapfelmeier, G., Zieglgansberger, W., And Rammes, G. (2003). Alpha2-Adrenoreceptor Activation Inhibits LTP And LTD In The Basolateral Amygdala: Involvement Of Gi/O-Protein-Mediated Modulation Of Ca2+-Channels And Inwardly Rectifying K+-Channels In LTD. *Eur. J. Neurosci*, 17, 1411-1424.

Denny, J. B., Polan-Curtain, J., Wayner, M. J., And Armstrong, D. L. (1991). Angiotensin II Blocks Hippocampal Long-Term Potentiation. *Brain Res*, 567, 321-324.

Deolmos, J. S., Alheid, G. F., And Beltramino, C. A. (1985). Amygdala. In 'The Rat Nervous System'. (Ed G. Paxinos). Pp. 223-334. (Academic Press: Sydney).

Diamond, D. M., Branch, B. J., And Fleshner, M. (1996). The Neurosteroid Dehydroepiandrosterone Sulfate (DHEAS) Enhances Hippocampal Primed Burst, But Not Long-Term, Potentiation. *Neurosci. Lett*, 202, 204-208.

Dingledine, R., Borges, K., Bowie, D., And Traynelis, S. F. (1999). The Glutamate Receptor Ion Channels. *Pharmacol. Rev*, 51, 7-61.

Doyere, V., Schafe, G. E., Sigurdsson, T., And Ledoux, J. E. (2003) Long-Term Potentiation In Freely Moving Rats Reveals Asymmetries In Thalamic And Cortical Inputs To The Lateral Amygdala. *Eur. J. Neurosci*, 17, 2703-2715.

Drephal, C., Schubert, M., And Albrecht, D. (2006). Input-Specific Long-Term Potentiation In The Rat Lateral Amygdala Of Horizontal Slices. *Neurobiol. Learn. Mem*, 85, 272-282.

Duvarci, S., Nader, K., And Ledoux, J. E. (2005). Activation Of Extracellular Signal-Regulated Kinase- Mitogen-Activated Protein Kinase Cascade In The Amygdala Is Required For Memory Reconsolidation Of Auditory Fear Conditioning. *Eur. J. Neurosci*, 21, 283-289.

Farb, C. R., Aoki, C., And Ledoux, J. E. (1995). Differential Localization Of NMDA And AMPA Receptor Subunits In The Lateral And Basal Nuclei Of The Amygdala: A Light And Electron Microscopic Study. *J. Comp Neurol*, 362, 86-108.

Farb, C. R., And Ledoux, J. E. (1997). NMDA And AMPA Receptors In The Lateral Nucleus Of The Amygdala Are Postsynaptic To Auditory Thalamic Afferents. *Synapse*, 27, 106-121.

Farb, C. R., And Ledoux, J. E. (1999). Afferents From Rat Temporal Cortex Synapse On Lateral Amygdala Neurons That Express NMDA And AMPA Receptors. *Synapse*, 33, 218-229.

Fendt, M., And Schmid, S. (2002). Metabotropic Glutamate Receptors Are Involved In Amygdaloid Plasticity. *Eur. J. Neurosci*, 15, 1535-1541.

Frerking, M., And Nicoll, R. A. (2000). Synaptic Kainate Receptors. *Curr. Opin. Neurobiol*, 10, 342-351.

Frey, S., Bergado-Rosado, J., Seidenbecher, T., Pape, H. C., And Frey, J. U. (2001). Reinforcement Of Early Long-Term Potentiation (Early-LTP) In Dentate Gyrus By Stimulation Of The Basolateral Amygdala: Heterosynaptic Induction Mechanisms Of Late-LTP. *J. Neurosci*, 21, 3697-3703.

Fu, Y., Pollandt, S., Liu, J., Krishnan, B., Genzer, K., Orozco-Cabal, L., Gallagher, J. P., And Shinnick-Gallagher, P. (2007). Long-Term Potentiation (LTP) In The Central Amygdala (Cea) Is Enhanced After Prolonged Withdrawal From Chronic Cocaine And Requires CRF1 Receptors. *J. Neurophysiol*, 97, 937-941.

Gean, P.W., Chang, F.-C., Huang, C.C., Lin, J.H., And Way, L.J. (1993). Long-Term Enhancement Of EPSP And NMDA Receptor-Mediated Synaptic Transmission In The Amygdala. *Brain Res. Bull*, 31, 7-11.

Goddard, G. V., Mcintyre, D. C., And Leech, C. K. (1969). A Permanent Change In Brain Function Resulting From Daily Electrical Stimulation. *Exp. Neurol*, 25, 295-330.

Goussakov, I., Chartoff, E. H., Tsvetkov, E., Gerety, L. P., Meloni, E. G., Carlezon, W. A., Jr., And Bolshakov, V. Y. (2006). LTP In The Lateral Amygdala During Cocaine Withdrawal. *Eur. J. Neurosci*, 23, 239-250.

Guarraci, F. A., Frohardt, R. J., And Kapp, B. S. (1999). Amygdaloid D1 Dopamine Receptor Involvement In Pavlovian Fear Conditioning. *Brain Res*, 827, 28-40.

Guterman, A., And Richter-Levin, G. (2006). Neuromodulators Of LTP And Ncams In The Amygdala And Hippocampus In Response To Stress. *EXS*, 98, 137-148.

Hall, J., Thomas, K. L., And Everitt, B. J. (2001). Fear Memory Retrieval Induces CREB Phosphorylation And Fos Expression Within The Amygdala. *Eur. J. Neurosci*, 13, 1453-1458.

Hamann, S. B., Ely, T. D., Grafton, S. T., And Kilts, C. D. (1999). Amygdala Activity Related To Enhanced Memory For Pleasant And Aversive Stimuli. *Nat. Neurosci*, 2, 289-293.

Hannesson, D. K., And Corcoran, M. E. (2000). The Mnemonic Effects Of Kindling. *Neurosci. Biobehav. Rev*, 24, 725-751.

He, Y., Janssen, W. G., And Morrison, J. H. (1999). Differential Synaptic Distribution Of The AMPA-Glur2 Subunit On Gabaergic And Non-Gabaergic Neurons In The Basolateral Amygdala. *Brain Res*, 827, 51-62.

Heinbockel, T., And Pape, H. C. (2000). Input-Specific Long-Term Depression In The Lateral Amygdala Evoked By Theta Frequency Stimulation. *J. Neurosci*, 20, RC68.

Hellner, K., Walther, T., Schubert, M., And Albrecht, D. (2005). Angiotensin-(1-7) Enhances LTP In The Hippocampus Through The G-Protein-Coupled Receptor Mas. *Mol. Cell. Neurosci*, 29, 427-435.

Huang, Y. C., Wang, S. J., Chiou, L. C., And Gean, P. W. (2003). Mediation Of Amphetamine-Induced Long-Term Depression Of Synaptic Transmission By CB1 Cannabinoid Receptors In The Rat Amygdala. *J. Neurosci*, 23, 10311-10320.

Huang, Y. Y., And Kandel, E. R. (1998). Postsynaptic Induction And PKA-Dependent Expression Of LTP In The Lateral Amygdala. *Neuron*, 21, 169-178.

Huang, Y. Y., And Kandel, E. R. (2007b). 5-Hydroxytryptamine Induces A Protein Kinase A/Mitogen-Activated Protein Kinase-Mediated And Macromolecular Synthesis-Dependent Late Phase Of Long-Term Potentiation In The Amygdala. *J. Neurosci*, 27, 3111-3119.

Huang, Y. Y., And Kandel, E. R. (2007a). Low-Frequency Stimulation Induces A Pathway-Specific Late Phase Of LTP In The Amygdala That Is Mediated By PKA And Dependent On Protein Synthesis. *Learn. Mem*, 14, 497-503.

Huang, Y. Y., Martin, K. C., And Kandel, E. R. (2000). Both Protein Kinase A And Mitogen-Activated Protein Kinase Are Required In The Amygdala For The Macromolecular Synthesis-Dependent Late Phase Of Long-Term Potentiation. *J. Neurosci.* 20, 6317-6325.

Huettner, J. E. (2003). Kainate Receptors And Synaptic Transmission. *Prog. Neurobiol*, 70, 387-407.

Humeau, Y., Herry, C., Kemp, N., Shaban, H., Fourcaudot, E., Bissiere, S., And Luthi, A. (2005). Dendritic Spine Heterogeneity Determines Afferent-Specific Hebbian Plasticity In The Amygdala. *Neuron*, 45, 119-131.

Humeau, Y., Reisel, D., Johnson, A. W., Borchardt, T., Jensen, V., Gebhardt, C., Bosch, V., Gass, P., Bannerman, D. M., Good, M. A., Hvalby, O., Sprengel, R., And Luthi, A. (2007). A Pathway-Specific Function For Different AMPA Receptor Subunits In Amygdala Long-Term Potentiation And Fear Conditioning. *J. Neurosci*, 27, 10947-10956.

Humeau, Y., Shaban, H., Bissiere, S., And Luthi, A. (2003). Presynaptic Induction Of Heterosynaptic Associative Plasticity In The Mammalian Brain. *Nature*, 426, 841-845.

Hurlemann, R., Wagner, M., Hawellek, B., Reich, H., Pieperhoff, P., Amunts, K., Oros-Peusquens, A. M., Shah, N. J., Maier, W., And Dolan, R. J. (2007). Amygdala Control Of Emotion-Induced Forgetting And Remembering: Evidence From Urbach-Wiethe Disease. *Neuropsychologia*, 45, 877-884.

Inglis, F. M., And Moghaddam, B. (1999). Dopaminergic Innervation Of The Amygdala Is Highly Responsive To Stress. *J. Neurochem*, 72, 1088-1094.

Izquierdo, I., Fin, C., Schmitz, P. K., Da Silva, R. C., Jerusalinsky, D., Quillfeldt, J. A., Ferreira, M. B., Medina, J. H., And Bazan, N. G. (1995). Memory Enhancement By Intrahippocampal, Intraamygdala, Or Intraentorhinal Infusion Of Platelet-Activating Factor Measured In An Inhibitory Avoidance Task. *Proc. Natl. Acad. Sci. USA*, 92, 5047-5051.

Izquierdo, I., And Medina, J. H. (1995). Correlation Between The Pharmacology Of Long-Term Potentiation And The Pharmacology Of Memory. *Neurobiol. Learn. Mem*, 63, 19-32.

Johnson, A. K., And Thunhorst, R. L. (1997). The Neuroendocrinology Of Thirst And Salt Appetite: Visceral Sensory Signals And Mechanisms Of Central Integration. *Front Neuroendocrinol*, 18, 292-353.

Johnson, L. R., Farb, C., Morrison, J. H., Mcewen, B. S., And Ledoux, J. E. (2005). Localization Of Glucocorticoid Receptors At Postsynaptic Membranes In The Lateral Amygdala. *Neuroscience*, 136, 289-299.

Josselyn, S. A., Kida, S., And Silva, A. J. (2004). Inducible Repression Of CREB Function Disrupts Amygdala-Dependent Memory. *Neurobiol. Learn. Mem*, 82, 159-163.

Kalynchuk, L. E. (2000). Long-Term Amygdala Kindling In Rats As A Model For The Study Of Interictal Emotionality In Temporal Lobe Epilepsy. *Neurosci. Biobehav. Rev*, 24, 691-704.

Kaminski, R. M., Banerjee, M., And Rogawski, M. A. (2004). Topiramate Selectively Protects Against Seizures Induced By ATPA, A Glur5 Kainate Receptor Agonist. *Neuropharmacology*, 46, 1097-1104.

Kantor, D. B., Lanzrein, M., Stary, S. J., Sandoval, G. M., Smith, W. B., Sullivan, B. M., Davidson, N., And Schuman, E. M. (1996). A Role For Endothelial NO Synthase In LTP Revealed By Adenovirus-Mediated Inhibition And Rescue. *Science*, 274, 1744-1748.

Kaschel, T., Schubert, M., And Albrecht, D. (2004). Long-Term Depression In Horizontal Slices Of The Rat Lateral Amygdala. *Synapse*, 53, 141-150.

Kaufmann, W. E., Worley, P. F., Pegg, J., Bremer, M., And Isakson, P. (1996). COX-2, A Synaptically Induced Enzyme, Is Expressed By Excitatory Neurons At Postsynaptic Sites In Rat Cerebral Cortex. *Proc. Natl. Acad. Sci. USA*, 93, 2317-2321.

Kavushansky, A., And Richter-Levin, G. (2006). Effects Of Stress And Corticosterone On Activity And Plasticity In The Amygdala. *J. Neurosci. Res*, 84, 1580-1587.

Kemp, N., And Bashir, Z. I. (1999). Induction Of LTD In The Adult Hippocampus By The Synaptic Activation Of AMPA/Kainate And Metabotropic Glutamate Receptors. *Neuropharmacology*, 38, 495-504.

Kerr, D. S., And Abraham, W. C. (1996). LTD: Many Means To How Many Ends? *Hippocampus*, 6, 30-34.

Kirkwood, A., And Bear, M. F. (1995). Elementary Forms Of Synaptic Plasticity In The Visual Cortex. *Biol. Res*, 28, 73-80.

Kiyama, Y., Manabe, T., Sakimura, K., Kawakami, F., Mori, H., And Mishina, M. (1998). Increased Thresholds For Long-Term Potentiation And Contextual Learning In Mice Lacking The NMDA-Type Glutamate Receptor Epsilon1 Subunit. *J. Neurosci*, 18, 6704-6712.

Kosaka, H., Omori, M., Murata, T., Iidaka, I., Yamada, H., Okada, T., Takahashi, T., Sadato, N., Itoh, H., Yonekura, Y., And Wada, Y. (2002). Differential Amygdala Response During Facial Recognition In Patients With Schizophrenia: An Fmri Study. *Schizophr. Res*, 57, 87-95.

Kostenis, E., Milligan, G., Christopoulos, A., Sanchez-Ferrer, C. F., Heringer-Walther, S., Sexton, P. M., Gembardt, F., Kellett, E., Martini, L., Vanderheyden, P., Schultheiss, H. P., And Walther, T. (2005). G-Protein-Coupled Receptor Mas Is A Physiological Antagonist Of The Angiotensin II Type 1 Receptor. *Circulation*, 111, 1806-1813.

Kramar, E. A., Armstrong, D. L., Ikeda, S., Wayner, M. J., Harding, J. W., And Wright, J. W. (2001). The Effects Of Angiotensin IV Analogs On Long-Term Potentiation Within The CA1 Region Of The Hippocampus In Vitro. *Brain Res*, 897, 114-121.

Krause, S., Schindowski, K., Zechel, S., And Von Bohlen Und Halbach, O. (2008). Expression Of Trkb And Trkc Receptors And Their Ligands Brain-Derived Neurotrophic Factor And Neurotrophin-3 In The Murine Amygdala. *J. Neurosci, Res* (In Press).

Krezel, W., Dupont, S., Krust, A., Chambon, P., And Chapman, P. F. (2001). Increased Anxiety And Synaptic Plasticity In Estrogen Receptor Beta -Deficient Mice. *Proc. Natl. Acad. Sci. USA*, 98, 12278-12282.

Lamprecht, R., Hazvi, S., And Dudai, Y. (1997). CAMP Response Element-Binding Protein In The Amygdala Is Required For Long-But Not Short-Term Conditioned Taste Aversion Memory. *J. Neurosci*, 17, 8443-8450.

Lamprecht, R., Margulies, D. S., Farb, C. R., Hou, M., Johnson, L. R., And Ledoux, J. E. (2006). Myosin Light Chain Kinase Regulates Synaptic Plasticity And Fear Learning In The Lateral Amygdala. *Neuroscience*, 139, 821-829.

Lanahan, A., Lyford, G., Stevenson, G. S., Worley, P. F., And Barnes, C. A. (1997). Selective Alteration Of Long-Term Potentiation-Induced Transcriptional Response In Hippocampus Of Aged, Memory-Impaired Rats. *J. Neurosci*, 17, 2876-2885.

Lang, E. J., And Pare, D. (1998). Synaptic Responsiveness Of Interneurons Of The Cat Lateral Amygdaloid Nucleus. *Neuroscience*, 83, 877-889.

Larson, J., And Lynch, G. (1988). Role Of N-Methyl-D-Aspartate Receptors In The Induction Of Synaptic Potentiation By Burst Stimulation Patterned After The Hippocampal Theta-Rhythm. *Brain Res*, 441, 111-118.

Ledoux, J. E. (2000). Emotion Circuits In The Brain. *Annu. Rev. Neurosci.* 23, 155-184.

Ledoux, J. E., And Muller, J. (1997). Emotional Memory And Psychopathology. *Philos. Trans. R. Soc. Lond B Biol. Sci*, 352, 1719-1726.

Lee, O., Lee, C. J., And Choi, S. (2002). Induction Mechanisms For L-LTP At Thalamic Input Synapses To The Lateral Amygdala: Requirement Of Mglur5 Activation. *Neuroreport*, 13, 685-691.

Lepicard, E. M., Mizuno, K., Antunes-Martins, A., Von Hertzen, L. S., And Giese, K. P. (2006). An Endogenous Inhibitor Of Calcium/Calmodulin-Dependent Kinase II Is Up-Regulated During Consolidation Of Fear Memory. *Eur. J. Neurosci*, 23, 3063-3070.

Li, H., Chen, A., Xing, G., Wei, M. L., And Rogawski, M. A. (2001). Kainate Receptor-Mediated Heterosynaptic Facilitation In The Amygdala. *Nat. Neurosci*, 4, 612-620.

Li, H., And Rogawski, M. A. (1998). Glur5 Kainate Receptor Mediated Synaptic Transmission In Rat Basolateral Amygdala In Vitro. *Neuropharmacology*, 37, 1279-1286.

Li, H., Weiss, S. R., Chuang, D. M., Post, R. M., And Rogawski, M. A. (1998). Bidirectional Synaptic Plasticity In The Rat Basolateral Amygdala: Characterization Of An Activity-Dependent Switch Sensitive To The Presynaptic Metabotropic Glutamate Receptor Antagonist 2S-Alpha-Ethylglutamic Acid. *J. Neurosci*, 18, 1662-1670.

Lin, C. H., Lee, C. C., And Gean, P. W. (2003a). Involvement Of A Calcineurin Cascade In Amygdala Depotentiation And Quenching Of Fear Memory. *Mol. Pharmacol*, 63, 44-52.

Lin, C. H., Yeh, S. H., Leu, T. H., Chang, W. C., Wang, S. T., And Gean, P. W. (2003b). Identification Of Calcineurin As A Key Signal In The Extinction Of Fear Memory. *J. Neurosci*, 23, 1574-1579.

Lin, C. H., Yeh, S. H., Lin, C. H., Lu, K. T., Leu, T. H., Chang, W. C., And Gean, P. W. (2001). A Role For The PI-3 Kinase Signaling Pathway In Fear Conditioning And Synaptic Plasticity In The Amygdala. *Neuron*, 31, 841-851.

Lin, H. C., Wang, S. J., Luo, M. Z., And Gean, P. W. (2000). Activation Of Group II Metabotropic Glutamate Receptors Induces Long-Term Depression Of Synaptic Transmission In The Rat Amygdala. *J. Neurosci*, 20, 9017-9024.

Lisman, J., And Raghavachari, S. (2006). A Unified Model Of The Presynaptic And Postsynaptic Changes During LTP At CA1 Synapses. *Sci. STKE*, 2006, Re11.

Little, H. J., Stephens, D. N., Ripley, T. L., Borlikova, G., Duka, T., Schubert, M., Albrecht, D., Becker, H. C., Lopez, M. F., Weiss, F., Drummond, C., Peoples, M., And Cunningham, C. (2005). Alcohol Withdrawal And Conditioning. *Alcohol Clin. Exp. Res*, 29, 453-464.

Lopez De, A. M., And Sah, P. (2007). Bidirectional Synaptic Plasticity At Nociceptive Afferents In The Rat Central Amygdala. *J. Physiol*, 581, 961-970.

Lynch, M. A. (2004). Long-Term Potentiation And Memory. *Physiol Rev*, 84, 87-136.

Mahanty, N. K., And Sah, P. (1998). Calcium-Permeable AMPA Receptors Mediate Long-Term Potentiation In Interneurons In The Amygdala. *Nature*, 394, 683-687.

Mahanty, N. K., And Sah, P. (1999). Excitatory Synaptic Inputs To Pyramidal Neurons Of The Lateral Amygdala. *Eur. J. Neurosci*, 11, 1217-1222.

Malenka, R. C. (2003). Synaptic Plasticity And AMPA Receptor Trafficking. *Ann. N. Y. Acad. Sci*, 1003, 1-11.

Maren, S. (2005). Synaptic Mechanisms Of Associative Memory In The Amygdala. *Neuron*, 47, 783-786.

Maren, S. (1995). Sexually Dimorphic Perforant Path Long-Term Potentiation (LTP) In Urethane-Anesthetized Rats. *Neurosci. Lett*, 196, 177-180.

Maren, S. (2001). Neurobiology Of Pavlovian Fear Conditioning. *Annu. Rev. Neurosci*, 24, 897-931.

Maren, S., De Oca, B., And Fanselow, M. S. (1994). Sex Differences In Hippocampal Long-Term Potentiation (LTP) And Pavlovian Fear Conditioning In Rats: Positive Correlation Between LTP And Contextual Learning. *Brain Res*, 661, 25-34.

Maren, S., And Fanselow, M. S. (1995). Synaptic Plasticity In The Basolateral Amygdala Induced By Hippocampal Formation Stimulation In Vivo. *J. Neurosci*, 15, 7548-7564.

Marsicano, G., Wotjak, C. T., Azad, S. C., Bisogno, T., Rammes, G., Cascio, M. G., Hermann, H., Tang, J., Hofmann, C., Zieglgansberger, W., Di, M. V., And Lutz, B. (2002). The Endogenous Cannabinoid System Controls Extinction Of Aversive Memories. *Nature*, 418, 530-534.

Matthies, H., Frey, U., Reymann, K., Krug, M., Jork, R., And Schroeder, H. (1990). Different Mechanisms And Multiple Stages Of LTP. *Adv. Exp. Med. Biol*, 268, 359-368.

Mcdonald, A. J., And Augustine, J. R. (1993). Localization Of GABA-Like Immunreactivity In The Monkey Amygdala. *Neuroscience*, 52, 281-294.

Mcgaugh, J. L. (2002). Memory Consolidation And The Amygdala: A Systems Perspective. *Trends Neurosci*, 25, 456.

Mcintyre, D. C., And Racine, R. J. (1986). Kindling Mechanisms: Current Progress On An Experimental Epilepsy Model. *Prog. Neurobiol*, 27, 1-12.

Mckernan, M. G., And Shinnick-Gallagher, P. (1997). Fear Conditioning Induces A Lasting Potentiation Of Synaptic Currents In Vitro. *Nature*, 390, 607-611.

Medina, J. F., Christopher, R. J., Mauk, M. D., And Ledoux, J. E. (2002). Parallels Between Cerebellum- And Amygdala-Dependent Conditioning. *Nat. Rev. Neurosci*, 3, 122-131.

Medina, J. H., And Izquierdo, I. (1995). Retrograde Messengers, Long-Term Potentiation And Memory. *Brain. Res. Rev*, 21, 185-194.

Merino, S. M., And Maren, S. (2006). Hitting Ras Where It Counts: Ras Antagonism In The Basolateral Amygdala Inhibits Long-Term Fear Memory. *Eur. J. Neurosci*, 23, 196-204.

Mitsushima, D., Yamada, K., Takase, K., Funabashi, T., And Kimura, F. (2006). Sex Differences In The Basolateral Amygdala: The Extracellular Levels Of Serotonin And Dopamine, And Their Responses To Restraint Stress In Rats. *Eur. J. Neurosci*, 24, 3245-3254.

Monyer, H., Sprengel, R., Schoepfer, R., Herb, A., Higuchi, M., Lomeli, H., Burnashev, N., Sakmann, B., And Seeburg, P. H. (1992). Heteromeric NMDA Receptors: Molecular And Functional Distinction Of Subtypes. *Science*, 256, 1217-1221.

Moore, C. I., Browning, M. D., And Rose, G. M. (1993). Hippocampal Plasticity Induced By Primed Burst, But Not Long-Term Potentiation, Stimulation Is Impaired In Area CA1 Of Aged Fischer 344 Rats. *Hippocampus*, 3, 57-66.

Moriya, T., Kouzu, Y., Shibata, S., Kadotani, H., Fukunaga, K., Miyamoto, E., And Yoshioka, T. (2000). Close Linkage Between Calcium/Calmodulin Kinase II Alpha/Beta And NMDA-2A Receptors In The Lateral Amygdala And Significance For Retrieval Of Auditory Fear Conditioning. *Eur. J. Neurosci*, 12, 3307-3314.

Mulkey, R. M., And Malenka, R. C. (1992). Mechanisms Underlying Induction Of Homosynaptic Long-Term Depression In Area CA1 Of The Hippocampus. *Neuron*, 9, 967-975.

Murray, H. J., And O'Connor, J. J. (2003). A Role For COX-2 And P38 Mitogen Activated Protein Kinase In Long-Term Depression In The Rat Dentate Gyrus In Vitro. *Neuropharmacology*, 44, 374-380.

Nakazawa, T., Komai, S., Watabe, A. M., Kiyama, Y., Fukaya, M., Rima-Yoshida, F., Horai, R., Sudo, K., Ebine, K., Delawary, M., Goto, J., Umemori, H., Tezuka, T., Iwakura, Y., Watanabe, M., Yamamoto, T., And Manabe, T. (2006). NR2B Tyrosine Phosphorylation Modulates Fear Learning As Well As Amygdaloid Synaptic Plasticity. *EMBO J*, 25, 2867-2877.

Neugebauer, V., Keele, N. B., And Shinnick-Gallagher, P. (1997). Loss Of Long-Lasting Potentiation Mediated By Group III Mglurs In Amygdala Neurons In Kindling-Induced Epileptogenesis. *J. Neurophysiol*, 78, 3475-3478.

O'Dell, T. J., Huang, P. L., Dawson, T. M., Dinerman, J. L., Snyder, S. H., Kandel, E. R., And Fishman, M. C. (1994). Endothelial NOS And The Blockade Of LTP By NOS Inhibitors In Mice Lacking Neuronal NOS. *Science*, 265, 542-546.

Oliet, S. H. R., Malenka, R. C., And Nicoll, R. A. (1997). Two Distinct Form Of Long-Term Depression Coexist In CA1 Hippocampal Pyramidal Cells. *Neuron*, 18, 969-982.

Orban, P. C., Chapman, P. F., And Brambilla, R. (1999). Is The Ras-MAPK Signalling Pathway Necessary For Long-Term Memory Formation? *Trends Neurosci*, 22, 38-44.

Orman, R., And Stewart, M. (2007). Hemispheric Differences In Protein Kinase C Betaii Levels In The Rat Amygdala: Baseline Asymmetry And Lateralized Changes Associated With Cue And Context In A Classical Fear Conditioning Paradigm. *Neuroscience*, 144, 797-807.

Ou, L. C., And Gean, P. W. (2007). Transcriptional Regulation Of Brain-Derived Neurotrophic Factor In The Amygdala During Consolidation Of Fear Memory. *Mol. Pharmacol*, 72, 350-358.

Paul, S., Olausson, P., Venkitaramani, D. V., Ruchkina, I., Moran, T. D., Tronson, N., Mills, E., Hakim, S., Salter, M. W., Taylor, J. R., And Lombroso, P. J. (2007). The Striatal-Enriched Protein Tyrosine Phosphatase Gates Long-Term Potentiation And Fear Memory In The Lateral Amygdala. *Biol. Psychiatry*, 61, 1049-1061.

Pikkarainen, M., Ronkko, S., Savander, V., Insausti, R., And Pitkanen, A. (1999). Projections From The Lateral, Basal, And Accessory Basal Nuclei Of The Amygdala To The Hippocampal Formation In Rat. *J. Comp Neurol*, 403, 229-260.

Pitkanen, A., Savander, V., And Ledoux, J. E. (1997). Organization Of Intra-Amygdaloid Circuitries In The Rat: An Emerging Framework For Understanding Functions Of The Amygdala. *Trends Neurosci*, 20, 517-523.

Pollandt, S., Drephal, C., And Albrecht, D. (2003). 8-OH-DPAT Suppresses The Induction Of LTP In Brain Slices Of The Rat Lateral Amygdala. *Neuroreport*, 14, 895-897.

Pollandt, S., Liu, J., Orozco-Cabal, L., Grigoriadis, D. E., Vale, W. W., Gallagher, J. P., And Shinnick-Gallagher, P. (2006). Cocaine Withdrawal Enhances Long-Term Potentiation Induced By Corticotropin-Releasing Factor At Central Amygdala Glutamatergic Synapses Via CRF, NMDA Receptors And PKA. *Eur. J. Neurosci*, 24, 1733-1743.

Popescu, A. T., Saghyan, A. A., And Pare, D. (2007). NMDA-Dependent Facilitation Of Corticostriatal Plasticity By The Amygdala. *Proc. Natl. Acad. Sci. USA*, 104, 341-6.

Post, R. M., Weiss, S. R., Li, H., Smith, M. A., Zhang, L. X., Xing, G., Osuch, E. A., And Mccann, U. D. (1998). Neural Plasticity And Emotional Memory. *Dev. Psychopathol*, 10, 829-855.

Pozzo-Miller, L. D., Inoue, T., And Murphy, D. D. (1999). Estradiol Increases Spine Density And NMDA-Dependent Ca2+ Transients In Spines Of CA1 Pyramidal Neurons From Hippocampal Slices. *J. Neurophysiol*, 81, 1404-1411.

Racine, R. J., Milgram, N. W., And Hafner, S. (1983). Long-Term Potentiation Phenomena In The Rat Limbic Forebrain. *Brain Res*, 260, 217-231.

Radwanska, K., Nikolaev, E., Knapska, E., And Kaczmarek, L. (2002). Differential Response Of Two Subdivisions Of Lateral Amygdala To Aversive Conditioning As Revealed By C-Fos And P-ERK Mapping. *Neuroreport*, 13, 2241-2246.

Rainnie, D. G., Asprodini, E. K., And Shinnick-Gallagher, P. (1991). Inhibitory Transmission In The Basolateral Amygdala. *J. Neurophysiol*, 66, 999-1009.

Rainnie, D. G., Holmes, K. H., And Shinnick-Gallagher, P. (1994). Activation Of Postsynaptic Metabotropic Glutamate Receptors By Trans-ACPD Hyperpolarizes Neurons Of The Basolateral Amygdala. *J. Neurosci*, 14, 7208-7220.

Rammes, G., Steckler, T., Kresse, A., Schutz, G., Zieglgansberger, W., And Lutz, B. (2000). Synaptic Plasticity In The Basolateral Amygdala In Transgenic Mice Expressing Dominant-Negative Camp Response Element-Binding Protein (CREB) In Forebrain. *Eur. J. Neurosci*, 12, 2534-2546.

Rattiner, L. M., Davis, M., And Ressler, K. J. (2005). Brain-Derived Neurotrophic Factor In Amygdala-Dependent Learning. *Neuroscientist*, 11, 323-333.

Richter-Levin, G., And Yaniv, D. (2001). Is LTP In The Hippocampus A Useful Model For Learning-Related Alterations In Gene Expression? *Rev. Neurosci*, 12, 289-296.

Ripley, T. L., Brown, G., Dunworth, S. J., And Stephens, D. N. (2003). Aversive Conditioning Following Repeated Withdrawal From Ethanol And Epileptic Kindling. *Eur. J. Neurosci*, 17, 1664-1670.

Rodrigues, S. M., Bauer, E. P., Farb, C. R., Schafe, G. E., And Ledoux, J. E. (2002). The Group I Metabotropic Glutamate Receptor Mglur5 Is Required For Fear Memory Formation And Long-Term Potentiation In The Lateral Amygdala. *J. Neurosci*, 22, 5219-5229.

Rodrigues, S. M., Farb, C. R., Bauer, E. P., Ledoux, J. E., And Schafe, G. E. (2004). Pavlovian Fear Conditioning Regulates Thr286 Autophosphorylation Of Ca2+/Calmodulin-Dependent Protein Kinase II At Lateral Amygdala Synapses. *J. Neurosci*, 24, 3281-3288.

Rodrigues, S. M., Schafe, G. E., And Ledoux, J. E. (2001). Intra-Amygdala Blockade Of The NR2B Subunit Of The NMDA Receptor Disrupts The Acquisition But Not The Expression Of Fear Conditioning. *J. Neurosci*, 21, 6889-6896.

Rogan, M. T., Staubli, U. V., And Ledoux, J. E. (1997). Fear Conditioning Induces Associative Long-Term Potentiation In The Amygdala. *Nature*, 390, 604-607.

Rogawski, M. A., Gryder, D., Castaneda, D., Yonekawa, W., Banks, M. K., And Lia, H. (2003). Glur5 Kainate Receptors, Seizures, And The Amygdala. *Ann. N. Y. Acad. Sci*, 985, 150-162.

Romeo, R. D., Mccarthy, J. B., Wang, A., Milner, T. A., And Mcewen, B. S. (2005). Sex Differences In Hippocampal Estradiol-Induced N-Methyl-D-Aspartic Acid Binding And Ultrastructural Localization Of Estrogen Receptor-Alpha. *Neuroendocrinology*, 81, 391-399.

Roozendaal, B., Lengvilas, R., Mcgaugh, J. L., Civelli, O., And Reinscheid, R. K. (2007). Orphanin FQ/Nociceptin Interacts With The Basolateral Amygdala Noradrenergic System In Memory Consolidation. *Learn. Mem*, 14, 29-35.

Royer, S., And Pare, D. (2002). Bidirectional Synaptic Plasticity In Intercalated Amygdala Neurons And The Extinction Of Conditioned Fear Responses. *Neuroscience*, 115, 455-462.

Royer, S., And Pare, D. (2003). Conservation Of Total Synaptic Weight Through Balanced Synaptic Depression And Potentiation. *Nature*, 422, 518-522.

Rumpel, S., Ledoux, J., Zador, A., And Malinow, R. (2005). Postsynaptic Receptor Trafficking Underlying A Form Of Associative Learning. *Science*, 308, 83-88.

Sah, P., Faber, E. S., Lopez De, A. M., And Power, J. (2003). The Amygdaloid Complex: Anatomy And Physiology. *Physiol Rev*, 83, 803-834.

Sah, P., And Lopez, D. A. (2003). Excitatory Synaptic Transmission In The Lateral And Central Amygdala. *Ann. N. Y. Acad. Sci*, 985, 67-77.

Samson, R. D., Dumont, E. C., And Pare, D. (2003). Feedback Inhibition Defines Transverse Processing Modules In The Lateral Amygdala. *J. Neurosci*, 23, 1966-1973.

Samson, R. D., And Pare, D. (2005). Activity-Dependent Synaptic Plasticity In The Central Nucleus Of The Amygdala. *J. Neurosci*, 25, 1847-1855.

Sato, T., Suzuki, E., Yokoyama, M., Watanabe, S., And Miyaoka, H. (2006). Auditory Fear Conditioning And Conditioned Stress Raise NO(3) Level In The Amygdala. *Neuropsychobiology*, 53, 142-147.

Schafe, G. E., Atkins, C. M., Swank, M. W., Bauer, E. P., Sweatt, J. D., And Ledoux, J. E. (2000). Activation Of ERK/MAP Kinase In The Amygdala Is Required For Memory Consolidation Of Pavlovian Fear Conditioning. *J. Neurosci*, 20, 8177-8187.

Schafe, G. E., Bauer, E. P., Rosis, S., Farb, C. R., Rodrigues, S. M., And Ledoux, J. E. (2005). Memory Consolidation Of Pavlovian Fear Conditioning Requires Nitric Oxide Signaling In The Lateral Amygdala. *Eur. J. Neurosci*, 22, 201-211.

Schafe, G. E., Nadel, N. V., Sullivan, G. M., Harris, A., And Ledoux, J. E. (1999). Memory Consolidation For Contextual And Auditory Fear Conditioning Is Dependent On Protein Synthesis, PKA, And MAP Kinase. *Learn. Mem*, 6, 97-110.

Schafe, G. E., Nader, K., Blair, H. T., And Ledoux, J. E. (2001). Memory Consolidation Of Pavlovian Fear Conditioning: A Cellular And Molecular Perspective. *Trends Neurosci*, 24, 540-546.

Schroeder, B. W., And Shinnick-Gallagher, P. (2004). Fear Memories Induce A Switch In Stimulus Response And Signaling Mechanisms For Long-Term Potentiation In The Lateral Amygdala. *Eur. J. Neurosci*, 20, 549-556.

Schubert, M., And Albrecht, D. (2008). Activation Of Kainate GLU(K5) Transmission Rescues Kindling-Induced Impairment Of LTP In The Rat Lateral Amygdala. *Neuropsychopharmacology*, (In Press).

Schubert, M., Drephal, C., And Albrecht, D. (2008). Gender-Dependent ATPA-Induced Changes In Long-Term Potentiation In The Rat Lateral Amygdala. *FASEB J* (In Press).

Schubert, M., Siegmund, H., Pape, H. C., And Albrecht, D. (2005). Kindling-Induced Changes In Plasticity Of The Rat Amygdala And Hippocampus. *Learn. Mem*, 12, 520-526.

Shaban, H., Humeau, Y., Herry, C., Cassasus, G., Shigemoto, R., Ciocchi, S., Barbieri, S., Van Der, P. H., Kaupmann, K., Bettler, B., And Luthi, A. (2006). Generalization Of Amygdala LTP And Conditioned Fear In The Absence Of Presynaptic Inhibition. *Nat. Neurosci*, 9, 1028-1035.

Shankar, S., Teyler, T. J., And Robbins, N. (1998). Aging Differentially Alters Forms Of Long-Term Potentiation In Rat Hippocampal Area CA1. *J. Neurophysiol*, 79, 334-341.

Shindou, T., Watanabe, S., Yamamoto, K., And Nakanishi, H. (1993). NMDA Receptor-Dependent Formation Of Long-Term Potentiation In The Rat Medial Amygdala Neuron In An In Vitro Slice Preparation. *Brain Res. Bull*, 31, 667-672.

Shumyatsky, G. P., Tsvetkov, E., Malleret, G., Vronskaya, S., Hatton, M., Hampton, L., Battey, J. F., Dulac, C., Kandel, E. R., And Bolshakov, V. Y. (2002). Identification Of A Signaling Network In Lateral Nucleus Of Amygdala Important For Inhibiting Memory Specifically Related To Learned Fear. *Cell*, 111, 905-918.

Slanina, K. A., Roberto, M., And Schweitzer, P. (2005). Endocannabinoids Restrict Hippocampal Long-Term Potentiation Via CB1. *Neuropharmacology*, 49, 660-668.

Smolders, I., Bortolotto, Z. A., Clarke, V. R., Warre, R., Khan, G. M., O'Neill, M. J., Ornstein, P. L., Bleakman, D., Ogden, A., Weiss, B., Stables, J. P., Ho, K. H., Ebinger, G., Collingridge, G. L., Lodge, D., And Michotte, Y. (2002). Antagonists Of GLU(K5)-Containing Kainate Receptors Prevent Pilocarpine-Induced Limbic Seizures. *Nat. Neurosci*, 5, 796-804.

Spezio, M. L., Huang, P. Y., Castelli, F., And Adolphs, R. (2007). Amygdala Damage Impairs Eye Contact During Conversations With Real People. *J. Neurosci*, 27, 3994-3997.

Stephens, D. N., Ripley, T. L., Borlikova, G., Schubert, M., Albrecht, D., Hogarth, L., And Duka, T. (2005). Repeated Ethanol Exposure And Withdrawal Impairs Human Fear Conditioning And Depresses Long-Term Potentiation In Rat Amygdala And Hippocampus. *Biol. Psychiatry*, 58, 392-400.

Sweeten, T. L., Posey, D. J., Shekhar, A., And Mcdougle, C. J. (2002). The Amygdala And Related Structures In The Pathophysiology Of Autism. *Pharmacol. Biochem. Behav*, 71, 449-455.

Tchekalarova, J., And Albrecht, D. (2007). Angiotensin II Suppresses Long-Term Depression In The Lateral Amygdala Of Mice Via L-Type Calcium Channels. *Neurosci. Lett*, 415, 68-72.

Teather, L. A., Packard, M. G., And Bazan, N. G. (2002). Post-Training Cyclooxygenase-2 (COX-2) Inhibition Impairs Memory Consolidation. *Learn. Mem*, 9, 41-47.

Tsvetkov, E., Carlezon, W. A., Benes, F. M., Kandel, E. R., And Bolshakov, V. Y. (2002). Fear Conditioning Occludes LTP-Induced Presynaptic Enhancement Of Synaptic Transmission In The Cortical Pathway To The Lateral Amygdala. *Neuron*, 34, 289-300.

Tsvetkov, E., Shin, R. M., And Bolshakov, V. Y. (2004). Glutamate Uptake Determines Pathway Specificity Of Long-Term Potentiation In The Neural Circuitry Of Fear Conditioning. *Neuron*, 41, 139-151.

Tully, K., Li, Y., Tsvetkov, E., And Bolshakov, V. Y. (2007). Norepinephrine Enables The Induction Of Associative Long-Term Potentiation At Thalamo-Amygdala Synapses. *Proc. Natl. Acad. Sci. U S A*, 104, 14146-14150.

Ullal, G., Fahnestock, M., And Racine, R. (2005). Time-Dependent Effect Of Kainate-Induced Seizures On Glutamate Receptor Glur5, Glur6, And Glur7 Mrna And Protein Expression In Rat Hippocampus. *Epilepsia*, 46, 616-623.

Von Bohlen Und Halbach, O., And Albrecht, D. (1998a). Angiotensin II Inhibits Long-Term Potentiation Within The Lateral Nucleus Of The Amygdala Through AT1 Receptors. *Peptides*, 19, 1031-1036.

Von Bohlen Und Halbach, O., And Albrecht, D. (1998b). Mapping Of Angiotensin AT1 Receptors In The Rat Limbic System. *Regul. Pept*, 78, 51-56.

Von Bohlen Und Halbach, O., And Albrecht, D. (1998c). Tracing Of Axonal Connectivities In A Combined Slice Preparation Of Rat Brains - A Study By Rhodamine-Dextran-Amine-Application In The Lateral Nucleus Of The Amygdala. *J. Neurosci. Methods*, 81, 169-175.

Von Bohlen Und Halbach, O., And Albrecht, D. (1998d). Visualization Of Specific Angiotensin II Binding Sites In The Rat Limbic System. *Neuropeptides*, 32, 241-245.

Von Bohlen Und Halbach, O., And Albrecht, D. (2000). Identification Of Angiotensin IV Binding Sites In The Mouse Brain By A Fluorescent Binding Study. *Neuroendocrinology*, 72, 218-223.

Von Bohlen Und Halbach, O., And Albrecht, D. (2002). Reciprocal Connections Of The Hippocampal Area CA1, The Lateral Nucleus Of The Amygdala And Cortical Areas In A Combined Horizontal Slice Preparation. *Neurosci. Res*, 44, 91-100.

Von Bohlen Und Halbach, O., And Albrecht, D. (2006). The CNS Renin-Angiotensin System. *Cell Tissue Res*, 326, 599-616.

Von Bohlen Und Halbach, O., Albrecht, D., Heinemann, U., And Schuchmann, S. (2002). Spatial Nitric Oxide Imaging Using 1,2-Diaminoanthraquinone To Investigate The

Involvement Of Nitric Oxide In Long-Term Potentiation In Rat Brain Slices. *Neuroimage*, 15, 633-639.

Von Bohlen Und Halbach, O., Schulze, K., And Albrecht, D. (2004). Amygdala-Kindling Induces Alterations In Neuronal Density And In Density Of Degenerated Fibers. *Hippocampus*, 14, 311-318.

Von Bohlen Und Halbach, O., Walther, T., Bader, M., And Albrecht, D. (2001). Genetic Deletion Of Angiotensin AT2 Receptor Leads To Increased Cell Numbers In Different Brain Structures Of Mice. *Regul. Pept*, 99, 209-216.

Von Bohlen Und Halbach, O., Walther, T., Bader, M., And Albrecht, D. (2000). Interaction Between Mas And The Angiotensin AT1 Receptor In The Amygdala. *J. Neurophysiol,* 83, 2012-2021.

Vouimba, R. M., Munoz, C., And Diamond, D. M. (2006). Differential Effects Of Predator Stress And The Antidepressant Tianeptine On Physiological Plasticity In The Hippocampus And Basolateral Amygdala. *Stress*, 9, 29-40.

Vouimba, R. M., Yaniv, D., Diamond, D., And Richter-Levin, G. (2004). Effects Of Inescapable Stress On LTP In The Amygdala Versus The Dentate Gyrus Of Freely Behaving Rats. *Eur. J. Neurosci*, 19, 1887-1894.

Vouimba, R. M., Yaniv, D., And Richter-Levin, G. (2007). Glucocorticoid Receptors And Beta-Adrenoceptors In Basolateral Amygdala Modulate Synaptic Plasticity In Hippocampal Dentate Gyrus, But Not In Area CA1. *Neuropharmacology*, 52, 244-252.

Walker, D. L., And Davis, M. (2000). Involvement Of NMDA Receptors Within The Amygdala In Short- Versus Long-Term Memory For Fear Conditioning As Assessed With Fear-Potentiated Startle. *Behav. Neurosci*, 114, 1019-1033.

Wang, S. J., And Gean, P. W. (1999). Long-Term Depression Of Excitatory Synaptic Transmission In The Rat Amygdala. *J. Neurosci*, 19, 10656-10663.

Watanabe, Y., Ikegaya, Y., Saito, H., And Abe, K. (1995a). Roles Of GABAA, NMDA And Muscarinic Receptors In Induction Of Long-Term Potentiation In The Medial And Lateral Amygdala In Vitro. *Neurosci. Res*, 21, 317-322.

Watanabe, Y., Saito, H., And Abe, K. (1995b). Nitric Oxide Is Involved In Long-Term Potentiation In The Medial But Not Lateral Amygdala Neuron Synapses In Vitro. *Brain Res*, 688, 233-236.

Wayner, M. J., Armstrong, D. L., Phelix, C. F., Wright, J. W., And Harding, J. W. (2001). Angiotensin IV Enhances LTP In Rat Dentate Gyrus In Vivo. *Peptides*, 22, 1403-1414.

Weisskopf, M. G., Bauer, E. P., And Ledoux, J. E. (1999). L-Type Voltage-Gated Calcium Channels Mediate NMDA-Independent Associative Long-Term Potentiation At Thalamic Input Synapses To The Amygdala. *J. Neurosci*, 19, 10512-10519.

Weisskopf, M. G., And Ledoux, J. E. (1999). Distinct Populations Of NMDA Receptors At Subcortical And Cortical Inputs To Principal Cells Of The Lateral Amygdala. *J. Neurophysiol*, 81, 930-934.

Wolfman, C., Fin, C., Dias, M., Bianchin, M., Da Silva, R. C., Schmitz, P. K., Medina, J. H., And Izquierdo, I. (1994). Intrahippocampal Or Intraamygdala Infusion Of KN62, A Specific Inhibitor Of Calcium/Calmodulin-Dependent Protein Kinase II, Causes Retrograde Amnesia In The Rat. *Behav. Neural Biol*, 61, 203-205.

Yaniv, D., Desmedt, A., Jaffard, R., And Richter-Levin, G. (2004). The Amygdala And Appraisal Processes: Stimulus And Response Complexity As An Organizing Factor. *Brain Res. Rev*, 44, 179-186.

Yaniv, D., Schafe, G. E., Ledoux, J. E., And Richter-Levin, G. (2001). A Gradient Of Plasticity In The Amygdala Revealed By Cortical And Subcortical Stimulation, In Vivo. *Neuroscience*, 106, 613-620.

Yee, B. K., Zhu, S. W., Mohammed, A. H., And Feldon, J. (2007). Levels Of Neurotrophic Factors In The Hippocampus And Amygdala Correlate With Anxiety- And Fear-Related Behaviour In C57BL6 Mice. *J. Neural Transm*, 114, 431-444.

Zhu, P. J., And Lovinger, D. M. (2005). Retrograde Endocannabinoid Signaling In A Postsynaptic Neuron/Synaptic Bouton Preparation From Basolateral Amygdala. *J. Neurosci*, 25, 6199-6207.

In: Synaptic Plasticity: New Research
Editors: Tim F. Kaiser and Felix J. Peters

ISBN: 978-1-60456-732-8

Chapter 10

SYNAPTIC PLASTICITY AND MNEMONIC ENCODING BY HIPPOCAMPAL FORMATION PLACE CELLS

M. Tsanov[1], J. R. Brotons-Mas[1,2], M. V. Sanchez-Vives[2,3] and S. M. O'Mara[1]

[1] Institute of Neuroscience, Trinity College, Dublin 2, Ireland
[2] Instituto de Neurociencias de Alicante, Universidad Miguel Hernandez-CSIC, San Juan de Alicante, Spain
[3]ICREA-Institut d'Investigacios Biomediques August Pi i Sunyer, Villarroel 170, 08036, Barcelona, Spain

ABSTRACT

In order to guide behavior, sensory information has to be analyzed in the context of previous memory and attention-related episodes. Such episodes can represent sequences of sensory items in space and time and the learning of such sequences is known as episodic memory. The formation of this memory is believed to be mediated in the hippocampal region, and is generated by the changes in neuronal efficacy known as long-term synaptic plasticity. In this chapter we will review some of the up-to-date models of synaptic plasticity and their relation to the structural and functional memory processes demonstrated by behavioral and electrophysiological experiments. The main aim of this chapter is to describe how neuroplastic mechanisms work together to create network representations of previous experiences. Here, we specifically consider experience-dependent modulation of hippocampal cell firing in the context of spatial memory formation. The information encoded by the firing patterns of these neurons represents sequences of events and places that will be stored in a long-term manner. However, the precise connection between the neuronal firing rate changes and long-term synaptic plasticity is still controversial. A significant challenge remains to reveal how the processing, encoding and storage of highly-integrated sensory information occurs within the circuitry of the hippocampus. Recent electrophysiological findings in combination with computational memory models have allowed us to obtain closer insight into how information is represented in the hippocampal formation and how this information is encoded.

In order to gain a better understanding of hippocampal experience-dependent synaptic plasticity we also will create parallels between the synaptic alterations in the declarative memory system and the equivalent synaptic changes throughout the functionally well-known perceptual and procedural memory systems. We review the development of hippocampus-dependent memory models and stress the importance of functional patterns that characterize the remodeling of the neural connectivity.

1. Experience-Dependent Changes of Synaptic Strength

A cardinal feature of neurons in the cerebral cortex comprises stimulus selectivity, and experience-dependent shifts in selectivity are a common correlate of memory formation. Many synapses in the hippocampus and neocortex are bidirectionally modifiable and depend on the recent history of cortical activity. For memory to occur, these modifications must persist long enough to contribute to long-term memory storage. This definitely appears to be the case for the forms of synaptic plasticity known as long-term potentiation (LTP) and long-term depression (LTD). Extensive research has been conducted to establish the contribution of LTP to spatial learning (Castro *et al.*, 1989; Barnes, 1995; Moser, 1995; Morris & Frey, 1997) and validate it as a mechanism encoding spatial learning.

Hippocampal synapses are known to respond with long-term potentiation, to a brief tetanus both in in vivo (Bliss & Lomo, 1973) and in vitro (Deadwyler *et al.*, 1975) . Electrophysiologically expressed, LTP was originally described by (Bliss & Lomo, 1973) as having two components: (1) synaptic, expressed by an increase in the synaptic efficacy, i.e., enhanced field excitatory postsynaptic potential (EPSP) with the same number of stimulated fibersand (2) non-synaptic, concerned with an increase in the probability that an EPSP will elicit an action potential. In some cases tetanic stimulation results in increased ability of an EPSP to fire an action potential, even when the EPSP amplitude is unchanged. This phenomenon is referred to as the non-synaptic component of LTP (Douglas & Goddard, 1975; Wilson, 1981; Taube & Schwartzkroin, 1988) and also as EPSP–spike or E–S potentiation (Andersen *et al.*, 1980; Wigstrom & Swann, 1980). The intracellular correlate of E–S potentiation is an increased probability of firing for a given EPSP amplitude (Chavez-Noriega *et al.*, 1990). The mechanisms underlying E–S potentiation are believed to be decrease in the ratio of inhibitory to excitatory drive (Wilson, 1981; Abraham *et al.*, 1987; Chavez-Noriega *et al.*, 1990) and/or an increase in the intrinsic excitability of the postsynaptic neuron through modulation of postsynaptic voltage-gated conductances (Hess & Gustafsson, 1990; Bernard & Wheal, 1996; Noguchi *et al.*, 1998) Frick et al., 2004 -Nature Neurosci, 7:126-135. Although non-synaptic mechanisms comprise important part of information processing in brain networks, we will focus further on the synaptic component of neuronal plasticity, as it is proposed to underline long-term memory processes.

LTD is a lasting activity-dependent decrease in synaptic efficacy (Lynch *et al.*, 1977). Both hetero- and homosynaptic forms of LTD can be induced in various pathways of the hippocampal formation in vitro (Dunwiddie & Lynch, 1978; Dudek & Bear, 1992) and in vivo (Levy & Steward, 1979; Thiels *et al.*, 1994; Doyere *et al.*, 1996; Heynen *et al.*, 1996; Thiels *et al.*, 1996). It has become apparent that LTD may be equally important for spatial information storage. Exposure of an animal to a novel spatial configurations, for example results in the expression of LTD in CA1 region (Manahan-Vaughan & Braunwell, 1999). It has been postulated that the mechanisms underlying long-term depression in the hippocampus, together with the mechanisms of long-term potentiation, are responsible for information storage by the hippocampus (Martin *et al.*, 2000). In the following section we will summarize the main models that explain the long-term changes in synaptic efficacy.

2. Models for Synaptic Plasticity Induction

Generally, synaptic plasticity can involve a presynaptic component as well as the postsynaptic one. Synaptic modifications also can be divided on homosynaptic, involving only one pre- and postsynaptic interaction, and heterosynaptic, where synaptic alterations involve more than one presynaptic component. Regarding the temporal effect, synaptic changes can be defined as short-lasting (seconds, minutes) and long-lasting (days, months). The most common object of plasticity research is the homosynaptic long-term change of synaptic strength as it is believed to be a necessary component in hippocampal network modifications. Here we will emphasize the two main models explaining how this type of synaptic plasticity can be induced.

2.1. Frequency-dependent plasticity

The BCM (Bienenstock, Cooper and Munro) rule states that synaptic strengths are increased when the activity of the pre- and post-synaptic neurons exceeds a particular threshold and weakened when activity is below it (Bienenstock *et al.*, 1982). Crucially, this modification of threshold varies according to the mean activity of both neurons, which prevents runaway scaling up or down of all the synapses (Bear *et al.*, 1987; Kirkwood *et al.*, 1995). In the BCM model, correlated pre- and postsynaptic activity evokes LTP when the postsynaptic firing rate is higher than the threshold value and LTD when it is lower (Fig 1A). To stabilize the model, the threshold is shifting as a function of the average postsynaptic firing rate. For example, the threshold increases if the postsynaptic neuron is highly active, making LTP more difficult and LTD easier to induce. Frequency-dependent plasticity relies on the natural fast and very fast cortical oscillations timed on a slower theta rhythm (Larson & Lynch, 1988, , 1989; Gray & McCormick, 1996).

Most forms of LTP are glutamatergic and the most prominent form is induced following activation of the *N*-methyl- D-aspartate (NMDA) receptor. NMDA-dependent LTP occurs only if there is both presynaptic firing and substantial postsynaptic depolarization sufficient to open the NMDA channel. Postsynaptic activity can occur with a delay, the duration of which is the time-constant of decay of the NMDA conductance (100–200ms) (Gustafsson *et al.*, 1987). Frequency-dependent models require repetitive firing for LTP induction. Scaling of the NMDA-mediated component has implications for Hebbian plasticity, because LTP and LTD are activated by calcium entry through NMDA receptors. It is accepted that large amounts of calcium entry induce LTP, while smaller amounts cause LTD (Lisman, 1994). If neurons scale down NMDA currents in response to enhanced activity, this may make it more difficult to evoke LTP and easier to induce LTD.

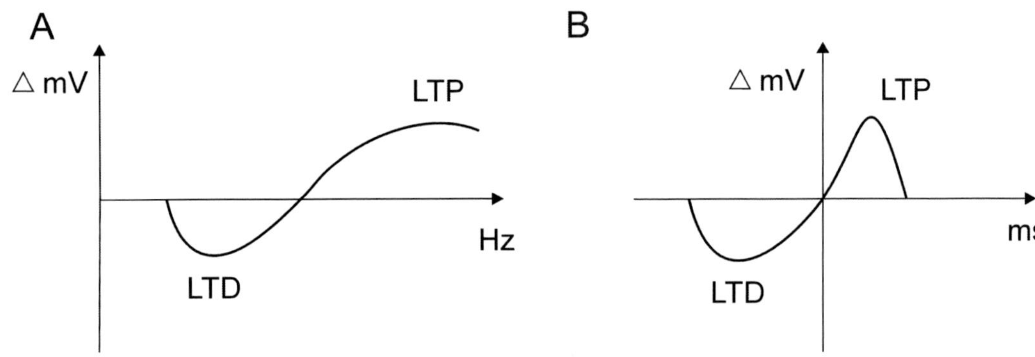

Figure 1. Models of synaptic plasticity induction. A. Frequency dependent synaptic plasticity. Diagram showing the dependence of synaptic plasticity, represented on the x-axis by the change of the measured neuronal response in mV, on the frequency (Hz) of homosynaptic interaction. A lower frequency, of ca. 1Hz, results in LTD, whereas higher frequencies will tend to evoke LTP. B. Spike-timing dependent plasticity. The diagram illustrates the importance of the sequence in pre- and postsynaptic activity as well as the significance of their temporal order. The timing is expressed in milliseconds on the x-axis, with the y-axis indicating the moment of coincident activity. If a presynaptic spike follows the postsynaptic response, LTD is induced and if presynaptic activity precedes the postsynaptic one, LTP is induced.

In an effort to more closely approximate endogenous conditions for synaptic plasticity many researchers have studied the relationship between hippocampal LTP and neuronal oscillations during exploratory behaviour. Long-term synaptic potentiation is optimal when the time interval between stimuli is approximately 200ms due to activation of NMDA receptor-mediated inward current or removal of the inactivation of T-type of Ca^{2+} channels followed by a rebound depolarization after 100–200ms. The timing corresponds ideally with the synchronized depolarization during theta oscillation, which considers the theta cycle as an information quantum. The specifically-expressed amplitude of the theta rhythm in the limbic system implies its involvement in memory formation. One of the more convincing links between learning and hippocampal LTP involves the use of theta-frequency stimulation, establishing a connection between theta rhythm and LTP (Larson & Lynch, 1986; Rose & Dunwiddie, 1986; Buzsáki *et al.*, 1987; Larson & Lynch, 1989). Patterned after the endogenous theta rhythm, one could effectively induce LTP extracellularly with short 100 Hz bursts delivered at 5 to 8 cycles per second (about 50 pulses total). LTP is more effectively induced in the dentate gyrus when tetanus was delivered on positive phases of theta in urethane anesthetized rats (Pavlides *et al.*, 1988). Similar results have been found in freely-moving animals with stimulation of the perforant path (Orr *et al.*, 2001). Thus the induction of synaptic plasticity in hippocampal regions after high-frequency firing activity coheres with naturally occurring spiking patterns. For the experience-dependent alterations of hippocampal place cells frequency-dependent plasticity is mediated by the complex-spike bursts (Muller *et al.*, 1987; Gothard *et al.*, 2001).

2.2. Spike timing-dependent plasticity

In addition to frequency-dependent Hebbian modifications, another mechanism also has been proposed to underlie adult functional plasticity (Dan & Poo, 2004; Yao & Dan, 2005). Changes in synaptic efficacy can be based also on the precise timing of presynaptic and postsynaptic activity (Levy & Steward, 1983; Markram *et al.*, 1997; Debanne *et al.*, 1998). This "spike-timing-dependent plasticity" (STDP) has several properties which are believed to transform changes in environmental inputs into changes in neural representations (Fu *et al.*, 2002; Sur *et al.*, 2002). The functional consequence of spike-timing plasicity is that synapses from a presynaptic neuron which contribute to the firing of the postsynaptic neuron will be strengthened, whereas synapses which are uncorrelated or negatively-paired with postsynaptic spike times will tend to be weakened (Fig 1B). The amount of LTP falls off roughly exponentially as a function of the difference between pre- and postsynaptic spike times with a time constant that is of the same order as a typical membrane time constant. This ensures that only those presynaptic spikes that arrive within the temporal range over which a neuron integrates its inputs are potentiated, further enforcing the requirement of causality. STDP appears to depend on interplay between the dynamics of NMDA receptor channel activation and the timing of action potentials back-propagating through the dendrites of the postsynaptic neuron (Magee & Johnston, 1997; Linden, 1999; Sourdet & Debanne, 1999). Repeated pairing of postsynaptic spiking after presynaptic activation results in larger calcium influx and LTP (EPSP precedes the back-propagating action potential), whereas postsynaptic spiking before presynaptic activation (EPSP follows the action potential) leads to a small calcium transient and LTD (Bell *et al.*, 1997; Markram *et al.*, 1997; Bi & Poo, 1998; Debanne *et al.*, 1998; Zhang *et al.*, 1998; Egger *et al.*, 1999; Feldman, 2000). This temporally-asymmetric Hebbian synaptic plasticity supports sequence learning because it tends to wire together neurons that form causal chains (Paulsen & Sejnovski, 2000). Thus, NMDAR-gated modification of synaptic efficacy is essential for creating and stabilizing activity patterns in neural networks. STDP can act as a learning mechanism for generating neuronal responses selective to input timing, order, and sequence. STDP-like rules have been applied to coincidence detection (Gerstner *et al.*, 1996), sequence learning (Abbott & Blum, 1996; Roberts, 1999), path learning in navigation (Blum & Abbott, 1996; Mehta *et al.*, 2000), and direction selectivity in visual responses (Schuett *et al.*, 2001; Yao & Dan, 2001). In general, STDP greatly expands the capability of frequency-dependent plasticity to address temporally sensitive computational tasks.

Given that the hippocampus is critical for spatial memory formation, and that its synapses undergo synaptic plasticity, an important question concerns how the functional activity and synaptic alterations in this region relate to one another. The first approach in this direction will be to define the rules under which hippocampal representations are modified with experience, an issue that we explore in the following section.

3. Experience-Dependent Alterations of Hippocampal Place Fields

Place cells are complex-spiking cells that fire in response to a rodent's spatial location (O'Keefe, 1976) and these cells are recorded in all areas of the hippocampus proper (Barnes *et al.*, 1990). Place-dependent complex spiking cells are found also in regions afferent to and efferent from hippocampus. Single units coding for spatial information are present in subiculum (Sharp & Green, 1994), entorhinal cortex (Quirk *et al.*, 1992; Hafting *et al.*, 2005), parasubiculum (Taube, 1995b) and postrhinal cortex (Burwell & Hafeman, 2003). Neurons with similar patterns are described in primate hippocampal region. The spatial cells there respond to a certain part of space - "view" neurons (Rolls & O'Mara, 1995). Cells in the human hippocampus are also shown to fire in correlation with spatial orientation tasks (Ekstrom *et al.*, 2003).

3.1. Place field plasticity for stable environment

Naturalistic studies demonstrate of how the place representation is modified by behavioral experience and the properties of such place cell plasticity share the principles of dynamic connectivity of synchronously active neurons. A substantial number of reports demonstrate systematic alterations in place fields in response to experiences that the animal has in an environment.

The simplest kind of experience is repeated entry into the same environment, and small but pronounced short-lasting changes in place fields have been observed when rats repeatedly run in the same direction along a linear track (Mehta *et al.*, 1997). Place fields undergo with experience asymmetrical expansion such that cells recorded over multiple laps around the same track displayed place fields that shifted backwards relative to the direction of motion and increased their both their firing rate and firing field size (Mehta *et al.*, 1997; Mehta *et al.*, 2000) (Fig 2). Hippocampal CA3 fields shift backward immediately after the environmental exposure and maintain these changes for several days, while CA1 fields shift backwards from the second day of exposure and fail to maintain the changes (Lee *et al.*, 2004). This feature favors CA3 region as a network that can store long-term sequential representations. The asymmetrical development of place fields is in accordance with the models of long-term potentiation which is suggested to occur only when the postsynaptic neuron is depolarised shortly after the depolarisation of the presynaptic neuron (Levy & Steward, 1983; Bi & Poo, 1998). As the cells with place fields are always activated in a particular temporal order, it is assumed that the synapses from early firing cells to later firing cells become selectively potentiated. Therefore each place cell will be driven to firing threshold progressively earlier with each lap around the track, resulting in a backwards shift along the track and increase of the field size. The development of place field expansion and backward shift is also dependent on NMDA receptors (Mehta *et al.*, 2000; Ekstrom *et al.*, 2001) in accordance with hippocampal models of NMDA-dependent synaptic plasticity (Bliss & Collingridge, 1993; Abraham & Bear, 1996; Jensen & Lisman, 1996).

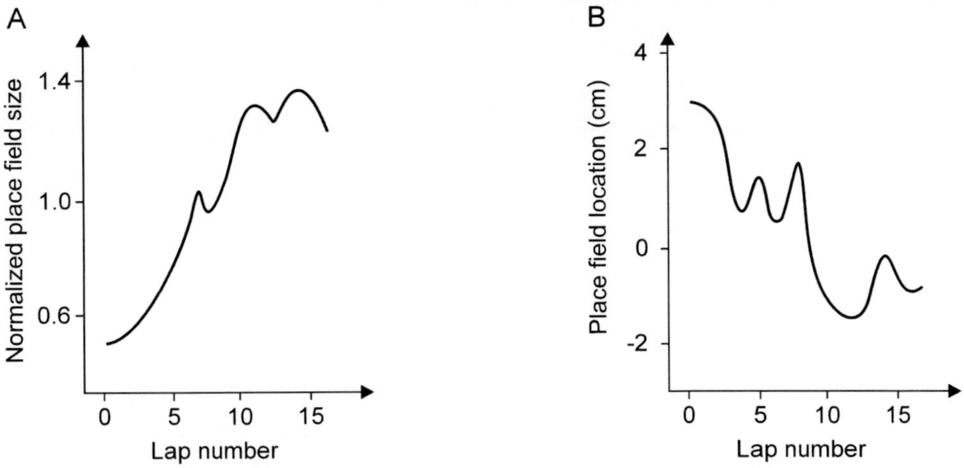

Figure 2. Experience-dependent asymmetrical expansion of place fields. A. The size of the place fields is gradually increasing with the number of laps. The relative place field size of the 43 place fields increased significantly and asymptotically by 124% over 17 laps on closed track (Adapted from Mehta et al., 1997). B. The location of the fields gradually is shifting backwards, towards the direction the rat is coming from, as the number of laps increased. The location of each place field on each lap was calculated relative to the center of mass of the corresponding average place field for all 17 trials. The place field location for 43 place fields is shown as a function of lap number. There was a significant, asymptotic backward shift in the relative field locations over the 17 laps on the track (adapted from (Mehta et al., 1997)).

3.2. Environmental manipulations and place fields

One of the first indications that memory modulates place fields is the finding that even after visual cues are removed, place cells firing persisted (O'Keefe & Speakman, 1987). Place field reorganization (or remapping) results from a variety of cue manipulations (O'Keefe, 1979; Young *et al.*, 1994; Cressant *et al.*, 1997; Shapiro *et al.*, 1997; Tanila *et al.*, 1997b). Plasticity of place cells has been observed as a remapping of either their firing rates or their receptive fields when cues in an environment (Bostock *et al.*, 1991), or the shape of an environment, are changed (Lever *et al.*, 2002; Fyhn *et al.*, 2007). Rotation of a cue card attached to the wall in a cylindrical arena is able to produce a rotation of the place field keeping the same angular relation as in the original configuration (Muller & Kubie, 1987). Removal of this cue card results in place field rotation to unpredictable positions. In contrast manipulations of the cue size did not affect place field. Placing a small barrier over the location of a previously recorded place field is enough to make the place field disappear. Doubling the size of the area and wall height is producing place field expansion of some cells or generation of completely new place fields (Bostock *et al.*, 1991). Context-specific responses of place cells emerge when rats are required to distinguish between contexts (Smith & Mizumori, 2006b, 2006a). The removal of a cue proximal to the place fields reduced their size, while removal of a distal cue would produce an enlargement of the place field size (Hetherington & Shapiro, 1997). The effect of visual cue manipulation differs also in the cases when the animal is present or absent during the manipulation. Place cells did not rotate their field if the cue was moved in their presence but if the cue was rotated while away, then the place field would also rotate (Jeffery & O'Keefe, 1999).

3.3. Learning-dependent modifications of place fields

Different learning experiences are able to change the firing fields of place cells, although the main environmental cues stay stable. Place field remapping can be triggered by a discrete learning event in the same, unchanged environment (Moita *et al.*, 2004) — in a form of Pavlovian conditioning called contextual fear conditioning. An electrical footshock is applied as an unconditional stimulus while the environment effectively acts as a conditional stimulus that, after training, can itself elicit a behavioral freezing response. The cell's place field remapped completely after contextual fear conditioning.

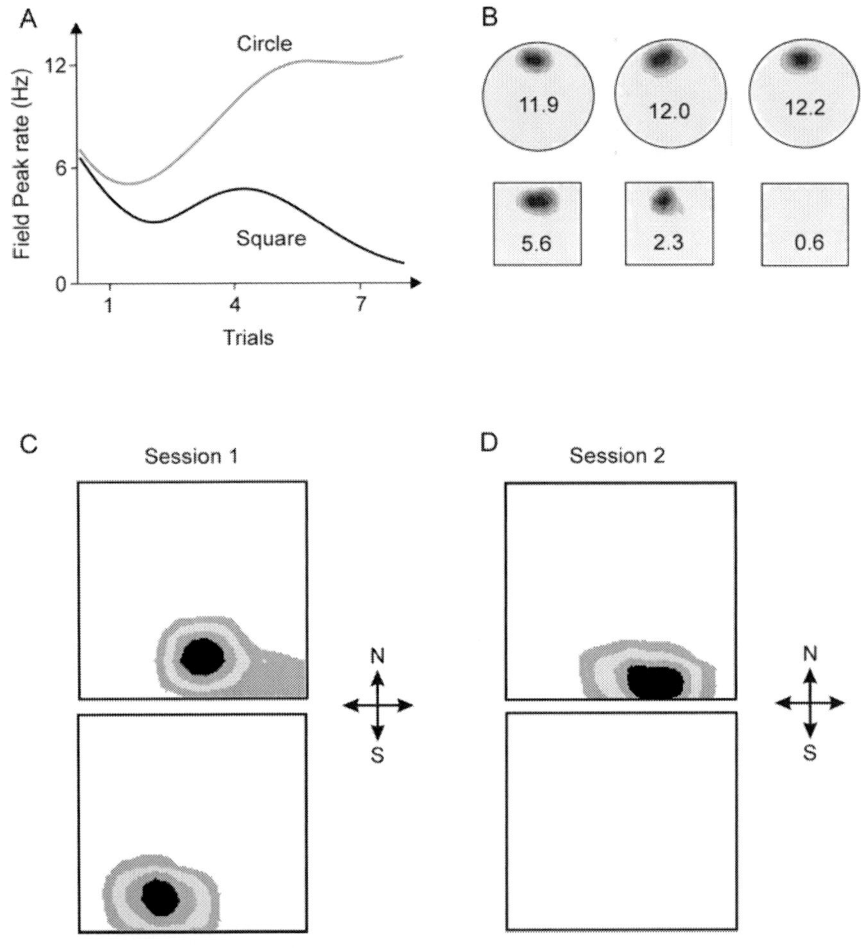

Figure 3. Learning-dependent pattern separation of place fields. A. Single place cell developed the ability to distinguish a square from a circular recording environment over the course of several sessions. B. Example of a place cell that is persisting to fire with the same frequency only in a circular, but not in a square recording box (Adapted from Lever et al., 2002 and Jeffery and Hayman, 2006). Higher intensity of grey color represents higher frequency of the unit discharge (Hz). C. Similarly, in two identical novel environments that differ only by their location in space the place cells fire in a similar pattern. D. Development of remapping by a single place cell is observed over the course of a single session. Learning-dependent experience resulted in pattern separation between the north- and south-located square. These observations show that individual cells can acquire the ability to discriminate environments (adapted from (Jeffery & Hayman, 2004)).

Place fields have been shown to become more selective as rats learn a maze (Mizumori & Kalyani, 1997). Place cells can gradually acquire diverging responses to two sets of similar but non-identical stimuli, a type of discriminative responding that is commonly known as "pattern separation" (Bostock *et al.*, 1991; Lever *et al.*, 2002; Hayman *et al.*, 2003). Over time, the place system considers the two "similar" environments as different and as a result a divergence of firing patterns in both environments occurs (Fig 3). Such experience-dependent change in responsiveness to environmental stimuli strongly implies experience-dependent synaptic plasticity of the place cell connections within the sequence-encoding network. LTP and LTD of the connections between the contextual inputs are proposed to mediate the long-term, experience-dependent divergence of place cell representations (Jeffery & Hayman, 2004). The coactivity of contextual inputs that are specific to that environment and the place cells is able to potentiate with time only those connections, which precisely represent the environment (Barry *et al.*, 2006). This idea is supported by the ability of place cells to acquire discriminations between closely similar environments that previously were undiscriminated, (Bostock *et al.*, 1991; Lever *et al.*, 2002; Hayman *et al.*, 2003; Jeffery & Anderson, 2003). Discrimination of similar environments appears often to involve the loss of a field in one or other of the two environments, sometimes with development of a new field (Lever *et al.*, 2002; Wills *et al.*, 2005). The observed phenomenon can be explained with a weakening of the link between inactive contextual inputs and the field-specifying inputs, by heterosynaptic LTD, so that this cell comes to be driven only by the relevant contextual elements (Abraham & Bear, 1996; Fazeli & Collingridge, 1996; Rolls & Deco, 2002). Additionally synaptic scaling models propose that LTP and LTD are always balanced, suggesting how place cells can learn to discriminate two environments (Turrigiano & Nelson, 2000): as inputs from the discriminative stimuli gradually increase in strength, the scaling process weakens the original inputs so that they are no longer able to induce complex-spiking of the cell (Jeffery & Hayman, 2004).

The anatomical candidate for pattern separation appears to be the CA3 hippocampal region. CA3 place cells are able to maintain distinct representations of two visually identical environments, and selectively reactivate either one of the representation patterns depending on the experience (Tanila, 1999). When rats experienced a completely different environment, CA3 place cells developed orthogonal representations of those different environments by changing their firing rates between the two environments, whereas CA1 place cells maintained similar responses (Leutgeb *et al.*, 2004).

3.4. Goal- and directionality-related plasticity of place fields

Not only sensory but also motivational factors can induce a reorganization of place fields (Mizumori, 2006). Changing the reward location within a single session can induce dramatic place field reorganization (Smith & Mizumori, 2006b, 2006a) (Fig 4). Units in the hippocampus have been shown to fire not only in relation to spatial location but also in relation with the different demands of the task (Eichenbaum *et al.*, 1999; Deadwyler & Hampson, 2004). Recording in a familiar room can induce remapping of the place fields toward new goal locations (Hollup *et al.*, 2001; Lenck-Santini *et al.*, 2001; Lenck-Santini *et al.*, 2002). The learning of rewarded locations in the environment can induce strengthening of the connections that associate certain places in the environment with the presence of goals and as a result to modify the episodic sequence in hippocampal network. Besides hippocampus proper the subiculum also plays a role in the performance of a delayed-nonmatch-to-sample short-term task (Hampson *et al.*, 2000).

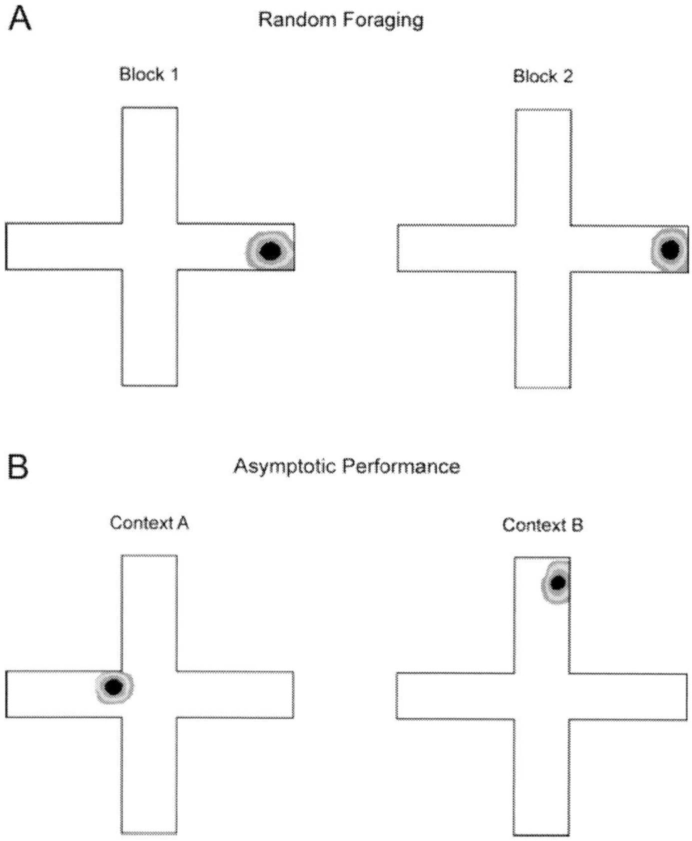

Figure 4. Experience-dependent, goal-related place field separation. A. Representation of the firing pattern of a neuron recorded during the first and second halves of the random reward session (Block 1 and Block 2). For each trial, rewards were placed at the end of randomly designated arms, and the rat started at one of the three non-rewarded arms. The random reward session was also divided into 2 blocks of trials, although all of the trials consisted of searching for randomly placed rewards, and the neuronal responses were compared across these blocks. Since the task demands did not differ across these 2 blocks, there was no context manipulation and the neuronal responses were not expected to differ. B. Illustration of the context-specific firing patterns of neurons recorded during asymptotic performance. In this experiment, rats were trained to retrieve rewards from one location on a plus maze during the first half of each training session and from a different location in the same environment during the second half of the sessions. The rats were given identical training sessions each day until they reached a behavioral criterion of 75% correct choices. The two session halves constituted separate contexts defined by their differing reward location. Left plot illustrates neuronal firing during the first half of the session (Context A) when the reward was always placed on the east arm, and during the second half (Context B) when the reward was always placed on the west arm. The differential responses developed only in rats that were given context training and not in rats that were given repeated random reward sessions, indicating that the context specific place fields could not have been due to factors unrelated to learning to distinguish the contexts (adapted from (Smith & Mizumori, 2006a)).

The firing frequency of the place cells has been shown to be higher in the radial arm maze and also in an open field arena whenever the animal had to move in a linear trajectory (Markus *et al.*, 1995). Similarly, place cell firing frequency was higher when the animal was running in an inwards direction in a radial arm maze (McNaughton *et al.*, 1983). Studies on the directionality of place cell demonstrated that the physical shape of the recording chamber can make place fields look directionally polarized (Muller *et al.*, 1994). As with the goal-related plasticity, although the environment is the same, the sequence of the encoded temporal events differs and this results in different firing patterns of the recorded place cells. The contribution of the head direction system to the direction-dependency of the place fields will be discussed in details later.

3.5. Aging and place field plasticity

Another approach in detecting the mnemonic experience-dependent features of hippocampal place cells is to compare the age-related differences in place field plasticity with the age-dependent alterations of synaptic plasticity machinery.

Place cells have been recorded from young and aged rats that often differ in their spatial learning abilities (Barnes *et al.*, 1983; Mizumori *et al.*, 1996; Barnes *et al.*, 1997; Tanila *et al.*, 1997a). Place cells in aged rats have a tendency to spontaneously remap in a familiar environment (Barnes *et al.*, 1997), a phenomenon termed "multistability." Also the place cells of aged animals often fail to remap in the face of salient environmental (Tanila *et al.*, 1997a; Wilson *et al.*, 2003), or task (Oler & Markus, 2000b, 2000a) change, where normal rats do. At the same time the threshold for LTP induction is increased (Deupree *et al.*, 1993; Moore *et al.*, 1993; Rosenzweig *et al.*, 1997), and the decay of LTP is accelerated in aged rats (deToledo-Morrell *et al.*, 1988). During old age, when memory function declines, hippocampal synapses exhibit alterations in calcium-dependent synaptic plasticity (Foster & Norris, 1997) due to impaired regulation of calcium homeostasis (Norris *et al.*, 1998). Impaired LTP and misbalance between potentiation and depression processes (Norris *et al.*, 1996; Foster & Norris, 1997) could be related to the decreased ability of hippocampal pattern separation (Oler & Markus, 2000a, 2000b).

Experience-dependent studies on place field plasticity provide insights of how dynamical place representations underline hippocampal mnemonic functions. Environmental manipulations demonstrate the ability of hippocampal network to discriminate differences in spatial configurations with time. This process of learning is dependent also on non-spatial and goal-related features, revealing the main function of hippocampus – to relate the temporal episodes with their context. To link experience-dependent alterations of place fields with experience dependent-synaptic plasticity we need to provide evidence for common mechanisms. Below, we review the data of how the place cell representation is modified by targeting cellular components and processes known to be crucial for plasticity induction.

4. Interventional Studies of Place Cells Plasticity

4.1. Pharmacological manipulations and place fields

For the induction of hippocampal synaptic plasticity, an elevation of postsynaptic calcium concentration is necessary (Bliss & Collingridge, 1993). The primary source of calcium influx during the induction of LTP in the CA1 region and dentate gyrus (DG) occurs through ionotropic receptors of the N-methyl-D-aspartate subtype (NMDA) (Collingridge *et al.*, 1983).

Systemic administration of the competitive NMDA channel blocker CPP had no effect on the established place fields in familiar environments (Kentros *et al.*, 1998). Similarly no effect was observed on the formation of new place fields in a novel environment and the short-term stability also remained unchanged. The result of NMDA blockade was expressed as lack of long-term preservation of the place field and demonstrated by different remapping of the place cells on the following day. The new remapping patterns of place cells firing showed no relation to those of the previous day (Kentros *et al.*, 1998). Therefore NMDA function mediates long-term stability of place fields.

Following NMDAR activation, intracellular calcium levels become elevated which results in the activation of different kinases and transcription factors that lead to protein synthesis-dependent morphological alterations of the involved synapses. Similarly to the NMDA studies, protein synthesis blockers impaired the long-term stability, but not the short-term maintenance of the place fields. Different maps are expressed on two days in the same novel environment after the protein-synthesis mechanisms were initially abolished (Agnihotri *et al.*, 2004).

4.2. Molecular genetic interventions on place field properties

Evidence that remapping requires hippocampal plasticity has come from analysis of subfield-specific knockouts. Place cell activity is disrupted in animals with CA1-specific knockout of the NMDA receptor subunit NR1, such that receptive fields do not retain strong location specificity and ensembles of cells with similar receptive fields are not correlated in their firing, consistent with the disruption of a functional representation of space (McHugh *et al.*, 1996). In CA3-specific knockouts of NR1, CA1 place cells have normal place fields in familiar environments but enlarged, unrefined place fields in novel environments (Nakazawa *et al.*, 2003), suggesting a role for plasticity at CA3 recurrent collateral synapses in remapping of place fields. Place cell remapping in area CA3 is also disrupted when NR1 expression is deleted in the dentate gyrus (McHugh *et al.*, 2007).

Other elements of the molecular cascade that starts with calcium influx have been targeted in various studies that examine the effect of these mechanisms on the activity of hippocampal place cells. Ca-calmodulin-dependent kinase II (CAMKII) is a kinase activated by increased intracellular calcium concentration and transducers the signal further to the nucleus. Mice expressing altered CaMKII displayed severely impaired spatial learning and degraded place-cell activity in CA1 (Cho *et al.*, 1998). Importantly these effects were combined with reduced stimulation-induced long-term plasticity.

4.3. Stimulation-induced modification of place fields

Another interventional strategy to explore place field plasticity is an external plasticity induction that mimics naturally occurring plasticity patterns.

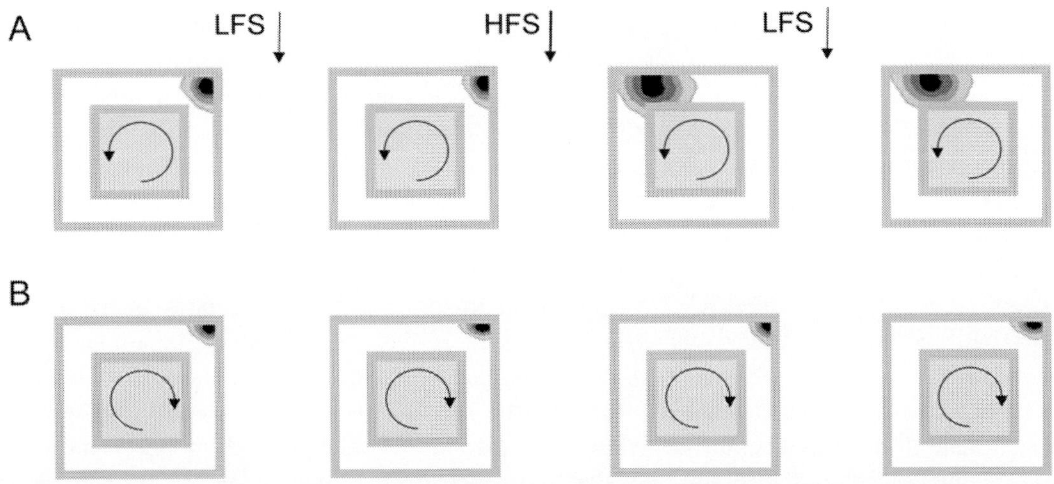

Figure 5. Place field representation can be modified by LTP-inducing stimulation. A. Example of place cell with unidirectional change of place field after LTP. Each map represents 10–20 min of counterclockwise or clockwise runs (curved arrows). Between run sessions the rat was placed back to the home cage. Low-frequency stimulation (LFS) or tetanic stimulation (HFS) were given. There is a decline of the initially recorded place field after the HFS protocol and also an emergence of a new place field during counterclockwise runs. B. The same cell has no significant change in place representation after LTP, when the animal is moving in a clockwise direction. Besides the unidirectional changed place fields LTP induction can lead to bidirectional changes as well as no place field changes in both directions (adapted from (Dragoi *et al.*, 2003)).

Hippocampal place cells are either silent or discharge with single spikes during behavioural arousal (O'Keefe, 1976). Complex spike bursts are also known to occur (Muller *et al.*, 1987; Gothard *et al.*, 2001) in the time course of the depolarizing theta oscillation due to the rhythmic decrease of perisomatic inhibition (Kamondi *et al.*, 1998). Consistent with this event, bursts of spikes significantly increase the effectiveness of synaptic transmission and at the same time induce frequency-dependent synaptic plasticity (Csicsvari *et al.*, 1998; Harris *et al.*, 2001; Hausser *et al.*, 2004). Pairing presynaptic activity with postsynaptic bursts in hippocampal pyramidal cells in vitro results in LTP of activated synapses (Magee & Johnston, 1997; Pike *et al.*, 1999). Pairing of presynaptic and postsynaptic activity of neurons, as modeled by long-term potentiation models, has been suggested to be the possible mechanism underlying synaptic weight changes in hippocampal network (Levy & Steward, 1979; Magee & Johnston, 1997; Markram *et al.*, 1997). The effect of LTP as means to explore the relations between the neurocognitive events underlying spatial representation and synaptic plasticity (O'Mara, 1995). Induction of long-term stimulation-evoked EPSP changes was associated with a "remapping" of the hippocampal representation of the environment (Fig 5), including creation of new place cells and abolition of preexisting place fields (Dragoi *et al.*, 2003), supporting the view that place features of pyramidal cells emerge within hippocampal circuits (McNaughton *et al.*, 1996; Lever *et al.*, 2002). LTP-induced effects have been shown to be context-dependent since place fields associated with one direction of movement were often selectively modified without affecting the neuron's place representation when moving in the opposite direction. Therefore single neurons can be part of several representations (O'Keefe & Nadel, 1978; Markus *et al.*, 1995; Wood *et al.*, 1999) and inputs from these representations can be modified selectively. Changes in place field representation did not affect the size and shape of place fields. No effect was observed on theta power and theta cycle compression of distances between place fields. Importantly the global firing rate of the network was preserved after the LTP protocol, suggesting that LTP rearranges the place representation in the hippocampus without altering the functional properties of the network (Dragoi *et al.*, 2003).

Interventional synaptic plasticity studies demonstrate that the persistence of the fields over a period of time greater than a few minutes or hours seems to depend on a mechanisms common with these underlying LTP-models. This suggests that spatial mnemonic functions recruit place fields in a non-NMDA-dependent process and then associates them, via an NMDAR- and protein synthesis-dependent processes, so that upon re-entry, the same map can be recalled. Experience-dependent plasticity of place field can be explained on a cellular level, but how these changes are mediated by the network connectivity remains difficult to reveal. The following section analyses the up-to-date computational models and their experimental substrates of how network dynamics define the functional properties of hippocamapl system.

5. Hipppocampal Network as a Memory System

The memory stored in any neuronal network can be represented by the firing rates of the population of neurons that are stored by the associative synaptic modification, and can be correctly recalled later (Treves & Rolls, 1991, 1992; Rolls & Kesner, 2006). Computational models suggest that autoassociation networks that undergo Hebbian modification can store the number of different memories, each one expressed as a stable attractor. An attractor network is one in which a stable pattern of firing is maintained once it has been started. In hippocampal region the CA3 neurons are proposed to operate as an attractor network (Treves & Rolls, 1991, 1992; Rolls *et al.*, 1997; Kesner & Rolls, 2001). Associative modification is mediated by long-term potentiation, and this synaptic modification appears to be involved in learning (Morris, 2003; Morris *et al.*, 2003; Lynch, 2004).

In order for most associative networks to store information efficiently, heterosynaptic long-term depression is required (Rolls & Treves, 1990; Treves & Rolls, 1991; Fazeli & Collingridge, 1996; Rolls & Treves, 1998; Rolls & Deco, 2002). Without heterosynaptic LTD, there would otherwise always be a correlation between any set of positively firing inputs acting as the input pattern vector to a neuron. LTD effectively enables the average firing of each input axon to be subtracted from its input at any one time (Rolls, 1996).

With its extensive recurrent collateral connectivity the CA3 region is suggested to act as an autoassociation memory which enables episodic memories to be formed and stored in hippocampus (Marr, 1971; McNaughton & Morris, 1987; Rolls, 1991; Treves & Rolls, 1992). The memory for sequences is then determined by the synaptic modifications in the recurrent collateral synapses (Rolls & Treves, 1998; Rolls & Deco, 2002). Subsequently the recurrent collateral activity allows for the retrieval of a whole representation to be initiated by the activation of some small part of the same representation. This property, known as "pattern completion", in principle allows a memory to be retrieved in full when the animal is presented with only some reminders of it. Therefore the Hebbian learning mechanisms occurring in the recurrent connections allow the full retrieval of a representation based on only a partial, fragmented input. An important property of the autoassociation model of the CA3 recurrent collateral network is that the retrieval can be symmetric - the whole memory sequence can be retrieved from any part. For example, in an object–place autoassociation memory, an object could be recalled from a place retrieval cue, and *vice versa.* As the hippocampus operates effectively as a single network, it can allow arbitrary associations between inputs originating from very different parts of the cerebral cortex to be formed. These might involve associations between information originating in the temporal visual cortex about the presence of an object, and information originating in the parietal cortex about where it is; hence hippocampus enables different memories to be stored in a certain sequence (Rolls & Kesner, 2006).

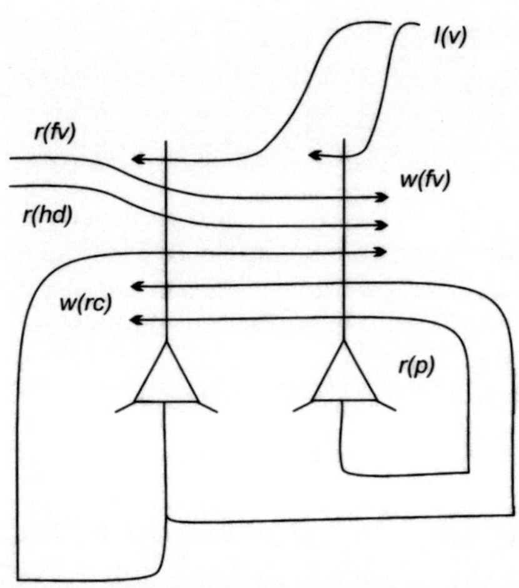

Figure 6. Neural network architecture for two-dimensional continuous attractor models of place cells. A recurrent network of place cells with firing rates r(p) receives external inputs from three sources: (1) visual system - I(v), (2) population of head direction cells with firing rates r(hd), and (3) population of forward velocity cells with firing rates r(fv). The recurrent weights between the place cells are denoted by w(rc), and the idiothetic weights to the place cells from the forward velocity cells and head direction cells are denoted by w(fv) (adapted from (Stringer *et al.*, 2004) and (Rolls & Kesner, 2006)).

Autoassociation models of the CA3 recurrent collateral network also implement the ability to maintain the firing of neurons using excitatory recurrent collateral connections. A stable attractor can maintain one memory active in this way for a considerable period, until a new input pushes the attractor to represent a new location or memory (Treves & Rolls, 1991, , 1992). There is evidence implicating the hippocampus in mediating associations across time

(Rawlins, 1985; Kesner, 1998) and also CA3 could bridge the temporal gap required for hippocampus-dependent temporal associations. The learning process therefore requires CA3 to hold one item active in continuing attractor state until the next item in the sequence arrives and then when both items are associated by temporally asymmetric synaptic plasticity (Rolls & Kesner, 2006).

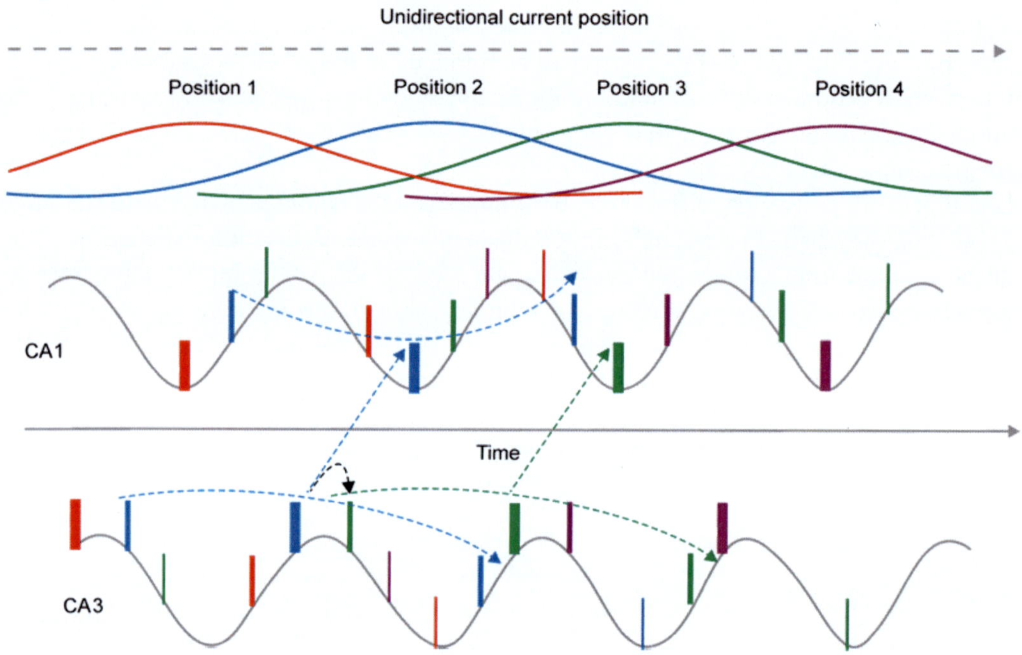

Figure 7. Phase precession of hippocampal place cells and sequences learning. Diagrammatic illustration of how phase precession occurs as an animal moves through the place field on a well-known path. On each successive theta cycle, firing occurs with an earlier phase, until the other end of the place field is reached. Each position (1 to 4, marked with curved solid lines) is defined by the most active cell assembly firing at each theta cycle (e.g., position 1 by the red assembly). The phase advance is marked by the curved, dotted arrows. The width of the bars indicates firing rates of the hypothesized assemblies while the theta time scale temporal differences between assemblies reflect distances of their spatial representations. Because each assembly contributes to multiple place representations, multiple assemblies are coactivated in each theta cycle. As a result, the current position is represented by the maximally active assembly at the cycle trough in CA1.
Assembly sequences within theta cycles could reflect strengthening of connections between adjacent places (e.g., position 2 – position 3). Cells encoding different items will fire with a temporal separation of one or several gamma cycles, a time that is within the window of NMDA-dependent LTP. Thus synaptic modification will occur at recurrent CA3 synapses that connect cells encoding sequential memory items. For example the place cells indicated with blue and green color will undergo synaptic potentiation (marked with black curved arrow) in the direction from blue to green as spike-timing plasticity rules postulate. In the CA3 recurrent system, the temporal differences among assembly members are assumed to be reflecting synaptic strengths between assembly members, resulting in a series of related phase precessions (e.g., the phase precession of the blue-marked cell will be followed by the phase precession of the green one). Similarly CA3 cells which fire earlier than CA1 cells for a given place field will strengthen the CA3-CA1 connections (marked with straight colored arrows). By this way is ensured a constant control between the predicted by the CA3 position and updated by the entorhinal cortex positions. This mechanism may allow distances to be translated into time and time into synaptic weights [adapted from (Dragoi & Buzsáki, 2006)].

The fact that spatial patterns, which imply continuous representations of space, are represented in the hippocampus has led to the application of continuous attractor models to help understand hippocampal function (Fig 6). A class of network that can maintain the firing of its neurons to represent any location along a continuous physical dimension such as spatial position and head direction is a ''Continuous Attractor'' neural network (Stringer *et al.*, 2004; Rolls & Kesner, 2006). It uses excitatory recurrent collateral connections between the neurons, as in the case with CA3, to reflect the distance between the neurons that represent allocentric spatial configuration.

The main function of an autoassociative network is to produce the correct firing of all cells that encode a memory when presented with only a partial or degraded form of that memory. Abstract theoretical models of sequence recall suggested that accurate sequence recall could be achieved by having autoassociative processes interact with heteroassociative processes (Kleinfeld, 1986; Sompolinsky & Kanter, 1986), and this concept was adapted to the specific circuitry of the hippocampus (Lisman, 1999; Lisman & Otmakhova, 2001). A possible CA3 recurrent network function is to store "heteroassociations" that link the cells encoding sequential memory items. The main function of a heteroassociative network is to recall the subsequent memory items in particular order when presented with a memory cue (Lisman & Otmakhova, 2001). In summary, it is proposed that the reciprocally interacting heteroassociative and autoassociative networks produce more accurate in learning and recalling sequences (Lisman, 1999).

6. Place Fields and Sequence Memory

Hippocampal circuity could store and recall memory sequences and a major line of evidence for sequence recall is the "phase precession" of hippocampal place cells. As the rat enters the receptive field of the neuron, the spikes occur on the peak of the theta cycle and may precede a full period as the rat passes through the entire receptive field of the cell (Dragoi & Buzsáki, 2006). Sequential activation of hippocampal place cells on a track can be represented by unique sets of cell assemblies (Fig 7), which are bound together by synaptic interactions into an episode (Jensen & Lisman, 1996; Tsodyks *et al.*, 1996). Such organization implies temporally-coordinated activity within and between anatomically distributed groups of sequential cell assemblies. Acting as an attractor dynamic system hippocampal formation induces phase precession of spikes within the theta cycle (Jensen & Lisman, 1996; Tsodyks *et al.*, 1996; Samsonovich & McNaughton, 1997; Wallenstein & Hasselmo, 1997; Wills *et al.*, 2005). Spike-phase variability of the place cells is temporally-correlated as the timing of neuronal action potentials depends on the activity of the synaptically-connected cell assemblies in which individual cells are embedded. The great majority of intrahippocampal synapses is established by the collateral system of CA3 neurons (Amaral & Witter, 1989; Li *et al.*, 1994), and it has been hypothesized that distances between place fields are encoded in the synaptic strengths between CA3-CA3 and CA3-CA1 neuron pairs (Muller *et al.*, 1996). Temporal encoding of spatial information, therefore, can be explained by the experience-dependent modification of synaptic strengths in these regions. It is hypothesized that the sequences are stored in the autoassociative CA3 recurrent and CA3-CA1 collateral systems (Jensen & Lisman, 1996; Muller *et al.*, 1996; Tsodyks, 1999; Dragoi

& Buzsáki, 2006) and are updated by entorhinal cortex-mediated environmental signals (Hafting *et al.*, 2005; Zugaro *et al.*, 2005). The sequence in which several temporally-linked cell assemblies, each representing spatial fields, will be recalled is triggered by the environmental input of the previous locations by way of the entorhinal cortex (Frank *et al.*, 2000; Hafting *et al.*, 2005). The temporal features of spike timing-dependent plasticity (Levy & Steward, 1979; Magee & Johnston, 1997; Markram *et al.*, 1997; Bi & Poo, 1998) ensure that the recalling of learned associations will be in the same sequence as it has been encoded during the learning experience (Mehta *et al.*, 1997). A consequence of the oscillatory temporal organization of cell assemblies is the theta phase precession of spikes of single place cells. Dynamic plasticity processes during theta cycles link continuously experience-dependent hippocampal assemblies in unidirectional sequence that represents spatial representations in time (Hasselmo *et al.*, 2002; Zugaro *et al.*, 2005; Dragoi & Buzsáki, 2006; Johnson & Redish, 2007). Synaptic strengths across assemblies, representing different spatial representations and discharging in different gamma cycles, can determine both their time order within the theta cycle and the distances between the respective place fields (Lisman & Idiart, 1995; Harris *et al.*, 2003). The phase shifts of cells assemblies in hippocampus indicate that hippocampal neurons do not just represent a highly processed image of the sensory environment, but generate sequence information that integrates subsequent episodes. The hippocampal formation can also encode relative spatial location, without reference to sensoy external cues, by the integration of linear and angular self-motion (path integration). This issue will be discussed next.

7. Path Integration

Place cells use environmentally-stable sensory stimuli as a directional reference to provide a rodent's orientation in space (Jeffery *et al.*, 1997; Goodridge *et al.*, 1998). Beside external sensory cues, and especially in the cases when these cues are unstable, the hippocampal network relies on an internal direction sense or idiothetic (body-, or head-motion) stimuli (Quirk *et al.*, 1992; Suzuki *et al.*, 1997; Young *et al.*, 1997; Xiang & Brown, 1998; Jeffery, 1999; Jeffery & O'Keefe, 1999; Mizumori *et al.*, 1999).

The head direction system is composed of neurons whose firing rate increases only whenever the animal head is pointed in a specific direction (Taube *et al.*, 1990). This type of cell, is found in different structures of the parahipocampal complex as well as in other subcortical structures (Taube, 1995a; Stackman & Taube, 1998; Taube, 1998). The firing of these neurons conveys information about where the animal's head is pointing. They seem to use environmental cues to calibrate their directional firing (Goodridge *et al.*, 1998) and they depend on vestibular input without which their firing disappears. Head-direction tuned neurons are present in the presubiculum and parasubiculum, regions that encode location and direction (Cacucci *et al.*, 2004). This region could synthesise spatial information and direction information, forming the bridge between both systems. Subiculum (Hartley *et al.*, 2000, our own unpublished observations), hippocampal CA1 (Leutgeb *et al.*, 2000) and entorhinal cortex (Hafting *et al.*, 2005) are also areas proposed to integrate place as well as head direction. Finally the sequence of idiothetic episodes, even in the absence of external sensory input is believed to be integrated within the hippocampus itself (Robertson *et al.*, 1998; Mizumori *et al.*, 1999).

An interaction between the head direction system and location information system is believed to be necessary for efficient spatial navigation. The head direction system would facilitate information to place cells to set their firing in relation to distal external cues, facilitating in this way efficient navigation under specific conditions. This interaction is clearly reflected in all proposed models of spatial navigation (McNaughton *et al.*, 1996; Redish & Touretzky, 1997; Sharp, 1999; McNaughton *et al.*, 2006). The external sensory cues are necessary to initialize this idiothetic representation of space (Quirk *et al.*, 1990; Markus *et al.*, 1994). Additionally it is demonstrated that motor input (Foster *et al.*, 1989; Bassett *et al.*, 2005) serves as another source for the internal reference to the spatial orientation. Several models have proposed the subicular region as a key structure that integrates movement, place information and direction (McNaughton *et al.*, 1996; Sharp, 1999; O'Mara, 2005; Barry *et al.*, 2006) (Fig 8). Subicular units seem to code for these three elements (Sharp and Green, 1994). Similarly the hypothetical 'boundary vector cells' in subiculum are believed to integrate different sources of spatial orientation in allocentric system that controls the development of hippocampal place fields (Hartley *et al.*, 2000; Barry *et al.*, 2006). Error-mediated repeated interaction between idiothetic representation and place fields is proposed to stabilize the path integration system, preventing place cells firing drift (Knierim *et al.*, 1995).

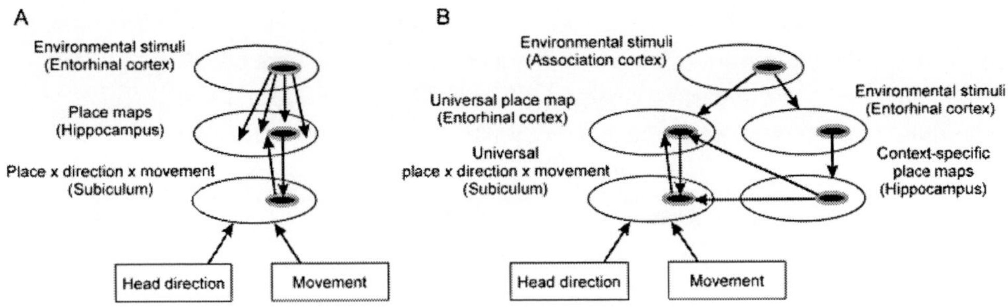

Figure 8. Path integration models. A. Diagram of a model proposed to explain hippocampal place cell firing properties. The hippocampal place cells are assumed to be linked through excitatory synapses to form a two-dimensional attractor surface. Each spatial configuration becomes attached to the stimuli in the environment it represents through Hebbian mechanisms. Path integration is accomplished through synaptic alterations of the input that receives information about place, directional heading, and movement. The entorhinal cortex integrates sensory information from different brain areas interacting with the internal map in the hippocampus which receives directional and motor information from the subiculum. In this way, the subiculum is seen as the bridge between different subsystems (Adapted from (McNaughton *et al.*, 1996) and (Sharp, 1999)). B. In the second path integration model, the entorhinal cortex and the subiculum are proposed as the anatomical bases of the universal spatial map. The subiculum integrates directional and motor input which is used by the system to implement path integration extrapolating similar spatial representation across different environments. Here, the entorhinal cortex and subiculum are assumed to work together to form a stable attractor and perform path integration, in the same way that the hippocampus and subiculum were assumed to work in A. Input from the universal map in the entorhinal cortex determines the hippocampal place field configuration. Environmental stimuli and events also play a role in defining which place cells will be active for particular location. Projections from the hippocampal place cells back to the place x direction x movement (subicular) layer assures the universal map to maintain the same rotational orientation each time the animal visits a environment with a familiar context (adapted from (Sharp, 1999)).

Entorhinal cortex also participates in path integration through a reciprocal connection with the subiculum (McNaughton *et al.*, 1996; Sharp, 1999). Entorhinal grid cells (Hafting *et al.*, 2005; Sargolini *et al.*, 2006) are accompanied by head direction cells and grid by direction cells in the entorhinal cortex (Hafting *et al.*, 2005; Sargolini *et al.*, 2006), suggesting that entorhinal cortex shares similar path integration functions with the anatomically-adjacent subiculum (McNaughton *et al.*, 2006).

In path integration, the updated information is a continuous variable representing position or head direction. A continuum of cell assemblies, or a continuous attractor (Amari, 1977; Droulez & Berthoz, 1991; Tsodyks, 1999; Stringer *et al.*, 2004), is therefore required to encode position or head direction. In such an attractor the strength of the excitatory connections between two cells could decrease with the distance between their respective preferred directions (Redish *et al.*, 1996; Zhang, 1996), which would result in a focused activity related to a particular direction (McNaughton *et al.*, 2006). A recurrent synaptic matrix with such architecture will ensure the strength of the excitatory connections between two cells decreases in proportion to the physical distance between the cells' respective place fields. Cells in such a direction-specific network will encode, conjointly, the rat's position and velocity vectors (McNaughton *et al.*, 1996; Zhang, 1996; Samsonovich & McNaughton, 1997), therefore, they would combine head direction and running speed inputs with location information from the attractor layer.

Finally, path integration research reveals that hippocampal place fields represent the changes of current location, environmental context, current and recent environmental sensory stimuli under the continuous reference of the idiothetic experience. Network connectivity alterations for path integration obey mechanisms of experience-dependent synaptic plasticity. As these mechanisms are to certain degree universal for all brain regions, a useful approach in understanding hippocampal learning is to compare medial temporal lobe with other regions known to undergo experience-dependent learning processes.

8. Plasticity in Other Systems

8.1. Cerebellar synaptic plasticity

The two main memory research directions, one involving declarative memory and the other – procedural memory reveal plasticity rules common for both explicit and implicit learning. Therefore comparison between the mechanisms that underline experience-dependent plasticity in both memory systems will give us better understanding of how brain networks are modified through experience. A central problem in the procedural memory studies is to demonstrate, both experimentally and theoretically, how neuronal networks of the cerebellum undergo synaptic plasticity after error-driven, LTD-based learning (Ito, 2001). Modern control system theories have been useful in accurately defining roles played by a microcomplex in motor control. In the usual design of a control system, precise control is secured by feedback (Fig 9). A two-degrees-of-freedom adaptive control system for voluntary movement proposed to combine feedback control by the cerebral cortex with feed-forward control by the cerebellum (Kawato *et al.*, 1987; Gomi & Kawato, 1992). In the cerebellum, there is a regularly organized circuit that delivers relatively unprocessed somatosensory and motor information to the Purkinje cells of the cerebellar cortex. It is believed that implicit motor learning is mediated by synaptic plasticity in the cerebellar cortex and/or the deep cerebellar nuclei (Marr, 1969; Ito & Kano, 1982; McCormick & Thompson, 1984; Attwell *et al.*, 2002). These structures are organized as two-dimensional topographical maps of the body, and it is possible to target specific microzones that mediate particular skeletal muscular responses (Andersson & Oscarsson, 1978; Garwicz & Ekerot, 1994). The best-studied example of this functional organization is probably classical conditioning of the nictitating membrane/eyeblink response in rabbits (Mauk *et al.*, 1986; Attwell *et al.*, 2002) Delgado-Garcia and Gruart, TINS 2006. With such regular, tractably organized and well-characterized circuitry, there will be a higher probability of demonstrating models of plasticity in learning paradigms in cerebellum than in the functionally-less understood hippocampal system. The knowledge about cerebellar error-dependent plasticity could be applied for other brain systems and particularly for hippocampal region through "vicarious trial and error" behaviors (Muenzinger, 1938; Tolman, 1939; Hu & Amsel, 1995; Hu *et al.*, 2006), which are mediated at least partially by hippocampal place fields (Johnson & Redish, 2007).

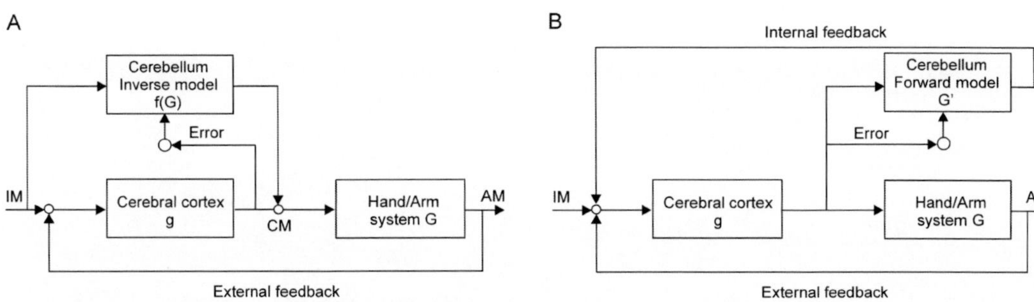

Figure 9. Motor control systems. A. Two-degrees-of-freedom control system. Two-degrees-of-freedom adaptive control system for voluntary movement combines feedback control by the cerebral cortex with feed-forward control by the cerebellum. Signal transfer characteristics of the controller (g) and of the controlled object (G); instruction of movement (IM); command signals for movement (CM) and actual movement performed (AM). AM becomes close to IM if g is sufficiently large if f(G) becomes equivalent to an inverse of G. In a typical feed-forward control, the controller converts instruction for a movement to command signals that act on the controlled object. The controlled object in turn converts the command signals to an actual movement. If the instruction/command conversion is inversely equivalent to the command/movement conversion by the controlled object, the actual movement becomes equivalent to the instruction (adapted from (Ito, 2000); (Kawato *et al.*, 1987) and (Ito, 2001)). B. Another way of performing a precise control in a seemingly feed-forward control system is to utilize an internal loop through a model that simulates the command/movement conversion by the controlled object and thereby predicts the movement to be produced by the controlled object. AM becomes equivalent to IM if the signal transfer characteristics of the forward model G' = G. If the internal loop contains not only dynamic properties of the controlled object but also the delay time involved in the external feedback, exactly the same effect as the external feedback from the actual movement will be reproduced. This model was applied to interpret functional meanings of the cerebrocerebellar communication loop (adapted from (Ito, 2000) and (Ito, 2001)).

8.2. Visual cortex plasticity

Episodic memories are encoded through the hippocampus, but the experimental tools to modulate synaptic weights at a spatially distributed set of hippocampal synapses are restricted by the difficulty of selecting which synapses to modify. The information that reaches the medial temporal lobe is highly integrated and episodic memory research faces methodological problems in decoding the informational content of hippocampal network. Conceivably, the functional effects of synaptic plasticity are more tractable for other forms of memory in the brain and particularly perceptual memory in sensory cortices.

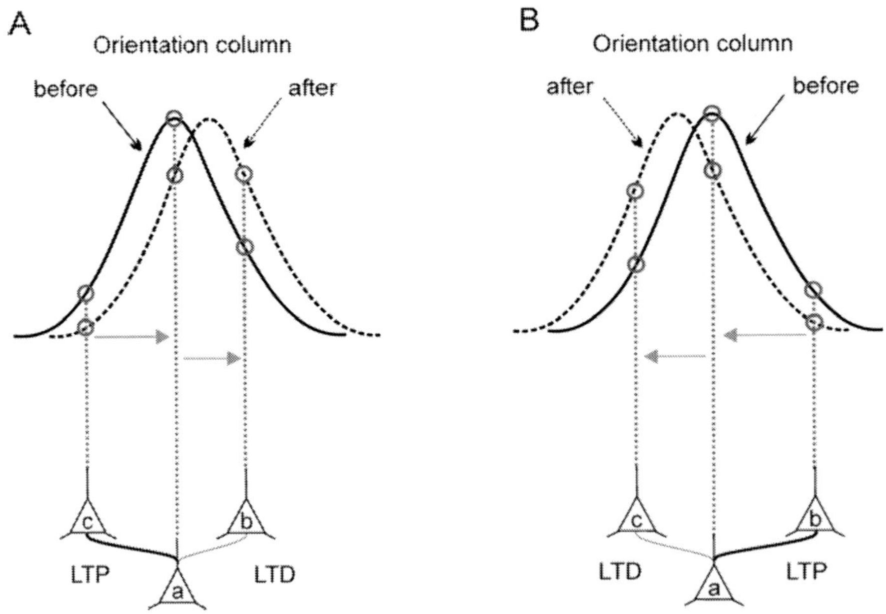

Figure 10. Shifts in perceived orientation and spike timing-dependent modification of the intracortical connections. A. The population profile of the orientation tuning response evoked by a visual test stimulus is shown before (solid lines) and after (dotted lines) conditioning. The colored circles represent the responses of a three neurons to the test stimulus, as predicted by their respective tuning curves. In this scheme, the perceived orientations are determined by the peak positions of the population response curves. Depending on the direction of the conditioning stimulus, the connections between the involved neurons will be affected differently. According to the spike timing-dependent rules the synaptic strength will increase if the presynaptic spike precedes postsynaptic activity and will decrease if the presynaptic spike follows the postsynaptic activity. Similarly if the orientation of the stimulus activates cell (a) after the cell (c), LTP of the projection from (c) to (a) will occur. At the same time (a) will be activated pror (b), which will lead to LTD of the projection from (b) to (a). The gray arrows indicate the temporal order of neuronal spikes. B. Test stimulus with the opposite orientation will activate the cells in reverse order, which will result in LTD of the projection from (c) to (a) and LTP of the projection from (b) to (a). The thickness of connecting lines represents the synaptic change, based on spike timing-dependent strengthening and weakening of the intracortical connections (adapted from (Yao & Dan, 2001)).

Plasticity is an integral part of information processing in visual cortex. In general, since it involves cortical areas at the early stages of visual processing, where most is known about neocortical circuitry, receptive field properties, and functional architecture, these cortical areas are therefore more tractable for learning the underlying mechanisms. Thus, the adult primary visual cortex has been the most used model up-to-date for exploring the phenomenon of neocortical synaptic plasticity, starting at the very early stages of visual processing understanding (Wiesel and Hubel, 1963). A striking aspect of the findings related to plasticity research is the apparent ability of the adult cortex to dynamically modify the processing of visual information according to immediate behavioral requirements (Crist *et al.*, 2001). The findings on orientation plasticity that involve spike timing-dependent rules demonstrate that these changes can be long-term and can continuously influence vision (Schoups *et al.*, 2001; Fu *et al.*, 2002; Sur *et al.*, 2002). Asynchronous visual stimuli flashed at two orientations (Yao & Dan, 2001; Yao *et al.*, 2004) have been found to induce rapid shifts in orientation tuning, suggesting a functional relevance for the cortical modifications (Fig 10). The dependence on the spiking sequence and interval has been demonstrated in visual cortical slices (Sjostrom *et al.*, 2001; Froemke & Dan, 2002) and in vivo (Yao & Dan, 2001; Fu *et al.*, 2002). Examining how visual cortical neurons adapt their response properties to patterned stimulation or to perceptual learning, and how the capacity for adaptive changes is mapped onto the cortex, is fundamental for understanding neuronal mechanisms of memory formation in general. Spike-timing dependent rules functionally demonstrated in visual cortex can be used to define experience-dependent asymmetric expansion of hippocampal place fields (Mehta *et al.*, 1997; Mehta *et al.*, 2000).

9. Overview: Integration of the Synaptic Plasticity and Place Field Mnemonic Functions

LTP and LTD are believed to underlie memory processes on a cellular level (Bliss & Collingridge, 1993; Bear, 1996; Martin *et al.*, 2000; Lynch, 2004). However, a significant challenge is precisely determining how LTP and LTD relate to experience-dependent place cells plasticity. During exploratory behaviour, exploration-associated complex-spike firing neurons in the hippocampus are shown to form assemblies of cells with similar spatial responses (O'Keefe, 1976). Together with spike timing-dependent plasticity (Levy & Steward, 1983), high-frequency spikes may provide a mechanism by which cell assemblies encode the same part of the environment (Lisman, 1997). Naturalistic and interventional experiments on place cell plasticity together with synaptic plasticity research and computational models of hippocampal function integrate the ideas of how place fields process experience-related mnemonic function. Place cell plasticity has different aspects which can be can be summarized as follows:

(1) Place cell activity is capable of stable representation of particular environment for continuous time even after the removal of place field-controlling sensory cues (Muller & Kubie, 1987) (O'Keefe & Speakman, 1987; Save *et al.*, 2005). This learning process is related to short-term synaptic plasticity and is believed to involve working memory mechanisms.
(2) In a stable environment place fields undergo with experience asymmetrical expansion (Mehta *et al.*, 1997; Mehta *et al.*, 2000). The change of firing rate and firing field size with time is also a form of plasticity which is expressed by the theta-related phase precession. The mechanisms responsible for this field development are believed to be common with spike-timing dependent plasticity rules.
(3) Place fields are able incrementally to discriminate different contexts and to undergo alterations with time due to discrete environmental cues. Therefore it is proposed that place cells appear to be a neural substrate for long-term incidental learning (Lever *et*

al., 2002). Pattern separation can be explained by heterosynaptic plasticity (Fazeli & Collingridge, 1996; Rolls & Deco, 2002) and/or synaptic scaling mechanisms (Turrigiano & Nelson, 2000). Synaptic scaling allows the total activity of a neuron to be maintained within a set range, while preserving the distribution of synaptic strengths.

The reviewed findings in this chapter are consistent with the proposal that the hippocampus is critical for rapid encoding of events that compose episodic representations. Different types of sensory and idiothetic information is integrated by hippocampal place cells and this information is encoded in sequences through short- and long-term alterations of the neuronal connectivity. Synaptic plasticity within hippocampal network mediates episodic memories and links them together through their common elements. Still the understanding of the cellular, synaptic and network plastic changes underlying most of place fields transformations is still lacking, and the wider question of how these memories become encoded in a form that is sustained after hippocampal damage, of course, remains unanswered.

Acknowledgments

This work was supported by the Wellcome Trust and the Higher Education Authority Programme for Research in Third-Level Institutions (SMOM) and the European Commission PRESENCCIA EU FP6-027731 and Synthetic Forager FP7- ICT-217148 (MVSV).

References

Abbott LF & Blum KI. (1996). Functional significance of long-term potentiation for sequence learning and prediction. *Cereb Cortex* **6,** 406-416.

Abraham WC & Bear MF. (1996). Metaplasticity: the plasticity of synaptic plasticity. *Trends Neurosci* **19,** 126-130.

Abraham WC, Gustafsson B & Wigstrom H. (1987). Long-term potentiation involves enhanced synaptic excitation relative to synaptic inhibition in guinea-pig hippocampus. *J Physiol* **394,** 367–380.

Agnihotri NT, Hawkins RD, Kandel ER & Kentros C. (2004). The long-term stability of new hippocampal place fields requires new protein synthesis. *Proc Natl Acad Sci USA* **101,** 3656-3661.

Amaral DG & Witter MP. (1989). The three-dimensional organization of the hippocampal formation: a review of anatomical data. *Neuroscience* **31,** 571–591.

Amari S. (1977). Dynamics of pattern formation in lateralinhibition type neural fields. *Biol Cybern* **27,** 77–87.

Andersen P, Sundberg SH, Sveen O, Swann JW & Wigstrom H. (1980). Possible mechanisms for long-lasting potentiation of synaptic transmission in hippocampal slices from guinea-pigs. *J Physiol* **302,** 463–482.

Andersson G & Oscarsson O. (1978). Climbing fiber microzones in cerebellar vermis and their projection to different groups of cells in the lateral vestibular nucleus. *Exp Brain Res* **32,** 565–579.

Attwell PJ, Cooke SF & Yeo CH. (2002). Cerebellar function in consolidation of a motor memory. *Neuron* **34,** 1011–1020.

Barnes CA. (1995). Involvement of LTP in memory: are we 'searching under the street light'? *Neuron* **15,** 751-754.

Barnes CA, McNaughton BL, Mizumori SJ, Leonard BW & Lin LH. (1990). Comparison of spatial and temporal characteristics of neuronal activity in sequential stages of hippocampal processing. *Prog Brain Res* **83,** 287-300.

Barnes CA, McNaughton BL & O'Keefe J. (1983). Loss of place specificity in hippocampal complex spike cells of senescent rat. *Neurobiol Aging* **4,** 113-119.

Barnes CA, Suster MS, Shen J & McNaughton BL. (1997). Multistability of cognitive maps in the hippocampus of old rats. *Nature* **388,** 272-275.

Barry C, Lever C, Hayman R, Hartley T, Burton S, O'Keefe J, Jeffery KJ & Burgess N. (2006). The boundary vector cell model of place cell firing and spatial memory. *Rev Neurosci* **17,** 71-97.

Bassett JP, Zugaro MB, Muir GM, Golob EJ, Muller RU & Taube JS. (2005). Passive movements of the head do not abolish anticipatory firing properties of head direction cells. *J Neurophysiol* **93,** 1304-1316.

Bear MF. (1996). A synaptic basis for memory storyge in the cerebral cortex. *Proc Natl Acad Sci* **93,** 13453–13459.

Bear MF, Cooper LN & Ebner FF. (1987). A physiological basis for a theory of synaptic modification. *Science* **237,** 42–48.

Bell CC, Han VZ, Sugawara Y & Grant K. (1997). Synaptic plasticity in a cerebellum-like structure depends on temporal order. *Nature* **387,** 278-281.

Bernard C & Wheal HVA. (1996). role for synaptic and network plasticity in controlling epileptiform activity in CA1 in the kainic acid-lesioned rat hippocampus in vitro. *J Physiol* **495,** 127–142.

Bi GQ & Poo MM. (1998). Synaptic modifications in cultured hippocampal neurons: dependence on spike timing, synaptic strength, and postsynaptic cell type. *J Neurosci* **18,** 10464-10472.

Bienenstock EL, Cooper LN & Munro PW. (1982). Theory for the development of neuron selectivity: orientation specificity and binocular interaction in visual cortex. *J Neurosci* **2,** 32-48.

Bliss TVP & Collingridge GL. (1993). A synaptic model of memory: long-term potentiationin the hippocampus. *Nature* **361,** 31–39.

Bliss TVP & Lomo T. (1973). Long-lasting potentiation of synaptic transmission in the dentate area of the anesthetized rabbit following stimulation of the perforant path. *J Physiol* **232,** 331-356.

Blum KI & Abbott LF. (1996). A model of spatial map formation in the hippocampus of the rat. *Neural Comput* **8,** 85-93.

Bostock E, Muller RU & Kubie JL. (1991). Experiencedependent modifications of hippocampal place cell firing. *Hippocampus* **1,** 93–205.

Burwell RD & Hafeman DM. (2003). Positional firing properties of postrhinal cortex neurons. *Neuroscience* **119,** 577-588.

Buzsáki G, Haas HL & Anderson EG. (1987). Long-term potentiation induced by physiologically relevant stimulus patterns. *Brain Res* **435,** 331-333.

Cacucci F, Lever C, Wills TJ, Burgess N & O'Keefe J. (2004). Theta-modulated place-by-direction cells in the hippocampal formation in the rat. *J Neurosci* **24,** 8265-8277.

Castro CA, Silbert LH, McNaughton BL & Barnes CA. (1989). Recovery of spatial learning deficits after decay of electrically induced synaptic enhancement in the hippocampus. *Nature* **342,** 545-548.

Chavez-Noriega LE, Halliwell JV & Bliss TV. (1990). A decrease in firing threshold observed after induction of the EPSP-spike (E-S) component of long-term potentiation in rat hippocampal slices. *Exp Brain Res* **79,** 633-641.

Cho YH, Giese KP, Tanila H, Silva AJ & Eichenbaum H. (1998). Abnormal hippocampal spatial representations in alphaCaMKIIT286A and CREBalphaDelta- mice. *Science* **279,** 867-869.

Collingridge GL, Kehl SJ & McLennan H. (1983). Excitatory amino acids in synaptic transmission in the Schaffer collateral-commissural pathway of the rat hippocampus. *J Physiol* **334,** 33-46.

Cressant A, Muller RU & Poucet B. (1997). Failure of centrally placed objects to control the firing fields of hippocampal place cells. *J Neurosci* **17,** 2531–2542.

Crist RE, Li W & Gilbert CS. (2001). Learning to see: experience and attention in primary visual cortex. *Nat Neurosci* **4,** 519–525.

Csicsvari J, Hirase H, Czurko A & Buzsáki G. (1998). Reliability and state dependence of pyramidal cell-interneuron synapses in the hippocampus: an ensemble approach in the behaving rat. *Neuron* **21,** 179-189.

Dan Y & Poo M. (2004). Spike timing-dependent plasticity of neural circuits. *Neuron* **44,** 23-30.

Deadwyler SA, Dudeck FE, Cotman CW & Lynch G. (1975). Intracellular responses of rat dentate granule cells in vitro: post-tetanic potentiation to perforant path stimulation. *Brain Res* **88,** 80-85.

Deadwyler SA & Hampson RE. (2004). Differential but complementary mnemonic functions of the hippocampus and subiculum. *Neuron* **42,** 465-476.

Debanne D, Gahwiler BH & Thompson SM. (1998). Long-term synaptic plasticity between pairs of individual CA3 pyramidal cells in rat hippocampal slice cultures. *J Physiol* **507,** 237–247.

deToledo-Morrell L, Geinisman Y & Morrell F. (1988). Age-dependent alterations In hippocampal synaptic plasticity: relation to memory disorders. *Neurobiol Aging* **9,** 581–590.

Deupree DL, Bradley J & Turner DA. (1993). Age-related alterations in potentiation in the CA1 region in F-344 rats. *Neurobiol Aging* **14,** 249 –258.

Douglas RM & Goddard GV. (1975). Long-term potentiation of the perforant path-granule cell synapse in the rat hippocampus. *Brain Res* **86,** 205-215.

Doyere V, Errington ML, Laroche S & Bliss TVP. (1996). Low-frequency trains of paired stimuli induce long-term depression in area CA1 but not in dentate gyrus of the intact rat. *Hippocampus* **6,** 52–57.

Dragoi G & Buzsáki G. (2006). Temporal encoding of place sequences by hippocampal cell assemblies. *Neuron* **50,** 145–157.

Dragoi G, Harris KD & Buzsáki G. (2003). Place representation within hippocampal networks is modified by long-term potentiation. *Neuron* **39,** 843-853.

Droulez J & Berthoz A. (1991). A neural network model of sensoritopic maps with predictive short-term memory properties. *Proc Natl Acad Sci USA* **88,** 9653-9657.

Dudek SM & Bear MF. (1992). Homosynaptic long-term depression and effects of Nmethyl-D-aspartate receptor blockade. *Proc Natl Acad Sci USA* **89,** 4363–4367.

Dunwiddie T & Lynch G. (1978). Long-term potentiation and depression of synaptic responses in the rat hippocampus: localization and frequency dependency. *J Physiol* **276,** 353–367.

Egger V, Feldmeyer D & Sakmann B. (1999). Coincidence detection and changes of synaptic efficacy in spiny stellate neurons in rat barrel cortex. *Nat Neurosci* **2,** 1098–1105.

Eichenbaum H, Dudchenko P, Wood E, Shapiro M & Tanila H. (1999). The hippocampus, memory, and place cells: is it spatial memory or a memory space? *Neuron* **23,** 209-226.

Ekstrom AD, Kahana MJ, Caplan JB, Fields TA, Isham EA, Newman EL & Fried I. (2003). Cellular networks underlying human spatial navigation. *Nature* **425,** 184-188.

Ekstrom AD, Meltzer J, McNaughton BL & Barnes CA. (2001). NMDA receptor antagonism blocks experience-dependent expansion of hippocampal ''place fields''. *Neuron* **31,** 631–638.

Fazeli MS & Collingridge GL. (1996). Cortical Plasticity: LTP and LTD. *Bios, Oxford.*

Feldman DE. (2000). Timing-based LTP and LTD at vertical inputs to layer II/III pyramidal cells in rat barrel cortex. *Neuron* **27,** 45–56.

Foster TC, Castro CA & McNaughton BL. (1989). Spatial selectivity of rat hippocampal neurons: dependence on preparedness for movement. *Science* **244,** 1580-1582.

Foster TC & Norris CM. (1997). Age-associated changes in Calcium-dependent processes: relation to hippocampal synaptic plasticity. *Hippocampus* **7,** 602– 612.

Frank LM, Brown EN & Wilson MA. (2000). Trajectory encoding in the hippocampus and entorhinal cortex. *Neuron* **27,** 169–178.

Froemke RC & Dan Y. (2002). Spike-timing-dependent synaptic modification induced by natural spike trains. *Nature* **416,** 433–438.

Fu YX, Djupsund K, Gao H, Hayden B, Shen K & Dan Y. (2002). Temporal specificity in the cortical plasticity of visual space representation. *Science* **296,** 1999-2003.

Fyhn M, Hafting T, Treves A, Moser MB & Moser EI. (2007). Hippocampal remapping and grid realignment in entorhinal cortex. *Nature* **446,** 190–194.

Garwicz M & Ekerot CF. (1994). Topographical organization of the cerebellar cortical projection to nucleus interpositus anterior in the cat. *J Physiol* **474,** 245–260.

Gerstner W, Kempter R, van Hemmen JL & Wagner H. (1996). A neuronal learning rule for sub-millisecond temporal coding. *Nature* **383,** 76-78.

Gomi H & Kawato M. (1992). Adaptive feedback control models of the vestibulocerebellum and spinocerebellum. *Biol Cybern* **68,** 105–114.

Goodridge JP, Dudchenko PA, Worboys KA, Golob EJ & Taube JS. (1998). Cue control and head direction cells. *Behav Neurosci* **112,** 749-761.

Gothard KM, Hoffman KL, Battaglia FP & McNaughton BL. (2001). Dentate gyrus and CA1 ensemble activity during spatial reference frame shifts in the presence and absence of visual input. *J Neurosci* **21,** 7284-7292.

Gray CM & McCormick DA. (1996). Chattering cells: superficial pyramidal neurons contributing to the generation of synchronous oscillations in the visual cortex. *Science* **274,** 109-113.

Gustafsson B, Wigstrom H, Abraham WC & Huang YY. (1987). Long-term potentiation in the hippocampus using depolarizing current pulses as the conditioning stimulus to single volley synaptic potentials. *J Neurosci* **7,** 774 –780.

Hafting T, Fyhn M, Molden S, Moser MB & Moser EI. (2005). Microstructure of a spatial map in the entorhinal cortex. *Nature* **436,** 801-806.

Hampson RE, Hedberg T & Deadwyler SA. (2000). Differential information processing by hippocampal and subicular neurons. *Ann N Y Acad Sci* **911,** 151-165.

Harris KD, Csicsvari J, Hirase H, Dragoi G & Buzsaki G. (2003). Organization of cell assemblies in the hippocampus. *Nature* **424,** 552–556.

Harris KD, Hirase H, Leinekugel X, Henze DA & Buzsáki G. (2001). Temporal interaction between single spikes and complex spike bursts in hippocampal pyramidal cells. *Neuron* **32,** 141-149.

Hartley T, Burgess N, Lever C, Cacucci F & O'Keefe J. (2000). Modeling place fields in terms of the cortical inputs to the hippocampus. *Hippocampus* **10,** 369-379.

mo ME, Bodelon C & Wyble BP. (2002). A proposed function for hippocampal theta rhythm: separate phases of encoding and retrieval enhance reversal of prior learning. *Neural Comput* **14,** 793–817.

Hausser M, Raman IM, Otis T, Smith SL, Nelson A, du Lac S, Loewenstein Y, Mahon S, Pennartz C, Cohen I & Yarom Y. (2004). The beat goes on: spontaneous firing in mammalian neuronal microcircuits. *J Neurosci* **24,** 9215-9219.

Hayman R, Chakraborty S, Anderson MI & Jeffery KJ. (2003). Context-specific acquisition of location discrimination by hippocampal place cells. *Eur J Neurosci* **18,** 2825-2834.

Hess G & Gustafsson B. (1990). Changes in field excitatory postsynaptic potential shape induced by tetanization in the CA1 region of the guinea-pig hippocampal slice. *Neuroscience* **37,** 61–69.

Hetherington PA & Shapiro ML. (1997). Hippocampal place fields are altered by the removal of single visual cues in a distance-dependent manner. *Behav Neurosci* **111,** 20-34.

Heynen AJ, Abraham WC & Bear MF. (1996). Bidirectional modification of CA1 synapses in the adult hippocampus in vivo. *Nature* **381,** 163-166.

Hollup SA, Molden S, Donnett JG, Moser MB & Moser EI. (2001). Accumulation of hippocampal place fields at the goal location in an annular watermaze task. *J Neurosci* **21,** 1635–1644.

Hu D & Amsel A. (1995). A simple test of the vicarious trial-and-error hypothesis of hippocampal function. *Proc Natl Acad Sci USA* **92,** 5506 –5509.

Hu D, Xu X & Gonzalez-Lima F. (2006). Vicarious trial-and-error behavior and hippocampal cytochrome oxidase activity during Y-maze discrimination learning in the rat. *Int J Neurosci* **116,** 265–280.

Ito M. (2000). Mechanisms of motor learning in the cerebellum. *Brain Res* **886,** 237–245.

Ito M. (2001). Cerebellar long-term depression: characterization, signal transduction, and functional roles. *Physiol Rev* **81,** 1143-1195.

Ito M & Kano M. (1982). Long-lasting depression of parallel fiber-Purkinje cell transmission induced by conjunctive stimulation of parallel fibers and climbing fibers in the cerebellar cortex. *Neurosci Lett* **33,** 253–258.

Jeffery KJ. (1999). Learning of landmark stability and instability by hippocampal place cells. *Neuropharmacology* **37,** 677-687.

Jeffery KJ & Anderson MI. (2003). Dissociation of the geometric and contextual influences on place cells. *Hippocampus* **13,** 868-872.

Jeffery KJ, Donnett JG, Burgess N & O'Keefe JM. (1997). Directional control of hippocampal place fields. *Exp Brain Res* **117,** 131-142.

Jeffery KJ & Hayman R. (2004). Plasticity of the hippocampal place cell representation. *Rev Neurosci* **15,** 309–331.

Jeffery KJ & O'Keefe JM. (1999). Learned interaction of visual and idiothetic cues in the control of place field orientation. *Exp Brain Res* **127,** 151-161.

Jensen O & Lisman JE. (1996). Theta/gamma networks with slow NMDA channels learn sequences and encode episodic memory: role of NMDA channels in recall. *Learn Mem* **3,** 264-278.

Johnson A & Redish AD. (2007). Neural ensembles in CA3 transiently encode paths forward of the animal at a decision point. *J Neurosci* **27,** 12176-12189.

Kamondi A, Acsady L, Wang XJ & Buzsáki G. (1998). Theta oscillations in somata and dendrites of hippocampal pyramidal cells in vivo: activity-dependent phase-precession of action potentials. *Hippocampus* **8,** 244-261.

Kawato M, Furukawa K & Suzuki R. (1987). A hierarchical neuronal network model for control and learning of voluntary movement. *Biol Cybern* **57,** 169–185.

Kentros C, Hargreaves E, Hawkins RD, Kandel ER, Shapiro M & Muller RV. (1998). Abolition of long-term stability of new hippocampal place cell maps by NMDA receptor blockade. *Science* **280,** 2121-2126.

Kesner RP. (1998). Neural mediation of memory for time: role of hippocampus and medial prefrontal cortex. *Psychol Bull Rev* **5,** 585–596.

Kesner RP & Rolls ET. (2001). Role of long term synaptic modification in short term memory. *Hippocampus* **11,** 240–250.

Kirkwood A, Lee H-K & Bear MF. (1995). Co-regulation of long-term potentiation and experience-dependent plasticity in visual cortex by age and experience. *Nature* **375,** 328–331.

Kleinfeld D. (1986). Sequential state generation by model neural networks. *Proc Natl Acad Sci USA* **83,** 9469 –9473.

Knierim JJ, Kudrimoti HS & McNaughton BL. (1995). Place cells, head direction cells, and the learning of landmark stability. *J Neurosci* **15,** 1648-1659.

Larson J & Lynch G. (1986). Induction of synaptic potentiation in the hippocampus by patterned stimulation involves two events. *Science* **232,** 985-988.

Larson J & Lynch G. (1988). Role of N-methyl-D-aspartate receptors in the induction of synaptic potentiation by burst stimulation patterned after the hippocampal theta-rhythm. *Brain Res* **441,** 111-118.

Larson J & Lynch G. (1989). Theta pattern stimulation and the induction of LTP: the sequence in which synapses are stimulated determines the degree to which they potentiate. *Brain Res* **489,** 49-58.

Lee I, Rao G & Knierim JJ. (2004). A double dissociation between hippocampal subfields: differential time course of CA3 and CA1 place cells for processing changed environments. *Neuron* **42,** 803-815.

Lenck-Santini PP, Muller RU, Save E & Poucet B. (2002). Relationships between place cell firing fields and navigational decisions by rats. *J Neurosci* **22,** 9035–9047.

Lenck-Santini PP, Save E & Poucet B. (2001). Evidence for a relationship between place-cell spatial firing and spatial memory performance. *Hippocampus* **11,** 377–390.

Leutgeb S, Leutgeb JK, Treves A, Moser MB & Moser EI. (2004). Distinct ensemble codes in hippocampal areas CA3 and CA1. *Science* **305,,** 1295–1298.

Leutgeb S, Ragozzino KE & Mizumori SJ. (2000). Convergence of head direction and place information in the CA1 region of hippocampus. *Neuroscience* **100,** 11-19.

Lever C, Wills T, Cacucci F, Burgess N & O'Keefe J. (2002). Long-term plasticity in hippocampal place-cell representation of environmental geometry. *Nature* **416,** 90–94.

Levy WB & Steward O. (1979). Synapses as associative memory elements in the hippocampal formation. *Brain Res* **175,** 233–245.

Levy WB & Steward O. (1983). Temporal contiguity requirements for long-term associative potentiation/depression in the hippocampus. *Neuroscience* **8,** 791-797.

Li XG, Somogyi P, Ylinen A & Buzsaki G. (1994). The hippocampal CA3 network: an in vivo intracellular labeling study. *J Comp Neurol* **339,** 181–208.

Linden DJ. (1999). The return of the spike, postsynaptic action potentials and the induction of LTP and LTD. *Neuron* **22,** 661-666.

Lisman JE. (1994). The CaM-kinase hypothesis for the storage of synaptic memory. *Trends Neurosci* **17,** 406−412.

Lisman JE. (1997). Bursts as a unit of neural information: making unreliable synapses reliable. *Trends Neurosci* **20,** 38-43.

Lisman JE. (1999). Relating hippocampal circuitry to function: Recall of memory sequences by reciprocal dentate/CA3 interactions. *Neuron* **22,** 233 -242.

Lisman JE & Idiart MA. (1995). Storage of 7 +/- 2 short-term memories in oscillatory subcycles. *Science* **267,** 1512–1515.
Lisman JE & Otmakhova NA. (2001). Storage, recall, and novelty detection of sequences by the hippocampus: elaborating on the SOCRATIC model to account for normal and aberrant effects of dopamine. *Hippocampus* **11,** 551-568.
Lynch GS, Dunwiddie T & Gribkoff V. (1977). Heterosynaptic depression: a postsynaptic correlate of long-term potentiation. *Nature* **266,** 737–739.
Lynch MA. (2004). Long-term potentiation and memory. *Physiol Rev* **84,** 87–136.
Magee JC & Johnston DA. (1997). Synaptically controlled, associative signal for hebbian plasticity in hippocampal neurons. *Science* **275,** 209-213.
Manahan-Vaughan D & Braunwell K-H. (1999). Novelty acquisition is associated with induction of hippocampal long-term depression. *Proc Natl Acad Sci* **96,** 8739-8744.
Markram H, Lubke J, Frotscher M & Sakmann B. (1997). Regulation of synaptic efficacy by coincidence of postsynaptic APs and EPSPs. *Science* **275,** 213–215.
Markus EJ, Barnes CA, McNaughton BL, Gladden VL & Skaggs WE. (1994). Spatial information content and reliability of hippocampal CA1 neurons: effects of visual input. *Hippocampus* **4,** 410-421.
Markus EJ, Qin YL, Leonard BW, Skaggs WE, McNaughton BL & Barnes CA. (1995). Interactions between location and task affect the spatial and directional firing of hippocampal neurons. *J Neurosci* **15,** 7079-7094.
Marr D. (1969). A theory of cerebellar cortex. *J Physiol* **202,** 437–470.
Marr D. (1971). Simple memory: a theory for archicortex. *Phil Trans R Soc, London B* **262,** 23–81.
Martin SJ, Grimwood PD & Morris RGM. (2000). Synaptic plasticity and memory: an evaluation of the hypothesis. *Annu Rev Neurosci* **23,** 649-711.
Mauk MD, Steinmetz JE & Thompson RF. (1986). Classical conditioning using stimulation of the inferior olive as the unconditioned stimulus. *Proc Natl Acad Sci USA* **83,** 5349–5353.
McCormick DA & Thompson RF. (1984). Cerebellum: essential involvement in the classically conditioned eyelid response. *Science* **223,** 296–299.
McHugh TJ, Blum KI, Tsien JZ, Tonegawa S & Wilson MA. (1996). Impaired hippocampal representation of space in CA1-specific NMDAR1 knockout mice. *Cell* **87,** 1339-1349.
McHugh TJ, Jones MW, Quinn JJ, Balthasar N, Coppari R, Elmquist JK, Lowell BB, Fanselow MS, Wilson MA & Tonegawa S. (2007). Dentate gyrus NMDA receptors mediate rapid pattern separation in the hippocampal network. *Science* **317,** 94-99.
McNaughton BL, Barnes CA, Gerrard JL, Gothard K, Jung MW, Knierim JJ, Kudrimoti H, Qin YL, Skaggs WE, Suster MS & Weaver K. (1996). Deciphering the hippocampal polyglot: the hippocampus as a path integration system. *J Exp Biol* **199,** 173-185.
McNaughton BL, Barnes CA & O'Keefe J. (1983). The contributions of position, direction, and velocity to single unit activity in the hippocampus of freely-moving rats. *Exp Brain Res* **52,** 41-49.
McNaughton BL, Battaglia FP, Jensen O, Moser EI & Moser MB. (2006). Path integration and the neural basis of the 'cognitive map'. *Nat Rev Neurosci* **7,** 663-678.
McNaughton BL & Morris RGM. (1987). Hippocampal synaptic enhancement and information storage within a distributed memory system. *Trends Neurosci* **10,** 408–415.
Mehta MR, Barnes CA & McNaughton BL. (1997). Experience-dependent, asymmetric expansion of hippocampal place fields. *Proc Natl Acad Sci USA* **94,** 8918-8921.
Mehta MR, Quirk MC & Wilson MA. (2000). Experience-dependent asymmetric shape of hippocampal receptive fields. *Neuron* **25,** 707–715.

Mizumori SJ. (2006). Hippocampal place fields: a neural code for episodic memory? *Hippocampus* **16,** 685-690.

Mizumori SJ & Kalyani A. (1997). Age and experience-dependent representational reorganization during spatial learning. *Neurobiol Aging* **18,** 651-659.

Mizumori SJ, Lavoie AM & Kalyani A. (1996). Redistribution of spatial representation in the hippocampus of aged rats performing a spatial memory task. *Behav Neurosci* **110,** 1006-1016.

Mizumori SJ, Ragozzino KE, Cooper BG & Leutgeb S. (1999). Hippocampal representational organization and spatial context. *Hippocampus* **9,** 444–451.

Moita MA, Rosis S, Zhou Y, LeDoux JE & Blair HT. (2004). Putting fear in its place: remapping of hippocampal place cells during fear conditioning. *J Neurosci* **24,** 7015–7023.

Moore CI, Browning MD & Rose GM. (1993). Hippocampal plasticity induced by primed burst, but not long-term potentiation, stimulation is impaired in area CA1 of aged Fischer 344 rats. *Hippocampus* **3,** 57– 66.

Morris RGM. (2003). Long-term potentiation and memory. *Philos Trans R Soc, London B Biol Sci* **358,** 643–647.

Morris RGM & Frey U. (1997). Hippocampal Synaptic Plasticity: Role in Spatial Learning or the Automatic Recording of Attended Experience? *Philos Trans R Soc Lond B Biol Sci* **352,** 1489-1503.

Morris RGM, Moser EI, Riedel G, Martin SJ, Sandin J, Day M & O'Carroll C. (2003). Elements of a neurobiological theory of the hippocampus: the role of activity-dependent synaptic plasticity in memory. *Philos Trans R Soc, London B Biol Sci* **358,** 773–786.

Moser EI. (1995). Learning-related changes in hippocampal field potentials. *Behav Brain Res* **71,** 11–18.

Muenzinger KF. (1938). Vicarious trial and error at a point of choice. I. A general survey of its relation to learning efficiency. *J Genet Psychol* **53,** 75– 86.

Muller RU, Bostock E, Taube JS & Kubie JL. (1994). On the directional firing properties of hippocampal place cells. *J Neurosci* **14,** 7235-7251.

Muller RU & Kubie JL. (1987). The effects of changes in the environment on the spatial firing of hippocampal complex-spike cells. *J Neurosci* **7,** 1951-1968.

Muller RU, Kubie JL & Ranck JBJ. (1987). Spatial firing patterns of hippocampal complex-spike cells in a fixed environment. *J Neurosci* **7,** 1935-1950.

Muller RU, Stead M & Pach J. (1996). The hippocampus as a cognitive graph. *J Gen Physiol* **107,** 663–694.

Nakazawa K, Sun LD, Quirk MC, Rondi-Reig L, Wilson MA & Tonegawa S. (2003). Hippocampal CA3 NMDA receptors are crucial for memory acquisition of one-time experience. *Neuron* **38,** 305-315.

Noguchi K, Saito H & Abe K. (1998). Medial amygdala stimulation produces a long-lasting excitatory postsynaptic potential/spike dissociation in the dentate gyrus in vivo. *Brain Res* **794,** 151–154.

Norris CM, Halpain S & Foster TC. (1998). Reversal of age-related alterations in synaptic plasticity by blockade of L-type Ca2+ channels. *J Neurosci* **18,** 3171-3179.

Norris CM, Korol DL & Foster TC. (1996). Increased susceptibility to induction of long-term depression and long-term potentiation reversal during aging. *J Neurosci* **16,** 5382–5392.

O'Keefe J. (1976). Place units in the hippocampus of the freely moving rat. *Exp Neurol* **51,** 78-109.

O'Keefe J & Speakman A. (1987). Single unit activity in the rat hippocampus during a spatial memory task. *Exp Brain Res* **68,** 1-27.

O'Mara S. (2005). The subiculum: what it does, what it might do, and what neuroanatomy has yet to tell us. *J Anat* **207,** 271-282.

O'Mara SM. (1995). Spatially selective firing properties of hippocampal formation neurons in rodents and primates. *Prog Neurobiol* **45,** 253-274.

O'Keefe J. (1979). A review of hippocampal place cells. *Prog Neurobiol* **13,** 419-439.

O'Keefe J & Nadel L. (1978). Hippocampus as a Cognitive Map. *(Oxford: Clarindon).*

Oler JA & Markus EJ. (2000a). Age-related deficits in episodic memory may result from decreased responsiveness of hippocampal place cells to changes in context. *Ann N Y Acad Sci* **911,** 465-470.

Oler JA & Markus EJ. (2000b). Age-related deficits in the ability to encode contextual change: a place cell analysis. *Hippocampus* **10,** 338-350.

Orr G, Rao G, Houston FP, McNaughton BL & Barnes CA. (2001). Hippocampal synaptic plasticity is modulated by theta rhythm in the fascia dentata of adult and aged freely behaving rats. *Hippocampus* **11,** 647-654.

Paulsen O & Sejnovski TJ. (2000). Natural patterns of activity and long-term synaptic plasticity. *Curr Opin Neurobiol* **10,** 172-179.

Pavlides C, Greenstein YJ, Grudman M & Winson J. (1988). Long-term potentiation in the dentate gyrus is induced preferentially on the positive phase of theta-rhythm. *Brain Res* **439,** 383-387.

Pike FG, Meredith RM, Olding AW & Paulsen O. (1999). Postsynaptic bursting is essential for "Hebbian" induction of associative long-term potentiation at excitatory synapses in rat hippocampus. *J Physiol* **518,** 571-576.

Quirk GJ, Muller RU & Kubie JL. (1990). The firing of hippocampal place cells in the dark depends on the rat's recent experience. *J Neurosci* **10,** 2008-2017.

Quirk GJ, Muller RU, Kubie JL & Ranck JBJ. (1992). The positional firing properties of medial entorhinal neurons: description and comparison with hippocampal place cells. *J Neurosci* **12,** 1945–1963.

Rawlins JNP. (1985). Associations across time: the hippocampus as a temporary memory store. *Behav Brain Sci* **8,** 479–496.

Redish AD, Elga AN & Touretzky DS. (1996). A coupled attractor model of the rodent head direction system. *Netw Comput Neural Syst* **7,** 671–685.

Redish AD & Touretzky DS. (1997). Cognitive maps beyond the hippocampus. *Hippocampus* **7,** 15-35.

Roberts PD. (1999). Computational consequences of temporally asymmetric learning rules, I. Differential Hebbian learning. *J Computational Neurosci* **7,** 235-246.

Robertson RG, Rolls ET & Georges-Francois P. (1998). Spatial view cells in the primate hippocampus: Effects of removal of view details. *J Neurophysiol* **79,** 1145–1156.

Rolls ET. (1991). Functions of the primate hippocampus in spatial and nonspatial memory. *Hippocampus* **1,** 258–261.

Rolls ET. (1996). Roles of long term potentiation and long term depression in neuronal network operations in the brain. *In: Fazeli, MS, Collingridge, GL (Eds), Cortical Plasticity Bios, Oxford,* , pp. 223–250.

Rolls ET & Deco G. (2002). Computational Neuroscience of Vision. *Oxford University Press, Oxford.*

Rolls ET & Kesner RP. (2006). A computational theory of hippocampal function, and empirical tests of the theory. *Prog Neurobiol* **79,** 1-48.

Rolls ET & O'Mara SM. (1995). View-responsive neurons in the primate hippocampal complex. *Hippocampus* **5,** 409–424.

Rolls ET & Treves A. (1990). The relative advantages of sparse versus distributed encoding for associative neuronal networks in the brain. *Network* **1,** 407–421.

Rolls ET & Treves A. (1998). Neural Networks and Brain Function. *Oxford, UK: Oxford Univ Press*, 418 pp.

Rolls ET, Treves A, Foster D & Perez-Vicente C. (1997). Simulation studies of the CA3 hippocampal subfield modelled as an attractor neural network. *Neural Netw* **10,** 1559–1569.

Rose G & Dunwiddie TV. (1986). Induction of hippocampal long-term potentiation using physiologically patterned stimulation. *Neurosci Lett* **69,** 244-248.

Rosenzweig ES, Rao G, McNaughton BL & Barnes CA. (1997). Role of temporal summation in age-related long-term potentiation induction deficits. *Hippocampus* **7,** 549 –558.

Samsonovich A & McNaughton BL. (1997). Path integration and cognitive mapping in a continuous attractor neural network model. *J Neurosci* **17,** 5900–5920.

Sargolini F, Fyhn M, Hafting T, McNaughton BL, Witter MP, Moser MB & Moser EI. (2006). Conjunctive representation of position, direction, and velocity in entorhinal cortex. *Science* **312,** 758-762.

Save E, Paz-Villagran V, Alexinsky T & Poucet B. (2005). Functional interaction between the associative parietal cortex and hippocampal place cell firing in the rat. *Eur J Neurosci* **21,** 522-530.

Schoups A, Vogels R, Quian N & Orban G. (2001). Practising orientation identification improves orientation coding in V1 neurons. *Nature* **412,** 549–553.

Schuett S, Bonhoeffer T & Hübener M. (2001). Pairing-induced changes of orientation maps in cat visual cortex. *Neuron* **32,** 325-337.

Shapiro ML, Tanila H & Eichenbaum H. (1997). Cues that hippocampal place cells encode: dynamic and hierarchical representation of local and distal stimuli. *Hippocampus* **7,** 624–642.

Sharp PE. (1999). Complimentary roles for hippocampal versus subicular/entorhinal place cells in coding place, context, and events. *Hippocampus* **9,** 432-443.

Sharp PE & Green C. (1994). Spatial correlates of firing patterns of single cells in the subiculum of the freely moving rat. *J Neurosci* **14,** 2339-2356.

Sjostrom PJ, Turrigiano GG & Nelson SB. (2001). Rate, timing, and cooperativity jointly determine cortical synaptic plasticity. *Neuron* **32,** 1149–1164.

Smith DM & Mizumori SJ. (2006a). Hippocampal place cells, context, and episodic memory. *Hippocampus* **16,** 716-729.

Smith DM & Mizumori SJ. (2006b). Learning-related development of context-specific neuronal responses to places and events: the hippocampal role in context processing. *J Neurosci* **26,** 3154-3163.

Sompolinsky H & Kanter I. (1986). Temporal association in asymmetric neural networks. *Phys Rev Lett* **57,** 2861–2864.

Sourdet V & Debanne D. (1999). The role of dendritic filtering in associative long-term synaptic plasticity. *Learn Mem* **6,** 422-447.

Stackman RW & Taube JS. (1998). Firing properties of rat lateral mammillary single units: head direction, head pitch, and angular head velocity [Erratum in: J Neurosci. 2003 Feb 15;23(4):1555-1556]. *J Neurosci* **18,** 9020-9037.

Stringer SM, Rolls ET & Trappenberg TP. (2004). Self-organising continuous attractor networks with multiple activity packets, and the representation of space. *Neural Netw* **17,** 5-27.

Sur M, Schummers J & Dragoi V. (2002). Cortical plasticity: time for a change. *Curr Biol* **12,** R168-170.

Suzuki WA, Miller EK & Desimone R. (1997). Object and place memory in the macaque entorhinal cortex. *J Neurophysiol* **78,** 1062–1081.

Tanila H. (1999). Hippocampal place cells can develop distinct representations of two visually identical environments. *Hippocampus* **9,** 235–246.

Tanila H, Shapiro M, Gallagher M & Eichenbaum H. (1997a). Brain aging: changes in the nature of information coding by the hippocampus. *J Neurosci* **17,** 5155-5166.

Tanila H, Shapiro ML & Eichenbaum H. (1997b). Discordance of spatial representation in ensembles of hippocampal place cells [Erratum in: Hippocampus 1998;8(1):83]. *Hippocampus* **7,** 613–623.

Taube JS. (1995a). Head direction cells recorded in the anterior thalamic nuclei of freely moving rats. *J Neurosci* **15,** 70-86.

Taube JS. (1995b). Place cells recorded in the parasubiculum of freely moving rats [published erratum in Hippocampus 1996;6(5):561]. *Hippocampus* **5,** 569-583.

Taube JS. (1998). Head direction cells and the neurophysiological basis for a sense of direction. *Prog Neurobiol* **55,** 225-256.

Taube JS, Muller RU & Ranck JBJ. (1990). Head-direction cells recorded from the postsubiculum in freely moving rats. II. Effects of environmental manipulations. *J Neurosci* **10,** 436-447.

Taube JS & Schwartzkroin PA. (1988). Mechanisms of long-term potentiation: EPSP/spike dissociation, intradendritic recordings, and glutamate sensitivity. *J Neurosci* **8,** 1632-1644.

Thiels E, Barrionuevo G & Berger TW. (1994). Excitatory stimulation during postsynaptic inhibition induces long-term depression in hippocamapus in vivo. *J Neurophysiol* **72,** 3009–3016.

Thiels E, Xie X, Yeckel MF, Barrionuevo G & Berger TW. (1996). NMDA receptor-dependent LTD in different subfields of hippocampus in vivo and in vitro. *Hippocampus* **6,** 43-51.

Tolman EC. (1939). Prediction of vicarious trial and error by means of the schematic sowbug. *Psychol Rev* **46,** 318 –336.

Treves A & Rolls ET. (1991). What determines the capacity of autoassociative memories in the brain? *Network* **2,** 371–397.

Treves A & Rolls ET. (1992). Computational constraints suggest the need for two distinct input systems to the hippocampal CA3 network. *Hippocampus* **2,** 189–199.

Tsodyks MV. (1999). Attractor neural network models of spatial maps in hippocampus. *Hippocampus* **9,** 481–489.

Tsodyks MV, Skaggs WE, Sejnowski TJ & McNaughton BL. (1996). Population dynamics and theta rhythm phase precession of hippocampal place cell firing: a spiking neuron model. *Hippocampus* **6,** 271–280.

Turrigiano GG & Nelson SB. (2000). Hebb and homeostasis in neuronal plasticity. *Curr Opin Neurobiol* **10,** 358-364.

Wallenstein GV & Hasselmo ME. (1997). GABAergic modulation of hippocampal population activity: sequence learning, place field development, and the phase precession effect. *J Neurophysiol* **78,** 393–408.

Wigstrom H & Swann JW. (1980). Strontium supports synaptic transmission and long-lasting potentiation in the hippocampus. *Brain Res* **194,** 181–191.

Wills TJ, Lever C, Cacucci F, Burgess N & O'Keefe J. (2005). Attractor dynamics in the hippocampal representation of the local environment. *Science* **308,** 873–876.

Wilson IA, Ikonen S, McMahan RW, Gallagher M, Eichenbaum H & Tanila H. (2003). Place cell rigidity correlates with impaired spatial learning in aged rats. *Neurobiol Aging* **24,** 297-305.

Wilson RC. (1981). Changes in translation of synaptic excitation to dentate granule cell discharge accompanying long-term potentiation. I. Differences between normal and reinnervated dentate gyrus. *J Neurophysiol* **46,** 324–338.

Wood ER, Dudchenko PA & Eichenbaum H. (1999). The global record of memory in hippocampal neuronal activity. *Nature* **397,** 613-616.

Xiang JZ & Brown MW. (1998). Differential neuronal encoding of novelty, familiarity and recency in regions of the anterior temporal lobe. *Neuropharmacology* **37,** 657–676.

Yao H & Dan Y. (2001). Stimulus timing-dependent plasticity in cortical processing of orientation. *Neuron* **32,** 315–323.

Yao H & Dan Y. (2005). Synaptic learning rules, cortical circuits, and visual function. *Neuroscientist* **11,** 206-216.

Yao H, Shen Y & Dan Y. (2004). Intracortical mechanism of stimulustiming- dependent plasticity in visual cortical orientation tuning. *Proc Natl Acad Sci* **101,** 5081–5086.

Young BJ, Fox GD & Eichenbaum H. (1994). Correlates of hippocampal complex-spike cell activity in rats performing a non-spatial radial maze task. *J Neurosci* **14,** 6553–6563.

Young BJ, Otto T, Fox GD & Eichenbaum H. (1997). Memory representation within the parahippocampal region. *J Neurosci* **17,** 5183–5195.

Zhang K. (1996). Representation of spatial orientation by the intrinsic dynamics of the head-direction cell ensemble: a theory. *J Neurosci* **16,** 2112–2126.

Zhang LI, Tao HW, Holt CE, Harris WA & Poo M. (1998). A critical window for cooperation and competition among developing retinotectal synapses. *Nature* **395,** 37–44.

Zugaro MB, Monconduit L & Buzsaki G. (2005). Spike phase precession persists after transient intrahippocampal perturbation. *Nat Neurosci* **8,** 67–71.

In: Synaptic Plasticity: New Research
Editors: Tim F. Kaiser and Felix J. Peters

ISBN: 978-1-60456-732-8

Chapter 11

REGULATION OF SYNAPTIC PLASTICITY BY THE SCAFFOLDING PROTEIN SPINOPHILIN

D. Sarrouilhe** *and T. Métayé
Institut de Physiologie et Biologie Cellulaires, Pôle Biologie Santé, Université de Poitiers, France

ABSTRACT

Spinophilin/neurabin 2 is a protein scaffold that targets protein phosphatase 1 catalytic subunit (PP1c) close to some of its substrates. Gene analysis and biochemical approaches have contributed to define in spinophilin a number of distinct modular domains, such as one F-actin-, a receptor- and a PP1c-binding domains, a PSD95/DLG/zo-1 (PDZ) and three coiled-coil domains, that govern protein-protein interactions. Spinophilin plays important functions in the nervous system where it is implicated in spine morphology and density regulation, neuronal migration and synaptic plasticity. Morphological studies and subcellular distribution analysis indicated that spinophilin was enriched in dendritic spines in the postsynaptic density (PSD). The spinophilin interactome includes the glutamatergic α-amino-3-hydroxy-5-methylisoxazole-4-propionic acid (AMPA) and N-methyl-D-aspartic acid (NMDA) receptors that interact with the PDZ domain of the scaffolding protein. Studies using spinophilin Knockout (KO) mice suggested that spinophilin serves to regulate excitatory synaptic transmission and plasticity by targeting PP1c in the proximity of AMPA and NMDA receptors, promoting their down-regulation by dephosphorylation and thus regulating the efficiency of post-synaptic glutamatergic neurotransmission. The use of spinophilin KO mice also provides evidence that spinophilin is a good candidate to serve as a link between excitatory synapse transmission and changes in spine morphology and density. The molecular mechanism that controls spine morphology was in part recently elucidated and involved another spinophilin partner protein, the Rho-guanine nucleotide exchange factor Lfc. This review presents the available data that are contributing to the

* Tel: +33 5 49 45 43 58; Fax: +33 5 49 45 43 58. E-mail address: Denis.Sarrouilhe@univ-poitiers.fr

appreciation of spinophilin functions in synaptic plasticity and compares these functions to those of the related structural protein neurabin 1.

ABBREVIATIONS

AMPA: α-amino-3-hydroxy-5-methylisoxazole-4-propionic acid; AR: adrenergic receptor; CaMKII: Ca^{2+}/calmodulin-dependent PK II; CCK: cholecystokinin; CD: circular dichroism; DARPP-32: dopamine- and cyclic AMP-regulated phosphoprotein, MW 32 kDa; DCX: doublecortin; ERK: extracellular-signal regulated protein kinase; GEF: guanine nucleotide exchange factors; KO: knockout; Lfc :Lbc[lymphoid blast crisis]'s first cousin; LTD: long-term depression; LTP: long-term potentiation; MAPK: mitogen-activated protein kinase; NMDA: N-methyl-D-aspartic acid; NMR: nuclear magnetic resonance; PDZ: PSD95/DLG/zo-1; PK: protein kinase; PP: protein phosphatase; PP1c: PP1 catalytic subunit; PSD: postsynaptic density; RGS: regulator of G-protein signalling; TGN: trans-Golgi network; TRP: the transient receptor potential.

1. INTRODUCTION

PP1 is a widespread expressed phosphoSerine/phosphoThreonine PP involved in many cellular processes [Ceulemans and Bollen, 2004]. There are four isoforms of PP1c: PP1α, PP1β, PP1γ1 and PP1γ2, the latter two arising through alternative splicing [Sasaki et al., 1990]. PP1c can form complexes with up to 50 regulatory subunits converting the enzyme into many different forms, which have distinct substrates specificities, restricted subcellular locations and diverse regulations [Cohen, 2002]. In the nervous system, PP1 regulates short term events such as the phosphorylation status of receptors, ion channels, and signalling proteins, as well as long term events requiring changes in protein synthesis, gene expression, and neuronal morphology that together modify neuronal plasticity. A novel PP1c binding protein that is a potent modulator of PP1 activity was characterized in rat brain ten years ago and named spinophilin [Allen et al., 1997]. In the same time, two novel actin filament-binding proteins were purified from rat brain and named neurabin 1 and neurabin 2. Neurabin 2 was further identified as spinophilin [Nakanishi et al., 1997] and neurabin 1 was shown to also bind PP1c and to inhibit PP1c activity [McAvoy et al., 1999]. Spinophilin exhibits the characteristics of scaffolding proteins with multiple protein interaction domains [Allen et al., 1997; Sarrouilhe et al., 2006]. Scaffolding proteins link signalling enzymes, substrates and potential effectors (such as channels, receptors) into a multiprotein signalling complex that may be anchored to the cytoskeleton. Spinophilin has emerged as important scaffold linking PP1c to a rapidly growing list of cellular proteins [Sarrouilhe et al., 2006]. Spinophilin and neurabin 1 are highly enriched at the synaptic membrane in dendritic spines, the site of excitatory neurotransmission, and thus may control PP1 functions during synaptic plasticity. Moreover, among the spinophilin interactome some partner proteins are involved in synaptic plasticity.

This review aims to outline the state of knowledge regarding spinophilin function in synaptic plasticity and compares these functions to those of neurabin 1.

2. Spinophilin Structure

The rat and human spinophilin proteins consist of 817 amino acids and shares 96% sequence identity [Allen et al., 1997; Vivo et al., 2001]. The protein contains one F-actin-, a receptor- and a PP1c- binding domains, a PDZ and three coiled-coil domains. Figure 1 provides a schematic diagram of the main neurabins structural domains.

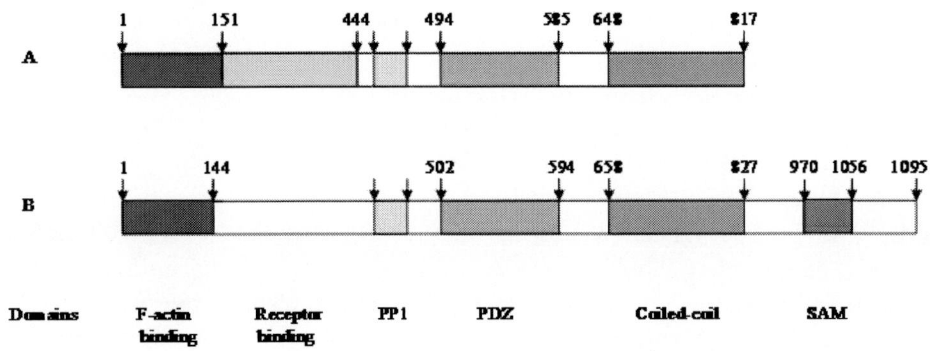

Figure 1. A schematic representation of the domain structure of full-length spinophilin (A) and neurabin 1 (B)

Spinophilin has been isolated from rat brain as a protein interacting with F-actin [Satoh et al., 1998]. Its F-actin-binding domain determined to be amino acids 1-154 is both necessary and sufficient to mediate actin polymers binding and cross-linking. Nuclear Magnetic Resonance (NMR) and circular dichroism (CD) spectroscopy studies showed that spinophilin F-actin-binding domain is intrinsically unstructured and that upon binding to F-actin it adopts a more ordered structure (a phenomenom also called folding-upon-binding). Another actin binding property, namely a F-actin pointed end capping activity was recently proposed for this domain [Schüler and Peti, 2007]. Spinophilin, PP1c and F-actin can form a trimeric complex in vitro.

A receptor-interacting domain, located between amino acids 151-444, interacts with the third intracellular loop (3i) of various seven transmembrane domain receptors [Smith et al., 1999; Richman et al., 2001] such as D2 dopamine and some subtypes of α-adrenergic receptors.

The primary PP1c-binding domain is located within residues 417-494 of spinophilin and this domain contains a pentapeptide motif (R/K-R/K-V/I-X-F) between amino acids 447 and 451 that is conserved in other PP1c regulatory subunits. This canonical PP1c-binding domain binds to the hydrophobic groove in the catalytic subunit. It was suggested that the canonical motif anchors PP1c to its binding proteins and facilitates diverse arrays of secondary interactions that play a role in modulating the overall strength of the interactions, regulating the activity of the associated catalytic subunit, and conferring PP1 isoform selectivity [Bollen, 2001].

Spinophilin also contains a single consensus sequence in PDZ, amino acids 494-585 [Allen et al., 1997]. The structure of the spinophilin and neurabin 1 PDZ domains have been recently solved by NMR spectroscopy. Both PDZ domains directly bind to carboxy-terminal peptides derived from glutamatergic AMPA and NMDA receptor [Kelker et al., 2007].

Sequence analysis predicted that the carboxy-terminal region of spinophilin (amino acids 664-814) forms 3 coiled-coil domains. Neurabins were observed as multimeric species in vitro and in vivo. Spinophilin and neurabin 1 homo- and hetero-dimerize via their carboxy-terminal coiled-coil domains [MacMillan et al., 1999; Oliver et al., 2002].

Consensus sequences for phosphorylation by several PKs, including cAMP-dependent PK (PKA), Ca^{2+}/calmodulin-dependent PK II (CaMKII), cyclin-dependent PK5 (Cdk5), extracellular-signal regulated PK (ERK) and protein tyrosine kinases were observed in spinophilin. Two major sites of phosphorylation for PKA (Ser-177 not conserved in human, and Ser-94) and two others sites for CaMKII phosphorylation (Ser-100 not conserved in neurabin 1, and Ser-116) were located within and near the F-actin-binding domain of spinophilin. Spinophilin is phosphorylated in intact cells by PKA at Ser-94 and Ser-177 and by CaMKII at Ser-100 [Hsieh-Wilson et al., 2003; Grossman et al., 2004]. Moreover neurabins can be phosphorylated in vitro and in intact cells by Cdk5 on Ser-17 and ERK2 (MAPK1) on Ser-15 and Ser-205, phosphoSer-17 being abundant in neuronal cells [Futter et al., 2005]. Two potential tyrosine phosphorylation sites lie within the coiled-coil regions of spinophilin and 2 others within a region adjacent to the PDZ domain.

Neurabin 1 consists of 1095 amino acids and contains one F-actin- and a PP1c-binding domains, a PDZ, a coiled-coil and a sterile alpha motif (SAM) domains at its [Nakanishi et al., 1997]. The structure of the neurabin 1 SAM domain was recently determined by NMR spectroscopy [Ju et al., 2007]. This SAM domain is a monomer in solution and must function via protein-protein interaction with other proteins. Primary sequence identity between spinophilin and neurabin 1 is: PDZ domain 86 %, PP1c binding domain 81 %, coiled-coil domain 63 % and F-actin binding domain 40 %.

3. Localization of Spinophilin in the Central Nervous System

Spinophilin expression in brain appeared to be differently regulated during mouse life, with high levels observed after birth and in the adult brain [Tsukada et al., 2003]. Spinophilin was enriched in cerebral cortex, caudatoputamen, hippocampal formation, and cerebellum [Ouimet et al., 2004]. Subcellular studies showed that spinophilin was localized predominantly in dendritic spines [Ouimet et al., 2004; Mully et al., 2004].

Dendritic spines are small membranous protusions from the central stalk of a dendrite, containing a bulbous head and a thin neck. Dendritic spines contain the majority of excitatory synapses and each spine has a single synapse. The localization of spinophilin within dendritic spines may be controlled by phosphorylation. Two localization domains of spinophilin were revealed within dendritic spines. One, consisting of the PSD and the subjacent 100 nm of spinoplasm, contained the highest density of label. Unphosphorylated spinophilin was enriched in PSD. The other, consisting of the deeper region of the spine, contained a lower density of spinophilin. No spinophilin labeling was found beyond 400 nm from the synapse [Mully et al., 2004]. A pool of phosphorylated spinophilin was found in the spinoplasm. Spinophilin phosphorylation by multiple kinase, in particular PKA and CaMKII [Hsieh-Wilson et al., 2003; Grossman et al., 2004] may modulate its localization within dendritic spines. CaMKII is synthesized locally in dendrites and is enriched in post-synaptic fractions enables phosphorylation of spinophilin.

Spinophilin was also found in dendrites, preterminal axons and glia suggesting that spinophilin's role in cellular processes is not exclusive to postsynaptic functions [Mully et al., 2004].

4. The Spinophilin Interactome

Spinophilin interactome includes cytoskeletal molecules (F-actin, doublecortin, neurabins), enzymes (like PP1), guanine nucleotide exchange factors and regulator of G-protein signalling protein (like Lfc, kalirin-7 and RGS2), membrane receptors (D2 dopamine, α-adrenergics, glutamatergic receptors), ions channels (TRP) and other proteins like TGN38 (Table I registered partner proteins involved in synaptic plasticity).

Shortly after the cloning of spinophilin as a novel PP1c-binding protein, another laboratory cloned this protein based on its ability to bind to F-actin [Satoh et al., 1998]. Recombinant spinophilin and neurabin 1 interacted with each other when co-expressed in cells. On the other hand, recombinant spinophilin was shown to form homodimers, trimers or tetramers by interaction between coiled-coil domains. Spinophilin homomeric complexes are thought to contribute to its actin-cross-linking activity [Satoh et al., 1998]. Doublecortin (DCX) is a microtubule-associated protein that can induce microtubule polymerization and stabilize microtubules filaments. Immunoprecipitation experiments with brain extracts show that spinophilin and DCX interact in cultured cells [Tsukada et al., 2003]. DCX is one of a number of proteins that is required for neuronal migration in the developing cerebral cortex [Dehmelt and Halpain, 2007].

Several studies have shown that spinophilin preferentially binds to PP1γ1 and PP1α isoforms in brain extracts [MacMillan et al., 1999; Terry-Lorenzo et al., 2002; Carmody et al., 2004]. Moreover spinophilin fragments potently inhibit native PP1γ1 in vitro [Colbran et al., 2003]. It was proposed that in vivo the PP1c/spinophilin complex exists in a dynamic equilibrium: 1) at the "resting" state spinophilin targets and inhibits PP1c in the vicinity of its physiological substrates, 2) in the "activating" state PP1c transiently dissociates from spinophilin to dephosphorylate its substrates [Yan et al., 1999].

Guanine nucleotide exchange factors (GEF) and regulator of G-protein signalling (RGS) proteins are regulators of monomeric and heteromeric G protein cycle respectively. Kalirin-7 is a neuronal GEF for Rac1. Spinophilin, through its carboxy-terminus containing the PDZ and coiled-coil domains interacts with kalirin-7. Neurabins target kalirin-7 to the PSD where it could regulate dendritic morphogenesis [Penzes et al., 2001]. Lfc (Lbc[lymphoid blast crisis]'s first cousin) is a Rho GEF that is highly expressed in neurons of the central nervous system. The coiled-coil domain of spinophilin (and neurabin 1) interacts with that of Lfc [Ryan et al., 2005]. Tiam1 is an ubiquitous expressed Rac-GEF and Ras-GRF1 is a dual exchange factor for both Ras and Rac. They both interact through their amino-terminal region with spinophilin [Buchsbaum et al., 2003]. The sequence spanning the PDZ and coiled-coil domains of spinophilin (amino acids 444-817) was shown to be implicated in interaction with Tiam1. RGS proteins play a crucial role in the shutting off process of G-protein-mediated responses and can be divided into five subfamilies [Ishii and Kurachi, 2003]. Spinophilin (and neurabin 1) binds to different members of the RGS familly (RGS1, RGS2, RGS4, RGS16 and GAIP) [Wang et al., 2007]. The binding between spinophilin and RGS2 occurs through the amino acids residues 480 to 525 of the scaffold protein and the amino-terminal domain of the RGS [Wang et al., 2005].

Spinophilin interacts with the D2 dopamin and α-adrenergic receptors (AR), that belong to the family of seven-transmembrane domain receptors, and with the ionotropic NMDA and AMPA-type glutamate receptors. Using the 3i of the D2 dopamine receptor, spinophilin (and not neurabin 1) was identified as a protein that specifically associates with the receptor in rat hippocampal [Smith et al., 1999]. The 3i of the α_{2A}-AR, α_{2B}-AR, and α_{2C}-AR subtypes interacted with spinophilin (and not neurabin 1). Furthermore, interactions occur in intact cells in an agonist-regulated fashion [Richman et al., 2001]. Sequences at the extreme amino-terminal and carboxy-terminal ends of the 3i are critical for interaction with spinophilin. Recently, it was shown that α_{1B}-AR can interact with spinophilin in vitro [Wang et al., 2005]. Moreover, spinophilin (but not neurabin 1) binds to the 3i of cholecystokinin (CCK) A, CCKB and M3 muscarinic receptors [Wang et al., 2007]. Both spinophilin and neurabin 1 PDZ domains directly bind to GluR2-, GluR3- (AMPA receptor) and NR1C2'-, NR2A/B- and NR2C/D- (NMDA receptor) derived peptides [Kelker et al., 2007].

The transient receptor potential canonical (TRPC) ion channels are Ca^{2+} /cation selective channels that are highly expressed in the central nervous system. Spinophilin was identified with other dendritic spines proteins as a protein partner of TRPC5 and TRPC6 channels [Goel et al., 2005]. TGN38 is an integral membrane protein that constitutively cycles between the trans-Golgi network (TGN) and plasma membrane via endosomal intermediates. TGN38 directly interacts with the coiled-coil region of spinophilin (and neurabin 1), preferentially with dimerized neurabins [Stephens and Banting, 1999].

5. Synaptic Plasticity

Excitatory synapses are localized on dendritic spines. In these protusions of the dendrites, F-actin is enriched in the vicinity of the PSD. Rearrangements of the spine's actin cytoskeleton are associated with synaptic transmission and plasticity. The Rho family of small GTPases are key regulators of the F-actin cytoskeleton and are involved in regulating the morphology of dendritic spines. The molecular mechanism that controls spine morphology was in part recently elucidated and involved Lfc a binding partner of neurabins [for a detailed discussion see Sarrouilhe et al., 2006]. The Rho-GEF Lfc is an upstream regulator that activates Rho through the exchange of bound GDP for GTP [Ryan et al., 2005]. Furthermore, phosphorylation by CaMKII, PKA and ERK2 reduced the affinity of spinophilin for F-actin and thus, could regulate spinophilin ability to reorganize actin cytoskeleton in spines [Hsieh-Wilson et al., 2003; Grossman et al., 2004; Futter et al., 2005]. Spinophilin and neurabin 1 represented two major PP1c-binding proteins concentrated in PSD fraction through their actin-binding domain. PP1γ1 and PP1α, but not PP1β, were enriched in dendritic spines and the selectivity of spinophilin for these PP1c isoforms suggests that the scaffold protein may contribute to the preferential targeting to PSD. Distinct populations of dendritic spines can be observed in the primate cortex, containing either PP1α alone or both PP1γ1 and PP1α suggesting different signalling properties. AMPA and NMDA glutamatergic receptors are also highly enriched in dendritic spines.

Table 1. The main partner proteins of spinophilin involved in synaptic plasticity

Partner protein	Spinophilin motif	Functional consequence of the interaction
F-actin	F-actin-binding domain	Actin polymer binding, cross-linking, capping
Spinophilin	coiled-coil domain	Actin cross-linking
Neurabin 1	coiled-coil domain	
PP1α, PP1γ1	R-K-I-H-F motif	Targetting, activity regulation
Lfc	coiled-coil domain	Control of spine morphology
AMPA- and NMDA-type	PDZ domain	Regulation of receptor phosphorylation
glutamate receptor		
TRPC5 and 6		Sculting electrical response to glutamate ?
TGN 38	coiled-coil domain	Post-synaptic membrane proteins trafficking

Glutamate receptor ion channels are abundantly expressed in the central nervous system and mediate the majority of excitatory responses. There are 3 majors types of ionotropic glutamate receptors called AMPA, NMDA and kainate. Four genes code for the AMPA receptors (GluR1-4) and 7 genes code for the NMDA receptors (NR1, NR2A-D, NR3A and NR3B). Alternative splicing from NR1 gene generates 8 different NR1 subunits. The gene products can coassemble within families to generate a large number of heteromeric receptor subtypes in vivo. Functional NMDA receptor is likely to be a tetramer composed most often of two NR1 and two NR2 subunits of the same or different subtypes. In receptors containing NR3 subunit, NR3 forms heterotetrameric complexes with NR1 and NR2 subunits [Mayer, 2005; Paoletti and Neyton, 2007]. AMPA receptor is a tetrameric assembly of dimers of the GluR1-4 subunits. The composition of the receptor is not static and could be altered during synaptic plasticity [Greger et al., 2007].

Long-lasting synaptic plasticity has been associated with brain development, learning and memory. NMDA receptor-dependent long-term potentiation (LTP) and long-term depression (LTD) in the CA1 region of the hippocampus have been the most extensively studied forms of synaptic plasticity [Malenka and Bear, 2004]. It is now well accepted that in hippocampus the triggering of the NMDA receptor-dependent form of LTP requires activation of the receptor, the influx of Ca^{2+} through the channel, a rise in Ca^{2+} within the spine and an activation of the CaMKII. The major mechanism for the expression of LTP involves changes in the AMPA receptor trafficking allowing an increase of the number of receptor at synaptic membrane. Another mechanism is modification of the AMPA channel's activity via its phosphorylation. LTP was found to be associated with phosphorylation of GluR1 on Ser-831 (CaMKII) and on Ser-845 (PKA) [Barria et al., 1997; Derkach et al., 2007]. The longer-lasting components of LTP require new protein synthesis, gene transcription, regulated protein degradation, changes in spine morphology and density involving actin cytoskeletal reorganization. The triggering of the NMDA receptor-dependent form of LTD requires also Ca^{2+} entering the dendritic spine through the NMDA channel, Ca^{2+} release from intracellular stores and PP activity. LTD expression is associated with dephosphorylation of Ser-845 which decreases AMPA receptor channel open probability [Banke et al., 2000]. A loss of AMPA receptor at the synapse plasma membrane is also observed [Beattie et al., 2000]. The maintenance of LTD, like the one of LTP, requires protein synthesis and regulated protein degradation. Long-lasting synaptic plasticity is a widespread phenomenon expressed at possibly every excitatory synapse, with identical but also different mechanisms compared to those of the hippocampus.

In initial experiments spinophilin and PP1 have been implicated in the regulation of AMPA-type glutamate receptor [Yan et al., 1999]. In spinophilin KO mice, whole-cell patch-clamp recording of dissociated cells showed that the ability of PP1 to regulate AMPA (medium spiny neurons prepared from the striatum) and NMDA (dissociated hippocampal neurons) glutamatergic receptor channels, which are highly enriched in dendritic spines is reduced [Feng et al., 2000]. AMPA receptor currents were more persistent and the enhancement of NMDA receptor currents by PP1 inhibitors was attenuated in spinophilin KO mice. These results suggested that spinophilin by targeting PP1c to AMPA and NMDA channels promotes their down regulation by dephosphorylation. The laboratory of W. Peti has recently proposed a model in which a dimer of spinophilin bind via the PDZ domain of one of its molecule to either the GluR2/GluR3 subunits of AMPA receptor or to the NR1C2' of NMDA receptor while the second molecule of spinophilin targets PP1c either to Ser-845 of GluR1 or to Ser-897 of NR1 (two PKA phosphorylation sites). This organization brings PP1c in the vicinity of the carboxy-terminal phosphorylation sites in its substrates and allows catalytic efficiency [Kelker et al., 2007].

Electrophysiological studies in hippocampal slices from spinophilin null mice note reduced LTD but normal LTP, in agreement with previous observations [Mulkey et al., 1993; Blitzer et al., 1998; Feng et al., 2000]. On the other hand, studies using mutant neurabin 1 showed that the wild-type neurabin 1/PP1c complex promotes lasting synaptic depression on LTD stimuli, inhibits LTP and prevents synaptic depression under basal conditions in hippocampal CA1 neurons [Hu et al., 2006]. The complex stimulates multiple signalling pathways involved in AMPA receptors subunits (GluR1 and GluR2) trafficking, depending on the pattern of synaptic activity [Hu et al., 2007]. Studies using neurabin 1 KO mice provide different evidence. In neurabin 1 KO mice, whole-cell patch clamp studies with hippocampal CA1 neurons showed that the deletion of the scaffolding protein abolished LTP whereas LTD was unaltered [Wu et al., 2008]. Moreover, an increased AMPA receptor- (but not NMDA-) mediated synaptic transmission was observed. Deletion of neurabin 1 regulated GluR1 phosphorylation in a site-specific manner. Phosphorylation of the main PKA site (Ser-845) was decreased whereas the one of CaMKII (Ser-831) was unaltered. Neurabin 1 KO mice showed a deficit in contextual fear conditioning, a form of associative memory, but not in auditory fear memory [Wu et al., 2008].

Medium spiny neurons are inhibitory GABAergic cells of the striatum with numerous small spines. These medium size neurons mainly received glutamatergic inputs from the neocortex and the thalamus. Moreover, immunoelectron microscopy studies have shown that dopamine D1 and D2 receptors are localized in dendritic spines of the striatum [Bergson et al., 1995; Yung et al., 1995]. Dopamine is a transmitter that modulates fast excitatory glutamatergic transmission. In acutely dissociated neostriatal medium spiny neurons, constitutively active PP1c, anchored in the vicinity of AMPA receptors by spinophilin, keeps the channel in the dephosphorylated ("low activity") state. At glutamatergic corticostriatal synapses, dopamine can have modulatory effects on synaptic plasticity [Calabresi et al., 2007]. In response to D1 receptor stimulation, PKA phosphorylates a PP1c binding protein DARPP-32 (dopamine- and cyclic AMP-regulated phosphoprotein, MW 32 kDa), and phosphoDARPP-32 potently inhibits PP1c [Greengard et al., 1999]. Activation of the D1 receptor/PKA/DARPP-32 cascade converts AMPA channels to the phosphorylated ("high activity") state [Yan et al., 1999]. Likewise, spinophilin Ser-94 phosphorylation alone by PKA reduces the ability of the scaffolding protein to associates with F-actin in mouse neurons. In striatonigral medium spiny neurons, D1 receptors stimulation activates spinophilin Ser-94 phosphorylation via PKA/DARPP32 dependent inhibition of PP1c. A_{2A} adenosine receptor stimulation has the same effect in striatopallidal medium spiny neurons. It was proposed that in medium spiny neurons, dopamine and adenosine could modulate spinophilin Ser-94 phosphorylation resulting in a dissociation of the spinophilin/PP1c complex from F-actin within the spines. Modulation of the localization of the spinophilin/PP1c complex could contribute to regulate excitatory neurotransmission mediated by AMPA (and NMDA) receptors [Uematsu et al., 2005]. Phosphorylation by CaMKII also reduced the affinity of spinophilin for F-actin and brought an additional level of regulation of AMPA channel [Grossman et al., 2004]. Both spinophilin and neurabin 1 are required for dopamine-mediated plasticity in striatum but with distinct roles [Allen et al., 2006]. D1-mediated regulation of AMPA receptor was deficient in striatal neurons from both spinophilin and neurabin 1 KO mices. LTP was deficient in neurabin 1 KO mice but not in spinophilin KO mice. LTP was rescued at the corticospinal synapses following D1 receptor activation. In contrast to these observations, LTD was deficient in spinophilin KO mice but not in neurabin 1 KO mice, and this form of synaptic plasticity was rescued following D2 receptor activation. D1 receptor stimulation results in PKA-mediated phosphorylation of GluR1 subunit at Ser-845 [Snyder et al., 2000] and NR1 subunit at Ser-897 [Snyder et al., 1998]. In both KO mices an increase in GluR1 Ser-845 phosphorylation was observed following D1 receptor stimulation while in contrast NR1 Ser-897 phosphorylation was unchanged. The authors suggested an indirect effect in which spinophilin and neurabin 1 are involved in dopamine-mediated control over AMPA receptor trafficking to the synaptic membrane [Allen et al., 2006].

It is interesting to note that α-adrenergic signalling regulated NMDA receptor function in the central nervous system [Liu et al., 2006]. Most α_1- and α_2-AR subtypes are highly expressed in various regions of the central nervous system. α_1-AR activation reduced NMDA receptor-mediated currents in prefrontal cortex pyramidal neurons. The α_1-AR effect depended on the phospholipase C-IP_3-Ca^{2+} pathway and is down-regulated by RGS2 and RGS4. The regulating effects of RGS2 and RGS4 were lost in spinophilin KO mice suggesting that the effect of α_1-AR signalling on NMDA receptor-current is attenuated by

RGS2/RGS4 that are recruited to the seven-transmembrane domain receptor complex by spinophilin [Liu et al., 2006].

Plasticity in dendritic spines may underlie learning and memory. Conditioned taste aversion learning (CTA) is a form of associative learning. CTA acquisition and retention has been previously associated to several regions of the central nervous system but not with hippocampus. Spinophilin KO mice had intact sensory processing whereas CTA is significantly impaired compared to wild-type littermates. These observations have shown that spinophilin plays a role in associative learning ability in vivo [Stafstrom-Davis et al., 2001].

Among the members of the spinophilin interactome two others proteins were suggested to be involved in synaptic plasticity. TRPC5 and TRPC6 Ca^{2+}/cation selective channels may play a critical role in sculpting the electrical response to neurotransmitter in dendritic spines [Goel et al., 2005]. TGN38 is a putative cargo receptor that may transport proteins between dendritic spine compartments and post-synaptic membrane. Direct interaction of spinophilin with TGN38 may be essential for the trafficking of spine's proteins and so for plasticity of glutamatergic synaptic transmission [Stephens and Banting, 1999; McNamara et al., 2004].

Conclusion

Spinophilin is a multifunctional protein that regulates excitatory synaptic transmission and plasticity at PSD by targeting PP1c to AMPA and NMDA channels, promoting their down regulation by dephosphorylation and also by modulating the structural organisation of dendritic spines. In spinophilin, domains fulfill joint functions. PP1-binding and PDZ domains target and anchor PP1c close to its synaptic substrates (AMPA and NMDA receptors), the F-actin-binding domain concentrates spinophilin in PSD and coiled-coil domain is involved in spinophilin multimerization.

Studies using KO mices provide evidence that spinophilin and neurabin 1 play different roles in hippocampal synaptic plasticity. Spinophilin is involved in hippocampal LTD and not in LTP whereas neurabin 1 contributes selectively to LTP but not LTD [Feng et al., 2000; Wu et al., 2008]. Experiments made with KO mices established the same distinct roles for spinophilin and neurabin 1 in dopamine-mediated plasticity in striatal neurons [Allen et al., 2006].

One open question is what is the structural difference upon which the functional difference observed in synaptic plasticity is based. An emerging notion is that spinophilin and neurabin 1 may differentially affect their target proteins and perform quite distinctive function in cell. For example, the two scaffolding proteins forms a functional pair of opposing regulators that reciprocally regulate signalling intensity by seven-transmembrane domain receptors [Wang et al., 2007].

Spinophilin has been implicated in the pathophysiology of several illness associated with striatum or hippocampal formation. A number of illness are associated with abnormalities of dopaminergic neurotransmission including Parkinson's disease. In a rat model, striatal spinophilin levels decreased during normal ageing, phenomena that can contribute to Parkinson's disease progression [Brown et al., 2005]. Spinophilin expression was significantly altered in the hippocampal formation in patients with schizophrenia and mood disorders [Law et al., 2004]. This result suggested the involvement of a postsynaptic component of glutamatergic synaptic pathology in the hippocampal formation in these illness. More studies are necessary to confirm this result that is a subject of debate [Dwork et al., 2005].

Synaptic plasticity is thought to be important for learning and memory. Spinophilin may play a role in CTA, a form of associative learning [Stafstrom-Davis et al., 2001] while neurabin 1 seems to be involved in contextual fear conditioning [Wu et al., 2008]. It could be interesting to thoroughly investigate the function of spinophilinin in hippocampal-independent learning and memory mechanisms.

Learning and memory are higher-order brain functions involving several signalling pathways and multiple partner proteins. Conditional transgenic and gene targeting methodologies allowing spatial and temporal control over gene manipulations [Baumgartel et al., 2007] may offer valuable tools for appropriate study of spinophilin and neurabin 1 functions in a specific brain area and in distinct temporal phases of synaptic plasticity.

References

Allen, P. B., Ouimet, C.C., and Greengard, P. (1997). Spinophilin, a novel protein phosphatase 1 binding protein localized to dendritic spines. *Proc. Natl. Acad. Sci*, USA. 94, 9956-9961.

Allen, P. B., Zachariou, V., Svenningsson, P., Lepore, A. C., Centonze, D., Costa, C., Rossi, S., Bender, G., Chen, G., Feng, J., Snyder, G. L., Bernardi, G., Nestler, E. J., Yan, Z., Calabresi, P., and Greengard, P. (2006). Distinct roles for spinophilin and neurabin in dopamine-mediated plasticity. *Neuroscience*, 140, 897-911.

Banke, T. G., Bowie, D., Lee, H. K., Huganir, R. L., Schousboe, A., and Traynelis, S. F. (2000). Control of GluR1 AMPA receptor function by cAMP-dependent protein kinase. *J. Neurosci*, 20, 89-102.

Barria, A., Muller, D., Derkach, V., Griffith, L. C., and Soderling, T. R. (1997). Regulatory phosphorylation of AMPA-type glutamate receptors by CaM-KII during long-term potentiation. *Science*, 276, 2042-2045.

Baumgartel, K., Fernandez, C., Johansson, T., and Mansuy, I. M. (2007). Conditional transgenesis and recombination to study the molecular mechanisms of brain plasticity and memory. *Handb. Exp. Pharmacol.* 178, 315-345.

Beattie, E. C., Carroll, R. C., Yu, X., Morishita, W., Yasuda, H., von Zastrow, M., and Malenka, R. C. (2000). Regulation of AMPA receptor endocytosis by a signaling mechanism shared with LTD. *Nature Neurosci*, 3, 1291-1300.

Bergson, C., Mrzljak, L., Smiley, J. F., Pappy, M., Levenson, R., and Goldman-Rakic, P. S. (1995). Regional, cellular, and subcellular variations in the distribution of D1 and D5 dopamine receptors in primate brain. *J. Neurosci*, 15, 7821-7836.

Blitzer, R. D., Connor, J. H., Brown, G. P., Wong, T., Shenolikar, S., Iyengar, R., and Landau, E. M. (1998). Gating of CaMKII by cAMP-regulated protein phosphatase activity during LTP. *Science*, 280, 1940-1943.

Bollen, M. (2001). Combinatorial control of protein phosphatase-1. *Trends Biochem. Sci.*, 26, 426-431.

Brown, A. M., Deutch, A. Y., and Colbran, A. J. (2005). Dopamine depletion alters phosphorylation of striatal proteins in a model of Parkinsonism. Eur. *J. Neurosci*, 22, 247-256.

Buchsbaum, R. J., Connolly, B. A., and Feig, L. A. (2003). Regulation of p70^{S6} kinase by complex formation between the Rac guanine nucleotide exchange factor (Rac-GEF) Tiam1 and the scaffold spinophilin. *J. Biol. Chem*, 278, 18833-18841.

Calabresi, P., Picconi, B., Tozzi, A., and Di Fillipo, M. (2007). Dopamine-mediated regulation of corticostriatal synaptic plasticity. *Trends Neurosci*, 30, 211-219.

Carmody, L. C., Bauman, P. A., Bass, M. A., Mavila, N., DePaoli-Roach, A. A., and Colbran R. J. (2004). A protein phosphatase-1γ1 isoform selectivity determinant in dendritic spine-associated neurabin. *J. Biol. Chem*, 279, 21714-21723.

Ceulemans, H., and Bollen, M. (2004). Functional diversity of protein phosphatase-1, a cellular economizer and reset button. *Physiol. Rev*, 84, 1-39.

Cohen, P. T. (2002). Protein phosphatase 1-targeted in many directions. *J. Cell Sci*, 115, 241-256.

Colbran, R. J., and Shenolikar, S. (2002). Targeting protein phosphatase 1 (PP1) to the actin cytoskeleton, the neurabin 1/PP1 complex regulates cell morphology. *Mol. Cell. Biol*, 22, 4690-4701.

Colbran, R. J., Carmody, L. C., Bauman, P. A., Wadzinski, B. E., and Bass, M. A. (2003). Analysis of specific interactions of native protein phosphatase 1 isoforms with targeting subunits. *Methods Enzymol*, 366, 156-175.

Dehmelt, L., and Halpain, S. (2007). Neurite outgrowth: a flick of the wrist. *Current Biol*, 17, R611-R614.

Derkach, V. A., Oh, M. C., Guire, E. S., and Soderling, T. R. (2007). Regulatory mechanisms of AMPA receptors in synaptic plasticity. *Nature Rev. Neurosci*, 8, 101-113.

Dwork, A. J., Rosoklija, G., and Jones, L. B. (2005). Reduced spinophilin in schizophrenia. Am. *J. Psychiatry*, 162, 1389.

Feng, J., Yan, Z., Ferreira, A., Tomizawa, K., Liauw, J. A., Zhuo, M., Allen, P. B., Ouimet, C. C., and Greengard, P. (2000). Spinophilin regulates the formation and function of dendritic spines. *Proc. Natl. Acad. Sci*, USA. 97, 9287-9292.

Futter, M., Uematsu, K., Bullock, S. A., Kim, Y., Hemmings, Jr. H. C., Nishi, A., Greengard, P., and Nairn, A. C. (2005). Phosphorylation of spinophilin by ERK and cyclin-dependent PK5 (Cdk5). *Proc. Natl. Acad. Sci*, USA. 102, 3489-3494.

Goel, M., Sinkins, W., Keightley, A., Kinter, M., and Schilling, W. P. (2005). Proteomic analysis of TRPC5- and TRPC6-binding partners reveals interaction with the plasmalemmal Na^+/K^+-ATPase. *Pflügers Archiv*, 451, 87-98.

Greengard, P., Allen, P. B., and Nairn, A. C. (1999). Beyond the dopamine receptor: the DARPP-32/protein phosphatase-1 cascade. *Neuron*, 23, 435-447.

Greger, I. H., Ziff, E. B., and Penn, A. C. (2007). Molecular determinants of AMPA receptor subunit assembly. *Trends Neurosc*, 30, 407-416.

Grossman, S. D., Futter, M., Snyder, G. L., Allen, P. B., Nairn, A. C., Greengard, P., and Hsieh-Wilson, L. C. (2004). Spinophilin is phosphorylated by Ca^{2+}/calmodulin-dependent protein kinase II resulting in regulation of its binding to F-actin. *J. Neurochem*, 90, 317-324.

Hsieh-Wilson, L. C., Benfenati, F., Snyder, G. L., Allen, P. B., Nairn, A. C., and Greengard, P. (2003). Phosphorylation of spinophilin modulates its interaction with actin filaments. *J. Biol. Chem*, 278, 1186-1194.

Hu, X. D., Huang, Q., Roadcap, D. W., Shenolikar, S. S., and Xia, H. (2006). Actin-associated neurabin-protein phosphatase-1 complex regulates hippocampal plasticity. *J. Neurochem*, 98, 1841-1851.

Hu, X. D., Huang, Q., Yang, X., and Xia, H. (2007). Differential regulation of AMPA receptor trafficking by neurabin-targeted synaptic protein phosphatase-1 in synaptic transmission and long-term depression in hippocampus. *J. Neurosci*, 27, 4674-4686.

Ishii, M., and Kurachi, Y. (2003). Physiologial actions of regulators of G-protein signalling (RGS) proteins. *Life Sci*, 74, 163-171.

Ju, T., Ragusa, M. J., Hudak, J., Nairn, A. C., and Peti, W. (2007). Structural characterization of the neurabin sterile alpha motif domain. *Proteins*, 69, 192-198.

Kelker, M. S., Dancheck, B. B., Ju, T., Kessler, R. P., Hudack, J., Nairn, A. C., and Peti, W. (2007). Structural basis for spinophilin-neurabin receptor interaction. *Biochemistry*, 46, 2333-2344.

Law, A. J., Weickert, C. S., Hyde, T. M., Kleinman, J. E., and Harrison, P. J. (2004). Reduced spinophilin but not microtubule-associated protein 2 expression in the hippocampal formation in schizophrenia and mood disorders: molecular evidence for a pathology of dendritic spines. *Am. J. Psychiatry*, 161, 1848-1855.

Liu, W., Yuen, E. Y., Allen, P. B., Feng, J., Greengard, P., and Yan, Z. (2006). Adrenergic modulation of NMDA receptors in prefrontal cortex is differentially regulated by RGS proteins and spinophilin. *Proc. Natl. Acad. Sci*, USA. 103, 18338-18343.

McAvoy, T., Allen, P. B., Obaishi, H., Nakanishi, H., Takai, Y., Greengard, P., Nairn, A. C., and Hemmings, Jr. H. C. (1999). Regulation of neurabin 1 interaction with protein phosphatase 1 by phosphorylation. *Biochemistry*, 38, 12943-12949.

MacMillan, L. B., Bass, M. A., Cheng, N., Howard, E. F., Tamura, M., Strack, S., Wadzinski, B. E., and Colbran, R. J. (1999). Brain actin-associated protein phosphatase 1 holoenzymes containing spinophilin, neurabin, and selected catalytic subunit isoforms. *J. Biol. Chem*, 274, 35845-35854.

McNamara, II J. O., Grigston, J. C., VanDongen, H. M. A., and VanDongen, A. M. J. (2004). Rapid dendritic transport of TGN38, a putative cargo receptor. *Mol. Brain Res*, 127, 68-78.

Malenka, R. C., and Bear, M. F. (2004). LTP and LTD, an embarrassment of riches. *Neuron*, 44, 5-21.

Mayer, M. L. (2005). Glutamate receptor ion channels. Curr. Opin. *Neurobiol*, 15, 282-288.

Mulkey, R. M., Herron, C. E., and Malenka, R. C. (1993). An essential role for protein phosphatases in hippocampal long-term depression. *Science*, 261, 1051-1055.

Muly, E. C., Smith, Y., Allen, P., and Greengard, P. (2004). Subcellular distribution of spinophilin immunolabeling in primate prefrontal cortex: localization to and within dendritic spines. *J. Comp. Neurol*, 469, 185-197.

Nakanishi, H., Obaishi, H., Satoh, A., Wada, M., Mandai, K., Satoh, K., Nishioka, H., Matsuura, Y., Mizoguchi, A., and Takai, Y. (1997). Neurabin: a novel neural tissue-specific actin filament-binding protein involved in neurite formation. *J. Cell Biol*, 139, 951-961.

Oliver, C. J., Terry-Lorenzo, R. T., Elliot, E., Bloomer, W. A. C., Li, S., Brautigan, D. L., Colbran, R. J., and Shenolikar, S. (2002). Targeting protein phosphatase 1 (PP1) to the actin cytoskeleton : the neurabin I/PP1 complex regulates cell morphology. *Mol. Cell. Biol*, 22, 4690-4701.

Ouimet, C. C., Katona, I., Allen, P., Freund, T. F., and Greengard, P. (2004). Cellular and subcellular distribution of spinophilin, a PP1 regulatory protein that bundles F-actin in dendritic spines. *J. Comp. Neurol*, 479, 374-388.

Paoletti, P., and Neyton, J. (2007). NMDA receptor subunits: function and pharmacology. *Curr. Opin. Pharmacol*, 7, 39-47.

Penzes, P., Johnson, R. C., Sattler, R., Zhang, X., Huganir, R. L., Kambampati, V., Mains, R. E., and Eipper, B. A. (2001). The neuronal Rho-GEF kalirin-7 interacts with PDZ domain-containing proteins and regulates dendritic morphogenesis. *Neuron*, 29, 229-242.

Richman, J. G., Brady, A. E., Wang, Q., Hensel, J. L., Colbran, R. J., and Limbird, L. E. (2001). Agonist-regulated Interaction between alpha2-adrenergic receptors and spinophilin. *J. Biol. Chem*, 276, 15003-15008.

Ryan, X. P., Alldritt, J., Svenningsson, P., Allen, P. B., Wu, G.Y., Nairn, A. C., and Greengard, P. (2005). The Rho-specific GEF Lfc interacts with neurabin and spinophilin to regulate dendritic spine morphology. *Neuron*, 47, 85-100.

Sarrouilhe, D., Di Tommaso, A., Métayé, T., and Ladeveze, V. (2006). Spinophilin: from partners to functions. *Biochimie*, 88, 1099-1113.

Sasaki, K., Shima, H., Kitagawa, Y., Irino, S., Sugimura, T., and Nagao, M. (1990). Identification of members of the protein phosphatase 1 gene family in the rat and enhanced expression of protein phosphatase 1α gene in rat hepatocellular carcinomas. Jpn. *J. Cancer Res*, 81, 1272-1280.

Satoh, A., Nakanishi, H., Obaishi, H., Wada, M., Takahashi, K., Satoh, K., Hirao, K., Nishioka, H., Hata, Y., Mizoguchi, A., and Takai, Y. (1998). Neurabin-II/spinophilin. An actin filament-binding protein with one pdz domain localized at cadherin-based cell-cell adhesion sites. *J. Biol. Chem*, 273, 3470-3475.

Schüler, H., and Peti, W. (2007). Structure-function analysis of the F-actin binding domain of the neuronal scaffolding protein spinophilin: induced folding-upon-binding and novel capping function. *FEBS J*, 275, 59-68.

Smith, F. D., Oxford, G. S., and Milgram, S. L. (1999). Association of the D2 dopamine receptor third cytoplasmic loop with spinophilin, a protein phosphatase-1-interacting protein. *J. Biol. Chem*, 274, 19894-19900.

Snyder, G. L., Fienberg, A. A., Huganir, R. L., and Greengard, P. (1998). A dopamine/D1 receptor/protein kinase A/dopamine- and cAMP-regulated phosphoprotein (Mr 32 kDa)/protein phosphatase-1 pathway regulates dephosphorylation of the NMDA receptor. *J. Neurosci*, 18, 10297-10303.

Snyder, G. L., Allen, P. B., Fienberg, A. A., Valle, C. G., Huganir, R. L., Nairn, A. C., and Greengard, P. (2000). Regulation of phosphorylation of the GluR1 AMPA receptor in the neostriatum by dopamine and psychostimulants in vivo. *J. Neurosci*, 20, 4480-4488.

Stafstrom-Davis, C. A., Ouimet, C. C., Feng, J., Allen, P. B., Greengard, P., and Houpt, T. A. (2001). Impaired conditioned taste aversion learning in spinophilin knockout mice. *Learn. Mem*, 8, 272-278.

Stephens, D. J., and Banting, G. (1999). Direct interaction of the trans-Golgi network membrane protein, TGN38, with the F-actin binding protein, neurabin. *J. Biol. Chem*, 274, 30080-30086.

Terry-Lorenzo, R. T., Carmody, L. C., Voltz, J. W., Connor, J. H., Li, S., Smith, F. D., Milgram, S. L., Colbran, R. J., and Shenolikar, S. (2002). The neuronal actin-binding proteins, neurabin I and neurabin II, recruit specific isoforms of protein phosphatase-1 catalytic subunits. *J. Biol. Chem*, 277, 27716-27724.

Tsukada, M., Prokscha, A., Oldekamp, J., and Eichele, G. (2003). Identification of neurabin II as a novel doublecortin interacting protein. *Mech. Dev*, 120, 1033-1043.

Uematsu, K., Futter, M., Hsieh-Wilson, L. C., Higashi, H., Maeda, H., Nairn, A. C., Greengard, P., and Nishi, A. (2005). Regulation of spinophilin Ser94 phosphorylation in neostriatal neurons involves both DARPP-32-dependent and independent pathways. *J. Neurochem*, 95, 1642-1652.

Vivo, M., Calogero, R. A., Sansone, F., Calabro, V., Parisi, T., Borrelli, L., Saviozzi, S., and La Mantia, G. (2001). The human tumor suppressor arf interacts with spinophilin/neurabin II, a type 1 protein-phosphatase-binding protein. *J. Biol. Chem*, 276, 14161-14169.

Wang, X., Zeng, W., Soyombo, A. A., Tang, W., Ross, E. M., Barnes, A. P., Milgram, S. L., Penninger, J. M., Allen, P. B., Greengard, P., and Muallem, S. (2005). Spinophilin regulated Ca^{2+} signalling by binding the N-terminal domain of RGS2 and the third intracellular loop of G-protein-coupled receptors. *Nat. Cell Biol*, 7, 405-411.

Wang, X., Zeng, W., Kim, M. S., Allen, P. B., Greengard, P., and Muallem, S. (2007). Spinophilin/neurabin reciprocally regulate signalling intensity by G protein-coupled receptors. *EMBO J*, 26, 2768-2776.

Wu, L. J., Ren, M., Wang, H., Kim, S. S., Cao, X., and Zhuo, M. (2008). Neurabin contributes to hippocampal long-term potentiation and fear memory. *Plos ONE*, 3, e1407.

Yan, Z., Hsieh-Wilson, L., Feng, J., Tomizawa, K., Allen, P. B., Fienberg, A. A., Nairn, A. C., and Greengard, P. (1999). Protein phosphatase 1 modulation of neostriatal AMPA channels: regulation by DARPP-32 and spinophilin. Nat. *Neurosci*, 2, 13-17.

Yung, K. K. L., Bolam, J. P., Smith, A. D., Hersch, S. M., Ciliax, B. J., and Levey, A. I. (1995). Immunocytochemical localization of D1 and D2 dopamine receptors in the basal ganglia of the rat: light and electron microscopy. *Neuroscience*, 65, 709-730.

In: Synaptic Plasticity: New Research
Editors: Tim F. Kaiser and Felix J. Peters
ISBN: 978-1-60456-732-8

Chapter 12

DOPAMINE-DEPENDENT SYNAPTIC PLASTICITY IN THE CORTICO-BASAL GANGLIA-THALAMOCORTICAL LOOPS AS MECHANISM OF VISUAL ATTENTION

Isabella Silkis *
Institute of Higher Nervous Activity and Neurophysiology, Moscow, Russia

ABSTRACT

A hypothesis is advanced that dopamine-dependent synaptic plasticity (LTP, LTD) and subsequent activity reorganization in the cortico-basal ganglia-thalamocortical loops underlies attentional selection and processing of a visual stimulus. Both effects are the result of opposite modulatory action of dopamine on strong and weak cortico-striatal inputs that synergistically leads to disinhibition and inhibition via the basal ganglia of thalamic cells projected to those neocortical neurons, in which initial visual activation was strong and weak, respectively. Thus, the output basal ganglia projections to the thalamus could play a role of "attentional filter" that amplifies cortical responses to attended stimulus, and suppresses reactions to ignored stimuli. A proposed model based on cortico-striatal synaptic plasticity allows explanation of some experimentally revealed effects of which mechanisms were unclear from points of view of commonly accepted models that are based on feedback connections from higher to lower cortical areas and to the thalamus. We assume that proposed necessity of sensory activation of dopaminergic cells for switching the attentional part of processing and known latency of sensory activation of dopaminergic cells (which is about 100 ms) explain the experimentally-

* I.G. Silkis PhD, Doctor of Biological Sciences, Lab. Neurophysiology of Learning, Institute of Higher Nervous Activity and Neurophysiology, Russian Academy of Sciences, 117485, 5a Butlerova str., Moscow, Russia Tel. +7 (495) 7893852 Fax. +7 (495) 3388500
Email: isa-silkis@mail.ru

obtained absence of attentional modulation of neocortical responses with latencies that do not exceed 100 ms. This model can also help understanding of the mechanisms underlaying attentional disorders.

Keywords: attention, visual processing, basal ganglia, synaptic plasticity, dopamine

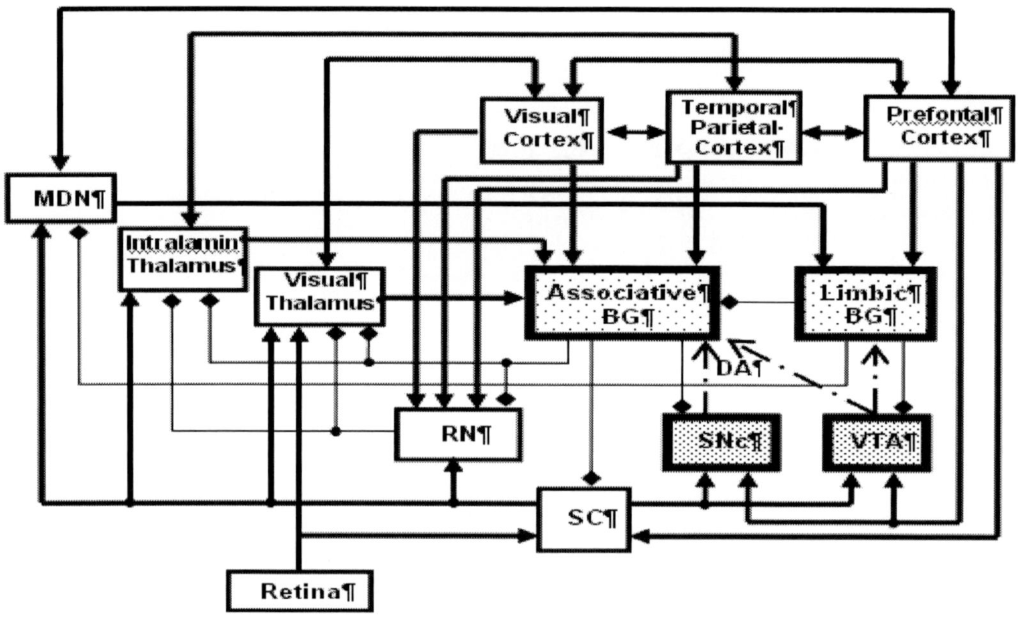

Figure 1. Simplified scheme of associative and limbic cortico – basal ganglia –thalamocortical loops involved in processing of visual information. BG, basal ganglia nuclei; MDN and RN, mediodorsal and reticular thalamic nuclei; Intralam, intralaminar; SC, superior colliculus; SNc, substantia nigra pars compacta; VTA, ventral tegmental area; DA-dopamine. Arrows – excitatory inputs; thin lines with rhomb – weak inhibitory inputs; chain lines with arrow - dopaminergic inputs

INTRODUCTION

Visual attention is necessary for selection of high priority information and filtering out irrelevant information since many different visual objects cannot all be processed simultaneously. The role of visual attention consists of not so much in the exact and full description of the world, as in intensifying a hierarchical ascending of signals in visual cortical fields (Treue, 2003). Attention that influences both ascending and descending streams of visual processing is controlled by a distributed network wherein the higher order areas in the prefrontal cortex (PfC) generate top-down signals that are transmitted via feedback connections to the visual areas and then to the first stage in visual processing, lateral geniculate nucleus (LGN) (Kastner and Pinsk, 2004). According to commonly accepted mechanism, focus of attention generates a column of the enlarged cortical inputs to the LGN, and simultaneously suppresses surrounding activity by GABA inhibition (Montero, 2000; Zikopoulos and Barbas, 2006). This inhibition is performed by the reticular thalamic nucleus that plays a role of inhibitory interface or "attentional gate", regulating a stream of information from the thalamus to neocortex (Montero, 2000).

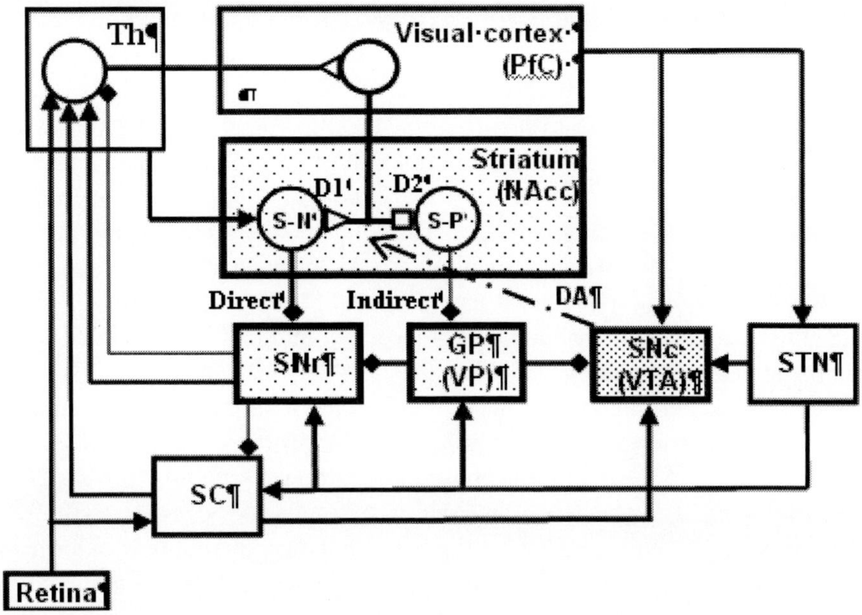

Figure 2. Dopamine-dependent selection of neocortical pattern by the cortico - basal ganglia - thalamocortical loop. Selection is the result of amplification of activity of cortical cells that "strongly" activate striatum and suppression of activity of cortical cells that "weakly" activate striatum during visually-evoked dopamine release (suppression is not shown). PFC, prefrontal cortex; Th, thalamus; NAcc, nucleus accumbens; SNr, substantia nigra pars reticulata; GP, external part of the globus pallidus; VP, ventral pallidum; SN and SP, GABAergic striatonigral and striatopallidal cells that express D1 and D2 receptors, and give rise to the "direct" disinhibitory and "indirect" inhibitory pathways through BG, respectively; cells in the SNr and GP/VP are GABAergic, large grey circles dopaminergic cells; small triangles and square, potentiated (LTP), and depressed (LTD) synapses, respectively; thick and thin lines, strong and weak inputs, respectively. Other abbreviations as in Figure 1.

However, accepted models mostly do not take into account that thalamic nuclei (including the reticular nucleus) are also under inhibitory influence from the output basal ganglia (BG) nucleus, the substantia nigra pars reticulata (SNr) (Parent and Hazrati, 1995) (Fig. 1, 2). In turn, neurons in the SNr are inhibited by spiny cells of the input BG nucleus striatum (caudatum/putamen) that receives excitation from the neocortex and thalamus (Fig. 2). The involvement of striatum in attentional precesses is evident from the data that that spiny cells discharge in relation to cues reorienting spatial attention (Kermadi and Boussaoud, 1995). Participation of the cortico-striatal inputs in attention is specified by the data that disconnection between the medial PfC and the ventral striatum named nucleus accumbens (NAcc), or bilateral lesion of the NAcc produces a significant reduction in the accuracy of performance of attentional task (Christakou et al., 2001; Christakou et al., 2004). Remarkably, that during voluntary attention neuronal activity is strengthened before the real stimulus appearance not only in the prefrontal and visual cortical areas but also in the striatum

(Kermadi and Boussaoud, 1995; Kimura et al., 2004; Mechelli et al., 2004; Saenz et al., 2003). Except for that, attention activates other BG nuclei, including the globus pallidus, as well as the medial thalamic nuclei and superior colliculus (SC) connected with the BG (Corbetta et al., 1991; Kermadi and Boussaoud, 1995; Kimura et al., 2004; Nakamura et al., 2000). On the contrary, activity in the frontal cortical areas, striatum and globus pallidus are suppressed during attentional deficiency (Booth et al, 2005). The role of dopamine in attention is specified by the data that patients with attention deficit hyperactivity disorder have abnormal dopaminergic function in multiple brain regions especially in the input BG nuclei, accumbens and putamen (Forssberg et al., 2006). Low dopamine concentration in the BG plays an important role in attentional deficits in patients with Parkinson's disease (Filoteo et al., 1997), but deficit of attention in nigrostriatal lesioned rats could be improved by dopamine receptor agonists (Nieoullon and Coquerel, 2003; Turle-Lorenzo et al., 2006). Known data led to a hypothesis that dopamine-dependent modulation of cortico-striatal inputs could participate in attentional effects (Miller, 1993).

Earlier we pointed out that dopamine-dependent modulation of cortico-striatal synaptic inputs in the motor cortico – basal ganglia – thalamocortical (C-BG-Th-C) loop might underlie a selection of a movement in response to conditioned stimulus (Sil'kis, 2006). Based on the similarity of the functional organizations of motor and visual C-BG-Th-C loops (Middleton and Strick, 1996), and taking into account that attention is a form of activity directed to selection of a stimulus for processing (Naatanen, 1998), we assumed that visual cue evoked dopamine release and subsequent activity reorganizations in visual C-BG-Th-C loops may underlie visual attention. A goal of the present work was to determine the role of C-BG-Th-C loops and dopamine in attentional modulation of visual processing.

A Hypothetical Role of Dopamine-Dependent Modulation of Cortico-Striatal Synaptic Transmission in Attentional Modulation of Visual Processing

According to our hypothesis, visually evoked dopamine release and subsequent dopamine-dependent reorganizations of neuronal activity in the C-BG-Th-C loops that lead to amplification of firing in neocortical neuronal patterns representing diverse properties of stimulus underlies the attentional enhancement of visual perception. Earlier we pointed out that each visual C-BG-Th-C loops could include a thalamic nucleus connected with corresponding visual cortical area that projects to one of striatal loci (Silkis, 2007). This striatal locus projects to corresponding loci in different BG nuclei, including the globus pallidus and SNr, which projects to the same thalamic nucleus (Fig. 1, 2). Limbic C-BG-Th-C loop includes the mediodorsal thalamic nucleus (MDN) or the pulvinar of thalamus connected with one of frontal cortical areas, which projects to the NAcc. This ventral part of the striatum is connected with the ventral pallidum and dorsomedial part of the SNr that send projections to the MDN or pulvinar.

Advances in neuroscience implicate reentrant signaling as the predominant form of communication between brain areas and mechanism subserving conscious sensory perception. According to the conventional view, this reentrance is the result of activity circulation in the cortico-cortical and cortico-thalamocortical loops (Crick and Koch, 1995; Edelman, 2003).

We assume that reentrance of information into the cortex could be also realized by diverse C-BG-Th-C loops. In these loops, BG–thalamic influence is not only disinhibitory but also excitatory since a large part of the SNr neurons projected to the thalamus is glutamatergic (Kha et al., 2001). SNr neurons can receive excitation from the neocortex via the subthalamic nucleus (Fig. 2). Some of the output SNr cells have visual receptive fields that are similar to those of superior colliculus cells (Nagy et al., 2005). Thus, reentrant excitation of the neocortex through the visual part of the BG and thalamus can participate in conscious visual perception.

Under our assumption, realization of involuntary visual attention requires a fulfilment of two conditions: release of dopamine in response to visual stimulus, and modulatory action of dopamine on cortico-striatal synaptic efficacy. The fulfilment of the first condition is supported by the data that dopaminergic neurons in the substantia nigra pars compacta (SNc) and ventral tegmental area (VTA) are activated not only by conditioned stimulus (Schultz, W., 1997) but also by non-conditioned visual stimuli (Domett et al., 2005; Horvitz et al., 1997). The primary source of visual excitation of dopaminergic cells is the SC (Dommett et al., 2005). However, dopaminergic cells become visually responsive only after disinhibition of the SC, whereas disinhibition of the visual cortex was ineffective (Dommett et al., 2005). We proposed that visual activation (via the thalamus) of GABAergic striatonigral cells projected onto GABAergic SNr neurons could lead to SC disinhibition thus promoting excitation of dopaminergic cells (Fig. 2) (Silkis; 2007). In addition, visual stimulus passing through the SC and MDN to the PfC can lead to both direct excitation of dopaminergic cells and descending prefrontal influence on dopaminergic cells through the NAcc. On the one hand, PfC excites striatonigral cells of the NAcc, projected to the VTA (Fig. 2) (Berendse et al., 1992). On the other hand, PfC acts on striatopallidal cells of the NAcc, projected to the ventral pallidum, which GABAergic neurons also innervate the VTA (Fig. 2). Thus, the PfC activating one group of dopaminergic cells and inhibiting others generates a pattern of firing dopaminergic cells in response to a visual stimulus.

The fulfilment of the second necessary condition is supported by the data that visual stimuli cause a greater than five-fold rise in the probability of burst firing of dopaminergic cells (Horvitz et al., 1997). By this reason, visually evoked enlargement in dopamine concentration might be sufficient for modulation of cortico-striatal synaptic transmission.

Earlier we pointed out that dopamine oppositely modulates the efficacy of cortical inputs that "strongly" and "weakly" excite striatal spiny cells (inputs that allow and do not allow, respectively, open postsynaptic NMDA channels) (Sil'kis, 2003). The character of dopamine-dependent modulation of synaptic inputs to striatonigral and striatopallidal cells that mainly express D1 and D2 receptors, respectively, is also opposite (Silkis, 2000; 2001). Due to such character of modulation of striatal cell firing, signals passing through the BG could disinhibit (via the SNr and thalamus) cortical neurons that initially were strongly excited by visual stimulus (Fig. 2), and simultaneously inhibit activity of cortical neurons, that initially were weakly excited by this stimulus. Thus in each visual cortical area, a contrasty amplified neural pattern could be selected that represents a certain attribute of attended visual stimulus. In the absence of dopamine, signals passing through the BG could inhibit activity of those cortical neurons, which initially visual response was strong, and simultaneously disinhibit those cortical neurons which response was weak. Such reorganization must disturb the initial neural pattern representing non-attended visual stimulus (or its feature).

Usually, attention is divided onto the involuntary one caused by ascending (bottom-up) excitation of visual cortical areas, and voluntary one (top-down), which source is descending excitation of visual areas by voluntary activated PfC (Naatanen, 1992). Remarkably, that dopamine modulates both types of attention (Kahkonen et al., 2001). In our model, diverse pathways for dopaminergic cell excitation contribute to mentioned types of attention. Involuntary attention is triggered by dopamine release in response to visual stimulus, whereas voluntary attention is initiated by dopamine release in response to voluntary activation of the PfC before appearance of a real stimulus (Fig. 3). In parallel, the PfC excites neurons in different visual cortical areas via feedback projections.

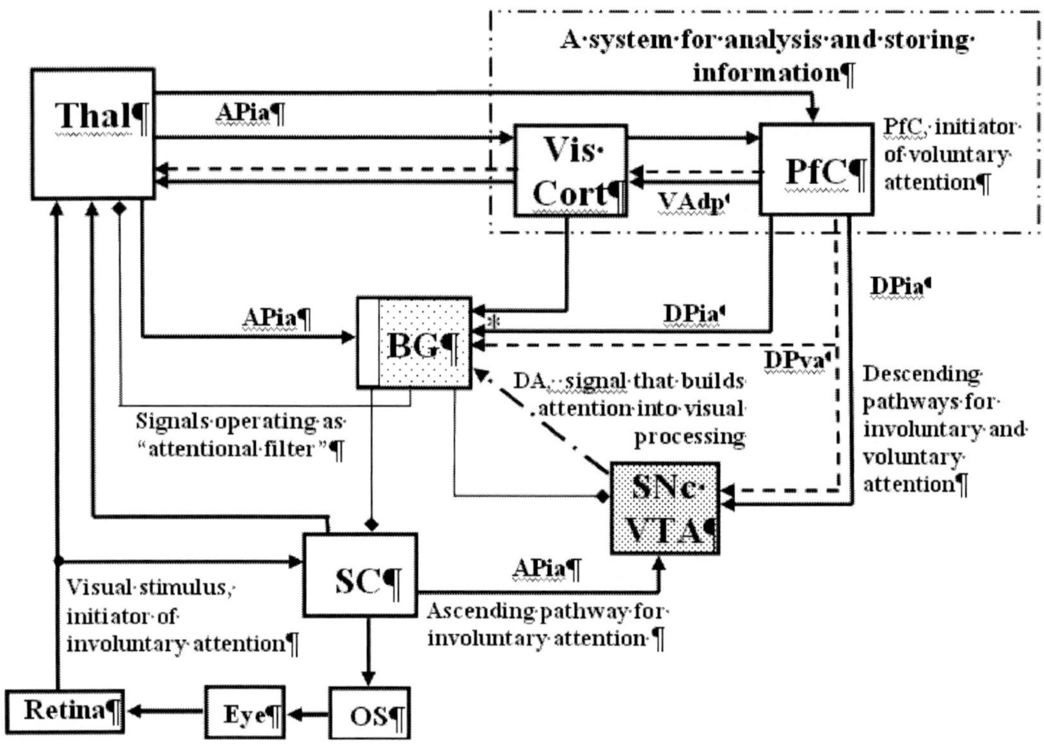

Figure 3. A model of contribution of cortico-basal ganglia-thalamocortical loop and dopamine to involuntary and voluntary visual attention. Processes in hatched part of the basal ganglia (BG) are dopamine-dependent; Thal, thalamus; OS, oculomotor structures. APia and DPia, ascending and descending pathways for initiating involuntary attention, respectively; DPva, descending pathways for initiating voluntary attention, are marked by broken lines; a star – modifiable inputs. Other abbreviations as in Figures 1 and 2.

It is possible that PFC represents relatively coarse visual information that can mediate between-category decisions (Bar, 2003). In spite of prefrontal representations of objects are not detailed, they are sufficient to activate anticipated activity in specific visual areas based on coarse information (Bar, 2003). During the expectation period preceding the attended presentations, regions within visual areas with a representation of the attended location are activated (Kastner et al., 1999). This activity is related to directing attention to the target location in the absence of visual stimulation, and the increase in activity during expectation is topographically specific. In areas that preferentially process a particular stimulus feature (e.g., color or motion), increases in baseline activity were shown to be stronger during the expectation of a preferred compared to a nonpreferred stimulus feature (Chawla et al., 2000). Interestingly, patterns of neocortical activity evoked by real visual stimulus and its voluntary imagination are similar (Mechelli et al., 2004). Even in early visual cortical areas, visual mental imagery could evoke activity with precise visual field topography (retinotopy) (Slotnick et al., 2005). Therefore, C-BG-Th-C loops that participate in involuntary and voluntary attentional modulation of visual processing are overlapped. This is consistent with known experimental data and general theories of attention that assume involuntary and voluntary attentional processes converge on a common neural architecture (Hunt and Kingstone, 2003; Kincade et al., 2005).

After the appearance of visual stimulus neural pattern representing this stimulus is superimposed with the neuronal representation of imagined stimulus. Then contrasted selection of total pattern is performed by C-BG-Th-C loops based on dopamine release in response to real stimulus. If real and imagined objects have similar properties, initial cortical representation of real stimulus becomes stronger, and its subsequent contrasted selection requires smaller number of cycles of circulation in the C-BG-Th-C loops. Thus the perception of the voluntary attended stimulus, which is similar to expected one, can be faster, in comparison with its perception without attention. Since processing of visual information occurs in the same neural networks, irrespective of a pathway of dopaminergic cell excitation, dopamine-dependent effects caused by top-down activation of dopaminergic cells can maintain and develop effects cased by their bottom-up excitation. Remarkably, the analysis of experimental data also led to assumption that top-down processes could modulate involuntary attention (Arnott et al., 2001).

In our model, mechanism of visual attention is built into the mechanism of visual processing. It becomes apparent in selection of a stimulus (its attribute) for the best processing and contrasted amplification of neuronal cortical representation of this stimulus (attribute). The output BG signal acting on the thalamus performs the role of "attentional filter" (Fig. 3). This signal depends on both the real stimulus, and traces of previous processing of similar stimuli in diverse C-BG-Th-C loops.

Earlier it was proposed that the interaction between cortical and dopaminergic inputs to striatal neurons and disinhibition of the SC via the striatum and SNr (i.e. via the direct pathway through the BG) may underlie purposeful saccades (Hikosaka et al., 2000). Saccades could be inhibited via the striatum, globus pallidus and SNr (i.e. via the indirect pathway through the BG) (Hikosaka et al., 2000). As distinct from mentioned model, we assume that in presence of dopamine, both direct and indirect pathways through the BG synergistically disinhibit SC, whereas in the absence of dopamine, SC are synergistically inhibited via direct and indirect pathways through the BG. Therefore, voluntary or involuntary evoked dopamine release and subsequent disinhibition (through the BG) of SC projected onto oculomotor structures, can promote focusing of eyes on attended stimulus (Fig. 3), and thus additionally strengthen responses of thalamic and neocortical neurones.

According to known experimental data, visual brain areas separately and asynchronously process different features of the same object (Zeki, 2001). However, vision produces unified perceptual experience indicating the solution of the "binding problem". Several lines of data support and evolve the idea that attention enhances the binding (Neri, 2004; Paul and Schyns, 2003; Saenz et al., 1990). Without attention, binding is less effective (Reeves et al., 2005).

There is an opinion that binding is performed by cortico-cortical connections in the "global workspace", which consists of the sensory upstream unimodal, downstream unimodal, heteromodal and limbic neocortical zones (Baars, 2002; Mesulam, 1998). We assume that C-BG-Th-C loops and dopamine favours the binding and its attentional enhancement due to following reasons. Release of dopamine lasts during 100-200 ms. Therefore it might support asynchronous selection and simultaneous conjunction of neuronal patterns representing different features of visual stimulus in numerous cortical areas. Interdepending changes in all stages of processing in diverse C-BG-Th-C loops is promoted by existence of not only reciprocal but also non-reciprocal connections between dopaminergic cells and striatal loci that belongs to different cortico-BG circuits (Haber, 2003). Based on the non-reciprocal projections dopaminergic cells, which influence processing in the higher-order C-BG-Th-C loops, could also influence activity reorganization in the lower-order C-BG-Th-C loops. In addition, dopaminergic neurons from both VTA and SNc are projected as into the NAcc, as into the dorso-lateral striatum (Lynd-Balta and Haber, 1994) (Fig. 1). Thus divergent dopaminergic projections can simultaneously promote processing in C-BG-Th-C loops that analyze diverse attributes of visual stimulus even though the attention was not especially attracted to all attributes.

Interpretation of Some Attentional Effects by Proposed Mechanism

Elaboration of a new attentional model is reasonable, if it allows explain some experimentally revealed effects which mechanisms were unclear from point of view of commonly accepted mechanism of attention, that is based on feedback connections from higher to lower cortical areas and then to reticular thalamic nucleus. For example, this mechanism cannot explain data denoting the disinhibition as a mechanism of attentional strengthening of visual cortical responses (Mehta et al., 2000) since disinhibition requires a chain of inhibitory cortical interneurons but their number is very small (less than 5%). Except for that, it is unclear how targets for disinhibition or inhibition could be chosen by attention taking into account significant convergence and divergence of interconnections between interneurons and pyramidal cells. In our model, attentional strengthening of visual cortical responses is in principle the result of disinhibition of thalamic cells that increases excitation of neocortical neurons, and initial neuronal response itself determines the choice of cells which activity must be increased.

From common point of view it is unclear why the attention directed on a certain attribute of a stimulus strengthens responsivity of neurons preferring this attribute, and suppresses reactions of neurons for which other attributes are preferable (Martinez-Trujillo and Treue, 2004). It was also obscured, why responses to ignored stimuli are attenuated (O'Connor et al., 2002; Treue and Maunsell, 1999). There is an opinion that various mechanisms underlie these effects (Hillyard et al., 1998). In contrast, in our model, the unified mechanism underlies both these effects. If stimulus evokes dopamine release and thus can attract attention, dopamine-dependent synaptic modifications promote disinhibition of the thalamus and subsequent increase of neocortical responses, while the lack of dopamine and therefore the absence of attention leads to rise of thalamic inhibition by the BG and subsequent suppression of neocortical responses. This mechanism explains experimentally obtained attentional modulation of neural activity in the LGN, wherein neural responses to attended stimuli were enhanced and responses to ignored stimuli were attenuated (Kastner and Pinsk, 2006; O'Connor et al., 2002). Thus LGN may serve as a "gatekeeper" in attentional control of visual responses.

It was shown that the cortical areas modulated by attention correspond closely to those showing activation during passive visual stimulation (Martinez et al., 2001), and that attention to a particular attribute of a visual stimulus (e.g. color, orientation, motion) enhances activity in the visual area specialised for processing the selected attribute (Corbetta et al., 1991). We suppose that attention influences neuronal firing in those cortical areas that are anatomically recruited by attended stimulus because only those cortico-striatal inputs could be modified that are active during dopamine release (Silkis, 2000), and because this modification is necessary for attentional filtering.

The real stimulus with expected properties should cause strong initial cortical reaction due to summing up real excitation with anticipating activity. Since in this case cortical response is strong the neuronal pattern could be further contrasty selected by the C-BG-Th-C loops. For the same reason visual attention to a stimulus feature could facilitate the processing of other stimuli sharing the same feature. Such effect is often obtained (Saenz et al., 2003). According to our model, the attention directed on a certain property of stimulus strengthens responses of those cortical neurons for which this property is preferable because their reactions are initially large and cortico-striatal input is strong. Simultaneously attention suppresses responses of neurons for which this stimulus property is not preferable since their responses are initially poor and cortico-striatal input is weak.

Remarkably, the earliest component of visual responses enhanced by attention was obtained in the extrastriate cortex in the time range of 80-130 ms after stimulus onset (Hillyard and Anllo-Vento, 1998; Martinez et al., 2001), whereas neuronal responses with latencies of 20-30 ms and 50-55 ms were not influenced by attention (Anllo-Vento et al., 1998; Di Russo et al., 2003; Maunsell and Gibson, 1992; Vidyasagar, 1998). If the attention is based only on recurrent cortico-cortical and/or cortico-thalamic projections as it is commonly proposed (Woldorff et al., 2002), the short latency components of responses should be also amplified since time lags of mentioned connections are small. Our model explains these results by necessity of activation of dopaminergic cell for attentional effects. By this reason, attention can increase only those components of reactions in different cortical areas whose onset exceeds the latency of visual responses of dopaminergic cells, which is about 100 ms (Dommett et al., 2005; Schultz et al., 1997).

It was found that identification of the second of two targets is impaired if it is presented less than about 500 ms after the first (Di Lollo et al., 2005). It was assumed that this effect, known as attentional blink, is more probably the result of temporary loss of control over the prevailing attentional set (Di Lollo et al., 2005). From point of view of our model, attentional blink could be explained by temporal characteristics of dopaminergic cell responses and release of dopamine in the striatum. Light flashes cause release of dopamine in the striatum with the mean latency 154 ms and mean duration about 331 ms (Domett et al., 2005). Since increase of excitation of dopaminergic cells in response to a light flash is followed by a decrease of firing rate that lasts about 150 ms (Domett et al., 2005), more than 500 ms is necessary for the normal response of dopaminergic cell to the second visual stimulus (i.e. for a large increase in striatal dopamine level) that is required for attentional perception of this stimulus.

Experimental data suggest that at least for low-level tasks each of visual and auditory modality is under separate attentional control, rather than under a supramodal attentional control (Alais et al., 2006). We suppose that this effect could be the consequence of processing the diverse features of visual and auditory information in different C-BG-Th-C loops. Since different populations of dopaminergic cells project to striatal loci connected with low-order visual and auditory cortical areas attentional influencing visual and auditory processing could be independent. The same mechanism can underlie commonly known distinction between object and spatial attention that reflects the organization of visual cortex into parallel "what" and "where" processing streams. We assume that object attention could be performed by C-BG-Th-C loop, which includes inferotemporal cortex, whereas spatial attention could be performed by C-BG-Th-C loop, which includes parietal cortex. This assumption is based on the data that mentioned cortical areas categorizes, respectively, what objects are in the world and where these objects are in space (Goodale and Milner, 1992).

It is known, that new unexpected stimuli involuntarily capture attention thus increasing neocortical responses. However even new objects do not attract attention unless they created a strong local changes (Franconeri et al., 2005). From our model follows, that only strong stimulus could switch on attention since only it can lead to discharges of striatonigral cells and thus provide disinhibition of the SC, which activates dopaminergic cells (Fig. 2).

According to experimental data, at least some different processes are involved into involuntary and voluntary attention (Fu et al., 2005). From our point of view, this difference could be the consequence of diverse pathways for dopaminergic cells excitation.

It was found that disruption of connections between medial PfC and STN or bilateral STN damage lead to attentional deficiency (Chudasama et al., 2003). On the contrary, high-frequency stimulation of STN neurons improved attention in parallel with dopamine medications (Brusa et al, 2001). Known models do not explain mechanisms of these effects, whereas it is directly follows from our models that STN activated by the PfC is necessary for attention since it directly excites dopaminergic cells (Fig. 2).

It was shown that the attention strengthens the binding of asynchronously perceived properties of stimulus due to acceleration of processing of each of these properties whereas perceptual asynchrony between attributes remains constant across attended and unattended conditions (Paul and Schyns, 2003). In the view of our model, this asynchrony remains constant because processing of different properties of stimulus is performed mainly in the separate C-BG-Th-C loops and in each loop dopamine promotes acceleration of processing due to reduction of number of circulation for selection of neural representation of each attribute of stimulus.

If the two stimuli share properties, processing of the second stimulus is more efficient than of a similar stimulus not preceded by the first stimulus (Dehaene et al., 1998). This typical attentional priming situation was explained by a short-term or iconic memory trace. Due to existence of such trace, activity of firstly excited neocortical neurons could be additionally amplified by C-BG-Th-C loop in comparison with none activated neurones. However, continued training abolishes the attentional effect (Chirimuuta et al., 2007). From point of view of our model, this abolishment could be the result of decrement and subsequent disappearance of responses of dopaminergic cells on repeating stimuli (Schultz, 1993).

THE MAIN DISTINCTIONS BETWEEN PROPOSED AND OTHER MODELS OF ATTENTION

It was proposed that attention to an object requires the simultaneous activity of three interconnected brain regions: the cortical site of attentional expression, the thalamic enhancement structure, and the prefrontal area of control (LaBerge, 1997). Unlike, in our model, attention requires the simultaneous interdependent activity in all regions of the C-BG-Th-C loops. Reentrant signaling realizes by signal circulation in these loops but not only in the cortico-cortical and cortico-thalamocortical loops. Formation of neural patterns representing visual stimulus is based not only on interactions between the prefrontal and visual cortical areas (Mechelli et al., 2004), but also on dopamine-dependent changes in signal transductions through the C-BG-Th-C loops.

In spite of the known role of dopamine in attentional effects (Nieoullon and Coquerel, 2003; Turle-Lorenzo et al., 2006), known models of attention do not include mechanism of dopaminergic cell activation by sensory stimulus. We have suggested such mechanism, and proposed that excitation of dopaminergic cell requires sensory activation of the direct pathway through the BG (Silkis, 2007).

In recent model of attention (Paul and Schyns, 2003), thalamic complex functionates in two directions: ascending activity promotes switching of attention to significant external signals, and descending activity supervises selection of signals participating in cognitive perception through the network cortex - BG. Unlike, in our model the BG nuclei, which influence transmission of signals through the thalamic complex to the neocortex, participate in both descending and ascending pathways for attentional switching.

There is a hypothesis that signals generated by "detectors of transient processes" switch on involuntary attention (Naatanen, 1992). These signals are determined by properties of sensory stimulus, its novelty and intensity, and "detectors of transient processes" exist in addition to detectors of sensory attributes. It is however unclear, what structures play the role of such "detectors", where and how the switching signal is generated and what is the character of this signal. From the point of view of our model, a network that includes striatonigral cells could execute detections of "transient processes". A release of dopamine in the striatum could play a role of a signal that switches on the attention. This signal is generated by dopaminergic neurons of the SNc and VTA in response to sensory stimulation.

It was proposed (Naatanen, 1992) that selection of stimulus for voluntary attentional perception occurs in primary cortical areas owing to comparison of a sensory input with the representation of physical properties of stimulus - “attentional trace”. We suppose that selection of stimulus for the best analysis occurs not only in primary, but also in other cortical areas where the diverse stimulus attributes are processed.

CONCLUSION

In our model, as well as in other models, the attention is a selective action directed on searching a stimulus for the best processing. We advanced a hypothesis that this action is the result of dopamine-dependent plastic reorganizations of neuronal activity in the visual and limbic cortico - basal ganglia - thalamocortical loops. Owing to opposite sign of dopamine-dependent modulation of the efficacy of strong and weak cortical inputs to the input basal ganglia nucleus, striatum, and subsequent activity reorganizations in all basal ganglia nuclei, the output basal ganglia signals ("attentional filter") exert disinhibitory and inhibitory influence on thalamic cells projected to neocortical neurons which initial visual activation was strong and weak, respectively. This "filter" simultaneously favours increase of responses of cortical neurons to attended stimulus, and decrease of responses to other stimuli. Divergent dopaminergic projections promote the attentional enhancement of perception of different features of the same stimulus and their binding into the entire object.

In proposed model, attention requires a release of dopamine in the striatum. Involuntary attention is initiated by stimulus-evoked dopamine release, which is promoted by visual activation of disinhibitory pathway through the basal ganglia to the superior colliculus that excites dopaminergic cells. Voluntary activation of the prefrontal cortex that excites dopaminergic cells initiates voluntary attention. Both involuntary and voluntary attention as well as processing of visual stimulus are performed in the same loops. Attention represents a part of sensory processing which improves its quality. However, this part of processing starts with a time lag of approximately 100 ms from the appearance of stimulus, due to the necessity of sensory activation of dopaminergic cells. This condition explains experimentally obtained absence of attentional modulation of neocortical responses with latencies that do not exceed 100 ms.

Experimental findings led to an assumption, that the role of basal ganglia in processing of information is nonspecific in terms of stimulus modality and the cognitive context of the task (Rektor et al., 2005). We suppose that the absence of modal specificity is the result of uniform character of signal processing in different cortico- basal ganglia – thalamocortical loops irrespective of the parts of cortical area, thalamic and basal ganglia nuclei included in these loops. In our opinion, divergent dopaminergic projections may underlie well established cross-modal attentional effects and attentional enhancement of binding. Proposed model that provides a new insight into the role of dopamine-dependent synaptic plasticity in the networks that include neocortex, basal ganglia and thalamus in mechanisms of visual perception and attention can help to understand mechanisms underlaying disorders in visual perception. For example, it explains why a lesion or degeneration of the visual striatum causes some deficits in visual perception (Jacobs et al., 1995).

This work was supported by the Russian Foundation for Basic Research, Grant 08-04-00218a

References

Alais, D., Morrone, C., and Burr, D. (2006). Separate attentional resources for vision and audition. *Proceedings of the Royal Society B: Biological Sciences*, 273, 1339-1345.

Anllo-Vento, L., Luck, S. J., and Hillyard, S. A. (1998). Spatio-temporal dynamics of attention to color: evidence from human electrophysiology, *Human Brain Mapping*, 6, 216-238.

Arnott, S. R., Pratt, J., Shore, D. I., and Alain, C. (2001). Attentional set modulates visual areas: an event-related potential study of attentional capture. *Cognitive Brain Research*, 12, 383-395.

Baars, B. J. (2002). The conscious access hypothesis: origins and recent evidence. *Trends in Cognitive Science*, 6, 47-52.

Bar, M. (2003). A cortical mechanism for triggering top-down facilitation in visual object recognition. *Journal of Cognitive Neuroscience*, 15, 600-609.

Berendse, H. W., Galis-de Graaf, Y., and Groenewegen, H. J. (1992). Topographical organization and relationship with ventral striatal compartments of prefrontal cortico-striatal projections in the rat. *Journal of Comparative Neurology*, 316, 314-347.

Booth, R. J., Burman, D. D., Meyer, J. R., Lei, Z., Trommer, B. L., Davenport, N.D., Li, W., Todd, B., Parrish T. B., Gitelman, D. R., and Mesulam, M. (2005). Larger deficits in brain networks for response inhibition than for visual selective attention in attention deficit hyperactivity disorder (ADHD). *Journal of Child Psychology and Psychiatry*, 46, 94-111.

Brusa, L., Pierantozzi, M., Peppe, A., Altibrandi, M. G., Giacomini, P., Mazzone, P., and Stanzione, P. (2001). Deep brain stimulation (DBS) attentional effects parallel those of l-dopa treatment. *Journal of Neural Transmission*, 108, 1021-1027.

Chawla, D., Rees, G., and Friston, K. J. (1999). The physiological basis of attentional modulation in extrastriate visual areas. *Nature Neuroscience*, 2, 671-676.

Chirimuuta, M., Burr D., and Morrone, M. C. (2007). The role of perceptual learning on modality-specific visual attentional effects. *Vision Research*, 47, 60-70.

Christakou, A., Robbins, T. W., and Everitt, B. J. (2004). Prefrontal cortical-ventral striatal interactions involved in affective modulation of attentional performance: implications for cortico-striatal circuit function. *Journal of Neuroscience*, 24, 773-780.

Christakou, A., Robbins, T. W., and Everitt, B. J. (2001). Functional disconnection of a prefrontal cortical-dorsal striatal system disrupts choice reaction time performance: implications for attentional function. *Behavioral Neuroscience*, 115, 812-825.

Chudasama, Y., Baunez, C., and Robbins, T. W. (2003). Functional disconnection of the medial prefrontal cortex and subthalamic nucleus in attentional performance: evidence for corticosubthalamic interaction. *Journal of Neuroscience*, 23, 5477-5485.

Corbetta, M., Miezin, S., Dobmeyer, S., Shulman, G. L., and Petersen, S. E. (1991). Selective and divided attention during visual discriminations of shape, color, speed: functional anatomy by positron emission tomography. *Journal of Neuroscience*, 11, 2383–2402.

Crick, F., Koch, C. (1995). Are we aware of neuronal activity in primary visual cortex? *Nature*, 375, 121-123.

Dehaene, S., Naccache, L., Le Clec'H, G., Koechlin, E., Mueller, M., Dehaene-Lambertz, G., van de Moortele, P.F., and Le Bihan, D. (1998). Imaging unconscious semantic priming. *Nature*, 395, 597-600.

Di Lollo, V., Kawahara, J., Shahab Ghorashi, S. M., and Enns, J. T. (2005). The attentional blink: resource depletion or temporary loss of control? *Psychological Research*, 69, 191-200.

Di Russo, F., Martinez, A., and Hillyard, S. A. (2003). Source analysis of event-related cortical activity during visuo-spatial attention. *Cerebral Cortex*, 13, 486-499.

Dommett, E., Coizet, V., Blaha, C. D., Martindale, J., Lefebvre, V., Walton, N., Mayhew, J. E., Overton, P. G., and Redgrave, P. (2005). How visual stimuli activate dopaminergic neurons at short latency. *Science*, 307, 1476-1479.

Edelman, G. M. (2003). Naturalizing consciousness: A theoretical framework. *Proceedings of the National Academy of Science USA*, 100, 5520-5524.

Filoteo, J. V., Delis, D. C., Salmon, D. P., Demadura, T., Roman, M. J., and Shults, C. W. (1997). An examination of the nature of attentional deficits in patients with Parkinson's disease: evidence from a spatial orienting task. *Journal of International Neuropsychological Society*, 3, 337-347.

Forssberg, H., Fernell, E., Waters, S., Waters, N., and Tedroff, J. (2006). Altered pattern of brain dopamine synthesis in male adolescents with attention deficit hyperactivity disorder. *Behavioral Brain Function*, 2, 40.

Franconeri, S. L., Hollingworth, A., and Simons, D. J. (2005). Do new objects capture attention? *Psychological Science*, 16, 275-281.

Fu, S., Greenwood, P. M., and Parasuraman, R. (2005). Brain mechanisms of involuntary visuospatial attention: An event-related potential study. *Human Brain Mapping*, 25, 378-390.

Goodale, M. A., and Milner, D. (1992). Separate visual pathways for perception and action. *Trends in Neuroscience*, 15, 10-25.

Haber, S. N., (2003). The primate basal ganglia: parallel and integrative networks. *Journal of Chemical Neuroanatomy*, 26, 317-330.

Hikosaka, O., Takikawa, Y., and Kawagoe, R. (2000). Role of the basal ganglia in the control of purposive saccadic eye movements. *Physiological Review*, 80, 954-978.

Hillyard, S. A., and Anllo-Vento, L. (1998). Event-related brain potentials in the study of visual selective attention. *Proceedings of the National Academy of Science USA*, 95, 781-787.

Hillyard, S. A., Vogel, E. K., and Luck, S. J. (1998). Sensory gain control (amplification) as a mechanism of selective attention: electrophysiological and neuroimaging evidence. *Philosophical Transactions of the Royal Society B: Biological Sciences*, 353, 1257-1270.

Horvitz, J. C., Stewart, T., and Jacobs, B. L. (1997). Burst activity of ventral tegmental dopamine neurons is elicited by sensory stimuli in the awake cat. *Brain Research*, 759, 251-258.

Hunt, A. R., and Kingstone, A. (2003). Covert and overt voluntary attention: linked or independent? *Cognitive Brain Research*, 18, 102-105.

Jacobs, D. H., Shuren, J., and Heilman, K. M. (1995). Impaired perception of facial identity and facial affect in Huntington's disease. *Neurology*, 45, 1217–1218.

Kahkonen, S., Ahveninen, J., Jaaskelainen, I. P., Kaakkola, S., Naatanen, R., Huttunen, J., and Pekkonen, E. (2001). Effects of haloperidol on selective attention: a combined whole-head MEG and high-resolution EEG study. *Neuropsychopharmacology*, 25, 498-504.

Kastner, S., and Pinsk, M. A. (2004). Visual attention as a multilevel selection process. *Cognitive Affective and Behavioral Neuroscience*, 4, 483-500.

Kastner, S., Pinsk, M. A., De Weerd, P., Desimone, R., and Ungerleider, L. G. (1999). Increased activity in human visual cortex during directed attention in the absence of visual stimulation. *Neuron*, 22, 751-761.

Kermadi, I., and Boussaoud, D. (1995). Role of primate striatum in attention and sensorimotor processes: comparison with pre-motor cortex. *Neuroreport*, 6, 1177–1181.

Kha, H. T., Finkelstein, D. I., Tomas, D., Drago, J., Pow, D. V., Horne, M. K. (2001). Projections from the substantia nigra pars reticulata to the motor thalamus of the rat: single axon reconstructions and immunohistochemical study. *Journal of Comparative Neurology*, 440, 20-30.

Kimura, M., Minamimoto, T., Matsumoto, N., and Hori, Y. (2004). Monitoring and switching of cortico-basal ganglia loop functions by the thalamo-striatal system. *Neuroscience Research*, 48, 355-360.

Kincade, J. M., Abrams, R. A., Astafiev, S. V., Shulman, G. L., and Corbetta, M. (2005). An event-related functional magnetic resonance imaging study of voluntary and stimulus-driven orienting of attention. *Journal of Neuroscience*, 25, 4593-4604.

LaBerge, D. (1997) Attention, awareness, and the triangular circuit. *Consciousness and Cognition*, 6, 149-181.

Lynd-Balta, E., and Haber, S. N. (1994). The organization of midbrain projections to the striatum in the primate: sensorimotor-related striatum versus ventral striatum. *Neuroscience*, 59, 625-640.

Martinez, A., DiRusso, F., Anllo-Vento, L., Sereno, M. I., Buxton, R. B., and Hillyard, S. A. (2001). Putting spatial attention on the map: timing and localization of stimulus selection processes in striate and extrastriate visual areas. *Vision Research*, 41, 1437-1457.

Martinez-Trujillo, J. C., and Treue, S. (2004). Feature-based attention increases the selectivity of population responses in primate visual cortex. *Current Biology*, 14, 744-751.

Maunsell, J. H., and Gibson, J. R. (1992). Visual response latencies in striate cortex of the macaque monkey. *Journal of Neurophysiology*, 68, 1332-1344.

Mechelli, A., Price, C. J., Friston, K. J., and Ishai, A. (2004). Where bottom-up meets top-down: neuronal interactions during perception and imagery. *Cerebral Cortex*, 14, 1256-1265.

Mehta, A. D., Ulbert, I., and Schroeder, C. E. (2000). Intermodal selective attention in monkeys. II: physiological mechanisms of modulation. *Cerebral Cortex*, 10, 359-370.

Mesulam, M. M. (1998). Dopamine agonists reorient visual exploration away from the neglected hemispace. *Neurology*, 51, 1395-1398.

Middleton, F. A., and Strick, P. L. (1996). The temporal lobe is a target of output from the basal ganglia. *Proceedings of the National Academy of Science USA*, 93, 8683-8687.

Miller, R. (1993). Striatal dopamine in reward and attention: A system for understanding the symptomatology of acute schizofrenia and mania. *International Review of Neurobiology*, 35, 161-278.

Montero, V. M. (2000). Attentional activation of the visual thalamic reticular nucleus depends on 'top-down' inputs from the primary visual cortex via corticogeniculate pathways. *Brain Research*, 864, 95-104.

Naatanen, R. (1992). Attention and Brain Function, Lawrence Erlbaum, Hillsdale, NJ.

Nagy, A., Eordegh, G., Norita, M., and Benedek, G. (2005). Visual receptive field properties of excitatory neurons in the substantia nigra. *Neuroscience*, 130, 513-518.

Nakamura, K., Honda, M., Okada, T., Hankawa, T., Fukuyama, H., Konishi, J., and Shibasaki, H. (2000). Attentional modulation of parieto-occipital cortical responses: implications for hemispatial neglect. *Journal of the Neurological Sciences*, 176, 136-143.

Neri, P. (2004). Attentional effects on sensory tuning for single-feature detection and double-feature conjunction. *Vision Research*, 44, 3053-3064.

Nieoullon, A., and Coquerel, A. (2003). Dopamine: a key regulator to adapt action, emotion, motivation and cognition. *Current Opinion in Neurology*, 16, S3-S9.

O'Connor, D. H., Fukui, M. M., Pinsk, M. A., and Kastner, S. (2002). Attention modulates responses in the human lateral geniculate nucleus. *Nature Neuroscience*, 5, 1203-1209.

Parent, A., and Hazrati, L.N. (1995). Functional anatomy of the basal ganglia. I. The cortico-basal ganglia-thalamo-cortical loop. *Brain Research Review*, 20, 91-127.

Paul, L., and Schyns, P. G. (2003). Attention enhances feature integration. *Vision Research*, 43, 1793–1798.

Reeves, A., Fuller, H., and Fine, E. M., (2005). The role of attention in binding shape to color. *Vision Research*, 45, 3343-3355.

Rektor, I., Bares, M., Brazdil, M., Kanovsky, P., Rektorova, I., Sochurkova, D., Kubova, D., Kuba, R., and Daniel, P. (2005). Cognitive- and movement-related potentials recorded in the human basal ganglia. *Movement Disorders*, 20, 562-568.

Saenz, M., Buracas, G. T., and Boynton, G. M. (2003). Global feature-based attention for motion and color. *Vision Research*, 43, 629-637.

Schultz, W. (1997). Dopamine neurons and their role in reward mechanisms. *Current Opinion in Neurobiology*, 7, 191–197.

Schultz, W., Apicella, P., and Ljungberg, T. (1993). Responses of monkey dopamine neurons to reward and conditioned stimuli during successive steps of learning a delayed response task. *Journal of Neuroscience*, 13, 900–913.

Silkis, I. (2000). The cortico-basal ganglia-thalamocortical circuit with synaptic plasticity. I. Modification rules for excitatory and inhibitory synapses in the striatum. *Biosystems*, 57, 187-196.

Silkis, I. (2001). The cortico-basal ganglia-thalamocortical circuit with synaptic plasticity. II. Mechanism of synergistic modulation of thalamic activity via the direct and indirect pathways through the basal ganglia. *Biosystems*, 59, 7-14.

Sil'kis, I. (2003). The involvement of dopamine in strengthening cortical signals activating NMDA receptors in the striatum (a hypothetical mechanism). *Neuroscience and Behavioral Physiology*, 33, 379-386.

Sil'kis, I. (2006). Possible mechanisms of the involvement of dopaminergic cells and cholinergic interneurons in the striatum in the conditioned-reflex selection of motor activity. *Neuroscience and Behavioral Physiology*, 36, 163-175.

Silkis, I. (2007). A hypothetical role of cortico - basal ganglia - thalamocortical loops in visual processing. *Biosystems*, 89, 227-235.

Slotnick, S.D., Thompson, W.L., and Kosslyn, S.M. (2005). Visual mental imagery induces retinotopically organized activation of early visual areas. *Cerebral Cortex, 15,*1570-1583.

Treue, S. (2003). Visual attention: the where, what, how and why of saliency. *Current Opinion in Neurobiology*, 13, 428-432.

Treue, S., and Maunsell, J. H. (1999). Effects of attention on the processing of motion in macaque middle temporal and medial superior temporal visual cortical areas. *Journal of Neuroscience*, 19, 7591-7602.

Turle-Lorenzo, N., Maurin, B., Puma, C., Chezaubernard, C., Morain, P., Baunez, C., Nieoullon, A., and Amalric, M. (2006). The dopamine agonist piribedil with L-DOPA improves attentional dysfunction: relevance for Parkinson's disease. *The Journal of Pharmacology and Experimental Therapeutics*, 319, 914-923.

Vidyasagar, T. R. (1998). Gating of neuronal responses in macaque primary visual cortex by an attentional spotlight. *Neuroreport*, 9, 1947-1952.

Woldorff, M. G., Liotti, M., Seabolt, M., Busse, L., Lancaster, J. L., and Fox, P.T. (2002). The temporal dynamics of the effects in occipital cortex of visual-spatial selective attention. *Cognitive Brain Research*, 15, 1-15.

Zeki, S. (2001). Localization and globalization in conscious vision. *Annual Review of Neuroscience, 24,* 57-86.

Zikopoulos, B., and Barbas, H. (2006). Prefrontal projections to the thalamic reticular nucleus form a unique circuit for attentional mechanisms. *Journal of Neuroscience*, 26, 7348-7361.

INDEX

#

6-OHDA, ix, 114, 116, 126, 128, 129, 130, 131, 132, 133, 134, 140, 206

A

Aβ, vii, 1, 3, 5, 6, 7, 9, 10, 18, 20, 26, 27, 30, 31, 34, 35, 96
AA, 81
aberrant, 3, 4, 17, 33, 119, 170, 338
abnormalities, 5, 20, 39, 184, 185, 249, 250, 354
absorption, 9, 36
abstinence, 178, 184, 185, 186, 195, 199, 202, 208
AC, 80
access, 126, 270, 289, 373
accuracy, 363
ACE, 293
ACE inhibitors, 293
acetylation, 11, 31
acetylcholine, 15, 21, 89, 104, 235, 245
acetylcholinesterase, 11, 139
acid, 10, 23, 27, 35, 37, 46, 79, 99, 101, 145, 166, 221, 222, 224, 225, 244, 257, 262
acidic, 38
acidic fibroblast growth factor, 38
acoustic, 254
actin, xii, 4, 14, 19, 20, 27, 28, 51, 59, 60, 72, 73, 74, 345, 346, 347, 348, 349, 350, 351, 352, 353, 354, 356, 357, 358, 359
action potential, 58, 84, 90, 132, 144, 146, 196, 226, 228, 229, 236, 255, 275, 277, 280, 310, 313, 325, 336, 337
activators, 61, 68, 283
active site, 50, 58
activity level, 54
acute, 18, 40, 133, 184, 189, 191, 192, 206, 209, 242, 244, 258, 287, 375
acute stress, 191, 192, 242, 258
AD, vii, 1, 2, 3, 4, 5, 6, 7, 8, 9, 11, 15, 17, 18, 20, 23, 32, 46, 63, 166, 167, 335, 336, 340
Adams, 22, 169, 170, 174, 243, 246, 259, 262
adaptation, 53, 135, 151, 152, 184, 185, 218
adaptive control, 328, 329
addiction, x, 92, 105, 177, 178, 179, 182, 184, 185, 186, 187, 188, 189, 191, 193, 194, 195, 196, 198, 199, 200, 201, 204, 205, 207, 208, 211, 212, 214, 215, 216, 217, 218, 220, 262, 288
adenosine, 206, 210, 244, 353
adenylyl cyclase, 80, 149
ADHD, 373
adhesion, 13, 22
administration, 7, 40, 43, 153, 178, 187, 188, 189, 190, 191, 192, 197, 198, 200, 201, 206, 208, 210, 215, 216, 217, 220, 244, 254, 260, 267, 281, 320
adolescents, 374
adrenoceptors, 235, 241, 258
adult, 2, 3, 16, 17, 20, 22, 27, 28, 34, 37, 42, 43, 50, 51, 52, 54, 63, 70, 83, 101, 115, 133, 135, 137, 138, 140, 171, 174, 209, 216, 258, 260, 266, 275, 276, 285, 286, 292, 313, 330, 336, 340, 348
adulthood, 14, 239
adults, 7, 39, 52, 53, 164, 199
AEA, 79, 80, 81, 82, 85, 87, 91, 93, 94
affective disorder, 174
age, xi, 3, 4, 7, 9, 20, 23, 24, 29, 52, 116, 137, 184, 213, 269, 275, 285, 286, 291, 319, 337, 339, 341
ageing, 354
agents, 10, 96, 168
aggregates, 3
aggression, 270
aging, vii, 1, 2, 3, 4, 7, 32, 34, 115, 116, 121, 131, 140, 286, 339, 342
agonist, 13, 23, 80, 82, 87, 95, 96, 99, 103, 106, 108, 188, 227, 228, 231, 236, 237, 238, 251, 259, 285, 293, 350
aid, 96
AIDS, 78

air, 152
AJ, 334, 336
alanine, 3, 69
alcohol, 78, 96, 207, 289, 290
alcohol abuse, 96
alcohol consumption, 289
alcohol dependence, 207
alcohol withdrawal, 289, 290
alcoholics, 219, 289
alcoholism, 96, 98
alertness, 264
allele, 11, 37
alpha, 67, 68, 69, 70, 71, 73, 235, 257, 281, 348, 357
alternative, 8, 95, 346
alternative energy, 8
alters, 18, 23, 53, 62, 111, 220, 247, 249, 260, 282, 356
Alzheimer, vii, 1, 2, 3, 6, 21, 22, 23, 24, 25, 26, 27, 28, 29, 30, 31, 32, 33, 34, 35, 36, 37, 38, 39, 40, 41, 42, 46, 63, 74, 77, 138, 140, 241, 245, 247, 294
Alzheimer disease, 21, 26, 33, 34, 36, 37, 40, 41, 42
AM, 221, 329, 339
American Association for the Advancement of Science, 16
amide, 80, 82, 100, 101
amine, 81, 222, 224
amino, xii, 3, 46, 53, 56, 61, 62, 67, 133, 139, 145, 166, 198, 214, 220, 221, 222, 224, 225, 257, 258, 274, 275, 334, 345, 346, 347, 348, 350
amino acid, 3, 53, 56, 133, 139, 214, 220, 258, 275, 334, 347, 348, 350
amino acids, 3, 56, 133, 139, 214, 220, 258, 334, 347, 348, 350
amnesia, 255, 266
amorphous, 60
AMPA, xii, 10, 17, 20, 24, 26, 32, 33, 34, 38, 39, 46, 61, 62, 66, 67, 69, 104, 132, 136, 142, 145, 146, 148, 150, 151, 153, 166, 183, 189, 190, 191, 198, 208, 211, 215, 218, 220, 221, 224, 230, 233, 237, 254, 255, 257, 265, 268, 274, 275, 279, 282, 297, 298, 299, 301, 345, 346, 348, 350, 351, 352, 353, 354, 355, 356, 357, 358, 359
amphetamine, 211, 217, 218, 219, 220, 244, 254, 262, 266, 281
amphetamines, 191
amplitude, 14, 55, 85, 100, 151, 153, 193, 206, 271, 293, 310, 312
Amsterdam, 135, 137
AMT, 81, 82, 83
amygdala, xi, 31, 54, 87, 94, 98, 102, 104, 121, 167, 168, 169, 174, 178, 179, 181, 182, 186, 188, 191, 194, 195, 202, 205, 210, 211, 212, 214, 217, 221, 224, 231, 232, 234, 238, 243, 244, 246, 247, 248, 252, 256, 257, 258, 259, 261, 262, 263, 267, 269, 270, 271, 272, 273, 274, 275, 276, 277, 279, 280, 281, 282, 283, 284, 285, 287, 288, 289, 290, 291, 292, 293, 339
amyloid, vii, 1, 3, 5, 22, 23, 24, 25, 27, 28, 29, 30, 31, 32, 34, 35, 37, 38, 39, 40, 41, 42, 63, 106, 110, 141, 241
amyloid beta, 32
amyloid deposits, 28
amyloid plaques, 5, 24, 63, 141
amyloid precursor protein, 3, 24, 25, 28, 35, 39, 241
AN, 153, 340
anaesthesia, 126, 127, 230
analgesia, 287
analog, 38, 204
anatomy, 21, 134, 180, 263, 373, 376
angiogenesis, 135
angiotensin, 288, 292, 293, 294, 296, 298, 299, 300, 306, 307
angiotensin II, 288, 292, 294, 296, 299, 306
angiotensin receptor antagonist, 293
anhedonia, 184, 215
animal learning, 218
animal models, 19, 126, 140, 174, 184, 191, 192, 195, 197, 204, 242
animal tissues, 78
animals, x, 7, 52, 54, 114, 126, 127, 129, 143, 152, 163, 164, 165, 166, 167, 169, 170, 183, 187, 189, 191, 192, 196, 199, 200, 206, 218, 226, 230, 233, 238, 244, 270, 272, 275, 280, 286, 290, 291, 312, 319, 320
antagonism, 335
antagonist, 11, 80, 87, 90, 92, 94, 95, 96, 102, 108, 153, 166, 168, 170, 183, 188, 189, 191, 192, 206, 207, 216, 225, 226, 227, 228, 231, 233, 236, 237, 238, 240, 241, 244, 274, 275, 276, 281, 285, 293
antagonistic, 292
antagonists, x, 85, 87, 92, 171, 174, 178, 191, 192, 197, 207, 210, 226, 227, 229, 273, 276, 278, 288, 291, 293
anterior cingulate cortex, 251
anterograde amnesia, 115
anthropological, 78
Antibodies, 159
antibody, 13
antidepressant, 242, 243, 263, 265, 266
antidepressants, 243, 262, 263
antipsychotic, 242
anxiety, 235, 241, 242, 245, 289,294, 300, 308
anxiety disorder, 235, 245
aorta, 127
AP, 58, 64, 126, 234

APOE, 23, 33, 42
Apolipoprotein E, 32, 37, 40
apoptosis, 11, 64, 73, 292
APP, 3, 7, 9, 35, 241
appetite, 292
application, 93, 168, 198, 206, 227, 228, 229, 237, 247, 273, 276, 287, 325
AR, 346, 350, 353
arachidonic acid, 80, 81, 82, 104, 107, 108, 279, 280
arbitrary associations, 323
Arctic, 7
arginine, 279
arousal, 185, 194, 253, 270, 321
arson, 228, 286, 311, 312
ascorbic, 126
ascorbic acid, 126
aspartate, 40, 69, 174, 181, 189, 258, 311, 334
assessment, 25, 38, 168
associations, 165, 186, 193, 197, 202, 210, 232, 289, 323, 326
astrocyte, 17, 24
astrocytes, 8, 9, 13, 17, 20, 22, 43
astrogliosis, 18
asymmetry, 117
asymptotic, 315, 318
asymptotically, 315
asynchronous, 368
atherosclerosis, 32
ATP, 30, 53, 58, 72, 133
ATPase, 356
atrophy, 7, 24, 32, 38, 242, 243
attachment, 170
attention, ix, xi, 17, 51, 78, 114, 126, 131, 165, 169, 209, 222, 226, 242, 244, 309, 334, 362, 363, 364, 366, 367, 368, 369, 370, 371, 372, 373, 374, 375, 376
attentional blink, 369, 373
attentional disorder, xiii, 362
atypical, 133, 242
audition, 372
auditory cortex, 246
auditory evoked potential, 271
auditory evoked potentials, 271
auditory modality, 272, 370
Australia, 221
autism, 270
autocrine, 97
autonomic, 137, 194, 243, 253, 271
autonomous, 53, 54
availability, 200, 204, 219, 237
avoidance, 218, 234
awareness, 375
axon, 4, 34, 58, 85, 87, 104, 116, 117, 118, 120, 123, 124, 133, 141, 144, 153, 180, 181, 212, 214, 259, 322, 374
axon terminals, 85, 87, 104, 133, 181, 212, 214
axonal, vii, 1, 2, 4, 12, 13, 30, 32, 35, 37, 39, 41, 42, 79, 116
axons, vii, 1, 15, 17, 19, 46, 55, 63, 119, 124, 130, 144, 149, 152, 153, 168, 182, 212, 224, 349

B

β-amyloid, 139
Baars, 368, 373
background information, x, 163
barrier, 315
basal forebrain, 2, 15, 21
basal ganglia, ix, xii, 19, 21, 113, 121, 122, 126, 134, 135, 136, 139, 140, 218, 359, 361, 362, 363, 364, 366, 371, 372, 374, 375, 376
basal nuclei, 275
basket cells, 143
BDNF, x, 13, 14, 18, 20, 24, 30, 31, 32, 33, 35, 43, 46, 55, 70, 131, 171, 172, 175, 177, 178, 179, 181, 182, 192, 193, 201, 202, 208, 209, 213, 215, 216, 217, 220, 222, 233, 247, 284, 295
behavior, vii, ix, x, xi, 48, 53, 92, 114, 122, 127, 178, 179, 180, 185, 190, 193, 195, 196, 197, 198, 199, 201, 202, 203, 204, 205, 206, 207, 208, 211, 213, 217, 219, 269, 285, 289, 309, 336
behavioral change, x, 177, 178, 179, 188, 190, 197, 202
behavioral disorders, 211
behavioral effects, 126, 187, 213, 263
behavioral models, 105
behavioral problems, 196
behaviours, 239
bell, 13
bell-shaped, 13
beta, 27, 35, 68, 69, 73, 103, 105, 106, 110, 233, 235, 241, 281
bias, 239
bilateral, 170, 218, 281, 363, 370
binding, xii, 5, 7, 9, 13, 26, 28, 40, 46, 47, 48, 49, 50, 52, 54, 55, 56, 58, 60, 62, 63, 67, 68, 69, 72, 73, 74, 97, 108, 118, 146, 147, 148, 153, 165, 171, 173, 204, 205, 215, 220, 222, 227, 259, 262, 279, 283, 345, 346, 347, 348, 349, 350, 351, 353, 354, 355, 356, 357, 358, 359, 367, 370, 372, 376
binge drinking, 289
biochemical, xii, 11, 19, 95, 116, 119, 133, 193, 280, 345
biochemistry, 101, 102
biogenesis, 25

biological, 5, 25, 79, 83, 85, 98, 178, 196, 247, 272, 280
biological activity, 83
biology, 5, 25, 65, 79
biomarker, 27, 28
biophysical, 84
biophysics, 250
biosynthesis, 8, 56, 66, 81, 82, 86, 99, 105, 107
bipolar, 64, 241
bipolar disorder, 64, 241
birth, 348
black, 6, 122, 190, 324
blocks, 50, 106, 133, 181, 207, 208, 210, 214, 228, 233, 236, 238, 243, 258, 262, 276, 318, 335
blood, 8, 292, 293
blood pressure, 292
blood-brain barrier, 8, 293
bottom-up, 366, 367, 375
boutons, 132, 137, 280
BP, 336
brain activity, 184, 247
brain damage, 115, 171, 179
brain development, 8, 83, 351
brain functions, 2, 97, 355
brain imaging techniques, 143
brain injury, 18, 42, 172
brain structure, 8, 115, 167, 186, 191, 199, 202, 239, 288
brain tumor, 101
brainstem, 51, 72, 110, 122, 144, 194, 223, 234, 235, 271
branching, 34, 60, 141, 243
breakdown, 64, 101
buffer, 127, 168
bundling, 60, 72
buttons, 125, 129, 130

C

Ca^{2+}, v, viii, 15, 19, 45, 46, 48, 50, 53, 54, 55, 58, 61, 62, 63, 66, 67, 68, 69, 70, 71, 72, 73, 74, 75, 80, 81, 82, 83, 85, 86, 87, 88, 89, 90, 91, 92, 94, 100, 102, 103, 105, 108, 111, 119, 132, 133, 140, 146, 147, 148, 149, 150, 151, 155, 156, 158, 159, 160, 173, 181, 253, 263, 275, 276, 277, 280, 281, 296, 303, 304, 312, 339, 346, 348, 350, 351, 353, 354, 356, 359
Ca^{2+} signals, 48
cadherin, 13, 37, 42, 358
caffeine, 206
calcium, 7, 12, 22, 35, 67, 68, 69, 70, 71, 72, 73, 74, 79, 81, 99, 105, 107, 108, 109, 118, 119, 132, 139, 142, 165, 170, 173, 220, 225, 227, 228, 229, 237, 241, 245, 249, 254, 259, 261, 263, 273, 274, 275, 276, 279, 281, 282, 284, 291, 311, 313, 319, 320
calcium channels, 12, 79, 99, 105, 108, 109, 119, 139, 165, 274, 276
calmodulin, viii, 45, 46, 47, 48, 49, 50, 51, 54, 61, 66, 67, 68, 69, 70, 71, 72, 73, 74, 75, 147, 281, 320, 346, 348, 356
CAM, 25, 42, 256
cAMP, 40, 46, 55, 62, 74, 75, 80, 81, 148, 149, 178, 222, 244, 262, 265, 283, 287, 348, 355, 358
Canada, 163
Cancer, 358
candidates, viii, 45, 48, 67, 146, 279
cannabinoids, viii, 77, 78, 85, 99, 101, 104, 105, 107, 108, 109, 110, 111, 227, 237, 238, 246, 257, 265
cannabis, 103, 266
capacity, 3, 22, 55, 114, 132, 169, 180, 289, 290, 331, 342
capsule, 272, 273
carbohydrates, 30
carbon, 279
carbon monoxide, 279
carboxyl, 61
cardiovascular, 9, 110, 293
cardiovascular disease, 9, 293
cardiovascular risk, 110
cargo, 354, 357
carrier, 8
case study, 263
caspase, 75
catalytic, xii, 47, 49, 345, 346, 347, 352, 357, 359
catecholamine, 126, 211, 254, 257
catecholamines, 56, 235
category d, 366
cation, 31, 350, 354
cats, 135
causality, 95, 172, 313
CB, 101, 107, 266
CBP, 30, 46, 55
CD, 346
CDK, 32, 46
CDKs, 32
cDNA, 79, 100
CE, 343
ceiling effect, x, 177, 189, 208
cell adhesion, 12, 13, 20, 23, 36, 38, 41, 60, 149, 222, 243, 358
cell assembly, 324
cell culture, 55, 85, 283
cell death, 63, 115
cell differentiation, 13
cell division, 10

cell line, 69
cell lines, 69
cell surface, 10
central nervous system (CNS), vii, viii, 2, 8, 11, 14, 17, 19, 20, 23, 24, 28, 31, 36, 39, 45, 46, 78, 80, 83, 87, 97, 101, 109, 116, 117, 135, 137, 154, 211, 292, 293, 296, 306, 349, 350, 351, 353, 354
cerebellar granule cells, 103
cerebellum, ix, 50, 53, 70, 71, 85, 87, 88, 89, 90, 95, 97, 100, 102, 104, 118, 143, 145, 149, 151, 152, 154, 328, 329, 333, 336, 348
cerebral blood flow, 186, 249, 267
cerebral cortex, 51, 60, 64, 118, 123, 124, 145, 217, 250, 252, 264, 310, 323, 328, 329, 333, 348, 349
cerebral ischemia, 31
cerebrospinal fluid, 5, 27
c-Fos, 209, 233, 234, 241, 244, 247, 266, 283
channel blocker, 90, 233, 320
channels, 15, 19, 21, 79, 80, 85, 86, 90, 100, 108, 133, 134, 147, 191, 282, 285, 288, 312, 336, 339, 346, 349, 350, 352, 353, 354, 359, 365
chemical, ix, x, 53, 80, 85, 114, 116, 143, 167, 169, 170, 227
chemistry, 115
chemotherapy, 78
Chicago, 213
childhood, 2, 258
children, 7, 26
China, 78
Chinese, 74
cholecystokinin, 346, 350
cholesterol, 8, 9, 30, 35, 36, 42
cholinergic, 2, 15, 21, 23, 25, 28, 29, 38, 51, 123, 124, 235, 250, 376
cholinergic neurons, 15, 21, 28, 29, 38, 124
chromaffin cells, 58
chromatin, 11, 24, 27
chronic, x, 40, 71, 98, 103, 139, 172, 177, 178, 181, 185, 198, 204, 205, 206, 209, 216, 242, 243, 260, 267, 291
chronic stress, 242
circular dichroism (CD), 346, 347
circulation, 364, 367, 370, 371
classes, 9, 13, 102, 131, 236, 252
classical, 17, 33, 39, 56, 95, 195, 271, 292, 329
classical conditioning, 33, 195, 271, 329
classification, 128, 167, 223
classified, 119, 121, 200, 236
cleavage, 3, 9, 81
clinical, vii, 1, 9, 15, 18, 28, 41, 78, 96, 97, 115, 121, 135, 142, 171, 185, 187, 204, 265, 289
clinical diagnosis, vii, 1
clinical symptoms, 265
clinical trial, 15, 41, 96
clinical trials, 96
clinician, 186
clone, 39
cloning, 42, 71, 78, 102, 111, 349
clozapine, 242, 258
clustering, 12, 62
clusters, 123
CNQX, 274
Co, 126, 276, 295, 298, 299, 337
cocaine, x, 177, 178, 179, 181, 182, 183, 184, 185, 186, 187, 188, 189, 190, 191, 192, 193, 194, 195, 196, 197, 198, 199, 200, 201, 202, 204, 205, 206, 207, 208, 209, 210, 211, 212, 213, 214, 215, 216, 217, 218, 219, 220, 244, 254, 262, 288
cocaine abuse, 184, 186, 205, 219
cocaine use, 184, 185, 187, 204, 206
codes, 256, 337
coding, 54, 218, 251, 252, 314, 335, 341, 342
cofilin, 27
cognition, 2, 23, 25, 33, 52, 68, 140, 165, 248, 250, 260, 261, 375
cognitive, viii, x, 2, 3, 5, 7, 9, 13, 15, 18, 20, 29, 30, 39, 40, 41, 96, 116, 121, 143, 185, 202, 204, 211, 219, 221, 222, 226, 237, 239, 241, 242, 243, 244, 245, 246, 249, 256, 258, 259, 260, 261, 264, 293, 333, 338, 339, 341, 371, 372
cognitive abilities, 245
cognitive alterations, 40
cognitive deficit, 2, 5, 9, 15, 20, 30, 116
cognitive deficits, 2, 5, 9, 15, 20, 30, 116
cognitive dysfunction, 3, 243, 293
cognitive function, x, 13, 15, 39, 41, 143, 221, 241, 242, 245, 258, 264
cognitive impairment, 7, 20, 39, 40, 41, 243, 249
cognitive map, 333, 338, 341
cognitive performance, 8, 29, 256, 293
cognitive process, 226, 244, 245
cognitive processing, 226, 244
coil, xii, 345, 347, 348, 349, 350, 351, 354
collateral, 53, 84, 124, 165, 286, 289, 320, 323, 325, 334
Columbia, 77
Columbia University, 77
combat, 247
communication, 17, 48, 115, 165, 270, 329, 364
competition, 69, 343
complement, 17, 39, 61, 121, 131
complement pathway, 17
complementary, 334
complexity, 115, 122, 125, 141, 168
complications, 135

components, 3, 8, 17, 20, 62, 84, 121, 174, 256, 265, 310, 319, 352, 369
composition, 4, 5, 6, 31, 65, 275, 282, 351
compounds, 79, 80, 166, 232, 233
compression, 322
compulsion, 211, 213, 216, 219
computation, 145
computational theory, 340
computed tomography, 184
computer, 203
Computer simulation, 226
concentrates, 354
concentration, 13, 18, 32, 52, 58, 66, 86, 119, 131, 133, 146, 147, 148, 150, 151, 211, 227, 277, 280, 281, 291, 320, 364, 365
conditioned response, 104, 152, 153, 201, 289
conditioned stimulus, 152, 153, 196, 197, 232, 233, 234, 238, 262, 271, 364, 365
conditioning, xi, 31, 54, 55, 56, 93, 94, 95, 152, 153, 181, 191, 196, 197, 201, 202, 203, 208, 216, 217, 232, 234, 238, 240, 241, 246, 251, 252, 261, 265, 267, 269, 271, 275, 277, 280, 281, 282, 283, 284, 285, 287, 289, 290, 316, 330, 335, 338, 339, 352, 355
conductance, 62, 67, 150, 311
configuration, 125, 248, 315, 325, 327
conflict, 240
conflict resolution, 240
conformational, 115
confounding variables, 198
Congress, iv
connectivity, xii, 6, 19, 31, 115, 123, 136, 164, 179, 223, 224, 242, 246, 267, 285, 310, 314, 322, 323, 328, 332
conscious awareness, 270
consciousness, 373
consensus, 236, 348
conservation, 32
consolidation, xi, 13, 23, 27, 30, 41, 53, 68, 71, 73, 94, 180, 195, 209, 215, 221, 223, 232, 234, 235, 240, 241, 244, 246, 256, 265, 266, 267, 270, 278, 280, 281, 283, 284, 287, 333
constraints, 342
consumption, x, 10, 98, 177, 178, 179, 185, 191, 195, 196, 198, 200, 207, 208
context-dependent, 64, 322
contiguity, 337
continuing, 33, 324
continuity, 133
continuous reinforcement, 195
contralateral hemisphere, 165
control, 4, 5, 9, 19, 23, 27, 29, 37, 38, 52, 55, 63, 97, 98, 104, 108, 109, 121, 131, 141, 171, 173, 178, 183, 184, 185, 186, 187, 188, 192, 194, 198, 199, 202, 203, 204, 213, 235, 249, 257, 260, 270, 278, 283, 289, 290, 292, 293, 324, 328, 329, 334, 335, 336, 346, 353, 355, 369, 370, 371, 374
control group, 131, 183, 184, 187, 192, 198, 199
controlled, 126, 151, 167, 190, 198, 208, 219, 257, 329, 338, 348, 362
convergence, 24, 252, 368
conversion, 81, 83, 107, 120, 329
copyright, iv
correlation, 152, 189, 259, 314, 322
correlations, 234
cortex, ix, xi, 14, 21, 25, 34, 52, 54, 69, 91, 92, 94, 97, 100, 106, 109, 114, 121, 122, 124, 132, 133, 135, 136, 138, 140, 141, 143, 144, 145, 148, 152, 153, 164, 167, 168, 188, 194, 198, 220, 221, 222, 224, 230, 232, 247, 249, 250, 253, 254, 258, 259, 260, 261, 262, 263, 264, 265, 266, 267, 269, 271, 272, 275, 314, 323, 326, 327, 328, 329, 330, 333, 334, 335, 336, 337, 338, 341, 351, 365, 369, 370, 371, 374, 375
cortical, x, xii, 3, 8, 15, 23, 29, 38, 53, 92, 94, 121, 122, 125, 132, 135, 139, 140, 141, 153, 172, 177, 180, 184, 185, 186, 188, 193, 195, 198, 199, 200, 205, 206, 208, 212, 216, 217, 218, 223, 224, 235, 239, 245, 246, 249, 250, 251, 252, 255, 256, 260, 262, 263, 264, 268, 272, 274, 275, 276, 277, 310, 311, 330, 335, 341, 343, 361, 362, 363, 364, 365, 366, 367, 368, 369, 370, 371, 372, 373, 375, 376
cortical inhibition, 263
cortical neurons, 4, 8, 29, 246, 260, 268, 331, 365, 369, 372
cortical processing, 343
corticospinal, 51, 73, 353
corticosteroids, 7
corticosterone, 267, 287, 288
Corticosterone, 299
couples, 150, 262
coupling, 40, 109, 228, 239, 274
covering, 47
COX-1, 93, 280
COX-2, 82, 83, 93, 280, 288, 293, 294, 299, 302, 306
COX-2 inhibitors, 280
CP, 79
CPCCOEt, 276
CR, 152, 153
craving, 178, 184, 185, 186, 187, 192, 195, 197, 202, 203, 204, 205, 211, 212, 215, 217, 219, 220, 244, 262
CREB, 5, 25, 46, 55, 74, 178, 210, 211, 222, 227, 237, 243, 245, 250, 254, 265, 283, 284, 297, 299, 303

cross-linking, 59, 347, 349, 351
crosstalk, 17
cross-talk, 61, 67, 181, 182, 280
CS, 152, 153, 196, 251, 334
CTA, 354, 355
C-terminal, 50, 62, 107
C-terminus, 146, 148
cues, 12, 185, 186, 187, 197, 201, 202, 205, 213, 220, 239, 289, 315, 316, 326, 327, 331, 336, 363
culture, 28, 78, 91, 105, 107
cycles, 39, 289, 312, 324, 326, 350, 367
cyclic AMP, 67, 148, 222, 227, 346, 353
cycling, 12, 32
cyclins, 12
cyclooxygenase, 93, 104, 108, 280
cyclooxygenase-2, 93, 104, 280
cytochrome, 82, 171, 336
cytochrome oxidase, 336
cytokine, 18
cytoplasm, 119, 146, 147
cytoskeleton, 12, 14, 20, 46, 51, 58, 59, 71, 346, 350, 356, 358
cytosol, 48, 60, 83
cytosolic, 51

D

DA, 87, 122, 125, 126, 132, 188, 189, 191, 192, 193, 194, 197, 198, 200, 204, 205, 207, 208, 222, 231, 242, 265, 334, 335, 338, 362
de novo, 83
death, vii, 1, 31, 34, 64, 133
decay, 84, 311, 319, 333
decisions, 337
declarative memory, xii, 180, 226, 310, 328
decoding, 155, 330
defects, 9, 21, 38
deficiency, 11, 53, 64, 211, 364, 370
deficit, 11, 24, 42, 54, 93, 96, 207, 241, 248, 275, 352, 364, 373, 374
deficits, 7, 9, 11, 12, 18, 20, 23, 24, 25, 28, 29, 35, 38, 64, 72, 116, 121, 153, 154, 217, 237, 241, 242, 283, 286, 290, 333, 340, 341, 364, 372, 373, 374
degenerate, 123
degenerative conditions, 21
degenerative disease, 121
degradation, 26, 64, 82, 83, 93, 109, 352
degree, 2, 3, 10, 12, 13, 132, 233, 278, 290, 328, 337
delays, 229, 239, 250
delivery, 8, 10, 33, 39, 55, 62, 70, 142, 218, 278, 290
delta, 106, 255
demand, viii, 77, 80
dementia, 3, 4, 6, 7, 21, 25, 27, 29, 35, 37, 39
dendrite, 3, 118, 119, 120, 129, 141, 225, 279, 348
dendrites, vii, ix, 1, 2, 4, 10, 15, 19, 33, 46, 51, 54, 55, 60, 71, 73, 85, 113, 117, 118, 119, 123, 124, 125, 127, 133, 139, 141, 144, 146, 150, 164, 181, 218, 224, 225, 228, 230, 236, 242, 245, 262, 264, 275, 282, 285, 287, 313, 336, 349, 350
dendritic spines, ix, xii, 4, 5, 6, 10, 13, 19, 24, 26, 27, 28, 33, 35, 60, 62, 73, 114, 117, 118, 119, 124, 127, 129, 133, 135, 137, 139, 140, 142, 165, 173, 213, 218, 224, 230, 236, 242, 262, 264, 275, 281, 287, 345, 346, 348, 350, 352, 353, 354, 355, 356, 357, 358
denervation, 64, 130, 131, 206, 210
density, viii, xii, 2, 5, 6, 9, 13, 15, 17, 19, 23, 24, 31, 34, 38, 42, 45, 46, 48, 68, 69, 70, 71, 72, 73, 74, 115, 116, 117, 119, 120, 121, 124, 127, 132, 133, 136, 185, 213, 215, 237, 244, 275, 280, 291, 345, 346, 348, 352
dentate gyrus (DG), 18, 26, 36, 41, 53, 55, 68, 85, 136, 164, 169, 170, 271, 285, 289, 312, 320, 334, 335, 338, 339, 340, 343
dephosphorylation, xii, 47, 59, 61, 62, 265, 345, 352, 354, 358
depolarization, 15, 22, 55, 85, 86, 87, 88, 90, 91, 97, 101, 105, 106, 107, 110, 146, 147, 149, 150, 151, 165, 182, 183, 197, 273, 275, 277, 311, 312
deposition, vii, 1, 3, 30
depressed, xi, 199, 249, 269, 278, 363
depression, vii, ix, x, xi, 10, 11, 41, 46, 53, 71, 84, 87, 89, 91, 99, 100, 102, 103, 104, 105, 108, 143, 145, 149, 165, 173, 177, 179, 181, 184, 198, 206, 209, 210, 213, 214, 215, 218, 219, 220, 221, 222, 225, 226, 233, 235, 241, 242, 243, 245, 246, 248, 249, 250, 253, 254, 255, 256, 257, 258, 261, 265, 269, 274, 287, 289, 310, 311, 319, 322, 334, 336, 337, 338, 339, 340, 342, 346, 351, 352, 357
depressive symptoms, 251
derivatives, 101, 280
desensitization, 62, 72
desire, 185, 187, 202, 203, 204
detection, 27, 73, 91, 95, 147, 180, 313, 334, 338, 375
detoxification, 289
developing brain, 17, 174
developmental change, 50
developmental process, 114
DG, 332
DHA, 9
DHT, 235
diabetes, 7, 8, 9, 28, 32, 35, 37, 39, 41
diabetes mellitus, 35, 37, 39
diacylglycerol, 82, 83, 88, 104, 108, 146

diagnostic, 187
Diagnostic and Statistical Manual of Mental Disorders, 184, 204
diagnostic criteria, 187
dialysis, 211
Diamond, 285, 296, 307
diet, 22, 31
dietary, 9, 29, 30
diets, 35
differentiation, 10, 15, 34, 56, 64, 73, 98, 136, 181, 202
diffusion, 103, 119, 148
dimer, 55, 352
dimerization, 55, 74
direct action, 90
direction control, 151
directionality, 317, 319
discharges, 167, 168, 265, 370
discontinuity, 128
discounting, 225
Discovery, 1, 74, 107
discrimination, 240, 336
discrimination learning, 336
discriminative stimuli, 317
disease model, 26
disease progression, 354
diseases, vii, 1, 5, 64, 67, 121
disinhibition, xii, 361, 365, 367, 368, 370
disorder, vii, 1, 3, 19, 20, 22, 63, 64, 178, 197, 206, 243, 250, 253, 287, 364, 373, 374
disposition, 117
dissociation, 50, 55, 62, 74, 79, 337, 339, 342, 353
distal, 10, 124, 264, 315, 327, 341
distortions, 4
distributed memory, 338
distribution, xii, 9, 10, 22, 36, 39, 50, 51, 52, 56, 68, 72, 74, 119, 205, 207, 220, 260, 282, 332, 345, 355, 357, 358
divergence, 317, 368
diversity, viii, 77, 226, 249, 356
division, 120, 121, 174
DNA, 40, 55, 100, 170
DNA damage, 40
Docosahexaenoic, 23
docosahexaenoic acid, 9, 27, 31, 32
domain structure, 47, 49, 347
dominance, 54, 56, 73, 119, 216
donor, 280
dopamine agonist, 376
dopamine antagonists, 263
dopaminergic, ix, xiii, 12, 19, 66, 92, 113, 114, 121, 123, 124, 125, 126, 130, 131, 138, 140, 141, 142, 181, 182, 183, 188, 191, 194, 195, 199, 204, 206, 209, 211, 212, 215, 216, 217, 218, 219, 229, 235, 236, 252, 253, 255, 259, 263, 287, 354, 361, 362, 363, 364, 365, 366, 367, 368, 369, 370, 371, 372, 373, 376
dopaminergic modulation, 263
dopaminergic neurons, 19, 92, 124, 142, 181, 183, 191, 199, 216, 217, 365, 368, 371, 373
dorsolateral prefrontal cortex, 194, 251, 252, 256, 261, 267
down-regulation, xii, 3, 60, 250, 291, 345
drinking, 96, 289
drinking pattern, 289
drinking patterns, 289
Drosophila, 28, 58
drug abuse, 96, 184, 207, 216, 220
drug addict, vii, x, xi, 96, 177, 178, 184, 185, 187, 190, 195, 196, 197, 204, 205, 206, 208, 211, 221, 241, 244, 245, 294
drug addiction, vii, x, xi, 96, 177, 178, 184, 185, 187, 190, 195, 196, 197, 204, 205, 206, 208, 211, 221, 241, 244, 245, 294
drug consumption, 182, 185, 186, 195, 202, 203, 204, 205, 208
drug dependence, 210
drug discovery, 211
drug exposure, 191, 197
drug targets, 164
drug treatment, 187
drug use, 202, 204, 212
drug withdrawal, 288
drug-induced, 178, 181, 195
drug-related, 185, 186, 197
drug-resistant, 167, 270
drugs, 78, 96, 133, 178, 179, 185, 189, 191, 192, 194, 195, 196, 197, 201, 203, 210, 215, 218, 219, 243, 265, 280, 288
DSE, 84, 86, 87, 93, 95, 150
DSM, 184, 204
DSM-II, 184
DSM-III, 184
DSM-IV, 204
duality, 18
duplication, 49
durability, 272
duration, 166, 259, 311, 369
dysfunctional, 2, 4, 15
dyskinesia, 110, 217
dysregulated, 64
dysregulation, 18, 19

E

E6, 64

EA, 82, 335
eating, 241
eating disorders, 241
ecology, 218
edema, 116, 130, 131
Eden, 236, 266
Education, 332
EEG, 166, 168, 209, 265, 374
efficacy, vii, xi, 1, 2, 16, 17, 24, 36, 63, 83, 84, 90, 96, 105, 115, 126, 133, 136, 145, 148, 151, 180, 193, 198, 206, 207, 234, 250, 252, 253, 309, 310, 313, 334, 338, 365, 372
EGF, 171
EI, 335, 336, 337, 338, 339, 341
Einstein, 5, 26
elaboration, 249
elderly, 7, 24, 25, 30, 41
electrical, 18, 115, 120, 131, 152, 165, 167, 168, 169, 174, 180, 182, 189, 247, 253, 266, 271, 289, 291, 316, 351, 354
electrodes, 182, 198, 199, 273
electron, 16, 27, 47, 49, 50, 60, 70, 116, 117, 118, 119, 127, 138, 246, 247, 266, 277, 287, 359
electron density, 116, 117, 118
electron microscopy, 16, 49, 50, 70, 119, 247, 277, 287, 359
electronic, iv
electrophysiological, xi, 91, 97, 131, 141, 152, 209, 238, 252, 260, 265, 277, 290, 309, 374
electrophysiological properties, 97, 141, 260
electrophysiological study, 252
electrophysiology, 125, 136, 372
electrostatic, iv
elongation, 119
embryo, 30
embryonic, 11, 13
emission, 184
emotion, 179, 193, 260, 270, 375
emotional, x, xi, 38, 177, 178, 179, 184, 185, 186, 187, 194, 195, 201, 207, 208, 223, 231, 237, 238, 241, 247, 254, 256, 259, 269, 270, 285, 287, 289, 291, 292, 294
emotional disorder, 241
emotional memory, 287
emotional processes, 194
emotional responses, x, 177, 178, 195, 201, 254, 292
emotional state, 186
emotions, 180, 223, 231
encoding, vi, x, xii, 3, 52, 79, 100, 163, 164, 165, 239, 248, 249, 257, 266, 270, 309, 310, 317, 324, 325, 332, 334, 335, 336, 340, 343
endocrine, 271
endocytosis, 10, 12, 24, 60, 146, 355
endogenous, viii, 18, 48, 58, 77, 78, 80, 82, 96, 99, 100, 101, 102, 103, 104, 105, 106, 109, 110, 141, 206, 226, 229, 237, 257, 258, 279, 281, 312
endoplasmic reticulum, 146, 147
Endothelial, 299, 302
energy, 8, 28, 133, 141
energy supply, 133
engineering, 53
English, 10, 26, 262
Enhancement, 14, 93, 189, 213, 296, 297, 298, 306
enlargement, 119, 120, 133, 315, 365
entorhinal cortex, 39, 164, 224, 270, 272, 274, 287, 314, 324, 326, 327, 328, 335, 341
environment, 126, 131, 179, 197, 201, 202, 213, 222, 242, 252, 314, 315, 316, 317, 318, 319, 320, 322, 326, 327, 331, 339, 342
environmental, ix, x, 113, 114, 115, 135, 177, 178, 180, 185, 195, 201, 208, 219, 313, 314, 316, 317, 319, 326, 328, 331, 337, 342
environmental change, 114
environmental conditions, 180
environmental context, 328
environmental stimuli, x, 177, 180, 195, 201, 208, 317
enzymatic, 82, 83, 99, 107, 277
enzyme, 50, 53, 57, 63, 64, 69, 81, 94, 280, 346
enzymes, viii, 28, 51, 56, 61, 66, 77, 81, 94, 95, 102, 346, 349
epidemiological, 9, 26
epidemiology, 10
epidermal, 171
epidermal growth factor, 171
epigenetic, 11
epigenetic mechanism, 11
epilepsy, x, xi, 17, 64, 68, 163, 164, 167, 168, 169, 170, 171, 172, 174, 269, 285, 289, 292
epileptic seizures, 171
epileptogenesis, 164, 167, 171, 172, 174, 175
episodic, xi, 238, 249, 263, 270, 309, 318, 323, 330, 332, 336, 339, 340, 341
episodic memory, xi, 238, 263, 270, 309, 330, 336, 339, 340, 341
epitopes, 7
equilibrium, 282, 349
ER, 146, 332, 337, 343
ERK1, 10, 38, 222, 235, 283
ES, 341
essential fatty acids, 9
ester, 279
esters, 83, 105, 108
estradiol, 21, 42
estrogen, 21, 23, 37, 138, 300, 304
ET, 337, 340, 341, 342

etanercept, 40
ethanol, 98, 304, 306
ethanolamine, 80, 82, 98
etiology, 126, 253
EU, 332
eukaryotic, 48
eukaryotic cell, 48
euphoria, 185
Europe, 22, 110
European, 22, 23, 24, 28, 36, 41, 160, 258, 332
European Commission, 332
event-related potential, 372, 374
evidence, vii, x, xii, 1, 3, 4, 5, 6, 8, 9, 13, 15, 18, 26, 30, 70, 78, 80, 81, 85, 90, 91, 94, 96, 101, 115, 116, 133, 135, 142, 165, 169, 174, 177, 179, 180, 181, 184, 185, 194, 201, 203, 211, 212, 213, 232, 233, 235, 238, 240, 241, 247, 248, 249, 251, 253, 254, 263, 267, 275, 278, 280, 281, 282, 283, 287, 293, 319, 323, 325, 345, 352, 354, 357, 372, 373, 374
evoked potential, 233
evolution, 73, 115, 130, 204
excitability, 62, 97, 100, 132, 153, 164, 167, 168, 171, 173, 191, 207, 211, 216, 251, 252, 260, 280, 287, 310
excitation, 84, 85, 86, 87, 106, 109, 139, 149, 150, 250, 251, 332, 343, 363, 365, 366, 367, 368, 369, 370, 371
excitatory postsynaptic potentials, 193, 224, 255, 275
excitatory synapses, 73, 92, 93, 95, 105, 118, 144, 151, 153, 181, 184, 189, 191, 193, 197, 198, 208, 209, 223, 253, 327, 340, 348
excitement, 85, 107
excitotoxic, ix, 114, 120, 133
excitotoxicity, 133, 173
execution, 121
executive function, 202, 205, 222, 223, 226, 240, 262, 264
executive functions, 202, 205, 222, 223, 262, 264
exocytosis, 10, 58, 66, 72
exogenous, 192, 193
experimental condition, 120, 131, 165
experimental design, 201
expert, iv
explicit memory, 53, 248
exposure, 14, 29, 71, 92, 103, 106, 167, 179, 187, 189, 191, 198, 200, 204, 209, 216, 218, 219, 228, 229, 232, 233, 234, 236, 242, 247, 252, 258, 289, 306, 311, 314
extinction, 93, 94, 95, 106, 192, 196, 230, 232, 233, 234, 235, 238, 240, 243, 246, 247, 248, 250, 251, 252, 253, 254, 257, 258, 259, 260, 262, 263, 264, 266, 267, 268, 280
extracellular, vii, 1, 3, 5, 7, 10, 15, 30, 35, 48, 52, 82, 87, 98, 132, 138, 188, 197, 204, 209, 214, 222, 235, 252, 254, 260, 265, 274, 275, 283, 285, 291, 346, 348
extrinsic, 16, 123
eye, 151, 152, 270
eye contact, 270
eye movement, 151
eyelid, 338
eyes, 367

F

facial expression, 270
FAD, 9, 12, 22
failure, 3, 16, 33, 36, 38, 115
FAK, 79, 101
false, 261
familial, 3, 9, 22, 26, 39
family, 9, 12, 13, 23, 29, 41, 48, 55, 62, 67, 72, 79, 132, 350, 358
family members, 12
fascia, 340
fatty acid, 9, 29, 31, 32, 34, 82, 100, 101, 108, 280
fatty acids, 29, 34
fax, 163
fear, xi, 31, 53, 54, 55, 94, 230, 231, 232, 233, 234, 235, 238, 240, 241, 243, 246, 247, 248, 250, 251, 252, 253, 254, 255, 257, 258, 259, 260, 261, 262, 263, 264, 267, 268, 269, 270, 271, 275, 277, 280, 281, 282, 283, 284, 285, 287, 289, 291, 316, 339, 352, 355, 359
fear response, 232, 234, 238, 263, 271, 276, 289
fears, 249
feedback, xiii, 62, 85, 122, 145, 328, 329, 335, 361, 362, 366, 368
feelings, 180, 184, 204
females, 36, 285
fertilization, 212
FES, 113, 114
fetal, 39, 220
FGF-2, 42
fiber, ix, x, 28, 53, 84, 138, 143, 144, 145, 146, 147, 148, 149, 150, 151, 152, 153, 163, 165, 169, 170, 171, 172, 174, 248, 286, 332, 336
fibers, ix, 3, 51, 88, 113, 124, 130, 144, 145, 147, 148, 149, 150, 151, 152, 164, 169, 197, 206, 207, 260, 270, 272, 274, 276, 278, 279, 280, 286, 291, 293, 336
fibrillar, vii, 1, 3
fibrils, 5
fibroblast, 13, 37, 42, 171
fibroblast growth factor, 13, 37, 42, 171

fibroblasts, 12, 15
filament, 46, 59, 346, 357, 358
filopodia, 4, 60
filters, 226
filtration, 48
fire, 132, 196, 234, 239, 310, 314, 316, 317, 324
fish, 10, 29, 34, 79, 111
flexibility, 28, 199, 226, 240, 242, 249, 274
flow, 122, 165, 179, 195, 200, 208
fluorescence, 279
fluoxetine, 189, 243, 250, 265, 266
fluvoxamine, 260
fMRI, 185, 202, 222, 243, 248, 255
focal adhesion kinase, 101
focusing, 116, 367
folding, 347, 358
food, 126, 196, 197, 198, 209, 219, 247
forebrain, 15, 21, 50, 51, 54, 71, 72, 73, 126, 235, 258, 263
forgetting, x, 178
fornix, 230
Fox, 69, 110, 343, 376
FP, 335, 338, 340
fragile X syndrome, 31, 34, 35, 37, 43, 256
Framingham study, 9
France, 345
freedom, 328, 329
freezing, 252, 267, 316
Freud, 180, 212
frontal cerebral cortex, 64
frontal cortex, 71, 132, 165, 210, 212, 215, 247, 251, 252, 255, 256, 257, 259, 260, 261, 267
frontal lobe, 255, 256, 257, 258, 263, 264
frontotemporal dementia, 264
fuel, 8
functional activation, 142
functional architecture, 257, 330
functional changes, 170, 197, 206, 208, 291
functional imaging, 270
functional magnetic resonance imaging, 185, 222, 375
functional memory, xi, 309
Fur, 99
fusion, 34, 57, 70, 282
FXS, 19

G

G protein, 79, 99, 107, 108, 150, 244, 349, 359
GABA, 8, 46, 79, 85, 86, 87, 88, 89, 90, 93, 103, 104, 105, 122, 123, 149, 150, 188, 207, 248, 264, 266, 273, 278, 295, 301, 362
$GABA_B$, 149, 168, 277
GABAergic, 5, 15, 79, 85, 89, 92, 94, 97, 100, 101, 102, 103, 104, 108, 109, 110, 123, 124, 131, 144, 148, 150, 195, 209, 226, 229, 230, 234, 247, 252, 255, 271, 274, 279, 292, 342, 353, 363, 365
game theory, 218
ganglia, xii, 121, 122, 136, 267, 361, 362, 366, 372, 376
Ganglia, vi, 137, 141, 217, 361
ganglion, 15, 16, 137
gastrin, 288
GC, 144, 153
GDP, 350
gel, 48
gender, xi, 9, 269, 285, 288
gender differences, 285
gene, x, xi, 3, 9, 11, 13, 19, 25, 27, 33, 36, 39, 40, 41, 42, 48, 49, 52, 55, 56, 64, 65, 66, 67, 71, 72, 74, 79, 91, 97, 134, 137, 163, 170, 171, 172, 175, 212, 233, 234, 237, 241, 247, 249, 252, 259, 260, 269, 279, 281, 282, 283, 346, 351, 352, 355, 358
gene arrays, 171
gene expression, x, xi, 3, 11, 14, 27, 36, 48, 55, 56, 66, 91, 134, 137, 163, 170, 171, 172, 212, 234, 252, 260, 269, 346
gene promoter, 40, 247
gene silencing, 19
gene targeting, 11, 355
gene therapy, 41
gene transfer, 39
generalization, 277, 289
generation, 55, 92, 98, 110, 121, 227, 230, 315, 335, 337
genes, 3, 30, 41, 43, 49, 52, 54, 64, 73, 79, 111, 170, 171, 244, 263, 351
genetic, x, 7, 11, 22, 29, 53, 55, 64, 65, 68, 126, 134, 136, 143, 152, 211, 236, 277, 320
genetic factors, 22
genetics, 136, 246
genomic, 287
genomics, 79
genotype, 26, 29, 31, 33
GFP, 147
GL, 333, 334, 335, 340
glass, 126
glaucoma, 78
GlaxoSmithKline, 1
glia, 2, 16, 18, 28, 36, 40, 41, 282, 287, 349
glial, 13, 15, 22, 28, 29, 34, 36, 39, 260
glial cells, 13, 15, 28, 29, 36
glioma, 100, 105
gliosis, 164
globalization, 377
globus, 121, 122, 363, 364, 367

glucocorticoid receptor, 287
glucocorticoids, 192
glucose, 7, 15, 24, 25, 28, 30, 39, 184, 255
glucose metabolism, 7, 25, 184, 255
glucose regulation, 7, 30
glucose tolerance, 7, 24, 39
glutamate, x, 5, 8, 12, 15, 17, 20, 21, 22, 29, 61, 62, 66, 67, 79, 86, 87, 88, 89, 90, 91, 93, 94, 97, 102, 110, 111, 118, 125, 126, 131, 132, 133, 138, 139, 141, 145, 146, 148, 150, 165, 173, 177, 178, 181, 182, 188, 189, 190, 198, 199, 200, 204, 206, 207, 208, 210, 213, 214, 220, 226, 230, 237, 242, 243, 248, 250, 254, 267, 274, 276, 277, 280, 282, 283, 285, 289, 342, 350, 351, 352, 355
glutamate receptor antagonists, 191
glutamatergic, xii, 2, 15, 19, 24, 25, 66, 70, 79, 87, 89, 91, 92, 93, 94, 98, 102, 103, 106, 119, 122, 124, 125, 126, 131, 132, 136, 137, 144, 181, 188, 189, 194, 195, 204, 205, 206, 207, 215, 219, 236, 246, 252, 253, 259, 261, 265, 273, 282, 289, 311, 345, 348, 349, 351, 352, 353, 354, 355, 365
glutaraldehyde, 127
glycerol, 83, 105, 106, 107, 150
glycine, 148, 165, 173, 274
glycogen, 25, 26, 29, 32, 42, 43
glycogen synthase kinase, 25, 26, 29, 32, 42, 43
glycoprotein, 13
goal-directed, x, 121, 178, 194, 199, 200, 202, 208, 212
goal-directed behavior, x, 178, 194, 199, 200, 202, 208, 212
goals, 202, 318
gold, 137
Golgi complex, 10
government, iv
GPCR, 79
G-protein, 60, 78, 79, 80, 87, 90, 292, 293, 346, 349, 357, 359
grants, 97
granule cells, 26, 85, 143, 144, 145, 172, 174, 334
graph, 339
gray matter, 51, 211
groups, 48, 85, 132, 141, 192, 195, 198, 199, 200, 233, 261, 274, 282, 325, 332
growth, ix, x, 2, 4, 8, 13, 26, 27, 28, 30, 33, 35, 37, 39, 41, 42, 55, 69, 71, 79, 91, 113, 134, 140, 163, 170, 171, 209, 242
growth factor, x, 8, 13, 27, 39, 55, 71, 163, 170, 171
growth factors, x, 55, 163
GSK-3, 11, 12, 22, 28, 29
guanine, xii, 283, 345, 346, 349, 356
guidance, 12, 13, 27, 34, 39, 41
Guinea, 154, 155, 160
gut, 82, 106
Gyrus, 39, 164, 295, 297, 302, 307

H

Haj, 102
half-life, 20
haloperidol, 374
handling, 52
head, ix, 4, 113, 115, 119, 124, 125, 151, 164, 195, 319, 323, 325, 326, 327, 328, 333, 335, 337, 340, 341, 343, 348, 374
head trauma, 164
health, 207
heart, 100, 107
heart failure, 100
heavy metal, 169
heavy metals, 169
height, 315
hemp, 78
hepatocellular, 358
hepatocellular carcinoma, 358
heroin, 214, 218
heterogeneity, 244
heterooligomers, 73
heterotrimeric, 150
heterozygote, 227, 228
heterozygotes, 54
high-frequency, 70, 92, 151, 165, 166, 180, 182, 197, 206, 207, 208, 209, 220, 268, 271, 285, 312, 331, 370
histochemistry, 67
histone, 11, 29, 30, 31
holoenzyme, 49
homeostasis, 27, 39, 292, 319, 342
homogeneity, 154
homogeneous, 22
homology, 10, 12, 13, 70, 274
Honda, 375
hormone, 36, 285
hormones, 215, 287
HPA, 192
HPC, 199, 200
human, vii, 1, 7, 9, 26, 32, 34, 36, 42, 64, 79, 102, 105, 108, 121, 126, 168, 172, 174, 184, 189, 193, 196, 197, 203, 204, 208, 211, 215, 222, 247, 248, 255, 261, 263, 264, 270, 314, 335, 347, 348, 359, 372, 374, 375, 376
human behavior, 193
human brain, vii, 1, 26, 215, 222, 248
human cognition, 64
human experience, 270

humans, 114, 115, 188, 191, 200, 202, 209, 216, 218, 226, 238, 239, 247, 270
Huntington disease, 135
hybrid, 100
hybridization, 67
hydrolysis, 9, 82, 83, 99, 104, 105, 108
hydrolyzed, 81, 83
hydrophobic, 347
hydroxyl, 67
hyperactivity, 7, 126, 131, 364, 373, 374
hyperphosphorylated tau protein, 3
hyperphosphorylation, 11, 32
Hypertension, 110
hypertensive, 292
hypertrophy, 119
hypothalamic, 23, 138, 192, 271
hypothalamic-pituitary-adrenal axis, 192
hypothalamus, 34, 223
hypothesis, xii, 5, 28, 71, 83, 119, 170, 173, 201, 209, 214, 243, 253, 272, 278, 290, 336, 337, 338, 361, 364, 371, 373

I

iconic memory, 370
ICT, 332
identification, 60, 341, 369
identity, 52, 92, 93, 94, 95, 275, 347, 348, 374
IGF, 21, 24
IGF-1, 21, 24
IGT, 7
imagery, 375
images, 6, 185, 187, 195, 197
imagination, 367
imaging, 24, 36, 119, 147, 184, 202, 213, 216, 220, 229, 238, 245
immune cells, 79
immunocytochemistry, 246
immunofluorescence, 260
immunoglobulin, 13, 41
immunoglobulin superfamily, 13, 41
immunohistochemical, 70, 72, 102, 220, 259, 374
immunoreactivity, 140, 264, 282
immunotherapy, 23
impaired glucose tolerance (IGT), 7, 20, 28
impairments, 5, 7, 9, 11, 12, 20, 43, 54, 55, 109, 164, 238, 241, 264, 265
implicit memory, 54
impregnation, 137
impulsive, 195, 200
impulsivity, 211
in situ, 216
in situ hybridization, 216
in vitro, 6, 7, 13, 15, 33, 36, 73, 82, 96, 103, 110, 139, 165, 167, 168, 182, 199, 215, 217, 220, 224, 228, 230, 236, 238, 244, 245, 250, 252, 253, 254, 255, 259, 267, 279, 281, 291, 293, 310, 321, 333, 334, 342, 347, 348, 349, 350
in vivo, 7, 13, 16, 39, 53, 80, 91, 92, 96, 110, 132, 133, 141, 149, 154, 165, 166, 168, 169, 170, 182, 198, 199, 206, 219, 224, 226, 228, 229, 230, 231, 232, 236, 238, 242, 243, 244, 245, 247, 248, 249, 250, 252, 253, 254, 255, 258, 260, 262, 263, 265, 281, 287, 291, 310, 331, 336, 337, 339, 342, 348, 349, 351, 354, 358
inactivation, x, 50, 62, 72, 82, 101, 102, 143, 152, 232, 233, 312
inactive, 50, 54, 148, 317
incentive, 178, 184, 191, 217, 262
incidence, 8, 224
incubation, 6, 212
Indazole, 296
independence, 174, 250
indication, 84
indirect effect, 353
inducible enzyme, 280
induction, x, xi, 5, 10, 11, 20, 21, 35, 37, 53, 55, 56, 62, 83, 91, 92, 94, 95, 99, 105, 106, 108, 120, 132, 133, 145, 146, 147, 148, 149, 150, 151, 163, 166, 170, 171, 173, 178, 181, 183, 190, 191, 192, 193, 199, 200, 206, 207, 208, 219, 226, 227, 228, 229, 231, 236, 237, 244, 245, 252, 254, 256, 258, 259, 261, 269, 270, 271, 272, 274, 276, 277, 278, 279, 280, 281, 286, 289, 290, 292, 293, 311, 312, 319, 320, 321, 334, 337, 338, 339, 340, 341
inductor, 193
inflammatory, 18
information processing, 84, 200, 247, 310, 330, 335
infusions, 193, 197, 201, 241
inhalation, 134, 237
inherited, 19, 241
inhibition, xii, 2, 7, 11, 17, 28, 32, 35, 41, 50, 54, 55, 64, 79, 84, 85, 86, 87, 90, 92, 93, 95, 96, 97, 98, 99, 100, 101, 103, 104, 105, 106, 107, 108, 109, 110, 111, 123, 138, 149, 150, 191, 206, 209, 210, 247, 250, 252, 258, 260, 277, 279, 290, 321, 332, 342, 353, 361, 362, 368, 373
inhibitor, 11, 15, 53, 55, 56, 72, 153, 201, 227, 231, 233, 240, 254, 279, 280, 281, 283
inhibitors, 10, 53, 92, 93, 94, 95, 96, 201, 280, 283, 352
inhibitory, viii, ix, x, 8, 11, 50, 54, 55, 75, 77, 80, 83, 85, 89, 91, 92, 94, 102, 105, 107, 109, 110, 119, 122, 143, 144, 145, 148, 149, 150, 153, 166, 177, 198, 222, 230, 231, 234, 237, 242, 244, 263, 273,

277, 279, 287, 292, 310, 353, 362, 363, 368, 372, 376
inhibitory effect, x, 55, 80, 177, 198, 292
initiation, 190, 214, 262
injection, ix, 8, 114, 116, 126, 132, 138, 187, 189, 192, 193, 201, 206, 224, 275
injections, 126, 190, 198, 213, 263, 289
injury, iv, vii, ix, 1, 2, 5, 20, 113, 133, 164, 209
inner ear, 151
innervation, 24, 125, 133, 141, 149, 197, 204, 257, 264, 287
inositol, 46, 51, 82, 146, 222, 227
insertion, 51, 56, 133, 215, 237, 265, 282
insight, 168, 185, 285, 293, 309, 372
instability, 336
instruction, 329
insulin, 7, 8, 20, 22, 23, 25, 27, 28, 36, 39, 41, 43, 104
insulin resistance, 8
insulin-like growth factor, 8, 22, 23
insulin-like growth factor I, 23
integration, 215, 253, 326, 327, 328, 338, 341, 376
integrin, 149
integrity, 207, 270
intensity, 167, 316, 354, 359, 371
interaction, 9, 13, 30, 53, 56, 58, 59, 60, 62, 67, 68, 69, 70, 73, 74, 79, 114, 132, 148, 155, 157, 160, 178, 182, 207, 208, 215, 250, 252, 293, 307, 311, 312, 327, 333, 335, 336, 341, 346, 348, 349, 350, 351, 354, 356, 357, 358, 359, 367, 373
interactions, xi, 14, 36, 37, 43, 48, 56, 83, 96, 98, 101, 132, 172, 199, 210, 211, 212, 221, 231, 246, 255, 261, 270, 283, 325, 337, 347, 350, 356, 371, 373, 375
interface, 53, 222, 263, 271, 363
interference, 58, 119, 209, 247, 263
interleukin, 18, 36, 37
interleukin-1, 18, 37
intermolecular, 170
interneuron, 101, 224, 334
interneurons, 79, 85, 87, 93, 97, 98, 104, 110, 123, 124, 144, 150, 188, 224, 229, 230, 231, 261, 264, 265, 274, 279, 287, 368, 376
interpretation, 192
interval, 152, 166, 170, 274, 275, 290, 312, 331
intervention, 171, 293
intoxication, 289
intracellular signaling, 12, 148, 165, 178, 179, 181, 182, 201, 208, 211
intracerebral, 190, 281
intracranial, 188, 289
intraperitoneal, 187, 198
intravenous, 187, 200, 217
intravenously, 291
intrinsic, 16, 123, 124, 168, 195, 199, 204, 208, 223, 257, 258, 259, 264, 273, 310, 343
invertebrates, 36
ion channels, 12, 61, 79, 173, 274, 346, 350, 351, 357
ionotropic glutamate receptor, 141, 145, 148, 166, 188, 351
ions, 147, 349
ipsilateral, ix, 114, 129, 130, 131, 132, 165, 230
IQ, 102
Ireland, 309
iron, 82
IRS, 46
ischemia, 30, 164, 172
ischemic, 41, 209
ischemic stroke, 41
isoenzymes, 89
isoforms, 10, 38, 47, 49, 50, 51, 55, 71, 72, 346, 349, 351, 356, 357, 359
isoleucine, 3
isozymes, 71
Ivan Pavlov, 179

J

Japan, 45, 127, 143
judgment, 256
Jun, 220
Jung, 104, 246, 338

K

K^+, 62, 72, 80, 90, 150, 296, 356
kainate receptor, 17, 274, 285, 291
kainic acid, 172, 333
ketamine, 243, 259
kinase, v, viii, 8, 11, 12, 20, 21, 22, 24, 25, 28, 29, 30, 31, 32, 33, 35, 38, 42, 45, 46, 48, 49, 50, 51, 53, 54, 55, 56, 61, 62, 63, 67, 68, 69, 70, 71, 72, 73, 74, 75, 79, 80, 81, 83, 94, 110, 146, 147, 149, 155, 156, 157, 178, 179, 201, 209, 222, 227, 233, 234, 235, 236, 245, 265, 266, 280, 281, 283, 287, 288, 291, 297, 298, 300, 301, 302, 304, 305, 307, 320, 337, 346, 349, 355, 356, 358
kinase activity, 50, 56, 68
kinases, 10, 12, 13, 23, 32, 48, 63, 67, 69, 79, 147, 227, 258, 261, 320, 348
Kinases, 10, 156
kinetics, 166, 252
King, 109
KL, 335

knockout, 11, 20, 27, 33, 35, 36, 53, 73, 81, 85, 87, 89, 91, 92, 94, 95, 98, 101, 110, 148, 149, 153, 201, 213, 217, 227, 228, 320, 338, 346, 358

L

L1, 13, 42, 256
LA, xi, 269, 271, 272, 273, 274, 275, 276, 277, 278, 279, 280, 281, 282, 283, 284, 285, 286, 287, 288, 289, 290, 291, 292, 293
labeling, 282, 337, 349
lack of control, 204
laminated, 223, 274
laminin, 256
land, 181
language, 143
large-scale, 4
latency, xiii, 153, 230, 361, 369, 373
late-onset, 9, 36
layered architecture, 273, 286
LC, 88
LDL, 9
lead, 9, 11, 20, 42, 55, 60, 115, 119, 136, 146, 150, 151, 167, 169, 171, 179, 204, 207, 208, 320, 321, 330, 364, 365, 370
learning disabilities, 169
learning efficiency, 339
learning process, 196, 201, 286, 324, 328, 331
learning task, x, 143, 238, 240
Lesion, 139, 152, 270, 295
lesioning, 18, 126, 127, 131, 133, 230, 231, 232, 233, 244
lesions, vii, ix, 1, 12, 114, 115, 128, 132, 197, 207, 213, 217, 218, 232, 233, 241, 242, 249, 250, 251, 252, 256, 257, 262, 264, 267, 270
leucine, 52, 71
levodopa, 110
LH, 333
life expectancy, 7
lifespan, 73, 186
lifestyles, 22
life-threatening, 287
lifetime, 8
ligand, 23, 80, 82, 96, 102, 107, 109, 148
ligands, viii, 5, 27, 31, 77, 78
likelihood, 94
limbic system, xi, 269, 287, 312
linear, 314, 319, 326
linkage, 281
links, viii, 6, 45, 48, 164, 165, 312, 332
lipase, 82, 83, 88, 101, 150
lipases, 104
lipid, viii, 9, 20, 27, 32, 36, 77, 80, 99, 279
lipid metabolism, 9, 20
lipids, 9, 10, 82
lipoid, 270
lipoprotein, 9, 35
lipoproteins, 9
lipoxygenase, 279
liquid chromatography, 60, 75
literature, x, xi, 7, 48, 131, 221, 223, 233, 269
liver, 43
LM, 335
LOAD, 9
localised, 237
localization, ix, 4, 8, 41, 51, 54, 62, 69, 72, 73, 85, 102, 103, 114, 140, 141, 252, 253, 264, 266, 334, 348, 353, 357, 359, 375
location, 83, 93, 132, 137, 164, 214, 257, 277, 315, 316, 317, 318, 320, 323, 325, 326, 327, 328, 336, 338, 366
location information, 327, 328
locomotion, 199
locomotor activity, x, 53, 177, 187, 188, 189, 192, 193, 195, 198, 213, 217, 219
locus, vii, 2, 20, 64, 207, 235, 247, 364
locus coeruleus, 235, 247
London, 135, 139, 174, 212, 217, 338, 339
Long Term Depression, 156
longitudinal study, 102
long-term memory, 10, 11, 38, 47, 223, 238, 251, 263, 264, 283, 310
loss of control, 205, 369, 373
low molecular weight, 58
low-level, 370
LPA, 83
LSD, 244
luteinizing hormone, 36
lymphoid, 346, 349
lysergic acid diethylamide, 260
lysophosphatidic acid (LPA), 83, 107
lysosomes, 10

M

M.O., 27
M1, 88, 89, 102, 107
machinery, viii, 30, 45, 48, 58, 61, 65, 90, 319
machines, 70
Mackintosh, 202, 215
macrophages, 81
macular degeneration, 29
Madison, 105
magnesium, 168, 274
magnetic, iv, 215, 263
magnetic resonance, 215

magnetic resonance imaging (MRI), 215, 251
maintenance, xi, 6, 8, 16, 29, 53, 55, 72, 121, 130, 131, 173, 191, 207, 231, 253, 269, 270, 272, 289, 320, 352
major depression, xi, 247, 255, 269
maladaptive, ix, x, 113, 178, 206, 248
males, 285
Mammalian, 161, 296, 298
mammalian brain, 136, 180, 181
mammalian cell, 247
mammalian cells, 247
mammals, 32, 116, 180
management, 8
mania, 253, 375
manifold, 39
manipulation, x, 17, 53, 68, 143, 293, 315, 318
manners, viii, 77
MAPK, 8, 10, 11, 12, 22, 25, 40, 70, 79, 147, 179, 267, 283, 302, 346
mapping, 247
marijuana, 78, 102, 237
Mas receptor, 293
masking, 229
mass spectrometry, 72, 74, 75
Massachusetts, 251, 264
maternal, 64
matrix, 123, 170, 218, 328
maturation, 24, 34, 136, 138
maze tasks, 251
MB, 333, 335, 336, 337, 338, 341, 343
MDA, 166
meanings, 329
measures, 24, 185, 188, 192, 193, 198, 203, 232
mechanical, iv
medial prefrontal cortex, x, 220, 221, 222, 223, 246, 247, 248, 249, 251, 252, 253, 254, 256, 257, 259, 260, 261, 262, 263, 264, 265, 266, 267, 337, 373
median, 246
mediation, 278, 285, 291, 293, 337
mediators, viii, 15, 77, 87, 217, 279
medication, 214
medications, 370
medicine, 38, 110
medulla, 87, 110, 144, 149
medulla oblongata, 144, 149
MEG, 374
MEK, 10, 201
membranes, 60, 100, 103, 116, 117, 132
memory capacity, 259
memory deficits, viii, 2, 7, 21, 26, 32, 169
memory formation, xi, 2, 11, 12, 21, 24, 31, 71, 83, 93, 115, 139, 152, 153, 218, 231, 232, 240, 257, 269, 270, 271, 281, 283, 310, 312, 331
memory loss, 27, 30
memory performance, 24, 291
memory processes, 8, 18, 179, 180, 181, 267, 270, 331
memory retrieval, 247, 251, 281, 283
men, 36
mental disorder, vii
mental illness, 246
mental image, 367, 376
mental imagery, 367, 376
mental retardation, 5, 19, 40, 41, 64, 74, 241, 245, 248
mental state, 78
mesencephalon, 141
mesocorticolimbic, x, 177, 208, 220
mesoderm, 42
messages, 38
messengers, 38, 91, 92, 97, 134, 182, 279
metabolic, 8, 11, 36, 185, 219, 226, 243, 252
metabolic changes, 185, 219
metabolism, 26, 28, 43, 82, 96, 99, 101, 107, 141, 184, 185, 219, 220, 233
metabolite, 108
metabolites, 279
metabotropic glutamate receptor, 34, 46, 61, 98, 99, 100, 101, 104, 106, 145, 222, 227, 246, 254, 259, 261, 274
metabotropic glutamate receptors, 61, 99, 100, 101, 104, 227, 261, 274
metazoa, 32
methamphetamine, 220, 244, 247, 254, 260
methylene, 252
methylphenidate, 220
Mexico, 113
Mg^{2+}, 83, 151
mGluR, 46, 61, 87, 89, 92, 93, 95, 106, 132, 147, 150, 222, 227, 228, 244, 259, 276, 277
mGluRs, 87, 89, 90, 95, 227, 228, 236, 244, 261, 274, 276, 277
mice, xi, xii, 7, 9, 10, 11, 18, 20, 21, 24, 25, 27, 30, 31, 33, 35, 36, 38, 52, 53, 54, 55, 64, 65, 70, 73, 81, 85, 89, 91, 92, 94, 95, 98, 101, 110, 115, 135, 139, 153, 154, 171, 173, 174, 184, 187, 200, 201, 207, 210, 211, 213, 217, 227, 228, 229, 251, 253, 254, 256, 259, 266, 267, 269, 273, 274, 276, 279, 280, 281, 282, 286, 292, 293, 334, 338, 345, 352, 353, 354, 358
microarray, 170
microdialysis, 108, 132, 141, 237, 241
microeconomics, 218
microglia, 17, 25
microglial, 99
microglial cells, 99

microscope, 60, 127
microscopy, 6, 39, 125, 353
microtubule, 46, 51, 56, 58, 59, 66, 74, 149, 349, 357
microtubules, 58, 59, 73, 74, 349
midbrain, 123, 138, 140, 178, 182, 183, 184, 188, 189, 191, 192, 193, 195, 197, 204, 206, 212, 216, 217, 375
middle-aged, 7, 37
migration, 13, 15, 35
mild cognitive impairment, vii, 1, 3, 25
mimicking, 13, 53, 226
minority, 225
misfolded, viii, 2
MIT, 105, 138, 251, 264
mitochondria, 133
mitogen, 8, 11, 22, 24, 26, 99, 147, 179, 222, 227, 254, 262, 283, 346
mitogen activated protein kinase, 222
mitogen-activated protein kinase, 8, 22, 26, 38, 40, 99, 147, 179, 227, 254, 262, 283, 346
MK-80, 166, 295
ML, 334, 336, 341, 342
mobility, 58, 73
modality, 372, 373
model system, 51, 169
modeling, x, 70, 163, 168
models, x, xi, xiii, 5, 18, 25, 34, 52, 64, 78, 110, 136, 142, 151, 163, 168, 171, 172, 182, 187, 191, 208, 223, 269, 309, 310, 311, 314, 317, 321, 322, 323, 325, 327, 329, 331, 335, 342, 361, 363, 370, 371
modulation, vii, viii, xii, xiii, 1, 12, 14, 15, 23, 32, 40, 48, 57, 78, 96, 98, 105, 109, 110, 111, 132, 139, 145, 171, 174, 196, 200, 212, 246, 247, 250, 251, 252, 253, 254, 255, 260, 261, 263, 264, 285, 309, 310, 342, 357, 359, 362, 364, 365, 367, 369, 372, 373, 375, 376
modules, 224
molecular biology, 65
molecular markers, 233, 234
molecular mechanisms, viii, ix, x, xi, 11, 12, 48, 56, 78, 109, 143, 145, 177, 179, 201, 208, 209, 221, 232, 240, 245, 263, 265, 272, 281, 355
molecular weight, 58
molecules, viii, xi, 2, 4, 5, 11, 13, 20, 22, 27, 38, 41, 45, 47, 65, 66, 68, 80, 83, 119, 147, 148, 164, 243, 269, 287, 349
monkeys, 215, 216, 256, 260, 263, 375
monoaminergic, 141, 235
monoclonal, 70
monoclonal antibodies, 70
monomer, 348
monomeric, 349
mood, 39, 116, 245, 250, 257, 260, 264, 354, 357
mood disorder, 116, 250, 257, 260, 354, 357
morphine, 64, 71, 209
morphogenesis, 12, 69, 349, 358
morphological, vii, 1, 19, 24, 117, 119, 120, 126, 133, 136, 170, 267, 320
morphology, xii, 2, 4, 5, 6, 14, 34, 48, 59, 115, 119, 140, 218, 241, 247, 249, 262, 267, 285, 345, 346, 350, 351, 352, 356, 358
morphometric, 25, 26, 138
Moscow, 361
motherhood, 138
moths, 185
motion, 151, 152, 314, 326, 367, 369, 376
motivation, x, 92, 177, 178, 179, 194, 197, 202, 210, 212, 214, 262, 264, 375
motor activity, 135, 188, 210, 214, 376
motor area, 145
motor behavior, 64, 203
motor control, ix, 92, 113, 143, 328
motor function, 135, 202, 209
motor neuron disease, 17
mouse, 4, 5, 9, 11, 20, 23, 24, 26, 28, 29, 30, 31, 32, 33, 34, 37, 42, 43, 53, 54, 74, 79, 81, 87, 97, 99, 100, 101, 109, 135, 136, 147, 148, 149, 152, 153, 218, 237, 247, 256, 258, 273, 287, 348, 353
mouse model, 4, 5, 9, 20, 23, 24, 26, 28, 29, 31, 32, 34, 42, 74, 135
mouth, 270
movement, 59, 60, 103, 121, 133, 136, 151, 266, 322, 327, 328, 329, 335, 336, 364, 376
movement disorders, 133, 136
mPFC, 222, 223, 224, 225, 226, 227, 228, 229, 230, 231, 232, 233, 234, 235, 236, 237, 238, 239, 240, 241, 242, 243, 244, 245, 258
MPTP, 110, 140
mRNA, 9, 51, 54, 63, 64, 70, 73, 106, 170, 209, 263, 282
MS, 15, 264, 333, 335, 338, 340
multidimensional, 75
multiple sclerosis, 17, 98
muscarinic receptor, 88, 89, 95, 108, 350
muscle, 102
mutant, 7, 9, 22, 52, 53, 54, 55, 70, 73, 147, 148, 153, 154, 200, 210, 276, 352
mutants, 52, 54, 56
mutation, 54, 68, 281
mutations, 3, 7, 12, 22, 28, 39
MV, 342
myosin, 60, 68, 288

N

NA, 279, 338

Na^+, 15, 356
NAc, x, 92, 97, 177, 178, 179, 182, 186, 188, 190, 191, 193, 194, 197, 198, 199, 200, 201, 203, 204, 208
National Academy of Sciences, 24, 27, 28, 29, 30, 31, 32, 34, 36, 41, 42
National Institutes of Health (NIH), 97
natural, 94, 187, 194, 197, 198, 206, 226, 311, 335
nausea, 78
neck, 4, 115, 119, 125, 195, 348
necrosis, 18, 31, 36
negative consequences, ix, 113
neglect, 375
neocortex, ix, 3, 4, 23, 95, 97, 111, 113, 135, 138, 169, 224, 241, 255, 257, 260, 263, 267, 310, 353, 363, 365, 371, 372
neonatal, 149, 242, 257
neonates, 52
neostriatum, 21, 42, 134, 135, 137, 138, 142, 209, 212, 213, 215, 358
nerve, ix, 13, 26, 29, 31, 37, 41, 46, 50, 55, 60, 65, 66, 90, 113, 132, 164, 166, 171, 222, 243, 263
nerve cells, ix, 60, 65, 113, 164, 166
nerve growth factor, 13, 26, 29, 31, 37, 41, 46, 55, 164, 171
nervous system, ix, xii, 12, 13, 40, 41, 48, 49, 52, 56, 66, 85, 114, 115, 116, 126, 140, 165, 167, 169, 180, 214, 258, 280, 345, 346, 353
network, xi, 48, 51, 52, 59, 60, 85, 102, 122, 140, 145, 194, 239, 249, 267, 268, 277, 279, 285, 309, 311, 314, 317, 318, 319, 321, 322, 323, 325, 326, 328, 330, 332, 333, 336, 337, 338, 340, 342, 346, 350, 359, 362, 371
neural development, 136
neural function, viii, 45, 77, 95
neural network, x, 18, 84, 95, 163, 164, 172, 249, 313, 325, 334, 337, 341, 342, 367
neural networks, x, 18, 84, 95, 163, 164, 249, 313, 337, 341, 367
neural stem cell, 18
neural systems, 181, 193, 211, 270
neural tissue, 357
neuritic plaques, 3, 26
neuroactive peptides, 56
neuroadaptation, 185
neuroadaptations, 216
neuroadaptive, 184, 185
neuroanatomy, 340
neurobiological, 116, 180, 183, 187, 189, 191, 192, 196, 202, 204, 212, 271, 339
neurobiology, 213, 250
neuroblastoma, 51, 55, 63, 68, 69, 71, 73, 75, 97, 99, 100, 105
neurodegeneration, vii, 1, 2, 4, 9, 12, 17, 28, 35, 37, 38, 40, 96, 115, 169
neurodegenerative, vii, 1, 2, 3, 5, 17, 19, 71, 116, 126, 133, 141, 164, 292
neurodegenerative disease, viii, 2, 17, 116, 126, 292
neurodegenerative diseases, viii, 2, 17, 116, 126, 292
neurodegenerative disorders, 5, 134, 141
neurodegenerative processes, 71
neuroendocrine, 242
neurofibrillary tangles, vii, 1, 3, 8, 22, 63
neurogenesis, vii, 1, 2, 18, 42, 171, 243, 263
neuroglia, 16
neuroimaging, 184, 185, 186, 187, 202, 204, 212, 238, 248, 257, 263, 270, 374
neuroimaging techniques, 184, 186, 187, 202, 204
neuroinflammation, 18
neuroleptic, 139
neuroleptics, 132
neurological disease, 57, 133, 173
neurological disorder, xi, 32, 48, 97, 221, 241, 242, 245
neuromodulation, 245
neuromodulator, 81, 235
neuron death, 31
neuronal apoptosis, 12
neuronal cells, 56, 85, 87, 195, 204, 348
neuronal circuits, 274
neuronal death, 133
neuronal degeneration, 12, 22, 30, 169
neuronal density, 141
neuronal excitability, 87, 172
neuronal loss, 42
neuronal migration, xii, 345, 349
neuronal plasticity, 2, 29, 48, 60, 61, 68, 193, 219, 256, 271, 285, 310, 342, 346
neuronal survival, 13, 23, 35
neuronal systems, 2
neuropathological, 3, 22
neuropathology, 141, 170, 172
neuropeptide, 58, 73, 142
neurophysiology, 95
neuroplasticity, 190, 199, 257, 283
neuroprotection, 24, 39, 97
neuroprotective, 22
neuropsychiatric disorders, 294
neuroscience, 114, 293, 364
neuroscientists, 114, 154
neurotoxic, 243
neurotoxicity, 42, 110, 243
neurotoxins, 5, 126, 142
neurotransmission, xii, 54, 78, 79, 91, 109, 110, 119, 133, 134, 246, 248, 253, 259, 289, 345, 346, 353, 354

neurotransmitter, vii, 14, 41, 48, 56, 57, 58, 66, 79, 85, 87, 89, 91, 94, 99, 100, 118, 122, 132, 145, 182, 197, 198, 199, 243, 271, 278, 279, 280, 285, 354
neurotransmitters, vii, ix, 113, 132, 178, 194, 260
neurotrophic, x, 8, 13, 14, 20, 21, 27, 30, 31, 32, 37, 38, 41, 46, 55, 130, 140, 170, 171, 174, 175, 177, 179, 181, 211, 212, 213, 217, 220, 222, 233
neurotrophic factors, 13, 20, 38, 170, 171, 174
neutral stimulus, 152, 196
New England, 37
New Frontier, 1
New York, iii, iv, 28, 31, 33, 38, 40, 77, 97, 105, 138, 139, 140, 141, 172, 173, 174, 213, 215, 218, 253
NFT, 46
Ni, 356, 359
nicotine, 229, 244, 249, 263
nifedipine, 100, 276
nigrostriatal, ix, 64, 114, 121, 124, 130, 131, 132, 136, 138, 142, 204, 206, 213, 364
nitric oxide (NO), 46, 63, 95, 109, 147, 279
nitric oxide synthase, 46, 63
nitric-oxide synthase, 69
Nixon, 247
NMDA receptors, xii, 5, 10, 25, 34, 61, 62, 69, 72, 95, 104, 119, 132, 134, 147, 151, 166, 171, 175, 183, 208, 211, 215, 219, 227, 229, 230, 231, 234, 235, 237, 238, 241, 245, 253, 258, 265, 266, 274, 276, 277, 279, 284, 290, 311, 314, 338, 339, 345, 351, 354, 357, 376
N-methyl-D-aspartate, 5, 42, 46, 51, 69, 72, 132, 140, 145, 173, 198, 214, 216, 222, 224, 250, 256, 260, 274, 320, 337
N-methyl-D-aspartic acid, xii, 165, 345, 346
NMR, 346, 347, 348
NO, 95, 147, 148, 279, 280, 288, 293, 294, 299, 304
non-human, 110, 131, 193
non-human primates, 131
noradrenaline, 235, 241, 245, 257, 258
norepinephrine, 23, 254
normal, ix, 3, 8, 16, 17, 20, 24, 25, 26, 53, 54, 56, 57, 64, 83, 93, 113, 114, 115, 116, 119, 165, 166, 170, 181, 184, 187, 202, 218, 233, 235, 245, 265, 275, 276, 287, 319, 320, 338, 343, 352, 354, 369
normal aging, 3, 26, 114
normal development, 115
NOS, 279, 302
novelty, 338, 343, 371
NR2A, 62, 69, 171, 175, 275, 276, 281, 350, 351
NR2B, 27, 61, 62, 72, 171, 175, 275, 276, 281, 302, 304
NS, 196, 280
NSE, 9
N-terminal, 359
nuclear, 11, 24, 52, 265, 283, 346
nuclear magnetic resonance, 346
nuclei, ix, xi, 51, 121, 122, 131, 139, 140, 143, 144, 145, 149, 152, 153, 182, 194, 195, 208, 235, 246, 269, 272, 329, 342, 362, 363, 364, 371, 372
nucleus, x, xi, 10, 21, 33, 89, 92, 94, 102, 103, 108, 121, 122, 130, 139, 140, 141, 152, 153, 177, 178, 183, 188, 194, 209, 210, 211, 212, 213, 214, 215, 216, 217, 218, 219, 220, 222, 223, 224, 233, 252, 256, 260, 261, 262, 269, 270, 271, 273, 284, 320, 332, 335, 362, 363, 364, 365, 368, 372, 373, 375, 377
nucleus accumbens, x, 92, 103, 108, 139, 177, 178, 194, 209, 210, 211, 212, 213, 214, 215, 216, 217, 218, 219, 220, 260, 262, 363
nucleus accumbens (NAc), x, 92, 177, 178, 194

O

obesity, 7, 22, 96
object recognition, 55, 240, 246, 247, 373
observations, 10, 12, 64, 87, 90, 92, 93, 95, 121, 130, 133, 245, 274, 276, 316, 326, 352, 353, 354
obsessive-compulsive, 241
obsessive-compulsive disorder, 241
occipital cortex, 376
occluding, 282
oculomotor, 152, 263, 366, 367
old age, 8, 319
olfactory, 25, 26, 43, 115, 139, 167, 238, 239, 266
olfactory bulb, 25, 26, 43, 167
oligomer, 6, 7, 18, 22, 30, 31
oligomeric, vii, 1, 7, 27, 49, 51, 285
oligomers, vii, 1, 5, 7, 28, 30, 31, 35, 41
olive, 338
omega-3, 31
Omega-3, 32
Oncogene, 37
open-field, 198
operant conditioning, 198, 238, 260
opioid, 65, 174, 219
opposition, 116, 207
optical, 28
orbitofrontal cortex, 219, 220
organ, 152
organelle, 60
organelles, 10, 59, 60, 119, 127, 287
organism, vii, ix, 113, 202, 239, 287
organization, ix, 61, 68, 70, 113, 116, 121, 123, 124, 180, 194, 195, 207, 220, 256, 264, 325, 329, 332, 335, 339, 352, 370, 373, 375

organizations, 364
orientation, 213, 260, 314, 326, 327, 330, 331, 333, 336, 341, 343, 369
oscillation, 268, 312, 321
oscillations, 102, 248, 264, 311, 312, 335, 336
oscillatory activity, 287
ovary, 74
overload, 133
overweight, 110
oxidative, 28, 43
oxide, 67, 97, 98, 148, 279
oxygenation, 83

P

p38, 11, 25, 283
PA, 83, 335, 336, 342, 343
packets, 341
pain, 64, 78, 110
pairing, 147, 151, 183, 229, 232, 275, 313
palpitations, 185
pancreatic, 104
pancreatic islet, 104
paper, 293
paracrine, 80
paradox, 139
paralysis, ix, 113
parasympathetic, 136
parietal cortex, 249, 263, 323, 341, 370
parietal lobe, 223
parietal lobes, 223
Paris, 98, 173, 253, 255
Parkinson, ix, 2, 19, 21, 25, 33, 38, 43, 46, 64, 96, 102, 110, 114, 116, 121, 131, 134, 135, 136, 137, 139, 140, 142, 194, 197, 199, 210, 217, 218, 242, 249, 256, 264, 354, 364, 374, 376
Parkinson disease, 25, 38, 43, 136, 142
parkinsonism, 19, 72, 110
Parkinsonism, 23, 64, 136, 356
paroxetine, 255
particles, 47
partition, 120
partnership, 16
parvalbumin, 231, 251, 264
passive, 187, 218, 369
pathogenesis, 29, 30, 33, 135
pathogenic, 27
pathology, 3, 5, 6, 9, 23, 25, 26, 31, 33, 34, 38, 139, 140, 172, 214, 241, 242, 245, 355, 357
pathophysiological, 18, 287, 288
pathophysiology, 96, 257, 294, 354
pathways, vii, x, 1, 9, 24, 35, 36, 39, 61, 78, 81, 82, 83, 89, 90, 95, 108, 122, 140, 142, 147, 165, 169, 177, 179, 183, 194, 195, 207, 211, 213, 260, 271, 272, 277, 283, 289, 291, 310, 352, 355, 359, 363, 366, 367, 370, 371, 374, 375, 376
patients, x, 7, 8, 9, 12, 15, 18, 20, 22, 25, 29, 39, 64, 78, 110, 130, 139, 163, 164, 168, 169, 171, 184, 185, 212, 216, 238, 242, 243, 247, 249, 256, 264, 270, 289, 291, 354, 364, 374
patterning, 174
Pavlovian, 180, 194, 196, 197, 201, 202, 203, 232, 247, 262, 271, 282, 287, 293, 297, 301, 304, 305, 316
Pavlovian conditioning, 194, 196, 201, 202, 293, 316
Pavlovian learning, 247
PCR, 282
PCs, 89, 90, 95
PD, 19, 46, 64, 96, 121, 123, 124, 126, 130, 133, 338, 340
PDZ domains, 348, 350, 354
PE, 83, 341
pediatric, 101
pentylenetetrazol, 174
PEPA, 268
peptide, vii, 1, 3, 8, 13, 23, 28, 32, 35, 36, 37, 58, 98, 102, 107, 288
peptides, 3, 68, 279, 348, 350
perception, 222, 237, 239, 364, 367, 370, 371, 372, 374, 375
perceptual learning, 331, 373
perforated synapses, ix, 114, 116, 120, 121, 126, 127, 128, 131, 133, 134, 135
perforation, 120, 121
performance, vii, ix, 15, 30, 53, 113, 196, 204, 211, 239, 240, 241, 249, 251, 256, 258, 260, 264, 265, 268, 318, 337, 363, 373
perfusion, 188
permeability, 274, 279
personality, 179
perturbation, 343
pertussis, 90, 100
PET, 36, 184, 185, 204, 216, 248, 266
PET scan, 184, 185, 204
PF, 89, 95, 144, 146, 153, 194
PFC, 94, 179, 182, 184, 188, 190, 191, 195, 199, 200, 204, 205, 222, 223, 224, 226, 227, 230, 231, 235, 236, 237, 238, 239, 240, 241, 242, 243, 244, 363, 366
pharmacological, 11, 17, 78, 80, 92, 96, 99, 101, 110, 152, 178, 199, 210, 260, 285, 293
pharmacology, 84, 101, 102, 236, 266, 274, 358
pharmacotherapies, 216
phase shifts, 326
phencyclidine, 210, 243, 246, 255, 259
phenomenology, vii, 1

phenotype, 23, 26, 64, 94
phenylalanine, 281
phosphatases, 12, 60, 148, 291, 357
phosphate, 62, 107, 127
phosphatidic acid, 81, 83
phosphatidylethanolamine, 81, 99, 105
phosphodiesterase, 82, 108
phospholipase C, 14, 82, 88, 146, 213, 222, 227, 237, 261, 353
phospholipids, 80, 81, 83, 103, 107, 108
phosphoprotein, 57, 149, 222, 265, 346, 353, 358
phosphorylates, 48, 55, 57, 62, 63, 66, 73, 146, 148, 237, 353
phosphorylation, 5, 8, 11, 12, 19, 23, 25, 37, 40, 42, 47, 48, 50, 52, 54, 55, 56, 58, 59, 61, 62, 63, 64, 66, 67, 68, 69, 70, 71, 72, 73, 74, 75, 79, 80, 146, 155, 227, 245, 250, 254, 257, 262, 265, 281, 283, 284, 297, 302, 346, 348, 350, 351, 352, 353, 355, 356, 357, 358, 359
photon, 184
physical activity, 7, 22
physical properties, 371
Physicians, 77
physiological, viii, x, xi, 10, 12, 18, 20, 32, 66, 78, 80, 83, 85, 89, 98, 99, 109, 115, 116, 126, 166, 178, 180, 182, 206, 210, 217, 221, 282, 293, 333, 349, 373, 375
physiological factors, 116
physiology, iv, 12, 48, 138, 263, 293
PI3K, 8, 11, 12, 14, 15, 22, 23, 80
pig, 174, 332, 336
pigs, 332
pilot study, 40
pitch, 341
pituitary, 7
PKC, 8, 11, 56, 62, 63, 146, 147, 149, 150, 222, 227, 235, 262
PKs, 348
PL, 222
planning, 222, 230, 264
plaque, 5, 7, 25, 27, 34
plaques, vii, 1, 3, 5, 33
plasma, 9, 18, 28, 58, 66, 146, 147, 287, 350, 352
plasma membrane, 58, 66, 146, 147, 350, 352
plastic, 3, 22, 114, 115, 172, 229, 238, 244, 332, 371
platelet, 279, 298
platelet-activating factor, 279
platelets, 108
play, xi, xii, 5, 9, 11, 13, 18, 47, 51, 57, 63, 79, 92, 93, 97, 130, 133, 147, 164, 165, 169, 178, 179, 187, 193, 208, 212, 235, 238, 244, 269, 281, 285, 327, 347, 350, 354, 355, 361, 371
PLC, 81, 82, 83, 88, 89, 92, 94, 95, 222
PLD, 81, 222
plus-maze, 199
PN, 144, 147, 153
point mutation, 54, 173
polarity, 12, 29, 68, 291
polarized, 319
polymer, 351
polymerization, 349
polymers, 347
polymorphisms, 36
polypeptides, 13
polyunsaturated fat, 35, 43
polyunsaturated fatty acid, 35, 43
polyunsaturated fatty acids, 43
poor, 24, 245, 369
population, 9, 28, 322, 323, 330, 342, 375
pore, 62, 70
positron, 247, 250, 255, 373
positron emission tomography, 247, 250, 255, 373
postmortem, 36, 64, 138
post-translational, 11
post-translational modifications, 11
posttraumatic stress, 247, 287
post-traumatic stress, 235, 242, 243, 250
posttraumatic stress disorder, 235, 242, 243, 247, 250, 287
potassium, 61, 79, 107
potassium channels, 79
power, 322
PP2A, 148
PPD, 84
preclinical, 215, 219
preconditioning, 276
prediction, 29, 202, 203, 332
pre-existing, 70, 180, 196
preference, 98, 190, 201, 206, 213
prefrontal cortex (PFC), x, 87, 90, 94, 98, 178, 181, 182, 184, 185, 186, 187, 188, 191, 194, 202, 208, 209, 210, 218, 221, 222, 241, 243, 246, 247, 248, 249, 250, 251, 252, 253, 254, 255, 256, 257, 258, 259, 260, 261, 262, 263, 264, 265, 266, 267, 268, 287, 353, 357, 362, 363, 372
preparation, iv, 7, 168, 186
preparedness, 335
presenilin 1, 27
presynaptic, viii, 4, 12, 15, 23, 40, 48, 56, 58, 65, 66, 72, 77, 83, 84, 85, 86, 87, 88, 89, 90, 93, 94, 95, 97, 99, 100, 105, 106, 107, 108, 109, 110, 111, 115, 116, 117, 120, 121, 125, 127, 129, 130, 133, 138, 141, 148, 150, 165, 180, 181, 182, 183, 193, 197, 206, 210, 225, 226, 227, 229, 240, 263, 273, 275, 277, 279, 280, 282, 287, 311, 312, 313, 314, 321, 330

prevention, 22, 29, 31, 32
primary visual cortex, 330, 334, 373, 375, 376
primate, 110, 213, 216, 223, 239, 247, 252, 261, 314, 340, 351, 355, 357, 374, 375
primates, 121, 200, 213, 223, 224, 238, 252, 267, 340
priming, 93, 228, 237, 248, 278, 370
probability, 100, 132, 147, 202, 225, 274, 277, 278, 280, 310, 329, 352, 365
procedural memory, xii, 310, 328
procedures, 152, 182, 198
production, 3, 9, 20, 35, 51, 71, 78, 87, 89, 92, 93, 94, 95, 279, 280
progenitor cells, 174
progesterone, 42
program, 187
progressive, 9, 63, 167, 187, 192, 197, 206, 217
proliferation, 4, 56, 99, 140
promote, 9, 10, 12, 13, 15, 17, 24, 34, 94, 114, 181, 188, 197, 367, 368, 372
promoter, 9, 36, 52, 68, 71, 72, 284
promoter region, 36
propagation, 18
property, iv, 16, 115, 149, 323, 347, 369
propionic acid, xii, 46, 61, 166, 181, 198, 274, 345, 346
prostaglandin, 21, 36, 105, 108
prostaglandins, 280
protection, 96
protein kinase C (PKC), 8, 32, 46, 56, 67, 146, 222, 227
protein kinases, viii, 45, 48, 49, 60, 61, 62, 63, 67, 70, 74, 181
protein synthesis, 19, 33, 51, 56, 63, 70, 91, 134, 233, 234, 239, 240, 245, 263, 266, 281, 283, 320, 322, 332, 346, 352
protein tyrosine phosphatases, 81
protein-protein interactions, xii, 345
proteins, viii, 2, 7, 8, 9, 10, 11, 12, 13, 17, 18, 19, 23, 24, 25, 40, 47, 48, 51, 52, 56, 57, 58, 59, 60, 61, 62, 63, 66, 70, 73, 74, 79, 80, 84, 138, 155, 244, 263, 279, 281, 282, 288, 346, 347, 348, 349, 350, 351, 354, 355, 356, 357, 358, 359
proteomics, 19, 79
protocol, 53, 85, 147, 166, 183, 184, 226, 227, 228, 229, 231, 245, 275, 290, 321, 322
protocols, xi, 85, 89, 166, 167, 169, 170, 173, 185, 189, 245, 269
protooncogene, 293
provocation, 250
proximal, 123, 124, 148, 282, 315
Prozac, 243
pruning, 24, 119
PSA, 222, 243, 266
PSD, viii, xii, 8, 45, 46, 48, 50, 51, 52, 54, 55, 59, 60, 61, 62, 63, 64, 65, 66, 67, 68, 69, 115, 116, 120, 133, 146, 345, 346, 348, 349, 350, 354
PSP, 342
psychiatric disorder, 245
psychiatric disorders, 245
psychiatry, 214
psychoactive, 78
psychoanalysis, 214
psychological, 242
psychopathology, 180
psychosis, 241
psychostimulants, 186, 191, 214, 358
psychotropic drug, 250
psychotropic drugs, 250
pulse, 84, 134, 166, 167, 227, 253, 255, 271, 274, 277, 280, 290
pulses, 15, 89, 92, 94, 166, 206, 231, 274, 279, 312, 335
Purkinje, ix, 37, 53, 67, 84, 85, 88, 99, 101, 105, 109, 110, 111, 118, 143, 144, 145, 146, 147, 148, 149, 150, 151, 152, 153, 154, 155, 156, 157, 158, 159, 160, 161, 329, 336
Purkinje cells, 85, 88, 101, 105, 109, 110, 111, 118, 143, 144, 145, 146, 147, 152, 153, 329
pyramidal, xi, 5, 15, 27, 34, 55, 85, 93, 95, 98, 108, 111, 118, 133, 164, 221, 223, 224, 225, 226, 229, 230, 231, 234, 236, 237, 241, 242, 244, 246, 248, 249, 250, 252, 253, 255, 257, 259, 261, 262, 263, 264, 267, 279, 321, 334, 335, 336, 353, 368
pyramidal cells, 27, 34, 85, 93, 108, 164, 249, 253, 255, 261, 263, 267, 279, 321, 334, 335, 336, 368
pyruvate, 8

Q

quality of life, 20
quantum, 312
questionnaire, 219
Quinones, 294

R

race, 242, 370
radiotherapy, 78
rain, 164, 193
Raman, 160, 336
random, 130, 137, 318
range, 12, 13, 54, 83, 150, 184, 216, 223, 226, 229, 231, 245, 270, 313, 332, 369
rapamycin, 12, 24, 29, 31

raphe, 89, 102, 121, 235, 246
RAS, 63, 292
RC, 335, 343
reaction time, 200, 373
reactivity, 32, 210
real-time, 282
recall, 3, 234, 241, 243, 247, 250, 254, 257, 259, 264, 325, 336, 338
recalling, 325, 326
receptive field, 315, 320, 325, 330, 338, 365, 375
receptor agonist, 35, 85, 87, 92, 98, 100, 107, 207, 227, 228, 238, 250, 291, 364
recognition, 18, 30, 38, 238, 240, 241, 256, 263, 267, 270
recombination, 355
reconditioning, 154
reconsolidation, 215, 216, 240, 246, 283
reconstruction, 119
recovery, 2, 126, 179, 262
recycling, 9, 10, 24, 35
redistribution, 39, 62, 218
reduction, 9, 25, 50, 55, 58, 59, 60, 85, 119, 132, 150, 173, 185, 206, 237, 243, 244, 247, 260, 267, 270, 279, 280, 283, 290, 291, 363, 370
reference frame, 335
reflexes, 151, 217
refractory, 166
regenerate, 17
regeneration, 32, 33, 135
regional, 186, 248, 249, 255
regression, 4, 26
regular, 224, 246, 329
regulation, ix, xi, xii, 8, 11, 12, 25, 27, 31, 35, 36, 40, 41, 42, 47, 50, 51, 54, 56, 57, 58, 60, 61, 62, 63, 65, 66, 67, 69, 74, 79, 93, 97, 101, 132, 138, 139, 141, 143, 149, 153, 164, 170, 171, 175, 210, 212, 220, 223, 234, 245, 246, 251, 254, 265, 269, 270, 281, 283, 285, 292, 319, 337, 345, 351, 352, 353, 354, 356, 357, 359
regulations, 346
regulators, 10, 11, 29, 349, 350, 354, 357
reinforcement, x, 177, 178, 194, 197, 202, 211, 214, 217
reinforcement learning, 197, 202, 214
reinforcers, 196
relapse, x, 177, 178, 184, 185, 186, 187, 189, 191, 192, 195, 196, 197, 202, 204, 205, 208, 218
relationship, 10, 131, 180, 188, 189, 200, 245, 246, 249, 312, 337, 373
relationships, 29, 36, 43, 140, 170, 218, 249
relevance, 3, 5, 7, 32, 85, 218, 220, 239, 255, 289, 331, 376
reliability, 338
Reliability, 334
REM, 231
remodeling, x, xii, 2, 3, 4, 11, 15, 24, 38, 72, 115, 136, 178, 193, 267, 310
remodelling, vii, 1, 22
renin, 292
renin-angiotensin system, 292
renin-angiotensin system (RAS), 292
repair, 9, 17, 39, 135
reperfusion, 31
repetitions, 226
research, iv, vii, viii, ix, 1, 45, 78, 79, 82, 97, 168, 171, 206, 216, 310, 311, 328, 330, 331
Research and Development, 1
researchers, xii, 48, 78, 312
reservoir, 17
residues, 347, 350
resilience, 257
resistance, 36, 196, 254
resistive, 121
resolution, 240, 374
resources, 372
respiratory, 133
responsiveness, x, 148, 167, 187, 189, 193, 209, 220, 221, 234, 247, 261, 292, 317, 340
restoration, 2
restructuring, 120, 138, 141
retardation, 19, 64
retention, 241, 265, 354
reticulum, 146, 147
retina, 51, 72, 151, 152
retinoic acid, 64
retrograde amnesia, 255, 281
Rett syndrome, 21
rewards, 187, 194, 196, 197, 198, 206, 318
Reynolds, 63, 71, 109, 125, 132, 140, 157
RF, 338
Rho, xii, 14, 35, 345, 349, 350, 358
rhythm, 42, 256, 311, 312, 336, 337, 340, 342
rhythms, 231, 255
rigidity, 342
risk, 7, 9, 34, 36, 37, 40
risk factors, 7
RNA, 43
RNAi, 60
rodent, 94, 168, 223, 228, 268, 273, 314, 326, 340
rodents, x, 20, 93, 96, 171, 178, 183, 187, 188, 189, 190, 193, 195, 196, 198, 199, 200, 206, 223, 226, 232, 247, 271, 275, 286, 340
Royal Society, 36, 372, 374
RP, 149, 337, 340
runaway, 311
Russia, 361

Russian, 361, 372
Russian Academy of Sciences, 361

S

SA, 140, 334, 335, 336
saccades, 367
saccadic eye movement, 374
saline, x, 126, 127, 178, 183, 184, 192, 198, 199, 206
salt, 292
sample, 318
SAP, 46, 61, 62, 69
saturated fat, 35
saturation, 181, 225, 289, 290, 291
savings, 252
scaffold, xii, 60, 61, 62, 345, 346, 350, 351, 356
scaffolding, xii, 8, 345, 346, 352, 353, 354, 358
scaling, 18, 39, 311, 317, 332
scavenger, 277
SCD, 100
schemas, 239
schizophrenia, 64, 71, 116, 138, 237, 241, 242, 247, 248, 249, 250, 253, 257, 258, 265, 266, 267, 270, 299, 354, 356, 357
Schmid, 107, 108, 209, 272, 276, 297
science, 48, 110
scientific, 212
sclerosis, 164
search, 13
searching, 64, 318, 333, 371
secrete, 17
secretion, 55, 56, 58, 70, 104, 192, 215, 292
seeding, 29
seizure, x, 53, 56, 163, 164, 167, 168, 169, 170, 171, 172, 174, 291
seizures, 40, 64, 167, 169, 171, 172, 174, 289, 291
selecting, 330
selective attention, 373, 374, 375, 376
selective serotonin reuptake inhibitor, 243
selectivity, 310, 313, 333, 335, 348, 351, 356, 375
Self, 214, 341
self-control, 212
self-organization, 22
self-regulation, 84
self-report, 186
self-reports, 186
SEM, 286, 290, 291
semantic, 373
semantic priming, 373
senescence, 38
senile, 27
sensitivity, 98, 101, 105, 107, 151, 212, 214, 236, 289, 342
sensitization, 184, 187, 188, 189, 190, 191, 192, 193, 194, 195, 198, 199, 201, 208, 209, 212, 214, 217, 218, 219, 220, 262
sensory cortices, 272, 330
separation, 117, 316, 317, 318, 319, 324, 332, 338
septum, 15, 29, 38, 251
sequencing, 74, 100, 222
series, 11, 170, 324
serine, 11, 12, 19, 23, 55, 68, 148, 278
serotonergic, 66, 260
Serotonin, 56, 102, 265, 274, 285, 288, 296, 302
serum, 9
services, iv
severity, 4, 21
sex, 29, 34, 184, 187, 196, 285
sex differences, 34, 285
sex hormones, 285
SH, 98, 332
shape, viii, xi, 2, 4, 6, 31, 115, 119, 133, 141, 179, 180, 221, 223, 227, 315, 319, 322, 336, 338, 373, 376
shaping, x, 221
shares, 49, 198, 328, 347
sharing, 369
shock, 218, 271
short period, 223
short term memory, 337
short-term, viii, xi, 18, 47, 77, 78, 83, 84, 85, 87, 89, 90, 91, 94, 97, 98, 99, 101, 105, 150, 221, 222, 223, 224, 225, 226, 231, 239, 240, 241, 244, 247, 250, 251, 253, 267, 268, 275, 318, 320, 331, 334, 338, 370
short-term memory, 18, 47, 240, 245, 251, 275, 334
side effects, 133
sign, 80, 87, 133, 264, 371
signal transduction, viii, 10, 45, 51, 52, 57, 58, 60, 61, 65, 79, 103, 104, 110, 201, 209, 214, 287, 336, 371
signaling, viii, xi, 2, 4, 8, 10, 12, 13, 14, 15, 20, 21, 22, 23, 29, 31, 34, 36, 37, 38, 39, 40, 41, 48, 51, 54, 55, 56, 60, 61, 62, 65, 67, 69, 70, 77, 78, 80, 83, 85, 87, 88, 89, 91, 92, 94, 95, 97, 98, 101, 102, 104, 105, 106, 110, 119, 125, 140, 146, 148, 149, 150, 165, 169, 171, 182, 201, 259, 260, 266, 269, 279, 281, 283, 287, 355, 364, 371
signaling pathway, 10, 12, 14, 23, 31, 36, 38, 54, 55, 67, 69, 88, 91, 146, 169, 201, 283, 287
signaling pathways, 14, 38, 67, 88, 91, 146, 169, 283, 287
signalling, 24, 36, 97, 98, 102, 107, 108, 111, 241, 246, 258, 280, 346, 349, 351, 352, 353, 354, 355, 357, 359

signals, ix, 2, 16, 52, 107, 114, 126, 145, 152, 195, 203, 215, 326, 329, 362, 365, 371, 372, 376
signal-to-noise ratio, 274
signs, 133, 135, 185, 289
similarity, 52, 245, 364
simulation, 147, 148
siRNA, 15
sites, 17, 50, 53, 63, 67, 68, 70, 73, 74, 96, 118, 124, 133, 152, 167, 170, 190, 257, 273, 287, 348, 352, 358
sleep, 231, 241
sleep disorders, 241
smoking, 96, 186, 204
smoking cessation, 96
SNAP, 58, 280
SNc, 121, 122, 123, 124, 126, 130, 131, 132, 362, 365, 368, 371
social, 242, 250, 270, 287, 289
social behavior, 270
social context, 287
social stress, 242
socially, 270
sodium, 103, 126, 127, 233, 292
somata, 15, 149, 153, 336
somatosensory, 272, 328
sorting, 9, 10, 26, 32
SP, 122, 363
Spain, 177, 309
spasticity, ix, 98, 113
spatial, xii, 8, 9, 11, 18, 22, 25, 32, 33, 34, 41, 42, 52, 53, 54, 55, 68, 72, 73, 90, 93, 106, 108, 121, 131, 173, 214, 216, 230, 231, 238, 239, 240, 242, 249, 255, 259, 260, 264, 266, 268, 309, 310, 313, 314, 317, 319, 320, 321, 322, 324, 325, 326, 327, 331, 333, 334, 335, 337, 338, 339, 340, 342, 343, 355, 363, 370, 373, 374, 375, 376
spatial information, 68, 173, 240, 311, 314, 325, 326
spatial learning, 8, 9, 11, 25, 34, 52, 73, 93, 108, 240, 310, 319, 321, 333, 339, 342
spatial location, 314, 317, 326
spatial memory, xii, 22, 32, 33, 41, 42, 55, 72, 93, 108, 121, 131, 216, 240, 242, 255, 264, 266, 309, 313, 333, 335, 337, 339
spatial representations, 324, 326, 334
spatiotemporal, 259
specialization, 125
species, 48, 82, 225, 281, 348
specificity, xi, 4, 5, 14, 48, 65, 110, 146, 210, 212, 269, 272, 277, 320, 333, 335, 372
SPECT, 184
spectroscopy, 347, 348
spectrum, 2, 115
speed, 328, 373
spinal cord, 51, 65, 73, 79, 82, 87, 106
spine, vii, xii, 2, 4, 5, 6, 10, 12, 13, 15, 17, 19, 20, 21, 23, 26, 29, 31, 34, 35, 36, 37, 39, 42, 60, 72, 115, 117, 118, 119, 120, 121, 123, 124, 125, 127, 128, 129, 131, 133, 136, 138, 139, 140, 141, 181, 218, 227, 236, 241, 243, 244, 259, 287, 345, 348, 350, 351, 354, 356, 358
spines, ix, 2, 4, 6, 10, 13, 15, 19, 20, 28, 38, 69, 71, 113, 114, 118, 119, 120, 123, 124, 130, 133, 140, 147, 181, 199, 207, 236, 245, 255, 275, 276, 282, 348, 350, 353
sporadic, 9, 26, 32, 195
Sprague-Dawley rats, 292
sprouting, vii, x, 1, 2, 4, 18, 29, 33, 119, 163, 169, 170, 171, 172, 174, 181
square wave, 166, 167
SR, 93, 96
stability, 28, 140, 320, 332, 336, 337
stabilization, 3, 71, 115, 278
stabilize, 267, 311, 327, 349
stages, 3, 4, 15, 36, 128, 130, 178, 189, 194, 195, 208, 218, 330, 333, 368
status epilepticus, 172, 174, 291
stellate cells, 143, 144, 147, 148
Stem cell, 17, 32
stem cells, 17, 32, 42
stereotypical, 117
sterile, 348, 357
steroid, 34, 258
steroid hormone, 34
steroid hormones, 34
steroids, 34, 285
stimulant, 198, 211
Stimuli, 201, 297
stimulus, xii, 84, 91, 93, 151, 152, 153, 167, 181, 182, 186, 196, 197, 201, 202, 206, 208, 223, 232, 233, 236, 239, 271, 273, 277, 278, 289, 290, 310, 316, 330, 333, 335, 338, 361, 363, 364, 365, 366, 367, 368, 369, 370, 371, 372, 375
stimulus generalization, 289
stimulus information, 271
storage, viii, xii, 7, 45, 53, 54, 71, 83, 94, 133, 193, 230, 232, 238, 239, 240, 259, 262, 263, 270, 283, 287, 309, 310, 311, 337, 338
strategies, 20, 172, 239, 266
strategy use, 259
streams, 207, 362, 370
strength, vii, 18, 55, 83, 115, 165, 180, 191, 192, 198, 224, 231, 253, 279, 290, 317, 328, 347
stress, xii, 11, 24, 25, 32, 191, 192, 209, 213, 214, 215, 217, 218, 242, 243, 247, 248, 249, 250, 254, 256, 259, 260, 262, 264, 265, 267, 285, 287, 310
stressors, 287

striatum, ix, x, 19, 54, 87, 91, 92, 97, 99, 102, 105, 109, 113, 114, 116, 118, 119, 121, 122, 123, 124, 125, 126, 127, 128, 129, 130, 131, 132, 133, 135, 139, 140, 141, 178, 181, 182, 185, 186, 187, 191, 193, 194, 195, 197, 200, 202, 204, 205, 206, 207, 208, 210, 213, 215, 217, 218, 219, 220, 239, 252, 258, 260, 352, 353, 354, 363, 364, 367, 368, 369, 371, 372, 374, 375, 376
stroke, vii, ix, 17, 108, 113
structural changes, 15, 59, 60, 136, 181
structural modifications, 13
structural protein, xii, 346
Subcellular, 51, 74, 348, 357
subcortical structures, 239, 326
subjective, 204
subjective experience, 204
subjectivity, 128
substances, 56, 189, 279
substantia nigra, ix, 87, 109, 113, 121, 122, 124, 189, 194, 195, 204, 213, 216, 362, 363, 365, 374, 375
substantia nigra pars compacta, 362, 365
substrates, vii, xii, 2, 8, 11, 12, 52, 56, 57, 58, 59, 61, 62, 66, 67, 73, 74, 178, 216, 233, 322, 345, 346, 349, 352, 354
sucrose, 192, 195
sugar, 8
Sun, 25, 69, 109, 136, 237, 247, 265, 339
supply, 8
suppression, 63, 84, 85, 86, 87, 89, 90, 91, 93, 97, 101, 102, 105, 106, 107, 108, 109, 149, 150, 226, 262, 289, 292, 363, 368
suppressor, 359
surface area, 119
Surgeons, 77
surgery, 128, 139, 168
surgical, x, 143, 152, 198
survival, 12, 13, 15, 28, 40, 131, 181
surviving, 17
susceptibility, 3, 36, 53, 56, 164, 169, 278, 339
swelling, 130, 133
switching, xiii, 226, 244, 361, 371, 375
symptom, 8, 242
symptoms, 19, 64, 121, 180, 185, 204, 246
synapse, vii, viii, xii, 2, 3, 4, 5, 6, 8, 13, 16, 17, 19, 24, 25, 31, 33, 36, 39, 40, 41, 42, 43, 46, 48, 54, 61, 62, 65, 69, 71, 77, 84, 85, 90, 99, 106, 116, 117, 118, 119, 120, 122, 124, 128, 132, 136, 137, 144, 149, 150, 151, 152, 153, 165, 170, 181, 195, 227, 236, 257, 261, 264, 272, 273, 277, 279, 282, 334, 345, 348, 352
synaptic strength, viii, x, 18, 22, 41, 55, 56, 61, 77, 78, 83, 91, 98, 133, 165, 177, 179, 180, 181, 189, 191, 198, 209, 211, 246, 274, 281, 282, 289, 290, 311, 324, 325, 330, 332, 333
synaptic transmission, vii, viii, xii, 2, 15, 16, 18, 20, 31, 32, 35, 38, 45, 46, 55, 79, 89, 91, 97, 99, 103, 104, 105, 110, 115, 120, 131, 132, 135, 138, 145, 147, 148, 165, 180, 198, 208, 209, 217, 236, 240, 243, 245, 246, 275, 276, 285, 289, 291, 321, 332, 333, 334, 342, 345, 350, 352, 354, 357, 365
synaptic vesicles, 3, 57, 58, 116, 118, 124
synaptogenesis, vii, 1, 2, 3, 8, 17, 23, 24, 79, 120, 135, 138, 170, 174
synaptophysin, 40, 243, 266
synchronization, 172
synchronous, 87, 169, 265, 335
syndrome, 19, 26, 29, 39, 64, 67, 74, 78, 207, 211, 241
synergistic, 147, 376
synthesis, 9, 17, 30, 36, 48, 54, 56, 63, 66, 73, 81, 83, 87, 91, 95, 96, 133, 138, 171, 281, 320, 352, 374
synthetic, 23, 28, 68
systematic, 54, 239, 314
systems, xi, xii, 67, 135, 178, 201, 211, 214, 217, 235, 249, 250, 269, 278, 281, 291, 293, 310, 325, 326, 328, 329, 342

T

tangles, 33, 63
targets, viii, xii, 11, 45, 48, 56, 62, 65, 66, 67, 87, 97, 127, 140, 141, 188, 212, 236, 248, 259, 280, 345, 349, 352, 368, 369
task demands, 318
taste, 283, 354, 358
taste aversion, 283, 354, 358
tau, vii, 1, 8, 11, 22, 27, 28, 32, 58, 63, 71, 73, 74, 75
tau pathology, 27
teaching, 144, 145
technology, 53
telencephalon, 266
temporal, 24, 25, 29, 50, 73, 90, 91, 139, 150, 152, 164, 166, 172, 187, 212, 223, 226, 229, 238, 247, 250, 251, 256, 264, 270, 311, 312, 313, 314, 319, 323, 324, 326, 328, 330, 333, 335, 341, 343, 355, 369, 372, 375, 376
temporal lobe, 24, 139, 172, 238, 256, 270, 328, 330, 343, 375
temporal lobe epilepsy, 172, 270
terminals, ix, 15, 48, 58, 66, 83, 85, 89, 90, 94, 105, 113, 123, 125, 132, 133, 134, 135, 138, 139, 140, 150, 169, 200, 236, 237, 248, 263, 264, 265, 280, 282, 287
ternary complex, 61, 73

territory, 140, 218
testis, 102
tetanus, 52, 182, 225, 228, 275, 276, 310, 312
Tetanus, 283
textiles, 78
thalamus, xii, 19, 92, 122, 124, 145, 224, 252, 256, 271, 275, 353, 361, 363, 364, 365, 366, 367, 368, 372, 374
theoretical, 325, 373
theory, 33, 217, 218, 259, 261, 262, 333, 338, 339, 340, 343
therapeutic, viii, 2, 64, 96, 133, 171, 172, 179, 243, 293
therapeutic agents, 133
therapeutic approaches, viii, 2
therapeutic interventions, 179
therapeutics, 28, 38, 98, 257
therapy, 11, 15, 35, 100, 133, 186
theta, 20, 42, 92, 166, 220, 231, 232, 256, 264, 265, 272, 274, 286, 290, 311, 312, 321, 324, 325, 331, 336, 337, 340, 342
thinking, 78
three-dimensional, 36, 50, 212, 332
three-dimensional reconstruction, 212
threonine, 11, 12, 19, 23, 50, 68, 69, 278
threshold, 20, 147, 150, 167, 173, 174, 226, 241, 249, 253, 259, 277, 278, 291, 311, 314, 319, 334
threshold level, 20, 253
thresholds, 187
thromboxane, 105
time, xi, 14, 15, 18, 29, 53, 66, 83, 84, 91, 92, 115, 130, 132, 150, 152, 166, 180, 181, 182, 184, 186, 187, 188, 190, 192, 193, 195, 196, 197, 203, 209, 223, 224, 236, 240, 247, 251, 272, 276, 278, 283, 290, 309, 311, 312, 313, 317, 319, 321, 322, 323, 324, 326, 327, 329, 330, 331, 337, 339, 340, 341, 346, 369, 372
time lags, 369
time periods, 92
timing, xi, 94, 100, 104, 151, 221, 222, 229, 245, 249, 255, 257, 259, 276, 277, 312, 313, 324, 325, 330, 331, 333, 334, 335, 341, 343, 375
tissue, viii, 45, 51, 65, 89, 138, 167, 168, 182, 185, 289
TJ, 333, 338, 340, 342
TLE, 164, 289, 291
TNF, 18, 21, 22, 36, 39, 40, 46
TNF-alpha, 21, 40
tobacco, 184
Tokyo, 45
tolerance, 7, 65, 92, 103, 197
tonic, ix, 93, 113, 167, 171, 200, 236, 252, 253
tonic-clonic seizures, 167, 171
top-down, 362, 366, 367, 373, 375
Topiramate, 299
topographic, 194
torture, 250
total cholesterol, 29
toxic, 3, 119, 247
toxicity, 103
toxin, 5, 100, 140
toxins, 31
TPA, 291
TPH, 46, 56, 66
trading, 104
traffic, 35, 263
training, 120, 131, 141, 152, 193, 197, 200, 209, 218, 233, 234, 239, 240, 241, 254, 259, 271, 281, 283, 289, 316, 318, 370
training block, 254
traits, 200
trajectory, 319
trans, 346, 350, 359
transcranial magnetic stimulation, 238, 263
transcription, 11, 12, 43, 51, 52, 55, 67, 74, 153, 170, 178, 212, 214, 227, 233, 237, 281, 283, 320, 352
transcription factor, 11, 52, 55, 67, 170, 178, 214, 320
transcription factors, 11, 55, 67, 170, 320
transcriptional, 9, 11, 52, 171, 283
transduction, 62, 66
transfection, 148
transfer, 81, 196, 329
transformations, 332
transgene, 54, 71
transgenesis, 355
transgenic, 4, 5, 7, 9, 18, 24, 28, 30, 33, 34, 35, 39, 42, 52, 53, 54, 67, 68, 241, 283, 292, 294, 303, 355
transgenic mice, 5, 7, 9, 10, 24, 28, 34, 35, 39, 42, 52, 53, 54, 68, 241, 283
transgenic mouse, 5, 7
transition, 202, 205, 236
transitions, 230
translation, 12, 31, 34, 41, 43, 51, 55, 63, 66, 71, 151, 343
translational, 8, 24, 37
translocation, 8, 50, 52, 60, 61, 65, 66, 283
transmembrane, 12, 26, 80, 347, 350, 354
transmission, x, xi, xii, 15, 55, 60, 83, 87, 90, 93, 99, 102, 104, 107, 120, 122, 131, 133, 137, 145, 177, 181, 182, 198, 200, 206, 209, 214, 219, 236, 237, 244, 247, 250, 252, 261, 269, 274, 275, 287, 292, 336, 345, 353, 371
transplantation, 18, 35, 41

transport, 7, 8, 9, 12, 28, 30, 32, 42, 48, 58, 82, 83, 96, 98, 99, 100, 108, 255, 354, 357
trauma, 172
traumatic brain injury, 17
traumatic events, 180
travel, viii, 77, 85
trees, 279
trial, 191, 318, 329, 336, 339, 342
trial and error, 329, 339, 342
trigeminal, 153
triggers, 86, 130, 230, 291
trophic support, 17
tryptophan, 46, 48, 56, 70, 74
tumor, 26, 41, 46, 359
tumor necrosis factor, 26, 41, 46
turnover, 260
two-dimensional, 323, 327, 329
type 2 diabetes mellitus, 22, 26
type II diabetes, 22, 26
tyrosine, 20, 23, 46, 56, 67, 70, 74, 135, 137, 147, 156, 264, 281, 283, 287, 302, 303, 348
tyrosine hydroxylase, 46, 56, 70, 135, 264

U

ubiquitin, 64
ubiquitous, 38, 85, 349
ultrastructure, 16
unconditioned, 152, 153, 196, 232, 271, 289, 338
unconditioned response, 152, 153
underlying mechanisms, vii, 223, 330
uniform, 18, 372
unilateral, ix, 114, 116, 126, 131, 132, 134, 138, 140, 142, 213
United Kingdom (UK), 1, 139, 172, 212, 217, 261, 341
unpredictability, 216
urethane, 285, 312

V

Valdez, v, 113, 134
valence, 270
values, 129, 286, 290, 291
vanadium, 134
variability, 325
variable, 172, 226, 328
variation, viii, 2, 4
vasodilation, 104, 110
vasopressin, 292
vector, 53, 322, 327, 333
velocity, 323, 328, 338, 341
Ventral tegmental area, 257
ventrolateral prefrontal cortex, 248
vertebrates, 36, 49, 84, 210
vesicle, 12, 40, 57, 58, 66, 67, 73
veterans, 247
video, 186, 204
Vietnam, 247
viral, 53, 282
visible, 54, 60
vision, 331, 367, 372, 377
visual, xii, 14, 21, 29, 34, 91, 94, 132, 140, 141, 151, 152, 204, 224, 238, 239, 250, 251, 261, 262, 272, 313, 315, 323, 330, 333, 335, 336, 337, 338, 341, 343, 361, 362, 363, 364, 365, 366, 367, 368, 369, 370, 371, 372, 373, 374, 375, 376
visual area, 362, 366, 369, 372, 373, 375, 376
visual attention, 362, 364, 365, 366, 367, 369, 373
visual field, 151, 367
visual perception, 364, 365, 372
visual processing, 330, 362, 364, 367, 376
visual stimuli, 261, 331, 365, 373
visual stimulus, xii, 361, 365, 366, 367, 368, 369, 371, 372
visual system, 323
visuospatial, 374
voltammetric, 252
vomiting, 78
vulnerability, 2, 4, 34, 200, 207, 218, 278

W

water, 53, 54, 93, 110, 126, 192, 240, 249, 292
water maze, 53, 54, 93, 110, 240, 249
Watson, 110, 126, 140, 212
WCST, 265
wealth, 52, 168
wear, 151
weight changes, 321
weight reduction, 110
Weinberg, 133, 136
wild type, 279
windows, 278
Wistar rats, 126, 272
withdrawal, x, 178, 184, 186, 187, 188, 192, 193, 195, 198, 199, 201, 202, 204, 212, 215, 216, 217, 256, 289
working memory, xi, 78, 205, 209, 221, 223, 224, 226, 230, 231, 235, 237, 238, 239, 240, 241, 242, 243, 244, 248, 250, 252, 255, 256, 257, 258, 259, 260, 263, 265, 266, 267, 268, 331
workspace, 368

Y

yang, 32
yeast, 32
yield, 7, 81, 83, 172
yin, 32, 73
Y-maze, 336
young adults, 102

Z

zinc, 52, 72, 169
ZO-1, 46, 61